Manual of Animal Tec

Edited by Stephen W. Barnett

Technical Education Consultant
Formerly Senior Lecturer, City of Westminster College
Vice President of the Institute of Animal Technology

With assistance from

Jasmine Barley
Roger Francis
Sarah Lane

Foreword by Prof. Sir Richard Gardner FRS

President of the Institute of Animal Technology
Edward Penley Abrahams Research Professor of the Royal Society

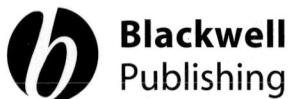

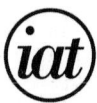

Blackwell Publishing editorial offices:
Blackwell Publishing Ltd, 9600 Garsington Road, Oxford OX4 2DQ, UK
Tel: +44 (0)1865 776868
Blackwell Publishing Professional, 2121 State Avenue, Ames, Iowa 50014-8300, USA
Tel: +1 515 292 0140
Blackwell Publishing Asia Pty Ltd, 550 Swanston Street, Carlton, Victoria 3053, Australia
Tel: +61 (0)3 8359 1011

First published 2007 by Blackwell Publishing Ltd

2   2008

ISBN: 978 06320 5593 7

Library of Congress Cataloging-in-Publication Data
The Institute of Animal Technology manual of animal technology/edited by Stephen W Barnett with Assistance
from Jasmine Barley, Roger Francis, Sarah Lane; foreword by Prof. Sir Richard Gardner. – 1st ed.
p. cm.
Includes bibliographical references and index.
ISBN-13: 978-0-632-05593-7 (pbk. : alk. paper)
ISBN-10: 0-632-05593-6 (pbk. : alk. paper) 1. Laboratory animals–Handbooks, manuals, etc. 2. Animal
experimentation–Handbooks, manuals, etc. I. Barnett, Stephen W.
SF406.I56 2006
636.088'5–dc22
2006017651

A catalogue record for this title is available from the British Library

Set in 10/12 pt Minion
by Graphicraft Limited, Hong Kong
Printed and bound in Singapore
by Markono Print Media Pte Ltd

For further information, visit our subject website: www.BlackwellVet.com

Contents

Foreword

by Prof. Sir Richard Gardner FRS
President of the Institute of Animal Technology
Edward Penley Abrahams Research Professor of the Royal Society

By the time this manual is published I shall have completed my term as President of the Institute of Animal Technology (IAT), having held this very special post for no less than twenty years. This period has been extremely educational for me since my understanding of the aims and aspirations of the Institute was woefully deficient when I took up the presidency. Through attending annual Congress and other more specialised meetings, I have learnt to appreciate just how much effort is devoted by the Institute to ensuring that those caring for the wide variety of animals now used in biomedical research are not only properly trained but also kept informed about current legislation and best practice.

The Institute's initiative in arranging the preparation of this impressively comprehensive manual is testimony to its continuing commitment to these goals. Moreover, it could not have assigned responsibility for this formidable undertaking to a more appropriate person than Steve Barnett. Steve has been responsible for training many generations of animal technicians, and clearly commands universal respect among those he has taught, for his dedication,

accessibility and sound judgement. Small wonder, therefore, that he has managed to secure the services of a formidable panel of experts to ensure that all relevant topics are covered in an up-to-date and authoritative way. The comprehensive coverage ranges from the general to the particular. Among the general contributions are chapters relating to the supply and production of protected animals, ethical and legislative matters, and the principles of good practice, surgery, anaesthesia, and many aspects of husbandry including reproductive physiology and disease prevention and containment. These provide invaluable background for more focused contributions, which include entire chapters devoted to each of the species of vertebrate in common use in biomedical research.

This manual, the product of an approximately six-year gestation, is an achievement of which both Steve Barnett and the IAT can justly be very proud. I have no doubt that it will prove indispensable as a source of information for all who are engaged in animal-based biomedical research, regardless of whether they are primarily involved with the science or the husbandry.

Preface

Using animals for scientific procedures is only morally acceptable if the care and welfare of the animals is ensured. Responsibility for providing this care, as well as carrying out experimental procedures, and the day-to-day operation of laboratory animal facilities is primarily that of animal technicians and technologists.

The *Manual of Animal Technology* aims to cover the topics which are important to technical staff in laboratory animal facilities. Approximately half the chapters cover the husbandry, environmental needs, nutrition and breeding requirements of a range of mammals, two species of bird, a commonly used fish and an amphibian.

The remaining chapters cover specific topics such as anaesthesia, surgical and experimental procedures, production of genetically altered animals, nutrition, disease and control of the environment.

The ethical aspects of the use of animals for scientific investigations are discussed, as well as the legal control of such work in the United Kingdom.

UK law will only be of immediate interest to UK readers but the principles discussed in the rest of the book should be of value wherever animals are used for experimental purposes. Therefore, the manual should be of use to laboratory animal staff wherever they work.

I am confident that the information in the Manual was up to date at the time of going to press but inevitably things change (for instance the Council of Europe Working Party is expected to publish new guidelines on cage and pen sizes very soon). Fortunately, with the advent of the World Wide Web, it is relatively easy to keep abreast of such developments, particularly those incorporated into law. The Home Office in the UK makes a large amount of information on the Animals (Scientific Procedures) Act 1986 available on its web site (www.homeoffice.gov.uk) and readers are encouraged to consult that site. The web addresses of other useful organisations are given in the text.

A number of DVDs, CD ROMs and videotapes which will be of interest to people who read this book are available from www.iat.org.uk.

The work of animal technologists, whichever country they live in, is vitally important in ensuring the wellbeing of laboratory animals and the integrity of scientific results. It is hoped that this manual will help them fulfil their responsibilities.

Stephen W. Barnett

Acknowledgements

I am grateful to all of the contributors to this manual, it would not have been finished without their efforts. I am delighted that Prof. Sir Richard Gardner FRS has agreed to write a foreword to the book. Sir Richard has a long record of support for the work of the Institute of Animal Technology and is held in great affection by its members.

This manual has taken a long time to complete. During its development many people have been of great help by reading parts of the manuscript, offering advice, answering questions and providing illustrations or arranging for me to take photographs.

Three people, Sarah Lane, Roger Francis and Jas Barley have been a great support throughout the project. I am very grateful to them for always being ready to offer assistance and for being ready to listen to my moaning.

Pilar Browne, Gary Childs, Steven Cubitt and Brian Lowe have also been willing to help whenever I have asked. These and many of the people listed below are ex or current students of mine from whom I have learned a great deal.

I am grateful for the patience of the Council of the Institute of Animal Technology and Richard Miles and Annie Choong of Blackwell Publishing.

People working on this book before I became involved produced some of the material in this version, particularly in Chapters 1, 2 and 4. They include Peter Hynes, Georgina Owen and Ted Wills.

I would also like to thank:

Sean Allen, Andy Bradwell, Clair Brazil, Gerry Bantin, Ian Bailey, Michael Brown, Claudine Chart, Gary Childs, Ben Clayton, Steven Cubitt, Adrian Deeny, Samantha Dinnage, Kevin Dolan, Stanley Done, Carley Flood, Robert Floyd, Carol Fox, David Green, David Gregory, Kevin Humphreys, Brian Howard, I.C. Johnson, Jessica Gruninger, Beverly Kennett, David Key, Nathan King, John Leslie, Alison Martin, Michael Martin-Short, Steven Meacham, Peter Morgan, Wendy Rudling, Diane Smith, Jeremy Smith, Douglas Stewart, Mandy Thorpe.

Pictures used in the manual have been supplied by chapter authors or the editor unless listed below. My thanks go to all the people who have contributed illustrations.

Sarah Lane for Figures 1.5 and 6.6. Roger J. Francis for Figures 1.4, 2.3, 2.4, 3.4, 19.3 and 28.4. B&K Universal Ltd for Figures 2.1, 3.1, 3.2, 4.1, 11.1, 11.5 and 11.7. Merck, Sharp Dohm Terlings Park for Figures 2.2, 3.3, 5.3, 5.4, 6.5 and 24.3. Peter Gerson for Figures 6.4 and 24.4. I.C. Johnson for Figures 7.2, 7.3 and 7.4. Pfizer Ltd for Figures 8.3, 8.4, 9.1, 9.3–9.9, 22.2, 22.3, 22.5, 22.6 and 22.8. Dstl, Porton Down for Figures 10.1, 11.3, 39.1 and 39.3. Martin Heath for Figures 5.1, 6.2, 6.3, 7.1 and 9.3. CRUK for Figure 14.1. NIMR, Mill Hill for Figures 13.1, 13.2 and 13.4. Fetch Europe for Figure 28.6. Jas Barley for Figures 21.1 and 21.7. Peter Morgan for Figures 18.1 and 19.4. Jeremy Smith for Figure 24.1. Harlan UK Ltd for Figures 34.1 and 34.7. Steven Cubitt for Figure 9.2. Michael Brown, MRC for Figure 13.3. Michael Martin-Short, Pfizer Veterinary Medicine for Figures 34.9–39.12. Royal Veterinary College for Figures 24.5 and 25.2–25.5. S.H. Done for Figure 34.1.

Stephen W. Barnett

Contributors

Jasmine B. Barley, MSc, FIAT, RAnTech: Facility Director.

Stephen W. Barnett, BA, MSc, Cert Ed, CBiol, MIBiol, RAnTech: Technical Education Consultant.

Pilar Browne, BSc (Hons), MIAT, FETC: Lecturer.

Gerald Clough, BSc, PhD, EurBiol, CBiol, MIBiol: Environmental Physiologist.

B. Curren, Edstrom Industries Inc., Waterford, WI, USA.

Adrian Deeny, BSc (Hons), CBiol, MIBiol: Harlan UK Ltd, Loughborough, Leics, LE12 9TE, UK.

Kevin P. Dolan, BD, SThL(JusCan), DipLaw, FIAT: Lecturer.

Eric Edstrom, Edstrom Industries Inc., Waterford, WI, USA.

Paul A. Flecknell, MA, VetMB, PhD, DLAS, Dip LECVA, MRCVS: Professor of Laboratory Animal Science, Comparative Biology Centre, The Medical School, Newcastle-Upon-Tyne, UK.

Roger J. Francis, MSc, FIAT, RAnTech: Director of Animal Care and Training, Bristol University.

Peter J. Gerson, MSc, FIAT, RAnTech: Facility Manager.

David Gregory, FIAT, RAnTech: Technical Sales Representative, Charles River Laboratories Research Models and Services UK.

Martin Heath, MSc, FIAT, FIScT, RAnTech: Learning Curve, PO Box 140, Ware, Herts, UK.

Sarah Lane, MSc, FIAT, RAnTech: Manager ACU, Novartis Horsham Research Centre.

Janice Lobb, BTech: Formerly Senior Lecturer.

Brian Lowe, MSc, FIAT: Lecturer.

Robert W. Kemp, FIAT (Hon), RAnTech: Chairman, Institute of Animal Technology.

Gerald McDonnell, BSc, PhD: Senior Director of Technical Affairs, STERIS Ltd, STERIS House, Basingstoke, UK.

R. Ian Porter, MSc, CBiol, MIBiol: Lecturer.

Barney Reed, MSc, RSPCA Laboratory Animal Department, Horsham, UK.

Victoria L. Savage, BSc (Hons), FIAT: Dstl, Porton Down, Wilts, UK.

Joanne C. Scott, BSc (Hons), FIAT: Facility Manager.

Jeremy Smith, MSc, CBiol, MIBiol, FIAT: MRC Head Office, 20 Park Crescent, London, UK.

Neil Vargesson, BSc, PhD: Lecturer, Imperial College, University of London, UK.

Bryan Waynforth, BSc, PhD, FIBiol: Laboratory Animal Scientist.

All contributors can be contacted through the IAT website (www.iat.org.uk).

1

The Supply and Production of Protected Animals

Stephen W. Barnett

This chapter covers the aspects of breeding which are common to all animals. Breeding systems used for individual species are discussed in Chapters 2–13 and 19–25.

Sources of animals

The Animals (Scientific Procedures) Act 1986 requires protected animals, listed on Schedule 2 of the Act, to be obtained from designated breeders or suppliers, unless the Home Secretary has authorised their purchase from another source (see Chapter 35). If designated scientific procedure establishments need to breed animals they must also be designated breeders. Protected animals not listed on Schedule 2 may be obtained from any source, but it is in the interest of animal welfare and good science that users satisfy themselves that the source provides clean, healthy and well cared for animals.

In practice most animals used for regulated procedures are purchased from specialist designated breeders who are able to supply a wide range of species and strains at various ages, together with documentation detailing health and genetic status (see Chapters 16 and 17). Designated breeders can provide animals at a cost which, in most cases, make it impractical for scientific procedure establishments to breed their own.

However there may be circumstances when it is necessary for scientific procedure establishments to produce their own animals, e.g.:

- work involving the use of foetuses or neonates;
- development of new transgenic strains;
- rarely used, or otherwise commercially unavailable species or strains;
- where there is a desire to have direct control over quality of animals.

An increasing number of protected animals are imported into the United Kingdom. This is largely due to the international cooperation in the use of genetically altered animals (see Chapter 14). The regulations covering the importation of animals into the UK are covered in Chapter 28.

Principles of breeding

The basic principles of breeding animals are the same whatever the species and whoever breeds them. Males and females must be brought together so that they can mate, produce and rear their young. Three main systems are used to do this, monogamous pairs, harems and arranged matings. The choice of which one is suitable will depend on the following:

- the behaviour of the animal (e.g. whether the male and female will tolerate being together permanently, or females object to the presence of the young of other females);
- the reproductive physiology of the animal (e.g. do they breed all year or seasonally, are they spontaneous or induced ovulators) (see Chapter 15);
- experimental requirements (e.g. demand for a specific genetic model, inbred or random bred strains, age of model);
- economic considerations.

Breeding systems

Monogamous pairs

Monogamous pairs (also referred to as permanent pairs) comprise one male and one female paired together, usually throughout their breeding lives. The system is most commonly used for small laboratory animals. The young stay with the parents until removed at the end of weaning.

Harems

Harems consist of one male and two or more females (small harems of one male to two females are called trios). Two variations are used.

(1) Permanent harems (also referred to as polygamous mating) where the male and females remain together with the young until they are removed at weaning.
(2) Discontinuous harems or 'boxing out' where the females are removed for parturition and are returned when their young have been weaned. Boxing out is used for animals which are sensitive to the presence of other females during parturition (e.g. rats) or when accurate records of parentage need to be kept.

Arranged mating

Arranged mating (sometimes referred to as hand mating) is the term used to describe the system where a male and female are placed together for a short time to mate and are then separated. Oestrus is identified in the female, she is taken to the male's cage and is removed either after mating has been observed (e.g. rabbits, dairy cattle) or after a suitable period (e.g. cats and ferrets).

The female must be taken to the male's cage, if the male is taken to the female's cage he will spend time scent marking and will not be interested in mating until he has made her cage his territory. This will waste time and may attract a hostile response from the female.

Table 1.1 compares the productivity and cost of the three breeding systems for rats and mice.

Artificial and assisted fertilisation

In addition to the natural mating systems described above, fertilisation can be achieved by artificial means. These include:

- artificial insemination;
- *in vitro* fertilisation;
- intra-cytoplasmic sperm injection.

Artificial insemination

Artificial insemination (AI) involves removing semen from a male and introducing it into the reproductive tract of a female, by means of a catheter, at a suitable stage in her reproductive cycle. AI is used extensively in agriculture and for research purposes. There are a number of collection techniques.

Table 1.1   Comparison of productivity, economics and ease of identification between monogamous pairs, harems and boxing out systems.

	Productivity	Cost	Identification
Monogamous pairs	In monogamous pairs the male is always present, so advantage can be taken of post-partum oestrus, minimising litter intervals. Pre-weaning loss is also low. These two factors result in a high productivity in terms of young per female per week.	Ratios of males to females is 1:1, whereas in a harem it could be 1:4 or greater. These extra males consume food, take up space and increase the service time of the colony, making monogamous pairs expensive to operate.	As there is only one male and one female in the cage, identification of the parentage of litters is straightforward.
Permanent harems	Productivity per cage is higher than in monogamous pairs, but productivity per female is lower because there is competition for milk and some young may be trampled by older animals in the cage. Post-partum oestrus can be used.	Permanent harems are less expensive to run than monogamous pairs as there are fewer males, more females can be housed in the same space and servicing a multi-occupied cage takes little, if any, extra time than a cage housing a single pair.	Accurate record keeping may be difficult as several litters can be born at the same time, making parentage difficult to determine.
Boxing out	Boxing out prevents the pre-weaning loss seen in permanent harems but post-partum oestrus is missed so litter intervals are longer.	Mating in harems but littering in single cages makes this system intermediate between harems and monogamous pairs in cost.	Accurate records of parentage can be kept because only one litter is present in the cage at a time.

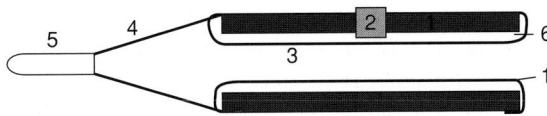

1. Rigid plastic or rubber tube
2. Stopper, where apparatus is filled with hot water
3. Rubber latex liner
4. Cone
5. Glass tube to collect semen
6. Space between rigid tube and liner, filled with water at 50 °C

Figure 1.1   Artificial vagina (AV).

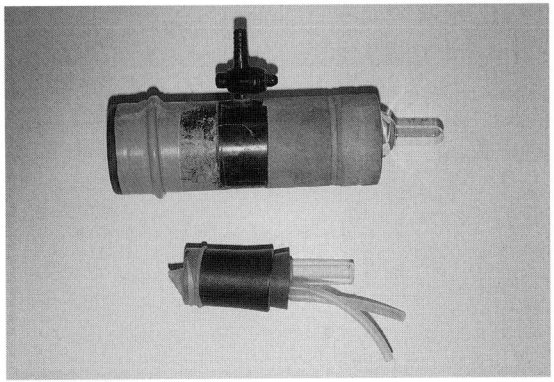

Figure 1.2   Sheep (top) and rabbit AVs.

Artificial vagina (AV)

The basic design of an AV is the same for all species but minor adaptations may be necessary to reflect the anatomical features of the female reproductive tract (see Figures 1.1 and 1.2).

A trained male will readily mount a teaser so that its erect penis can be directed into the AV. In animals such as the rabbit or bull the warm water and rubber liner provide enough stimulus to cause the animal to ejaculate with a single thrust. In other animals such as the boar and the dog the procedure is prolonged and greater stimulation is required. The AV used for these animals is adapted to include an air pump so that pressure can be built up around the penis. Semen is sensitive to the rubber latex which lines the AV so the length must be adjusted to minimise contact with the liner.

Teasers can be females (although care must be taken to ensure normal mating does not occur), castrated males or, in the case of well trained animals, fur covered gloves (suitable for rabbits) or padded frames (boars).

Hand collection

Some species will ejaculate when manipulated by hand. For instance if the distal end of an erect boar's penis is gripped tightly with a gloved hand the boar will ejaculate and the semen can be collected into a flask wrapped in an insulating material. Dogs and chickens will also ejaculate when their penis is manipulated by hand.

Invasive techniques

The techniques outlined above cannot be used with animals smaller than a rabbit. In small species sperm can be harvested from the epididymis (see *in vitro* fertilisation below, p. 4).

Electro-ejaculators can also be used to collect semen. The ejaculator is placed in the rectum and electrical stimulation applied to the structures and nerves of the lumbar region. This stimulates ejaculation, although not necessarily erection. Semen quality is low with electro-ejaculation. The technique is an unpleasant experience for the animal and should only be used in sedated animals.

Assessment of semen

One of the advantages of AI is that the quality of the semen can be assessed before it is used to inseminate a female. A small sample can be viewed under a microscope to assess motility and the presence of morphological abnormalities. The sperm can be counted using automatic counters or a haemocytometer, to determine concentration and can be stained in order to distinguish live from dead sperm.

In commercial cattle breeding sperm is diluted in a cryopreservative and placed in thin plastic tubes called 'straws', frozen and stored at −196 °C in liquid nitrogen. Dilution is possible as fewer sperm are required to ensure fertilisation. This is because the semen is deposited higher up in the female reproductive tract in AI than in natural mating and it therefore has a greater chance of reaching the egg. Frozen semen can be kept indefinitely.

Progeny testing

When semen from one male is diluted and used to inseminate large numbers of females there is a theoretical risk of genetic abnormalities being distributed quickly and widely. This could be particularly important in commercial breeding and is avoided by

carefully selecting AI males and instituting a programme of progeny testing.

Progeny testing is particularly advanced in cattle
breeding. After the initial semen collection has been
made the bull is not used for AI until his semen has
been used to inseminate a number of cows, the offspring of which have had calves of their own and have
been through one lactation. Any abnormalities or
poor productivity should be evident by the end of the
progeny testing period. The process could take up to
three years to complete. It is only after bulls have been
shown to produce good quality offspring that they
are used for routine insemination.

Insemination

Semen is introduced into the reproductive tract of a
female in oestrus by means of a catheter. In cattle the
cervix of the uterus is located by rectal palpation and
a long, thin catheter guided to this point through the
vagina. (For descriptions of AI in farm species see
Chapters 19–22.)

In vitro *fertilisation*

In vitro fertilisation is mainly used for small animals
such as mice. It involves collecting sperm and ova and
mixing them together in a Petri dish. To collect the
sperm the male is killed by cervical dislocation, the
epididymis is dissected out and the *cauda* part (tail) is
removed and placed in a suitable medium, such as
bovine serum albumin (BSA). The epididymis is then
cut into short sections so that the sperm can swim out
into the medium from where it can be harvested. In
addition to acting as a collecting medium, the BSA
activates the sperm to enable it to break through the
zona pellucida, attach themselves to and enter the ova.

Ova are collected from superovulated females prepared as described in Chapter 14, however, instead
of the female being mated her eggs are recovered by
flushing them from the uterine tube. The eggs and
sperm are mixed together *in vitro* and after a period of
external incubation are implanted into receptive
females (see Chapter 14).

Intra-cytoplasmic *sperm injection*

Intra-cytoplasmic sperm injection involves harvesting ova and sperm as described above but in this case
a spermatozoon, minus its tail, is injected into the ova

so that fertilisation can be achieved. The technique
is a difficult one and is only used in special circumstances, for instance where a valuable strain is at risk
of dying out due to low sperm production in the
males.

Indications of mating and confirmation of pregnancy

Whatever system is used to achieve fertilisation, pregnancy must be confirmed. Methods differ with species
and stage of pregnancy. Tables 1.2–1.4 list examples

Table 1.2   Method of confirming mating.

Method	Examples of animals
Observed mating	Any animal bred using arranged mating system
Copulation plugs	Mice, rats
Sperm in vaginal smears	Most species
Raddles	Sheep, cattle
Tail paint	Sheep, cattle

Table 1.3   Examples of signs indicating pregnancy.

Signs	Examples of animals
Non-return of oestrus	Most species
Increase in body weight	Most species
Change in behaviour, e.g. nest building	Rodents, rabbits, pigs, dogs
Change in body shape, enlarged abdomen, development of mammary tissue	Most species, in late pregnancy

'Indications' imply there could be reasons other than pregnancy for
the signs, e.g. pseudopregnancy resulting from sterile mating.

Table 1.4   Examples of methods to confirm pregnancy.

Method	Examples of animals
External palpation	Most animals*
Internal palpation: *via* rectum	Cattle, horses*
Internal palpation: *via* vagina	Old World primates*
Hormone analysis of blood or milk	Mainly used for farm animals
Ultrasound	All species

* There is a risk of damage to foetus and female with these methods,
so they should only be performed by trained people.

of methods for confirming mating, indicating pregnancy and confirming pregnancy. Specific methods are given in the chapters on each species.

Specific breeding techniques

Timed mating or dated mating

It is sometimes necessary to know exactly when a litter will be born. Foetuses at an exact stage of development, or pups of a particular age, on a particular day may be required for experimental reasons (for instance when deriving or re-deriving animals for barrier units and preparation for embryo transfer). Timed mating techniques are used to establish when the female was mated so the stage of development and date of birth can be calculated. A number of techniques can be used to do this:

- mating may be observed (e.g. rabbits, hamsters, dogs, pigs);
- oestrus can be established by external signs or by vaginal smears and an assumption made that females in oestrus will mate when they are placed with a male (e.g. rats, mice);
- vaginal smears may be taken after males and females have been together and examined for the presence of sperm (e.g. rats, mice);
- presence of a copulatory plug after mating (part of the contents in the semen in some species which solidifies), seen either in the vagina or in the bedding/tray (e.g. rats, mice) (see Figure 3.4, p. 22);
- determination of oestrus by electrical means, e.g. vaginal impedance.

Manipulation of oestrus to obtain young on a set day

Oestrus in mice can be manipulated by using a naturally occurring physiological process. If female mice are kept isolated from males their reproductive cycles will stop. If they are then housed where they can see and smell a male but are separate from him, approximately 60% of them will come into oestrus after a period of 48 hours. This technique, called the Whitten effect (named after the person who first identified it), can be useful in ensuring females are ready to mate on a set day (see Appendix 1).

Oestrus can also be manipulated by administering hormones as described in Chapter 14.

Identification of oestrus

Vaginal smears
The reproductive cycle of female mammals has four stages, pro-oestrus, oestrus, metoestrus and di-oestrus (see Chapter 15). Some mammals also have a stage called anoestrus where they appear to stop cycling altogether for a period. In many mammal species the stages can easily be identified by taking samples of cells from the vagina, whose cytology alters under the influence of hormones (see Chapter 15). The stages of the oestrous cycle in the mouse and rat are described in Table 1.5 (interpretation of vaginal smears may be slightly different in other mammals).

Smears can be taken in three ways:

(1) A blunt ended pipette containing a very small amount of sterile saline is placed into the vagina of the female and is flushed several times. The mixture is then placed on a microscope slide and allowed to dry in air.
(2) A small cotton bud soaked in sterile saline is introduced into the vagina. When removed the bud will hold cells from the vaginal lining which are then smeared onto a slide.
(3) A modified microbiological loop is dipped into sterile saline and is then introduced into the vagina to collect a small sample of cells from the lining of the wall. The sample is then transferred onto a slide.

Care must be taken to ensure the instrument used to take the smear is not pushed too far into the vagina, if it stimulates the cervix it may cause pseudopregnancy.

When completely dry, slides can be flooded with methylene blue stain for three minutes, after which

Table 1.5 Appearance of vaginal smears.

Pro-oestrus	Mainly nucleated epithelial cells
Oestrus	Cornified epithelial cells, appear as rafts (joined together)
Metoestrus	Many leucocytes (white blood cells) and cornified cells. Some nucleated epithelium
Di-oestrus	Many leucocytes some nucleated epithelial cells

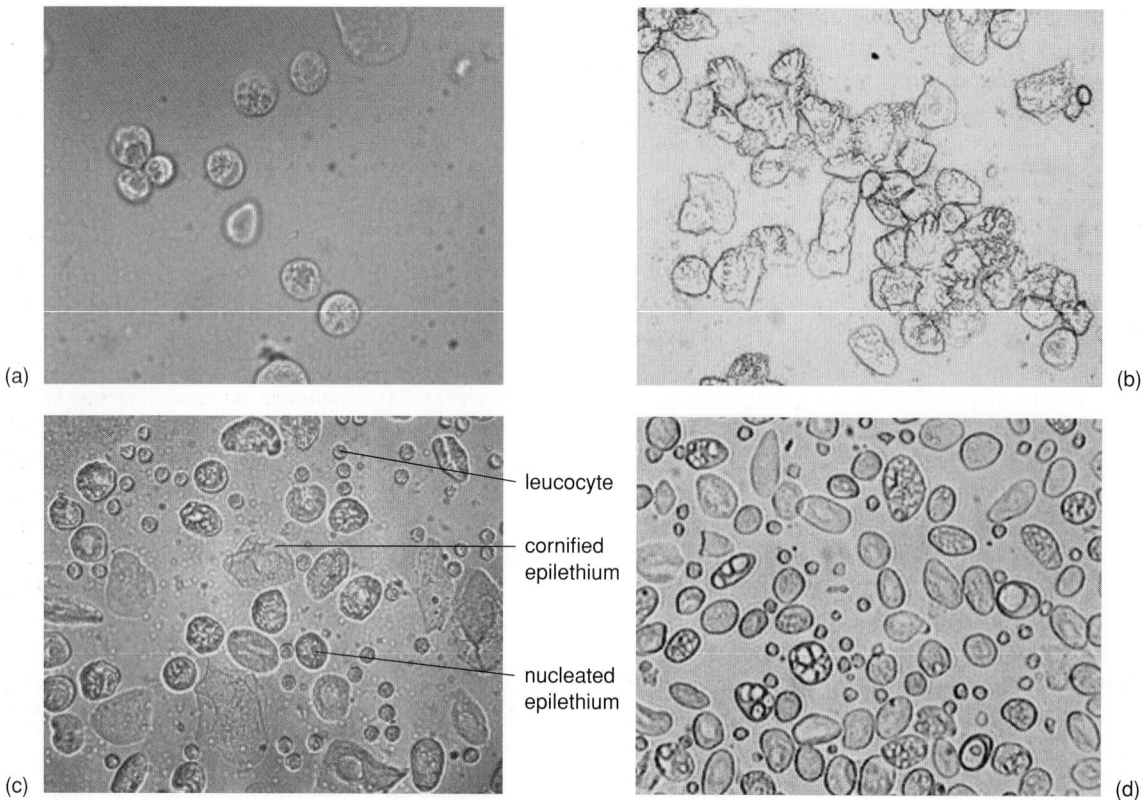

leucocyte

cornified
epilethium

nucleated
epilethium

Figure 1.3   Unstained vaginal smears: (a) pro-oestrus; (b) oestrus; (c) metoestrus; (d) di-oestrus. Images Courtesy of Sean Allen (a and b) and Sarah Lane (c and d).

the stain is washed off with gently running water and the slide can be viewed under the microscope. Nuclei of the cells stain dark blue and the cytoplasm light blue.

Experienced people can identify the stage of oestrus without staining the specimen (Figure 1.3 (a), (b), (c) and (d)), and some use more sophisticated stains (e.g. Papanicolaou or phase-contrast microscopes).

External signs of oestrus

The physiological changes which occur during oestrus result in enlarging and/or reddening of the vulva (e.g. rats, mice, dogs, sows). In some species the changes are obvious (e.g. sows) in others the changes are subtle and experience is needed to accurately identify oestrus.

Distinctive discharges from the vulva occur in some species (e.g. dogs, hamsters) and obvious oestral behaviour may also be evident (e.g. cows, cats). Detailed descriptions of these indications can be found in the species chapters.

Electrical impedance

It has been shown that the electrical impedance of the epithelial cells lining the vagina alters during the cycle, being highest during pro-oestrus. A probe is inserted deep into the vagina and the impedance is registered on a meter. The time of day the reading is taken is critical and should be between 13.00 and 15.00 hrs. A reading of 3 k ohms indicates pro-oestrus.

Genetically defined laboratory animals

A genetically defined animal is one which has been bred so that the arrangement of its genes are known, e.g. inbred, outbred.

Inbreeding

Inbreeding occurs when closely related animals are mated together. It occurs intentionally when an inbred strain is developed but it can also happen unintentionally where colony management is poor. In closed colonies it will eventually occur and minimal inbreeding techniques must be used in order to delay it as long as possible in non-inbred colonies.

Inbred strains

An inbred strain is produced as the result of twenty consecutive generations of brother × sister or youngest parent × offspring matings. Inbred strains have certain characteristics which make them valuable experimental animals. The two main ones are:

(1) Isogenisity, which means all individuals within the strain are genetically identical.
(2) Homozygosity, over 98.6% of the two genes (one copy from the male parent and one from the female parent) at each locus are identical.

Other characteristics of inbred strains follow from the two above:

- the strains are genetically stable (because of the high degree of homozygosity);
- they are more phenotypically uniform than non-inbred animals (because they are isogenic);
- each inbred strain is unique since only that strain has that particular combination of genes;
- strains can be identified using genetic monitoring techniques.

Using inbred strains for scientific study eliminates one of the major influences on experimental results – genetic variability. This means that statistically meaningful experimental results can be gained using fewer animals.

Inbreeding depression

Most genes which code for harmful characteristics (deleterious genes) are recessive. They can only affect the phenotype of the animal if the deleterious gene is homozygous. In non-inbred animals this situation rarely arises because deleterious genes, if present, are masked by dominant 'normal' genes. In the production of inbred strains the genes become progressively more homozygous so deleterious genes are more likely to be expressed. This often leads to inbreeding depression, characterised by:

- small litter sizes;
- small pup sizes;
- slow growth rates;
- high pre-weaning mortality;
- long litter intervals;
- increased susceptibility to disease and environmental change.

Coefficient of inbreeding

The degree of inbreeding in an individual is stated in terms of the coefficient of inbreeding. It is defined as the probability that the two genes at any locus are identical by descent (Falconer 1960). This means that both copies of the gene have descended from one gene carried by a common ancestor (Festing 1987). The coefficient is expressed as a percentage of all genes. It is assumed that when two animals are paired at the beginning of the establishment of a new inbred strain the coefficient of inbreeding is 0. The coefficient rises rapidly over the first few generations and it is at this stage that the effects of inbreeding depression become evident. If the strain survives at this point the depression gets no worse.

After twenty consecutive generations of brother × sister matings the coefficient of inbreeding reaches 98.6%. 100% is never achieved.

Hybrid vigour

For the reasons explained above, inbred strains often suffer from inbreeding depression. Experimental factors may require animals which are isogenic but which have the vigour associated with non-inbred animals. These characteristics can be produced by mating animals from two inbred strains and using their offspring for experiments. The first generation of such matings (the F1 hybrids) will be heterozygous but isogenic. Only the F1 hybrids can be used as subsequent generations will cease to be isogenic.

Production of inbred strains

Foundation stock

Inbred strains start from pairing one male and one female. The offspring produced from this mating are then paired up (brother × sister), this is called the F1 generation. The offspring from the F1 generation are paired to produce the F2 generation and so on. Only one b × s pair will be chosen to produce the strain, but as some pairings can be expected to die out due to inbreeding depression, as many b × s pairings are set up as possible at each generation. Accurate records are kept of the breeding performance of these pairs in the form of a pedigree chart. After every three or four generations the breeding performance of all pairs is assessed and the line which is most productive is chosen as the main line of descent. The other surviving lines are stopped from breeding. This goes on for twenty consecutive generations after which the strain can be said to be inbred.

Producing a new inbred strain is not a common thing to be asked to do. A more usual requirement is to maintain an established inbred strain. The same technique which has been described above to establish a new inbred strain has to be used to maintain the main line of descent, often called the primary line.

Expansion colony

The primary line maintains the inbred strain but does not produce many animals for experimental use; the number of animals produced has to be increased. This is achieved by removing animals produced in the primary colony, and not required for breeding within the primary colony, to an expansion colony. In the expansion colony they can be used for experimentation or can be used for breeding to increase the number of animals. However, breeding must not go on for more than three generations after they have left the primary colony. Up to three generations will not affect the inbred status of the animals but a greater number of generations away from the common ancestor in the primary colony will risk a genetic separation from it and the animals will no longer be considered inbred.

Systems have been developed to ensure this separation does not occur, without the need for complicated and time consuming record keeping. One such system is called the traffic light system.

All animals removed from the primary colony are placed in boxes with white labels. Animals in this box can be used for experiments or can be used for breeding. The offspring produced in boxes with white labels are placed in a box with a green label. Young produced in boxes with green labels can be issued for use or can be mated. The offspring produced in green boxes are placed in boxes with amber labels; these too can be used for experiments or used for breeding. The offspring from the amber box are placed in a box with a red label. All animals in the red box must be used for experiments.

Non-inbreeding techniques

Random breeding

Random breeding involves using animals for mating without any regard to their relationship. There are no selection criteria other than ensuring the animals are healthy and are of the opposite sex. In theory a random selection procedure should be used. With small numbers of animals this could involve giving all the animals a number, writing the numbers on pieces of paper and drawing them out of a hat. With larger numbers, random number tables or random number generators can be used.

Some animals set up by this method could be closely related, even brother and sister, others distantly related. However, at each generation the situation would change and separate lines of descent are prevented from being established. The coefficient of inbreeding differs at each generation.

Outbreeding

Outbreeding is the active avoidance of inbreeding. Only unrelated animals are paired. If the colony is an open one, new animals from other colonies can be introduced to prevent inbreeding. In closed colonies this is not possible and eventually a degree of inbreeding is inevitable. Minimal inbreeding techniques can be used to minimise the coefficient of inbreeding.

Minimal inbreeding requires the use of pairs because if one male is used with more than one female all the offspring will be related. It also requires that each pair in the colony contribute the same number of offspring to the next generation of breeders. Systems have been devised to make the avoidance of inbreeding simple to arrange. The most straightforward of these systems is as follows; each breeding pair is given a number and the offspring of the pair keep the number until they are selected for breeding (Falconer 1976). Pairing then follows the pattern described below:

(1) offspring from pair 1 are paired with offspring from pair 2, they make new pair 1;
(2) offspring from pair 3 are paired with offspring from pair 4, they make new pair 2 and so on.

This can be summarised as:

$$1 \times 2 = 1$$
$$3 \times 4 = 2$$

$$5 \times 6 = 3$$
$$7 \times 8 = 4$$

Specific genetic models

Co-isogenic strains

Co-isogenic strains are two strains which are genetically identical except for one gene. This can arise as a single mutation in an inbred strain which has then been maintained by breeding.

Congenic strains

These are two strains which are identical except for a short segment of chromosome bearing a gene of interest. They are produced when a gene of interest is identified in an animal. In order to study the effects of the gene it is useful to breed it into an established inbred strain. This is done by mating the animal with the gene (called the donor) to an animal from an inbred strain. Offspring which carry the gene are identified and backcrossed to the inbred strain. This is repeated for fifteen backcross generations. The result is a strain which carries the gene and a strain which is identical to it except that it does not carry the gene. The two strains can be compared to see the effect the gene has on the animal or how it affects experimental treatments. If the gene of interest is a recessive one, progeny testing (backcrossing offspring to the donor animals) has to be done between each generation in order to identify the animals carrying the gene.

Recombinant inbred strains

These are produced by mating a male from one inbred strain and a female from another inbred strain and pairing their offspring in the same way as an inbred strain, each of the pairings are continued for twenty consecutive generations. After this time a number of inbred strains will have been produced, each containing a set of genes which have originated from the two original inbred strains. When used in conjunction, recombinant inbred strains can be used to identify characteristics that are controlled by single genes or many genes (polygenic) and can be used for gene mapping studies.

Genetic mutants

Some strains of animal carry naturally occurring genetic mutations which cause them to develop diseases that

Table 1.6 Pattern of inheritance of nude gene. Homozygous nude = nu nu; Heterozygous nude (phenotypically normal) = nu +. The resulting offspring will be in the ratio of 2 × nu nu (homozygous nudes) and 2 × nu + (heterozygous nudes).

Male →	nu	nu
Female ↓		
nu	nu nu	nu nu
+	nu +	nu +

are similar to conditions seen in humans (e.g. diabetic rat, obese mouse) or make them useful in the study of physiological systems (e.g. the athymic (nude) mouse and the severe combined immunodeficient (SCID) mouse used in immunological studies). Animals homozygous for the characteristic are often poor breeders so it is necessary to breed from animals which are heterozygous for the characteristic.

In the case of nude mice the homozygous female has difficulty in rearing her young so pre-weaning mortality is high. Females carrying one copy of the nude gene (heterozygous nudes) have a normal phenotype. It is, therefore, common practice to mate heterozygous females with homozygous males to produce litters which, on average, will be 50% homozygous and 50% heterozygous animals (Table 1.6; Figure 1.4).

Successful breeding of animals with specific mutations does not always follow this pattern and therefore different breeding techniques will need to be used. In the case of diabetic rats for instance, homozygous diabetics can be bred from providing their diabetes is controlled by medication.

Breeding records and productivity measurements

Breeding colonies must be carefully monitored to ensure acceptable breeding performance is maintained. Productivity in the colony has obvious economic importance but more importantly is a gauge of the health and welfare of the animals. The Code of Practice for the Housing and Care of Animals in Designated Breeding and Supplying Establishments states, 'The appearance of pathogenic organisms in the animal breeding area, loss of environmental control, a poor batch of diet, or even an unsympathetic or poorly trained animal technician can affect the

Hairy pup   Nude pup   Hetrozygous female   Nude male   **Figure 1.4**   Breeding box of nude mice.

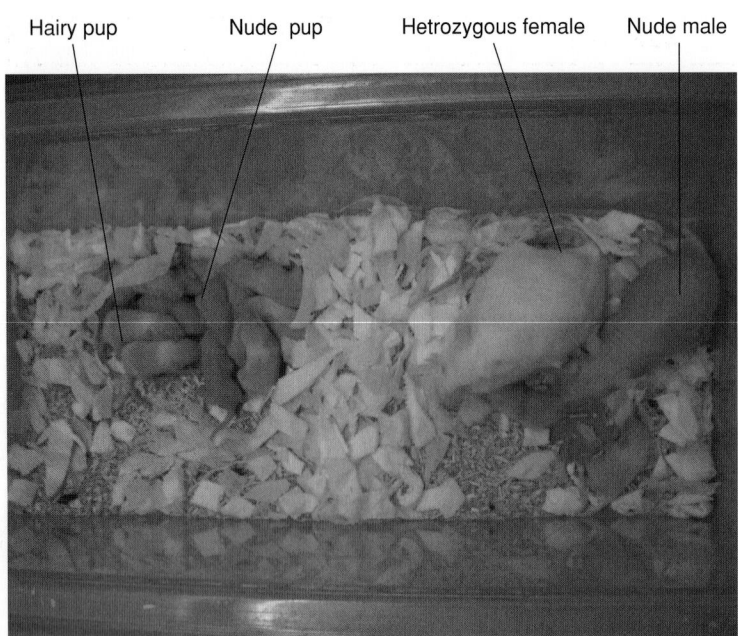

performance of the breeding colony, leading to re-duced fertility, an increase in pre- and post-weaning mortality and/or reduction in growth rates. These effects will often precede any obvious clinical signs of ill health.'

In addition to maintaining records of the source, use and final disposal of animals, the Code of Practice specifies the following information must be kept:

- colony size;
- individual performance per breeding female (in some cases for individual males);
- total output of the colony;
- litter size;
- number of litters in a given period;
- pre-weaning and post-weaning mortality.

The Code of Practice further requires that the information 'be averaged over appropriate periods so that any change in performance will be rapidly identified' (Home Office 1995).

Methods of maintaining records

The chosen method of keeping breeding records will depend on the species being bred, the size of the colony and local preferences. Most methods start by using pen and paper to make records in the breeding room and involve computers, at a later stage, to pro-vide calculated values, permanent records and to

speed up the retrieval of information, such as family relationships, which may be required in the future.

Any method of record keeping must ensure all the required information is collected as efficiently as pos-sible. This is usually achieved by using a predesigned card (Figure 1.5).

The information on the card allows important breeding indicators to be calculated, e.g.:

- % pre-weaning mortality

$$\frac{\text{column } 3 - \text{column } 7}{\text{column } 3} \times 100$$

- Average litter size $\dfrac{\text{total of column } 7}{\text{total number of litters}}$

- Litter interval   calculated in days from the date the animals were paired
                         or
                         grouped to the birth of last litter

- Sex ratio   column 5:6

- Economic   comparing   birth   dates   of
  breeding life   parents with number and dates
                        of birth of litters

An overall measure of productivity can be calcu-lated from this data. In small rodents it is usually quoted in terms of young per female per week. Animals with long gestation periods can be calculated

Figure 1.5   Breeding record card.

Pair Nos: 02/532							
Strain:			**Doe Nos:**			**Sire Nos:**	
			Date born: 3/6/02			**Date born:** 31/5/02	
Date paired: 18/7/02							
(1)	(2)	(3)	(4)	(5)	(6)	(7)	
Litter Nos	**Date born**	**Nos Born**	**Date weaned**	**Sexes at weaning** M	F	**Total**	**Remarks**
A	6/8/02	8	26/8/02	3	5	8	
B	30/8/02	9	19/9/02	4	4	8	1 pup dead 4/9/02
C	23/9/02	8	13/10/02	4	4	8	4 taken for breeding
D	17/10/02	7	7/11/02	4	3	7	
E	5/12/02	9	26/12/02	4	5	9	
F	21/1/03	7	10/2/03	3	4	7	
							male removed 6/2/03

over 100 days (called the Q value) (Lane-Petter & Pearson 1971):

young/female/week
$$= \frac{\text{number of young successfully weaned}}{\text{days male and female were together}} \times 7$$

Using the data on Figure 1.5 (above):

young successfully weaned = 47

number of days male and female were together = 168 days

$$= \frac{47}{168} \times 7$$

$$= 1.96$$

Young per female per week figures can be compared with expected figures to judge the productivity of the breeding animals. In the case of outbred mice an acceptable figure would be two but there will be strain variations.

This measure is useful because it takes into account all factors which could affect productivity, such as small litter sizes, long litter intervals and high pre-weaning loss.

Another useful indicator of productivity is the production index (PI):

$$\text{PI} = \frac{\text{number of young weaned}}{\text{number of females in colony}}$$

In very large colonies detailed records on cards are not always kept, although overall productivity in the colony will be carefully monitored. The performance of individual females is recorded by means of ear punches on the animal itself. If a female produces a litter of the required number and quality a punch is made in the right ear. If a litter falls below the quality required a hole is punched in the left ear. More than two substandard litters and the female is discarded. Future breeding stock will not be drawn from females with any holes in the left ear.

In addition to monitoring productivity, accurate breeding records enable the economic breeding life of an animal to be recorded. The economic breeding life is the period when the animal is producing litters of the acceptable quantity and quality with a reasonable litter interval. As animals get older their reproductive efficiency declines and it becomes uneconomic to breed from them. Economic breeding life is measured in terms of numbers of litters or age.

(1) Number of litters – if animals are bred continuously the number of litters is used to define economic breeding life. In mice and rats it is usually six litters (for other species see species chapters). First litters in these species are often low in numbers; litter size tends to peak at litter three to four and then declines again. After litter six they tend to have low productivity and the breeders are replaced.

(2) Age – if animals are not bred continuously then age determines the economic breeding life. In mice and rats this is approximately six months, in larger animals it may be over several years. As they age all animals become less productive. It is important that some species are not first bred too late as they may have difficulty in giving birth. Guinea pigs, for instance, should not be bred for the first mating time after seven months of age as their pubic symphysis becomes ossified and will not open wide enough to allow the large pups to pass through (see Chapter 5). Examples of breeding calculations are given in Appendix 1.

Factors which influence productivity and quality in a breeding colony

Genetic factors

For the reasons mentioned above, litters of inbred strains tend to be weak, low in numbers and have longer litter intervals than random bred or outbred animals. Some transgenic and genetic mutant strains may also show low productivity.

Dietary factors

Feeding during the reproductive period has to be carefully managed. During late pregnancy females have to build up nutritional reserves to support early lactation but they must not get too fat as this can make parturition more difficult. Lactation and growth are the most nutritionally demanding activities which animals carry out. In addition, the time when a female is producing most milk is the time when her appetite is low. Diets fed at this time must not only contain sufficient nutrients but may need to supply them in a more concentrated form than at other times. Small animals are usually left to manage their own nutrition. Breeding diets are available and must be fed if females and litters are not to be compromised; transgenic animals are often provided with wet diet or gel at weaning. Feeding in large animals such as dairy cows needs careful management (see Chapter 26 and Chapters 19–23).

Semen quality also falls if nutrition is inadequate but it is also important that males are not allowed to get overweight as this too has a detrimental effect on breeding performance.

Chapter 26 deals with nutrition in detail.

Health factors

Infectious disease always has a detrimental effect on breeding colonies. Mating frequency, fertility, litter numbers and litter quality all decline. The newborn animals are greatly at risk, therefore pre-weaning mortality is raised and it is possible that an infected female will die during parturition. Even if the colony survives the resulting animals will be weak and not suitable for experimental work. For these reasons breeders of protected animals use full barrier units and make every effort to prevent disease organisms entering.

The effect the disease has depends on its nature and on the strain of animals being bred, e.g. Sendai virus will kill all the young mouse pups of some strains but have a negligible effect on other strains.

Other environmental factors

Providing suitable caging, nesting material, nest boxes and breeding systems is of fundamental importance for successful breeding. These are described in the species chapters.

Light intensity and photoperiod, temperature, noise and humidity all have a large effect on breeding colonies. These are discussed in Chapter 33.

References and further reading

Falconer, D.S. (1960) *Introduction to Quantitative Genetics*. Oliver and Boyd, Edinburgh and London.

Festing, M.F.W. (1999) Introduction to laboratory animal genetics. In: T. Poole (Ed.) *The UFAW Handbook on the Care and Management of Laboratory Animals* (7th edn). Blackwell Science, Oxford.

2
The Mouse

Introduction

The modern laboratory mouse has been developed from the house mouse (*Mus musculus*). Classification is shown in Table 2.1. In the wild they inhabit holes and crevices in buildings, where they live in male-dominated groups. They have well-defined territories and are aggressive to strange males encroaching on their territory.

The predominant method of communication in the mouse is through the production and reception of odours. Scents are deposited in prepucial gland secretions, urine and faeces. Their sensitive olfactory mechanism is able to identify information such as sex, reproductively receptive females, group members, territory and food sources from scent marks.

Mice are able to hear over a wide range of frequencies (0.8–100 kHz) with peak sensitivity between 5–20 kHz in the audible range and 50 kHz in the ultrasound range (Sales & Milligan 1992). Vision is considered to be very poor.

Use in regulated procedures

Over half the procedures reported in Home Office statistics each year are performed on mice. The reasons for its popularity as a laboratory animal are its relatively small body size, ease of handling, low maintenance cost and the large amount of background data available (Figure 2.1) (Cunliffe-Beamer & Les 1987).

In addition to the many outbred strains of mice, several hundred strains of inbred mice have been developed, although only a relatively small number of these are in regular use. Many mutant strains are also available. Tables 2.2 and 2.3 provide examples of the major characteristics of some inbred and mutant strains. Several substrains of each strain may be available, each with the same major characteristic but with slight variations. Further information on inbred strains can be obtained from Festing (1999) and Jax Labs (www.jax.org).

A large number of transgenic strains have been developed and are being developed for use in biomedical research (see Chapter 14).

Environment

Environmental levels recommended in the *Home Office Code of Practice for the Housing and Care of Animals used in Scientific Procedures* (Home Office 1989) and for the *Housing and Care of Animals in Designated Breeding and Supplying Establishments* (Home Office 1995) are given in Table 2.4.

Mice, in common with all laboratory animals, must be provided with a stable environment. They are adversely affected by fluctuations in temperature and relative humidity. Once a temperature has been selected from the range it should not vary more than ± 2 °C. The temperature in the cage can be 3–6 °C above the room temperature, depending on the type of cage used (Home Office 1995). Relative humidity should not be allowed to drop below 40%. Air changes depend on the stocking density and types of caging used. A relatively high light intensity is required for staff to be able to inspect animals adequately and to ensure the room is kept clean. The

Table 2.1 Classification of the mouse *Mus domesticus domesticus*.

Kingdom	Animalia
Phylum	Chordata
Sub-phylum	Vertebrata
Class	Mammalia
Order	Rodentia
Family	Muridae
Generic and specific names	*Mus domesticus domesticus*

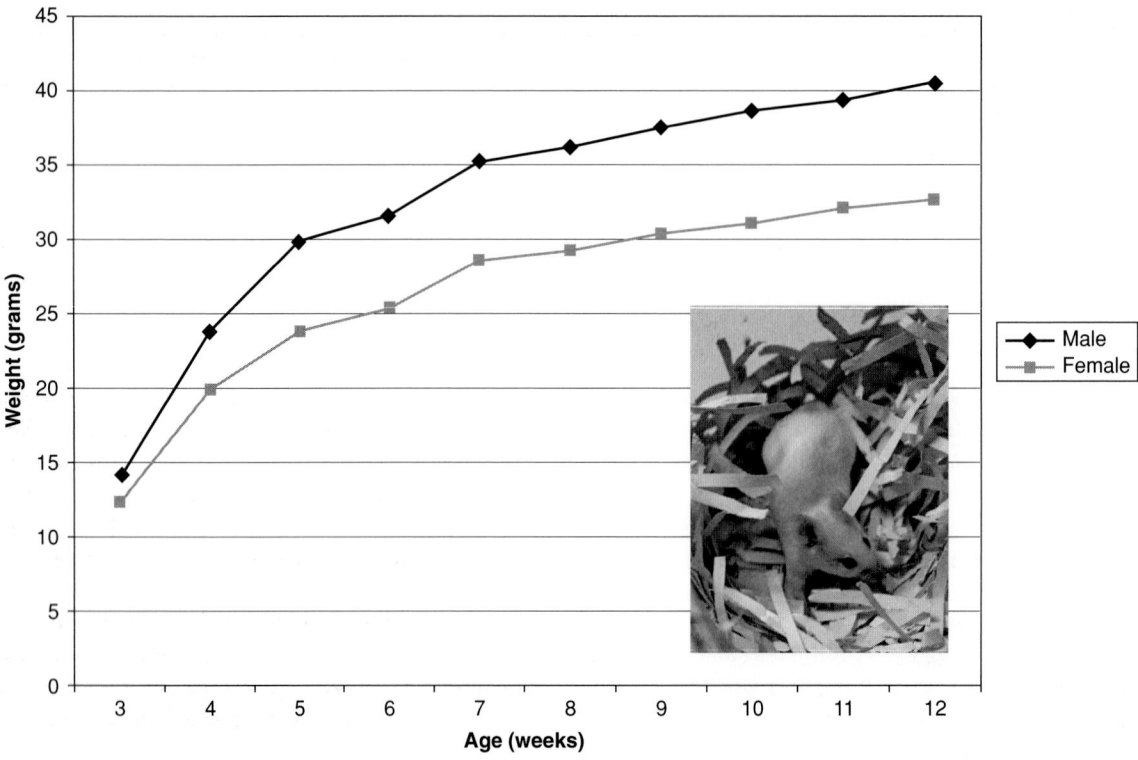

Figure 2.1   Balb/c growth curve.

Table 2.2   Examples of inbred strains.

Strain	Characteristics	Examples of use
C57BL/6J	Long lived, develops few spontaneous tumours. A large amount of background information is available.	One of the most widely used inbred strains. Used as a background for mutant strains.
STR/Ort	Develop severe non-inflammatory joint disease by the time they are one year old.	Used for osteoarthrosis studies.
C3H	Develop viral-induced mammary tumours. Carry retinal dystrophy gene.	Studies of mammary tumours and retinal degeneration.
129	High incidence of testicular tumours.	Cancer research.
DBA/IJ	Develop arthritis when treated with collagen.	Rheumatoid arthritis.

Table 2.3   Examples of mutant strains.

Strain	Characteristics	Examples of use
C57BL/Ks-*db*	Develop severe diabetes.	Diabetes research.
C57BL/6-*ob*	These become extremely obese, have elevated blood glucose levels, defective thermoregulation.	Develop non-insulin dependent diabetes mellitus and hypotension.
BALB/c-*nu*	Hairless, absence of thymus gland, causing depressed cellular immune response.	Cancer and disease studies.

animals themselves must be protected from exposure to this level of light, particularly if they are housed in the top of a rack.

Special conditions have to be provided for sensitive strains, for instance nude mice are kept at a slightly higher temperature (25 °C) than hairy ones.

Caging

Cages are usually constructed of polypropylene, polycarbonate, polysulfone or stainless steel. Cages

Table 2.4 Environmental levels for mice (Home Office 1989, 1995).

	Scientific procedure establishments	Breeding and supplying establishments
Room temperature	19–23 °C	19–23 °C
Relative humidity	55% ± 10%	55% ± 15%
Room air changes per hour	15–20	15–20
Photoperiod	12 hours light: 12 hours dark	12 hours light: 12 hours dark
Light intensity	350–400 lux at bench level	Adequate to allow staff to perform husbandry duties safely

with solid bottoms are preferred. Mesh floors are available but should only be used if there is no alternative. The lids of plastic cages are constructed of stainless steel with a preformed basket to hold food and a container for the water bottle.

Mice may be housed in a variety of containment systems, e.g. isolators or individually ventilated cage systems, depending on their health status or the type of procedures they are involved in, these are described in Chapter 33.

Guidance on stocking densities can be found in the current codes of practice (Home Office 1989, 1995).

Wherever possible mice should be group housed. The aggressive nature of some strains (e.g. Balb/c) may make this impossible, particularly when housing males. An assortment of materials is available to put into cages to provide a more stimulating environment for the animals. Environmental enrichment should reflect, as far as possible, the natural habitat of the animal. Tubes and 'des reses' can be used to mimic tunnels and holes used by mice in the wild (Figure 2.2).

Bedding and nesting materials

A wide range of materials are available for bedding. Corn cob, dust-free softwood sawdust, wood chips or shavings can be used in solid-bottomed cages and sawdust or absorbent paper can be used in trays beneath grid-bottomed cages. Shredded soft paper or nestlets are examples of suitable nesting materials (Figure 2.2) (Barnett 2001).

It is normal practice to provide clean cages at least once a week. The use of cage cleaning stations and individual ventilated cages minimises the spread of allergens and infectious organisms (see Chapter 33).

Food and water

Mice are fed commercially prepared diets in the form of expanded or traditional pellets, from baskets suspended or incorporated into the lid of the cage. Experimental powdered diets are fed in specially designed hoppers (see Chapter 26). Enrichment may

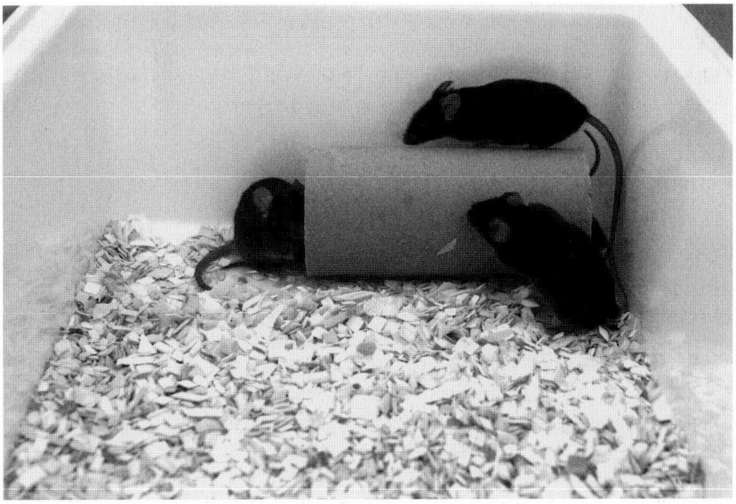

Figure 2.2 Mouse cage with tube used for environmental enrichment.

be achieved by providing forage food, e.g. peanuts and sunflower seeds, where this will not compromise the study.

Water is presented in plastic bottles with spouts which should both be changed regularly and sterilised once a week. Alternatively, water can be supplied from an automatic watering system (Chapter 27).

An average adult male mouse consumes approximately 5 g of food and 6 cm^3 of water daily.

Breeding

A summary of the breeding data for examples of outbred and inbred mouse strains is given in Table 2.5. This data must be interpreted with care as there are considerable strain differences.

Female mice are sexually mature by four weeks of age, although they are not used for breeding until they are at least six weeks old. Earlier use results in poor quality litters and affects the wellbeing of the female.

The female mouse is polyoestrus in the presence of the male (or male pheromones). The oestrous cycle occurs every four or five days in laboratory conditions, providing lighting is supplied for between twelve and fourteen hours per day. It has been reported that various factors can influence the length of the oestrous cycle, e.g. individually housed females

may have abnormally long cycles and group-housed females become di-oestrus, anoestrus, or pseudo-pregnant (Cunliffe-Beamer & Les 1987).

Pseudopregnancy can also occur following sterile mating or poor technique when taking vaginal smears. Pseudopregnancy lasts for thirteen to fourteen days in the mouse.

Oestrus can be manipulated by the use of the Whitten effect (see Chapter 1) or by the use of hormones (see Chapter 14).

Breeding systems

The gregarious nature of mice enables most strains to be bred from monogamous pairs or permanent harems. These systems allow post-partum oestrus to be taken advantage of. Successful post-partum mating will depend on strain and physiological condition of the female but can be expected to be at least 66%.

Monogamous pairs must be used for the primary line of inbred strains. Where more than one inbred strain is bred in one room there is a risk of genetic contamination. This risk can be minimised by appropriate genetic screening (see Chapter 16) and by instituting the following work practices:

- maintain each inbred strain in a separate room;
- if it is unavoidable to keep more than one strain in a room, only keep strains with different coat colour in the same room;
- institute a policy of killing escaped animals.

As a result of inbreeding depression, breeding productivity is usually lower in inbred strains than in outbred ones (Figure 2.3). Adult inbred animals are also smaller than outbred animals of the same age (Figure 2.4).

Figure 2.3 shows a comparison between number in litters and pup size of an inbred strain CBA/ca (top) and outbred strain CD1 (bottom).

Female mice will tolerate the presence of other females with their litters and can therefore be mated and housed permanently in larger groups. The ratio of females to males will vary between colonies and may be as low as two to one or as many as six females to one male. Responsibility for the care of the pups is shared by all of the females, which makes accurate recording of the productivity of individual females impossible in the harem. Where accurate identification of the parentage of young is necessary the boxing-out system can be used.

Table 2.5   Breeding data for outbred and inbred mouse strains.

	Typical outbred strain	Inbred strain Balb/c
Age when sexually mature	5 weeks	6 weeks
Age at first mating	6 weeks	6–8 weeks
Weight at first mating	20 g	18–20 g
Length of oestrous cycle	4–5 days	4–5 days
Duration of oestrus	12 hours	12 hours
Duration of pseudopregnancy	13–14 days	13–14 days
Gestation period	19–21 days	19–21 days
Birth weight	1 g	1 g
Average litter size	8	6
Return to oestrus post partum	Immediate then at end of lactation	Immediate then at end of lactation
Weaning age	21 days	21 days
Weight at weaning	10–12 g	10 g
Adult weight: male	45 g	30 g
Adult weight: female	40 g	25 g
Economic breeding life	6 litters	6 litters

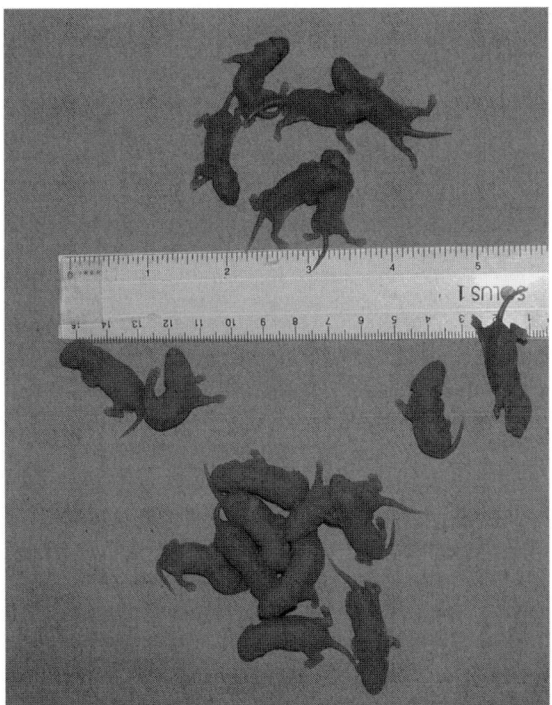

Figure 2.3 Comparison between number in litters and pup size of an inbred strain – CBA/ca (top) and outbred strain CD1 (bottom).

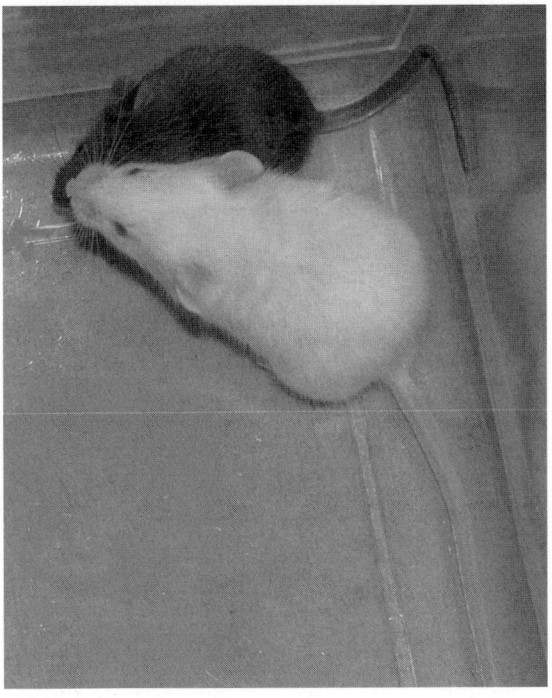

Figure 2.4 Inbred mouse CBA/ca (dark) and outbred CD1 of same age (white).

In both monogamous pair and permanent harem systems, weaning should be completed by twenty-one days. If this is not done the male parent will attack his sons and mate with his daughters when they reach sexual maturity.

Mating

Mating usually occurs at night and may be confirmed, if necessary, by making a wet preparation vaginal smear and examining it for the presence of sperm or by observing the presence of a cream-coloured, waxy plug (copulation plug) in the vagina. The vaginal plug is often retained deep in the vagina and a loop or small speculum may be needed to check for its presence.

Experienced people can confirm pregnancy, by external palpation, as early as day seven post copulation. An ultrasound scanning technique has been developed for mice; in experienced hands, pregnancy can be identified at about seven days post mating.

Pregnancy and parturition

Pregnancy in the majority of females is uncomplicated. As the female approaches full term she will augment her nest with whatever is available in her cage. Parturition usually occurs at night, one pup followed by its placenta with an interval of several minutes between the births of each pup. If the male is present at birth they will mate post partum thus reducing the litter interval to approximately twenty-five days.

Lactation

It is unusual for healthy females to have problems during lactation. If females suffer from a loss of milk, pups can be fostered onto other females. Cross fostering is used to make up litters of the same sex, same size, to obtain even litter numbers, etc. Hand rearing of newborn mice is not usually practical.

Health

Mice are affected by a large number of infectious and non-infectious diseases. Detailed consideration of these is beyond the scope of this chapter but a comprehensive summary can be found in Baumans

(1999). Rectal temperature of the mouse is in the range 36.5–38 °C.

Signs of ill heath in mice are similar to all animals, e.g.:

- obvious evidence of bleeding or discharge;
- abnormal movement;
- isolation from cage mates;
- piloerection and lack of grooming;
- lethargy;
- failure to eat and/or drink.

Identification

Permanent identification can be made by ear punching, tagging, tattooing the tail or with subcutaneous transponders. Temporary marking can be applied by the use of alcohol-based stains or inks (Barnett 2001).

References and further reading

Barnett, S.W. (2001) *Introduction to Animal Technology* (2nd edn). Blackwell Science, Oxford.

Baumans, V. (1999) The laboratory mouse. In: T. Poole (Ed.) *The UFAW Handbook on the Care and Management of Laboratory Animals* (7th edn). Blackwell Science, Oxford.

Cunliffe-Beamer, T.L. and Les, E.P. (1987) The laboratory mouse (pp. 275–308). In: T. Poole (Ed.) *The UFAW Handbook on the Care and Management of Laboratory Animals* (6th edn). Longman, Scientific & Technical, Harlow, UK.

Festing, M.F.W. (1993) *International Index of Laboratory Animals* (6th edn). PO Box 301, Leicester, LE1 7RU, UK.

Festing, M.F.W. (1999) Introduction to laboratory animal genetics. In: T. Poole (Ed.) *The UFAW Handbook on the Care and Management of Laboratory Animals* (7th edn). Blackwell Science, Oxford.

Home Office (1989) *Code of Practice for the Housing and Care of Animals used in Scientific Procedures.* HMSO, London.

Home Office (1995) *Code of Practice for the Housing and Care of Animals in Designated Breeding and Supplying Establishments.* HMSO, London.

Sales, G.D. and Milligan, S.R. (1992). Ultrasound and laboratory animals. *Animal Technology*, **43** (2).

3
The Rat

Introduction

The Norway rat was the first species to be domesticated primarily for scientific purposes; the first experimental work was published in the mid-nineteenth century. The rat is the second most commonly used laboratory mammal in the UK. Classification of the rat is to be found in Table 3.1.

Like the mouse, smell is the predominant sense in the rat; it can gain a wide range of information through perceiving odours. Both mice and rats have been observed spending up to ninety minutes scent marking a cage after being placed in a clean one (Barclay et al. 1988).

Table 3.1 Classification of the rat *Rattus norvegicus*.

Kingdom	Animalia
Phylum	Chordata
Sub-phylum	Vertebrata
Class	Mammalia
Order	Rodentia
Family	Muridae
Generic and specific names	*Rattus norvegicus*

Rats have the ability to perceive sounds at frequencies of 0.75–76 kHz. They have a peak sensitivity in the audible range (8–16 kHz) and another in the ultrasound range (35–40 kHz) (Sales & Milligan 1992). Communication in ultrasound has been shown to be important during courtship, between dam and offspring and during dominance disputes.

These sensitivities must be taken into consideration when designing a suitable environment for laboratory rats (see Chapter 33).

Use in regulated procedures

Many outbred strains of rat are available and a number of inbred strains have been produced. Examples are given in Tables 3.2 and 3.3.

Environment

Table 3.4 lists the Home Office codes of practice recommendations for the environment of rats.

Table 3.2 Examples of outbred rat strains.

Strain	Characteristics	Use
Lister Hooded	Good breeder, slow growth.	General purpose, good for lifetime studies.
Sprague Dawley (Figure 3.1)	Good breeder, easy to handle. Rapid weight gain.	General purpose.
Wistar (Figure 3.2)	Good breeder, moderate weight growth	General purpose.

Table 3.3 Examples of rat inbred strains.

Strain	Characteristic	Use
F334	Good breeder, medium life span. Susceptible to a range of tumours.	Cancer research, toxicology.
LEW	Docile, susceptible to the induction of a range of auto-immune diseases.	Immunology.
SHR	Spontaneous high blood pressure. High incidence of cardiovascular disease.	Cardio-vascular disease studies. This is a harmful mutation so it must be bred under a project licence.
WKY	Normal blood pressure.	Used with SHR in studies of cardio-vascular disease.

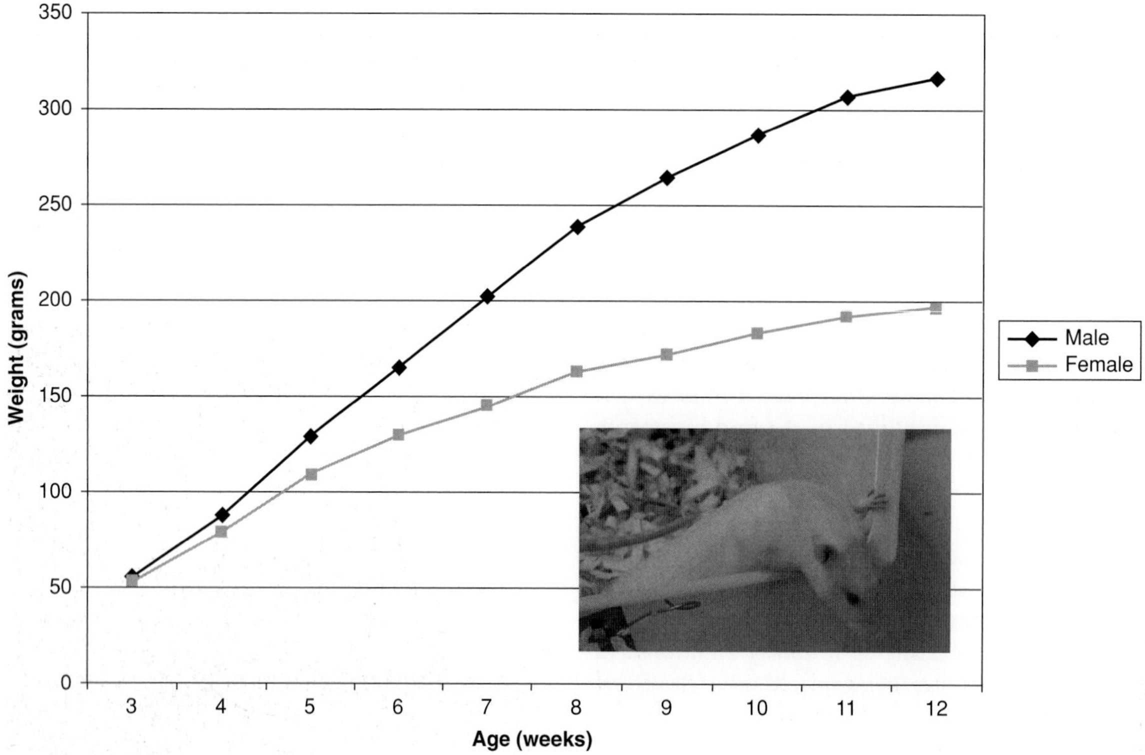

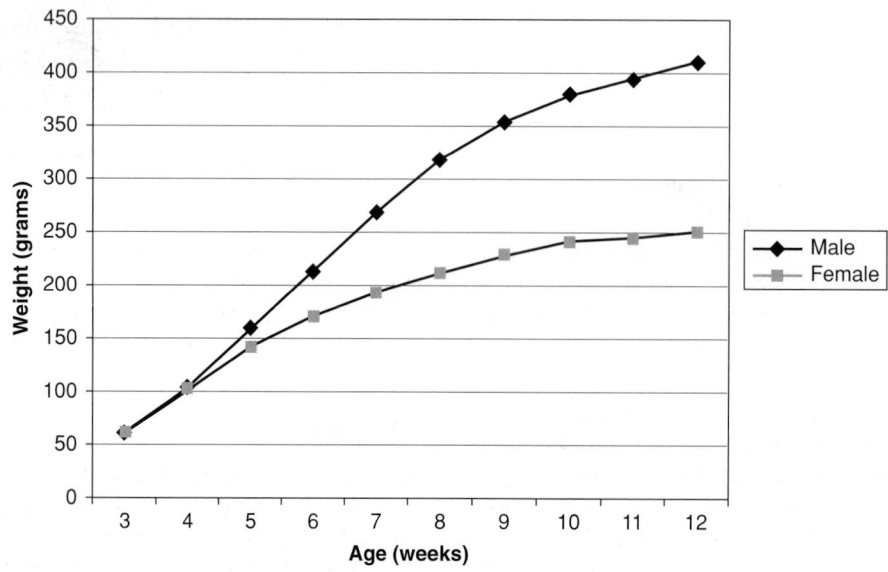

Figure 3.1   Sprague Dawley rat growth curve.

Figure 3.2   Wistar rat growth curve.

Table 3.4   Environmental levels for rats (Home Office 1989, 1995).

	Scientific procedure establishments	Breeding and supplying establishments
Room temperature	19–23 °C	19–23 °C
Relative humidity	55% ± 10%	55% ± 15%
Room air changes per hour	15–20	15–20
Photoperiod	12 hours light:12 hours dark	12 hours light: 12 hours dark
Light intensity	350–400 lux at bench level	Adequate to allow staff to perform husbandry duties safely

The comments made on environmental levels in Chapter 2 on the mouse apply equally to the rat. Young rats are particularly susceptible to ringtail if the relative humidity falls below 40% and when the temperature is high (see Chapter 33).

Caging

Cage sizes vary depending on group size and individual size of the rats. Guidance on stocking densities can be found in the current Home Office *Codes of Practice for the Care and Housing of Animals used in Scientific Procedures* (Home Office 1989) or the equivalent for designated breeding and supplying establishments (Home Office 1995).

Rats of both sexes are by nature gregarious animals and should not be housed singly unless it is an experimental requirement. Single housing compromises their welfare and may cause them to become nervous and/or aggressive, making them more difficult to handle and manipulate for the performance of experimental procedures. Rats housed on their own may develop stereotypies.

Cages for rats are constructed of both stainless steel and a range of plastic materials, such as polypropylene, polycarbonate and polysulfone.

Solid-floored cages with a bedding of wood shavings or other suitable substrate are the norm for rats. The presence of bedding and nesting materials and items of environmental enrichment allows the animals to have some control over their micro-environment (Figure 3.3).

Occasionally, it may be necessary to house rats in grid-bottomed cages where the substrate is placed in a tray below the grid (e.g. where timed mating is needed). Although these cages may be easier to clean than solid-bottomed cages the effect on the comfort and wellbeing of the rats is such that they should only be used when the experimental protocol demands

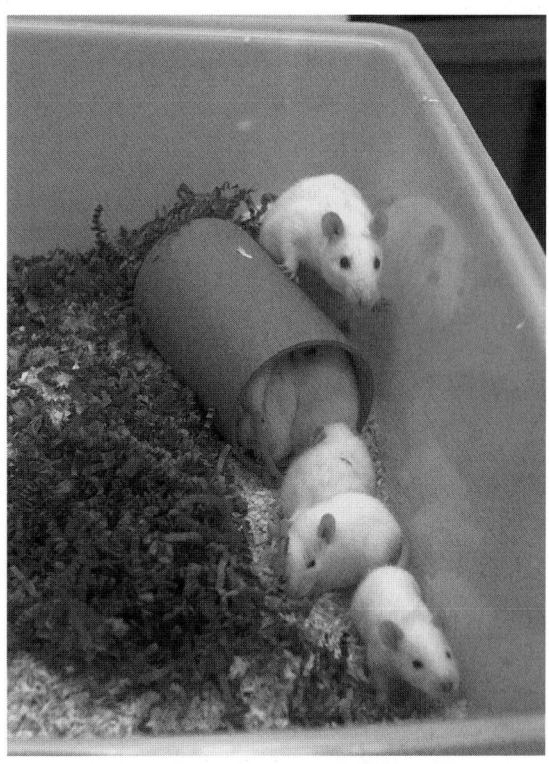

Figure 3.3   Rats in cage with bedding and nesting materials.

them, for instance with diabetic animals who consume large quantities of water and produce excessive amounts of urine. When grid-bottomed cages have to be used, small solid resting areas should be provided.

Routines

Rats are usually cleaned at least twice a week when the animals are to be placed in a clean cage with fresh substrate and nesting materials. It may be necessary to increase the frequency of cleaning, for instance with some diabetic models.

Control of allergens is particularly important when cleaning animals and a variety of techniques can be used to minimise their distribution. Cleaning systems implemented should aim to minimise the need for personal protection equipment by using dust-free bedding materials, cage cleaning stations and individual ventilated cages (see Chapter 33).

Food and water

Rats are accomplished gnawers whose teeth continue to grow; they will readily eat cubed diet through the bars of a basket-type hopper. The dietary requirements of rats and mice are similar and several different formulations are commercially produced which provide a balanced diet suitable for both species. Low energy diets are available for use in long-term studies (see Chapter 26). Bodyweight of long-term rats can be also be controlled by restricted feeding, where a set amount of food, approximately 85% of *ad libitum* intake, is fed every day. If powdered diets have to be fed for extended periods, rats should be provided with chew blocks or similar opportunities for gnawing. An adult rat eats approximately 15 g of diet a day.

The provision of water of high quality is essential for laboratory animals. It may be presented in water bottles or by an automatic piped system. Plastic or glass bottles may be used, fitted with either metal or melamine spouts. Automatic drinkers are normally mounted on the rack so that they project through a hole in the back of the cage. If flooding of the cage or tray is a problem, the drinker may be located outside the cage. A larger than normal hole in the rear of the cage allows the rat access to the drinker, any drips fall outside the cage or tray and are collected. Automatic systems must be checked daily to ensure they are functioning correctly as there is no obvious visual check for water consumption (see Chapter 27). A system of filters and regular flushing ensures the water is fresh when the rats drink it. An average adult male rat consumes approximately 35 cm^3 of water a day.

Breeding

The rat is poly-oestrous with a four- or five-day cycle. Ovulation is spontaneous and the female remains in oestrus for ten to twenty hours. There are no obvious visual indications of oestrus other than the willing-

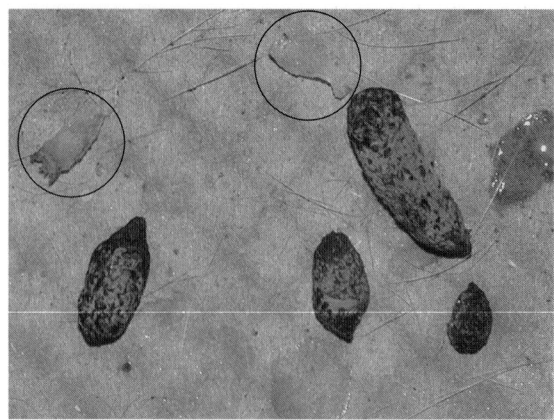

Figure 3.4 Vaginal plugs.

ness to mate. Copulation normally occurs during the night and can be confirmed the following day by the presence of a vaginal plug (Figure 3.4). A sterile mating leads to a pseudopregnancy lasting about fourteen days. Gestation lasts twenty-one to twenty-two days. Rats have a post-partum oestrus and mating at this oestrus has approximately 50% success rate. Litter size varies between the strains, with a typical outbred strain averaging around ten. Although puberty is reached earlier, rats are not normally mated until they are between ten and twelve weeks of age when non-inbred females will weigh 200–250 g and the males over 300 g.

The economic breeding life is usually measured in litters rather than months, five or six litters being the norm.

Breeding data is summarised in Table 3.5. There are strain differences so observed breeding data may differ from that stated here.

Breeding systems

Monogamous pairs

A male and female rat are paired together for their breeding life. Females are allowed to litter and rear their young in the presence of the male. With the male present at parturition post-partum mating may take place, thus reducing the litter interval. As the female will be lactating, implantation of the embryos may be delayed, effectively extending the gestation period by three to four days. Females conceiving post

Table 3.5 Breeding data of typical outbred strain.

	Typical outbred strain
Sexually mature	6–7 weeks
Age at first mating: male	12 weeks
Age at first mating: female	10 weeks
Weight at first mating: male	200 g
Weight at first mating: female	150 g
Oestrus cycle	4–5 days
Duration of oestrus	10–24 hours
Pseudopregnancy	14 days
Gestation	21–22 days
Birth weight	4–7 g
Litter size	10
Return to oestrus post partum	Immediate then end of lactation
Weaning age	21 days
Weight at weaning	40–60 g
Adult weight: male	Outbred 800 g Inbred 400 g
Adult weight: female	Outbred 600 g Inbred 300 g
Economic breeding life	6 litters

partum will, therefore, have a litter interval of approximately twenty-five days, whereas females not conceiving post partum will have an interval of approximately seven weeks. Using this system the colony litter interval averages about five and a half weeks. The monogamous pair system is used when accurate breeding records must be kept and for genetic reasons, for example in inbred colonies. It is not economic to maintain a large outbred colony using this system because of space. Larger cages have to be used and a large number of males must be kept (see Chapter 1).

Harem system

In this system two or more females are housed with one male. The size of the harem is governed by the size of the cage but one male to six females is an acceptable ratio. Since rats do not usually nurse well in a communal setting it is normal to box out the late-term pregnant females, allowing them to litter down individually. This reduces the possibility of young being trampled, but of course there will be no post-partum mating.

Timed mating

It may be necessary to produce rats of a known age or of a specified stage of pregnancy. It is always advisable to use proven animals, i.e. experienced males and females or mature virgin females.

There are two methods of ensuring matings on a particular night.

Method one

This method is particularly useful when large numbers of pregnant females are required. Ten females are placed with a male in the late afternoon and then separated the following morning. Each female is carefully examined for signs of a copulation plug which indicates that mating has taken place. The plug passes out of the vagina fairly soon after mating so mating is often arranged in grid-bottomed cages so that the plugs can be observed in the tray beneath the grid.

A vaginal smear is taken from any female without a plug, mounted on a slide as a wet preparation and examined under a microscope for evidence of sperm. To ensure a high success rate, females are only considered likely to be pregnant if large numbers of sperm are recovered. Using this method it is not unreasonable to expect a pregnancy success rate in excess of 80% of the mated females.

It is necessary to use at least five females for each positive required, i.e. twenty timed-mated animals require the mating of one hundred females (because only about one fifth of them are likely to be in oestrus on the night).

Females who do not appear to have mated should be put to one side, after two weeks any of these animals which are pregnant can be put into normal production, the remaining non-pregnant animals can be re-used for timed matings.

This method requires little preparation but it can take up considerable space.

Method two

Females can be examined for signs of oestrus by taking vaginal smears. This can be done five days before the animals are to be mated. If smearing is done immediately before mating, conception rates may be lowered. All females in oestrus are identified or removed to separate boxes. One or two females are placed with each male on the fifth night following smearing. At this time they will just be coming back into oestrus. It may be necessary to mate twice the number of females to ensure the required number of pregnancies. Experience will allow refinement of this method. Pregnancy is diagnosed as previously described.

This method is initially more time consuming but requires less space and is ideal for the production of relatively small numbers of time-mated animals at irregular intervals.

Oestrus can also be detected by the use of a device which measures vaginal impedance. The use of this type of equipment significantly reduces the number of animals required and the amount of labour needed.

Parturition/lactation

Pregnant females should be provided with suitable nesting materials such as shredded paper. Birth usually occurs at night with each pup being followed by its placenta, which the female eats. Litters should be disturbed as little as possible in the lactation period and should not be cleaned out in the week following the birth of the pups, thereafter they should be cleaned out once a week.

Cross fostering

The practice of cross fostering has been carried out for many years and can be used to maximise efficiency of animal production by ensuring that all litters being reared are of a standard size. If there is a bias in a scientific experiment for one sex, pups can be removed from all females, sexed and sorted into same-sex and same-size litters which are then redistributed to the females. Unwanted animals can then be killed and surplus dams can be put back for remating. Cross fostering is normally carried out shortly after birth.

Weaning

Young begin to take solid food at about fourteen days and weaning is complete at three weeks of age, when the young will weigh between 40–60 g. It is usual to select future breeders at this time.

Health

The general comments on signs of ill health in Chapter 2 on the mouse apply to the rat. The rectal temperature of the rat is 38 °C.

Identification

Rats can be identified for short periods by staining the fur using a histological stain. Permanent marker pens can be used to colour the fur, bands may be drawn around the tail or numbers may be written on the backs, the ears or the tail.

If rats are to be kept for long periods a more permanent method of identification may be needed. Ear punching or clipping to an established code is satisfactory but the skin tissue may occasionally regrow and there is a risk of damage to the ear through fighting and subsequent loss of identification.

Rats may be permanently identified by tattooing the tail or the ears. An electric tattoo pen may be used to write a freehand number or code down the tail or small tattooing pliers can be used to apply a pin-punched number or letter to the pinna.

Subcutaneous transponders can also be used for permanent identification.

References and further reading

Barclay, R.J., Herbert, W.J. and Poole, T.B. (1988) The disturbance index: a behavioural method of assessing the severity of common laboratory procedures on rodents. *UFAW Animal Welfare Report No. 2.* Potters Bar, UK.

Home Office (1989) *Code of Practice for the Housing and Care of Animals used in Scientific Procedures.* HMSO, London.

Home Office (1995) *Code of Practice for the Housing and Care of Animals in Designated Breeding and Supplying Establishments.* HMSO, London.

Sales, G.D. and Milligan, S.R. (1992) Ultrasound and laboratory animals. *Animal Technology,* **43** (2).

4

The Hamster

Roger J. Francis

Introduction

There are two main groups of hamster.

(1) Mouse-like hamsters (*Calomyscus* species), many of which have large ears, well-furred, long tails and no cheek pouches, e.g.:

- *Calomyscus mystax*: Afghan mouse-like hamster
- *Calomyscus hotsoni*: Hotson's mouse-like hamster.

(2) The group commonly known as the rat-like hamsters, comprising the genus *Cricetulus*.

Within group 2 are the hamsters most often used for research.

- *Mesocricetus auratus*: the Syrian hamster or the Golden hamster (Figure 4.1);
- *Cricetulus griseus*: the Chinese hamster (Figure 4.2);
- *Phodopus sungorus*: the Djungarian hamster.

The latter two are often referred to as dwarf hamsters. Table 4.1 lists the classification of hamsters.

The coat colours of the Syrian hamster range from white to black and piebald, the most common is a reddish brown (golden) with a lighter coloured underside. Certain colour forms, i.e. ruby-eyed cinnamon colour, are sex linked and males of this colour are frequently sterile.

The Syrian hamster has an undeserved reputation as being difficult to handle. It is nocturnal and should be allowed to wake up before being picked up. They can be picked up single handed by placing a hand over the back and lifting them up, or by cupping them up in both hands. They should not be 'scruffed' unless it is the only way to restrain them for a procedure. They have a very loose scruff and it is essential

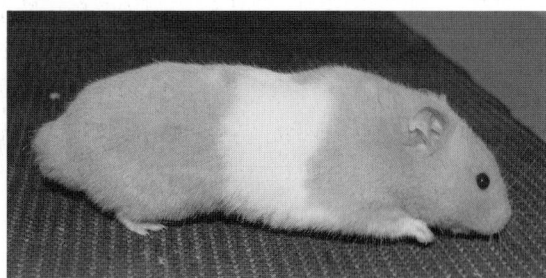

Figure 4.1   Syrian hamster.

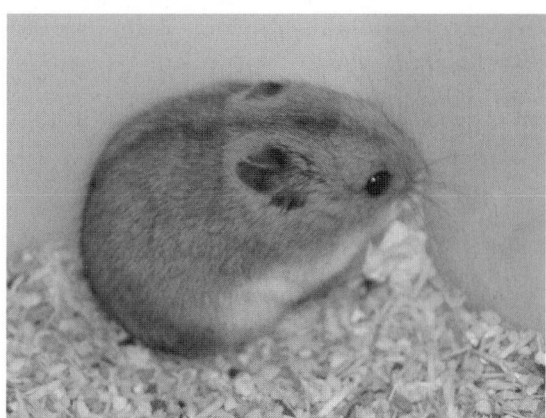

Figure 4.2   Chinese hamster.

Table 4.1   Classification of hamsters *Mesocricetus auratus, Cricetulus griseus* and *Phodopus sungorus*.

Kingdom	Animalia
Phylum	Chordata
Sub-phylum	Vertebrata
Class	Mammalia
Order	Rodentia
Family	Cricetidae
Generic and specific names	*Mesocricetus auratus*
	Cricetulus griseus
	Phodopus sungorus

to have a grip of the scruff from high in the neck and down the length of the back.

The Chinese and Djungarian hamsters are very similar in appearance, both being silver-grey with a black dorsal stripe and a white underside. Both are now available in a range of coat colours; in the wild both are known to moult into a white winter coat.

If ambient temperature remains below 10 °C and daylight is reduced, hamsters may go into hibernation. Hibernation is not an essential process in the hamster's life and forced hibernation may be detrimental to immature animals.

Use in regulated procedures

The short gestation period of the Syrian hamster makes them a suitable model for some types of reproduction and teratology studies. The immune system of the Syrian hamster is unlike most other animals' in that they are tolerant of implants of tissues, parasites, viruses and bacteria from other species, including humans. This makes them valuable for cancer studies and work with infectious organisms. They are used in dental research as their molar teeth are similar in structure to human teeth. Chinese hamsters are used for diabetes mellitus studies (Hobbs 1987).

Environment

The environmental values for hamsters quoted in the Home Office codes of practice (1989, 1995) are given in Table 4.2.

The comments made in the environment section of Chapter 2 on the mouse apply to hamsters. The reproductive cycle of Syrian hamsters is very sensitive to photoperiod. A minimum of twelve hours light is necessary to keep them in breeding condition.

Caging

In their natural environment hamsters are solitary animals and require single housing, but with docile and compatible strains it is possible to establish groups at weaning and keep them together throughout their lives. Some compatible strains can be housed as monogamous pairs throughout their breeding lives.

Guidance on stocking densities can be found in the current codes of practice (Home Office 1989, 1995). These guidelines are minimal levels and more generous space allocation is often necessary to accommodate items for environmental enrichment.

Hamsters should be housed in solid-floored cages. The solid floor should be covered with a suitable substrate, i.e. sawdust, wood shavings, Lignocel®, etc. They are prolific nest builders and should be offered adequate nesting material with which to build a nest. Refuges (e.g. cardboard tubes) should be provided where they can build a nest with material provided. Giving refuges and adequate nesting material may help to reduce food hoarding, animals with inadequate nesting material may break up all the food available to them and attempt to build a nest with it, failing this, they may heap all of the substrate into a corner to create a nest. Refuges also provide an escape for docile animals from more aggressive cage mates.

If grid floors must be used, the animal should be given a solid-floored resting area or nesting box.

Food and water

Hamsters can be fed standard rodent breeding or maintenance diet, which can be provided in hoppers;

Table 4.2   Environmental levels for hamsters (Home Office 1989, 1995).

	Scientific procedure establishments	Breeding and supplying establishments
Room temperature	19–23 °C	19–23 °C
Relative humidity	55% ± 10%	55% ± 15%
Room air changes per hour	15–20	Sufficient to ensure a supply of fresh air and level of ammonia in the cage at an acceptable level.
Photoperiod	12 light: 12 dark	12 light: 12 dark
Light intensity	350–400 lux at bench level	Adequate to allow staff to perform husbandry duties safely.

food hoppers should not be repeatedly filled if food has been hoarded in the cage. Hamsters will consume a wide range of seeds. Seeds such as sunflower, wheat and maize can be added to the substrate in small quantities, this will enable the animals to forage for the seeds. Chinese and Djungarian hamsters rarely come across fruits and vegetables in the wild, feeding these may cause diarrhoea so in this case only seeds should be provided as forage foods.

Water can be provided in water bottles. The hamster's tendency to gnaw can cause automatic watering systems to leak, leading to flooding, bottles are therefore more suitable for this species,

An average adult Syrian hamster will consume approximately 10–15 g of food and 10 cm^3 of water daily.

Breeding

A summary of the breeding data for hamsters is given in Table 4.3. This data must be interpreted with care as there may be strain differences.

The hamster is seasonally polyoestrous and has a four to five day oestrous cycle. The stages of the oestrous cycle can be identified by vaginal smears, however in the hamster it is easier to look for the post-ovulatory discharge. This is a thick, creamy vaginal discharge, which sticks to a gloved finger and forms a string as it is withdrawn (Figure 4.3). By recording the days of discharge it is possible to predict when the female will be in pro-oestrus and can be placed with the male.

Breeding systems

Monogamous pairs can be used as long as the animals are paired at weaning. If the strain is particularly aggressive or if strange adults are to be mated then arranged mating must be used. Normally breeding animals should be selected by about eight to ten weeks of age.

When using arranged mating a female in oestrus is placed into the cage of a stud male. If oestrus has been predicted correctly the receptive female will show lordosis as the male approaches, the male will mount her and mating will take place. The pair can then be left together for a short while. A female which is not receptive will be aggressive to the male and should be removed before the male is injured. The female hamster is most receptive approximately one to two hours after the onset of the dark period. To facilitate pairing within the working day, light cycles are often adjusted so that the animal's dark phase starts at mid-day, permitting cleaning, feeding etc. in the morning and pairing for mating in the early afternoon. A red light allows the animals to be seen without disturbing

Table 4.3   Summary of breeding data for hamsters.

	Syrian	Chinese	Djungarian
Sexually mature	6 weeks	7–14 weeks	6–9 weeks
Age at first mating	6 weeks	10–12 weeks	7 weeks
Weight at first mating: male	80 g	30 g	25 g
Weight at first mating: female	75 g	30 g	25 g
Oestrous cycle	4–5 days	4 days	4 days
Duration of oestrus	12 hours	6–8 hours	–
Pseudopregnancy	9–10 days	–	–
Gestation	16 days	21 days	18 days
Birth weight	1.5–2.5 g	1.5–2.5 g	1.5–2 g
Litter size	7–9	5	3
Return to oestrus post partum	Immediate	–	immediate
Weaning age	21 days	21 days	18 days
Weight at weaning	25–30 g	–	–
Adult weight: male	90–125 g	40 g	35 g
Adult weight: female	95–140 g	40 g	35 g
Economic breeding life	6 litters	–	–

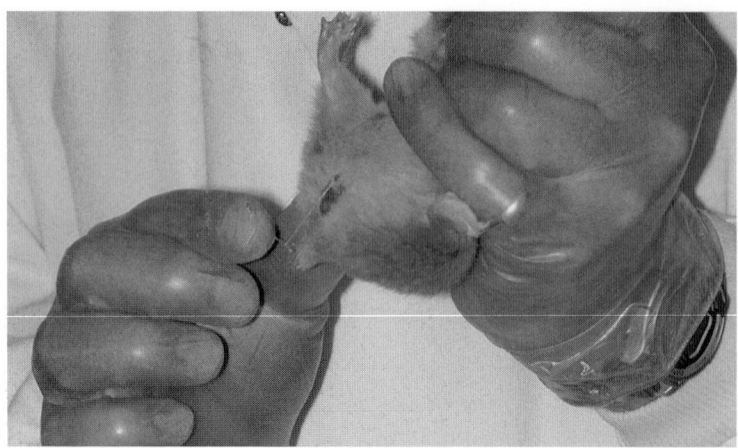

Figure 4.3   Post-ovulatory discharge.

them enabling selected animals to be paired. Pairs which are compatible and have mated can be left together for the afternoon and separated before leaving work at night. Those animals which are not compatible should be separated immediately.

Pregnancy and parturition

Pregnancy is not as obvious in hamsters as it is in some rodents. If the stock is handled regularly, checking for the lack of vaginal discharge should indicate a successful mating. Gestation is approximately sixteen days, parturition normally occurs within the dark phase and is usually trouble free. Although some hamsters will show a post-partum oestrus it is not usually fertile and the next oestrus is at the end of lactation. Litter size is usually seven to nine pups.

The litters of some strains can be handled from a very young age, but this should be avoided wherever possible. Although not generally practised, hamsters can be cross fostered. Care should be taken to handle all the pups within the newly created litter and they should be rubbed with the nesting material of the dam prior to her return to the cage.

Development of the hamster is very similar to the mouse and rat; the coat is apparent at seven to eight days, eyes are open at twelve to fourteen days, leaving the nest and feeding occurs at sixteen to seventeen days. Weaning is complete at twenty-one days. Unless the animals are to be used for breeding they should be separated into single-sex groups at this stage.

The economic breeding life of the hamster is ten to twelve months or six litters.

Health

The general points about signs of health listed in Chapter 2 on the mouse apply to hamsters. The rectal temperature of a hamster is 37–38 °C.

Identification

As with other rodents hamsters can be earmarked, ear tagged or injected with a microchip transponder.

References and further reading

Hobbs, K.R. (1987) Hamsters (pp. 275–308). In: T. Poole (Ed.) *The UFAW Handbook on the Care and Management of Laboratory Animals* (6th edn). Longmans, Scientific & Technical, Harlow, UK.

Home Office (1989) *Code of Practice for the Housing and Care of Animals used in Scientific Procedures.* HMSO, London.

Home Office (1995) *Code of Practice for the Housing and Care of Animals in Designated Breeding and Supplying Establishments.* HMSO, London.

Whittaker, D. (1999) Hamsters. In: T. Poole (Ed.) *The UFAW Handbook on the Care and Management of Laboratory Animals* (7th edn). Blackwell Science, Oxford.

5
The Guinea Pig

Introduction

Guinea pigs or cavies have their origins in South America. The strain in most common use as an experimental animal is the short-haired, albino, out-bred Dunkin Hartley (Figure 5.1), but coloured strains are available. Inbred strains have been established with Strains 2 (Figure 5.2) and 13 being the most popular.

Guinea pigs are normally docile but can be stressed easily and they respond to sympathetic handling. They react to being startled by freezing or scattering. Mature males can be aggressive and cause significant injuries to less dominant males, particularly in the presence of females. Table 5.1 lists the classification of guinea pigs.

Guinea pigs mark their territory with secretions from glands in the anal region. Dominant males are also known to urinate on members of their group to mark them. They communicate vocally, producing more individual sounds than any other small laboratory animal species. Although they have some hearing

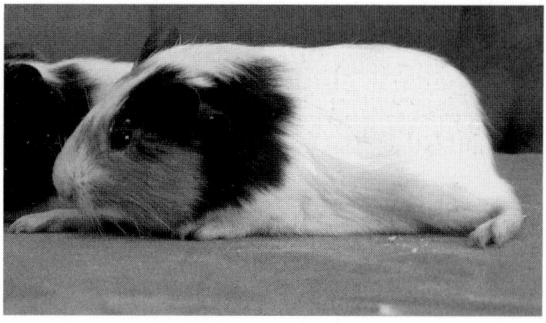

Figure 5.2 Guinea pig Strain 2.

Table 5.1 Classification of guinea pig *Cavia porcellus*.

Kingdom	Animalia
Phylum	Chordata
Sub-phylum	Vertebrata
Class	Mammalia
Order	Rodentia
Family	Caviidae
Generic and specific names	*Cavia porcellus*

Figure 5.1 Albino guinea pigs.

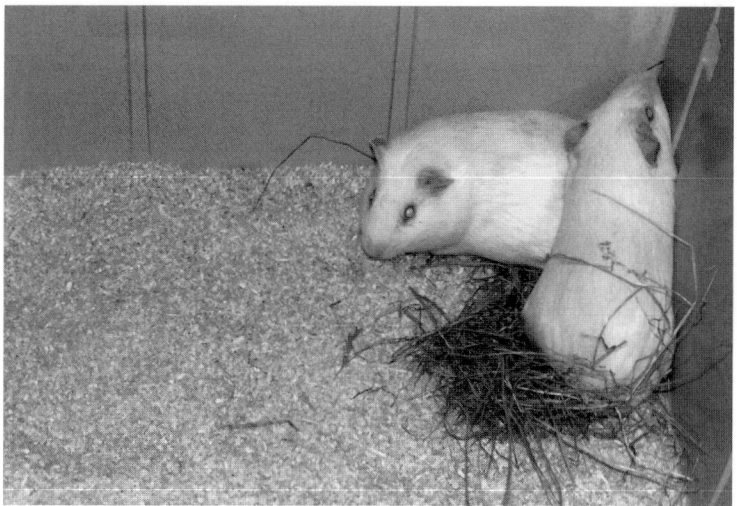

in the ultrasound range, their peak sensitivity appears to be at a much lower frequency, 0.5–8 kHz (Sales & Milligan 1992).

Use in regulated procedures

Guinea pigs are used for a variety of purposes, many related to the specific physiological differences they have when compared to rats and mice. Uses include:

- immunology – similar immunological response to man (Strains 2 and 13 particularly);
- biochemistry and pharmacology – isolated organs/ tissues rather than whole animal;
- skin sensitivity testing because they are less mobile than rats and mice and cannot get access to the treated site;
- mycobacterium research;
- vaccine testing;
- nutritional studies – vitamin C requirement.

Environment

Current recommended environmental values stated in the Home Office codes of practice can be found in Table 5.2 (Home Office 1989; 1995).

The comments on environment made in Chapter 2 are relevant to guinea pigs (see also Chapter 33).

Housing

Stock or experimental guinea pigs can be kept on either solid- or perforated-floored cages. Although a perforated floor aids the cage cleaning process, it increases the risk of legs becoming trapped or broken. This risk is highest during the animal's early life, from birth to about 300 g, and should be avoided for these animals. A covering of hay on the floor reduces the problem. Current stocking densities can be found in Home Office codes of practice (1989; 1995)

Cages may be in tiers on racks. As albino animals are sensitive to prolonged light exposed top cages must be covered (Figure 5.3).

Table 5.2   Environmental levels for guinea pigs (Home Office 1989, 1995).

	Scientific procedure establishments	Breeding and supplying establishments
Temperature	16–23 °C	15–24 °C
Relative humidity	55% ± 10%	55% ± 15%
Air changes per hour	15–20, depending on stocking density	15–20
Photoperiod	12 hours light:12 hours dark	
Light intensity	350–400 lux at bench level	Adequate to allow staff to perform husbandry duties safely

Figure 5.3   Tiered guinea pig cages.

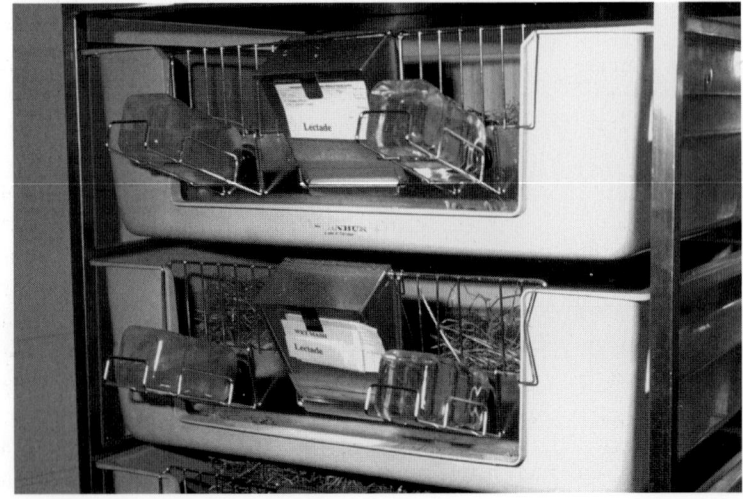

Figure 5.4   Young guinea pigs.

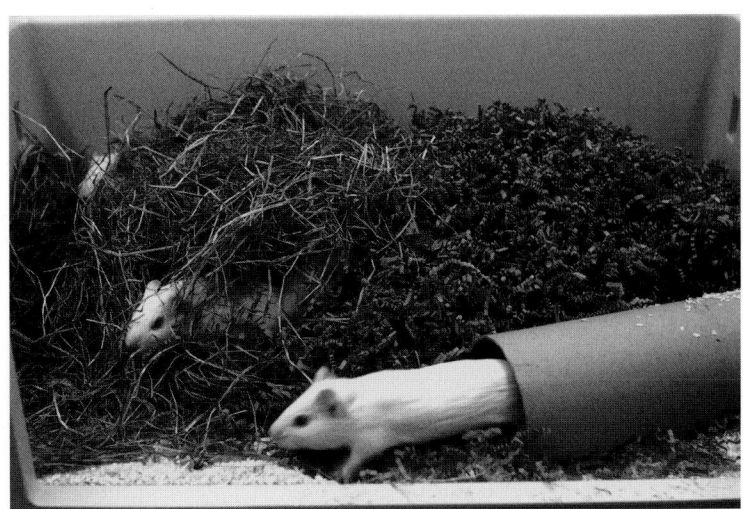

Breeding animals can also be maintained on per-forated floors, but in most animal units solid-floored cages or floor pens are used.

Bedding and nesting materials

The floor of solid-bottomed cages should be covered with sawdust or wood shavings with an overlay of good quality meadow hay. Hay appears to be important for guinea pigs, particularly in breeding colonies where efforts to eliminate it have met with disastrous losses in production. Hay provides a useful bedding material and also enriches the environment of the pigs, a fact that becomes obvious by the animals' behaviour when the 'hay barrow' begins its journey around the animal room. In addition it adds essential bulk roughage to the diet.

Untreated hay contains many pathogenic micro-organisms and therefore presents a risk of introducing disease organisms into the unit. It must be decontaminated before it is given to the animals; the methods available to do this are either auto-claving or irradiation. The more expensive option, irradiated hay, is preferred as it retains the natural texture of hay; autoclaved hay tends to be hard and caramelised.

Guinea pig bedding needs to be changed several times a week depending on stocking levels. Bedding can become wet very quickly because the pigs play with their water, so may need changing very often. The cage should be changed at regular intervals.

Environmental enrichment

Guinea pigs enjoy running through hay and clean deep litter (Figure 5.4).

If possible, hay should be provided up to three times a week, the old, soiled hay being removed.

Adult pigs will gnaw any exposed surface and can even chew through aluminium food hoppers. Chew sticks/blocks of wood are useful substitutes.

Feeding and watering

There are several commercially available pelleted guinea pig diets (see Chapter 26). These can be fed *ad libitum* in hoppers or open bowls. In addition to its value as a nesting material and for environment enrichment, hay has a digestive benefit. A regular supply decreases the incidence of digestive disorders such as impaction of the colon and rectum.

The guinea pig, like the primate, must be given a daily dietary source of vitamin C. The traditional method of providing fresh vegetables such as cabbage as a source of vitamin C has generally been discontinued because it is a source of pathogenic agents and because it takes time to prepare and to clean out any which has not been eaten. The most convenient method of providing vitamin C is to use a commercial diet specifically formulated for guinea pigs. This will contain the required amounts of the vitamin. If the diet is to be autoclaved much of the vitamin C will be destroyed, possibly leaving insufficient levels in the diet, however most laboratory animal diet manufacturers ensure sufficient vitamin C survives autoclaving. Irradiation is the preferred method of sterilising diets as with this method the nutrient value is virtually unaffected. Care must be taken to ensure guinea pig diet is used before its use-by date or the levels of vitamin C may be depleted. Vitamin C can be provided by the addition of ascorbic acid to the drinking water but this tends to be rather time consuming to prepare as the supply must be changed daily. Plastic bottle tops must be used because metal catalyses the oxidation reaction which causes vitamin C to be converted to an inactive compound.

Cages or pens can be fitted with automatic drinking systems but care must be taken if solid floors are used. The guinea pig is a notorious waster of water, playing with the drinkers or even sleeping against the drinker nipple. Positioning the drinkers so that any water spill falls outside the cage can prevent flooding. Even when using mesh-floored cages it is advisable to position the drinkers so that any drips fall outside the dirt-tray and are collected in special channels.

An adult guinea pig will consume approximately 40 g of diet and 100 cm^3 of water a day.

Breeding

Of the rodents commonly used in the laboratory the guinea pig has the longest gestation. The young are born fully furred with ears and eyes open, able to walk and capable of taking solid food from a very early stage. They are sensitive to cold and must be kept warm if pre-weaning death is to be avoided. The average litter size is three to four young and weaning can be completed at fourteen days of age, at which time they weigh about 160–200 g.

The optimum age to start to use females for breeding is around twelve weeks, by which time they will have achieved sufficient growth so that the pregnancy will not impair further development. At this age they weigh about 500–600 g. The guinea pig has a fourteen- to sixteen-day oestrous cycle, the oestrus stage lasting approximately twenty-four to forty-eight hours. They ovulate spontaneously and have an average gestation period of around 63 days,

Table 5.3 Breeding data for guinea pigs.

Age when sexually mature	68 days
Age at first mating: male	16 weeks
Age at first mating: female	12 weeks
Weight at first mating	500–600 g
Length of oestrous cycle	14–6 days
Duration of oestrus	24–48 hours
Average gestation period	63 days (range 59–72 days)
Birth weight	50–100 g
Litter size	3–4
Return to oestrus post partum	Immediate then at end of lactation
Weaning age	14 days
Weight at weaning	180–200 g
Adult weight: male	1 kg
Adult weight: female	800 g
Economic breeding life	8 litters or 2–3 years

although the range is 59–72 days. The economic breeding life is usually two to three years depending upon performance.

Male guinea pigs are normally twelve weeks of age (600 g) when first used for breeding.

Breeding data is summarised in Table 5.3. This data should be interpreted with care as there is considerable individual and strain variation.

In order to allow the passage of large pups, the pelvic cavity of the female must be able to expand. In the final stage of parturition a hormone is released (called relaxin) which causes the ligaments holding the two pelvic bones together, at the pubic symphysis, to relax. A gap between the two pelvic bones forms, which can be as large as 2.5 cm during birth. The pelvis returns to normal within twenty-four hours of parturition. As virgin female guinea pigs get older the pubic symphysis ossifies and therefore will not respond to relaxin, making it difficult for the young to pass down the birth canal. For this reason female guinea pigs should not be used for breeding for the first time if they are older than seven months.

Pregnant guinea pigs increase in size significantly and require careful handling to avoid miscarriages or high losses at birth; full support should be given to the rear quarters.

It is not unusual for breeding females to undergo temporary alopecia during gestation and lactation. The cause is suspected to be hormonal change and not due to nutritional deficiencies or parasites. Hair will regrow in most cases.

Breeding systems

Monogamous pairs

One male and one female are paired at ten weeks old and are housed together throughout their breeding life. This system takes advantage of post-partum oestrus, which may be up to 75% successful, thus reducing litter intervals and increasing production. Although the percentage of successful post-partum matings will be higher than in the harem system there is little to recommend monogamous pairs as they take up significantly more room and more males have to be kept. It is mainly used where the identity of the mother, the parentage, or birth dates must be known, e.g. inbred strains.

Harem system

Guinea pigs rear their young successfully in the presence of others; in fact the young are often shared by the lactating sows. Sizes of harems can vary from one male with four females to one male with twenty females. Smaller harems appear to give the best production figures – harems of four to five females may produce up to eighteen young per female per year.

It is not uncommon for females to synchronise their oestrous cycles and this may mean that there will be four healthy pregnant females together in a cage at the same time. This can give an increased risk of mortality from trampling. Guinea pigs do not have nest areas and startle easily; this can result in the heavily pregnant females running over newborn animals.

In some instances sows may need to be removed to a cage on their own to litter and return to the harem group after their young are weaned (boxing out), e.g. when individual breeding performance, records and identity of young are needed. The boxing-out system will extend the litter interval from ten to approximately fifteen weeks.

Timed mating

A female in oestrus is placed with a male. Signs of oestrus are:

- the sow has a hymen (a membrane across the vaginal opening) which breaks down just before oestrus and regrows during metoestrus – females in which the hymen has degenerated are therefore in or close to oestrus;

- behavioural changes, including lordosis and the mounting of other sows, may also be seen;
- mating can sometimes be observed, as oestrus lasts over twenty-four hours;
- copulation plugs can be used to confirm mating, but they are often missed, chances of identifying them is increased if the animals are kept on grid floors;
- vaginal smears may be taken after the male and female have been together to detect sperm.

As the gestation period is so long it is possible for barren females to escape notice.

Young are born in a very advanced state. They are ready to eat solid food, but will suck the female for up to two weeks.

Record keeping

Record keeping in monogamous pairs is straightforward and normal cage card information is easy to collect. In harems, when females may give birth together, it is not always possible to determine from which sow the young have been born. Similarly, in the event of stillborn litters they could be attributed to the wrong female. It is therefore necessary to check for litters daily (even twice a day) for accurate determination.

Health

The general points about signs of ill health in Chapter 2 on the mouse apply to guinea pigs. The rectal temperature of guinea pigs is 37.2–39.5 °C. Common diseases of guinea pigs are described by North (1999) and Huerkamp et al. (1996).

Identification

Guinea pigs are not easy animals to identify. Ear punching is not suitable for long term marking as pigs have a habit of chewing and damaging their cagemates' ears. Tattooing the inner ear with forceps and suitably sized numerals is perhaps the most effective method (one digit per ear). Stains/agricultural markers can be considered for short-term identification and can be refreshed at birth, weaning or cleaning. Small ear discs can also be used. Transponders are the most suitable method.

References and further reading

Home Office (1989) *Code of Practice for the Housing and Care of Animals used in Scientific Procedures.* HMSO, London.

Home Office (1995) *Code of Practice for the Housing and Care of Animals in Designated Breeding and Supplying Establishments.* HMSO, London.

Huerkamp, M.J., Murray, K.A. and Orosz, S.E. (1996) Guinea pigs. In: K. Laber-Laird, M.M. Swindle and P. Flecknell (Eds) *Handbook of Rodent and Rabbit Medicine.* (Pergamon Veterinary Handbook series). Butterworth Heinemann Ltd (now part of Elsevier).

North, D. (1999) The guinea pig. In: T. Poole (Ed.) *The UFAW Handbook on the Care and Management of Laboratory Animals* (7th edn). Blackwell Science, Oxford.

Sales, G.D. and Milligan, S.R. (1992) Ultrasound and laboratory animals. *Animal Technology,* **43** (2).

6

The Rabbit

David Gregory

Introduction

Rabbits belong to the order Lagomorpha, they differ from rodents in several ways. The most noticeable difference is that they have a second pair of upper incisors set behind the first pair (Figure 6.1). Table 6.1 sets out the classification of rabbits. A number of different breeds of rabbit are used in research – New Zealand White (Figure 6.2) is the most common but other breeds are used, e.g. the smaller Dutch (Figure 6.3). Laboratory strains have been developed from the large lop-eared breeds for work involving collection of blood from ear veins. A number of inbred strains of rabbit are available.

Use in regulated procedures

Rabbits are used in a range of regulated procedures. Their relatively large size and prominent ear veins make them suitable for antibody production. Other uses include research into teratology, hypotension and arteriosclerosis.

Table 6.1 Classification of rabbit *Oryctolagus cuniculus*.

Kingdom	Animalia
Phylum	Chordata
Sub-phylum	Vertebrata
Class	Mammalia
Order	Lagomorpha
Family	Leporidae
Generic and specific names	*Oryctolagus cuniculus*

Environment

Environmental levels recommended in the Home Office codes of practice (1989; 1995) are given in Table 6.2.

Figure 6.1 Rabbit skull showing second pair of upper incisors behind the main pair.

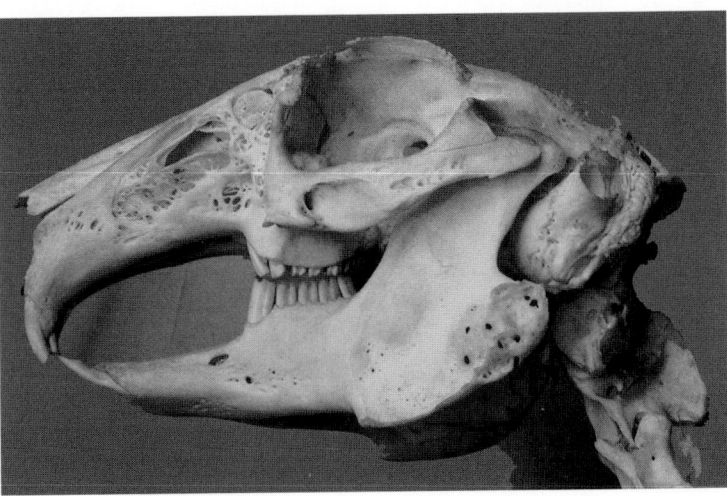

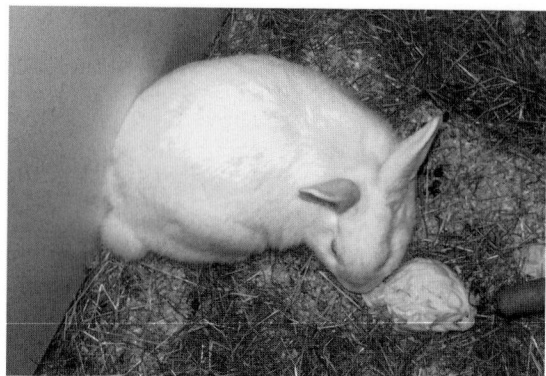

Figure 6.2   New Zealand White rabbit.

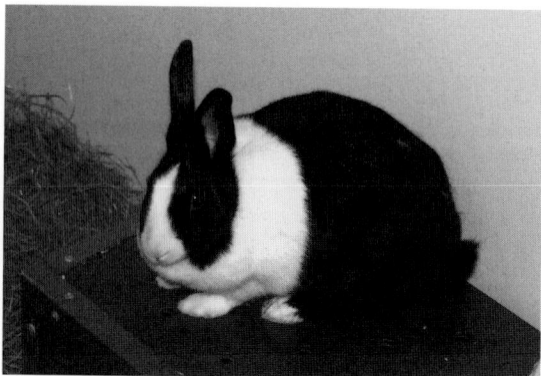

Figure 6.3   Dutch rabbit.

Rabbits are maintained at slightly lower temperatures than rodents, they will suffer if exposed to high temperatures. Sudden loud noises startle rabbits and may cause injury by making them jump and damage themselves on the cage. This is particularly evident after a period of quiet. A source of background noise from a radio has been suggested to reduce the startle factor from a loud noise.

Ventilation rates must provide all animals with good quality air. In order to do this, air changes may need to be higher in rooms where animals are housed in racks rather than in floor pens.

Housing

Guidance on stocking densities can be found in the current Home Office codes of practice (1989; 1995). The choice of housing used will be dictated by the purpose for which the animals are being kept and the space available. Commonly used systems are:

- single-housed in individual cages;
- group- or pair-housed in one or more inter-connected cages;
- floor-housed in pens either singly or in groups.

In addition to space requirements the other factors which must be considered when choosing a housing system are:

- duration of holding;
- experimental requirements/objectives;
- characteristics of the strain (e.g. not all rabbits are gregarious, it is quite common for adult animals to fight and inflict serious injury on one another);
- sex;
- growth rate/size of strain as adult;
- environmental enrichment.

All animals should be provided with an environment which is stimulating and where possible allows them to perform their full repertoire of natural behaviour. This can be enhanced by cage design and through socialising. Rabbits respond well to human interaction and therefore work routines should be designed to encourage close contact.

Cages

Cages can be manufactured in a wide range of materials, e.g. aluminium, stainless steel (either mesh or solid) and various plastics, e.g. polyethylene, polypropylene.

Table 6.2   Environmental levels for rabbits (Home Office 1989, 1995).

	Scientific procedure establishments	Breeding and supplying establishments
Room temperature	16–20 °C	15–24 °C
Relative humidity	55% ± 10%	55% ± 15%
Room air changes per hour	15–20	15–20
Photoperiod	12 hours light: 12 hours dark	–
Light intensity	350–400 lux at bench level	Adequate to allow staff to perform husbandry duties safely

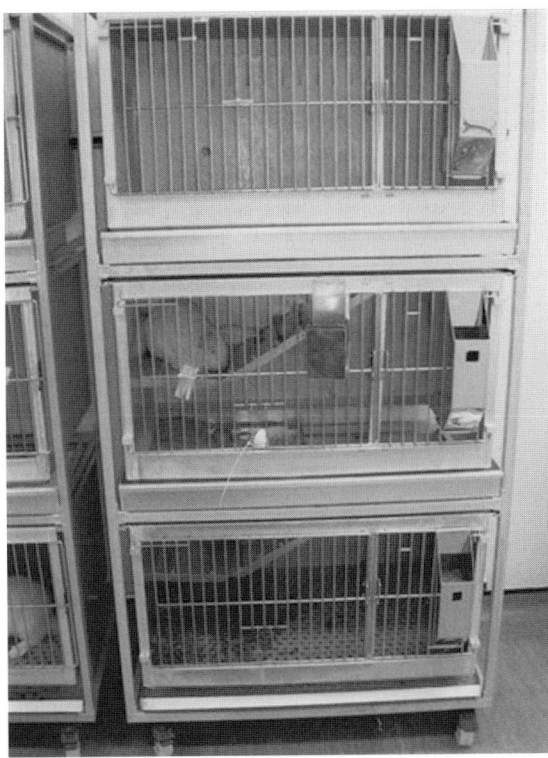

Figure 6.4 Multi-level rabbit housing.

Floors in cages are usually perforated rather than mesh, and shelves or solid areas are provided for comfort. Perforated flooring has almost eliminated the painful condition of sore hocks once common in caged rabbits. Faeces and urine pass through the perforated floor to a tray beneath which is a suitable substrate, e.g. sawdust or paper.

Modern cages provide shelves to allow vertical movement, and an area beneath the shelf for an added feeling of security for the animal. In spite of the extra cage furniture the rabbit must be able to be inspected by staff. Figure 6.4 shows an arrangement which allows a rabbit access to three cages via ladders (Gerson 2000).

Cleaning routines differ but as a guide the substrate in cages or cage trays should be cleaned at least twice a week, the whole cage being changed at regular intervals.

Pens

Housing in floor pens can be efficient and stimulating for rabbits, although it is not advisable to group house males over the age of ten weeks.

Pens can be permanent or temporary and are made in a variety of materials. They can be constructed to any size but the maximum number of animals in any pen should be approximately twenty. The need to observe and catch the rabbits is a more important consideration in pen design (Figure 6.5). Pens should be cleaned out weekly.

Rabbits produce a large amount of hair and this can block air extract filters therefore cleaning regimes must include regular replacement of filters.

Rabbits should be placed in same-sex groups at

Figure 6.5 Rabbit in floor pen with enrichment.

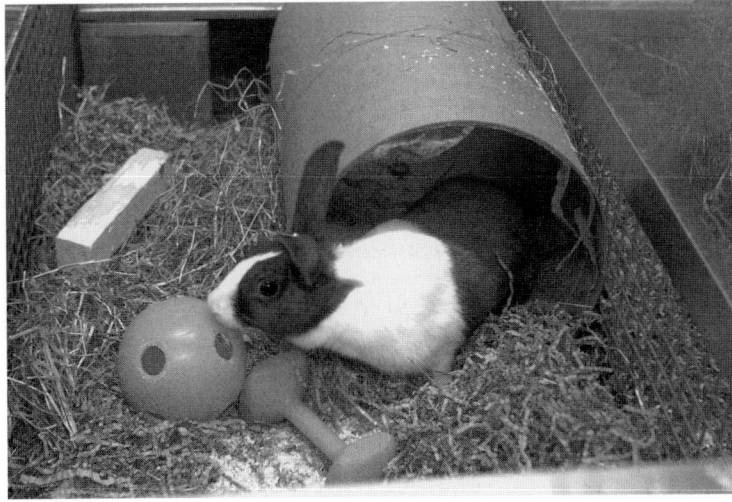

weaning. They should be checked physically and weighed weekly so that stocking densities can be adjusted. Once a group has been established, new animals should not be added as this will lead to fighting.

Pens give much more opportunity to provide shelves, tunnels, elevated ramps and hay racks than do cages.

Food and water

Laboratory rabbits are usually fed on a complete pelleted diet. Protein concentrations may be increased for breeding rabbits or reduced for stockholding (see Chapter 26). It is common to feed rabbits *ad libitum* but in some instances it is appropriate to restrict the amount provided (e.g. to prevent animals from becoming obese in long term studies). Approximately 190 g of food per day is usually sufficient for their needs. Pregnant or lactating does should not be put on restricted feeding regimens. Moistened diet may be beneficial to lactating does with litters leaving the nest box. Hay is usually fed to provide variation and to increase the fibre content of the diet.

Feed is normally provided in boot-shaped gravity feeders but bowls may also be used. Bowls increase the risk of the food being spoiled by the animals urinating or defecating in the container, so they must be checked regularly.

Mature rabbits can drink between 300–500 cm^3 of water a day, it must be provided *ad libitum*. Water can be provided in bowls, bottles or through automatic watering valves. Fresh water must be provided daily and must be checked and/or treated to ensure that there is no risk of contamination by water-borne pathogens. These may be reduced by chlorination, acidification, filtration or ultraviolet radiation (see Chapter 27). All food and water receptacles or systems should be cleaned and disinfected routinely.

Breeding

A summary of breeding data for New Zealand White and Dutch rabbits is given in Table 6.3. It should be interpreted with care as there are strain differences. The rabbit breeds throughout the year in laboratory

Table 6.3   Breeding data for New Zealand White and Dutch rabbits.

	New Zealand White	Dutch
Sexually mature	4–5 months	6 months
Age at first mating: male	9 months	8 months
Age at first mating: female	8 months	6 months
Weight at first mating: male	3–3.5 kg	2.5 kg
Weight at first mating: female	2.5–3 kg	2 kg
Oestrous cycle	Extensive in the absence of the male.	
Duration of oestrus	Extensive in the absence of the male.	
Pseudopregnancy	7–19 days	7–19 days
Gestation	31 days	28 days
Birth weight	70 g	40 g
Litter size	7	7
Return to oestrus post partum	Immediate then third to fourth week of lactation	
Weaning age	5–8 weeks	5–8 weeks
Weight at weaning	1–1.5 kg	0.85–1 kg
Adult weight: male	6 kg	3.5 kg
Adult weight: female	5 kg	2.5 kg
Economic breeding life	10–12 litters over 2–3 years	

conditions. The female New Zealand White rabbit is sexually mature at four to five months but is not used for breeding until eight months of age, the Dutch females are first used at six months. The males of both breeds are first used between eight and nine months of age. The doe is an induced ovulator and oestrus is extensive if she is not mated. Oestrus can be confirmed by observing a swollen, red vulva. The doe will return to oestrus immediately after giving birth but because rabbits are bred in arranged mating systems this is never taken advantage of. During their reproductive life laboratory rabbits will produce between ten and twelve litters over a two to three year period.

Breeding systems

Arranged mating is used because the possibility of aggression between males and females housed together make monogamous pairs and harems inappropriate for rabbits. The doe is placed in the buck's cage for mating. Established breeders will mate readily but occasionally virgin females can be reluctant and should not be forced. A mating is considered successful if the male rolls off the doe after copulation. As long as there is no sign of aggressive behaviour the pair may be left together for up to half an hour following the observed mating. During this time further matings may occur. After mating the female is returned to her home cage and the procedure is repeated a few hours later.

Although males can impregnate females on successive days, using them on alternate days appears to be most productive. In breeding units a ratio of one male to six females should be used.

Pregnancy

Pregnancy can be confirmed by external palpation at approximately ten days post mating. In inexperienced hands this procedure is dangerous to the foetus and to the doe therefore it should only be carried out after adequate training. Pregnancy can also be determined by progesterone assay from blood taken ten days after mating. The gestation period in the rabbit is thirty-one days in the New Zealand White and twenty-eight days in the Dutch.

Approximately one week before the anticipated parturition date (e.g. twenty-three days post mating in New Zealand White rabbits) the female should be provided with a nesting box. If the box is placed in the cage too soon the female may use it as a place to urinate and defecate. The nest box should provide security for the female. Covered nest boxes are preferable because they provide a warm, dark micro-environment. Material for nesting (e.g. wood shavings, shredded paper, hay) should be provided. The female will construct the nest and line it with hair from her abdomen.

Parturition

Complications at parturition are infrequent in healthy breeding stock. Any animal going past the expected date of parturition should be inspected and veterinary assistance called if necessary.

There is a persistent idea that does will eat their litters if disturbed but with good husbandry and regular handling the incidence of this is minimal. Some females are more protective than others but if treated well they are unlikely to destroy their litter.

Fostering and cross fostering is possible if the foster young are rubbed in soiled bedding from the cage of the foster doe. It is necessary to wash hands between handling each litter.

Does' milk is very concentrated and they only feed their young once a day. This should not be interpreted as neglect.

Weaning

Weaning is complete between five and eight weeks of age when New Zealand White rabbits should weigh 1–1.5 kg and Dutch rabbits 300–500 g.

If the young are left with the female too long after this time she will prevent them from sucking and this could result in injury to the young, particularly if the doe is pregnant.

Health

Signs of ill health in the rabbit are similar to those found in other animals. The normal rectal temperature of the rabbit is in the range of 38.5–39.5 °C.

In conventional units rabbits are at risk of pasteurellosis – a bacterial respiratory disease made evident by creamy discharges around the nose and medial aspect of the forelegs. Sore hocks used to be a problem when rabbits were housed on uneven grid floors; it is much less common now rabbits are housed on perforated floors.

Claws must be checked regularly and trimmed if necessary. In common with rodents, rabbits may suffer from malocclusion leading to overgrown teeth. Ingestion of hair can lead to hair ball (trichobezoars), resulting in anorexia and consequent weight loss. Diseases of rabbits are described by Stein and Walshaw (1996).

Identification

Commercially obtained rabbits should already be identified so that their parental histories can be checked. Ear tattoos, ear tags, electronic transponders or leg rings are used (Barnett 2001). Figure 6.6 shows rabbits, with different coat colours, group housed in a pen which eliminates the need for invasive identification techniques. These animals would have been grouped at weaning.

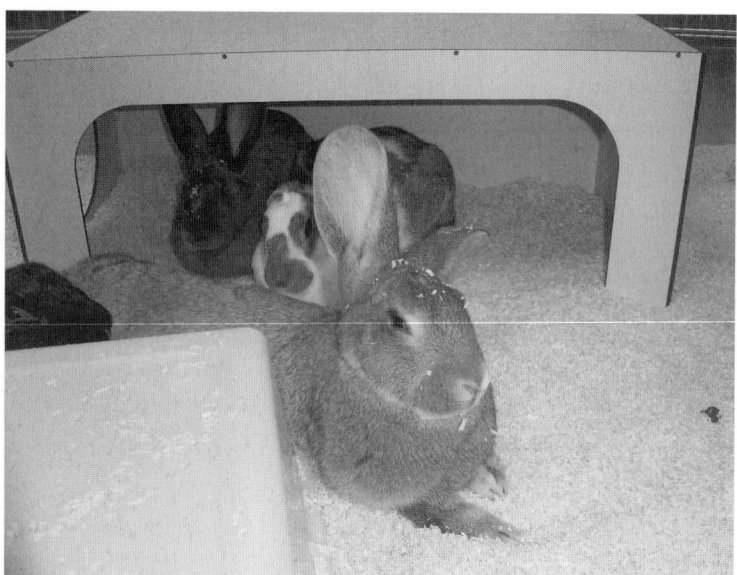

Figure 6.6   Group-housed rabbits identified by coat colour.

References and further reading

Barnett, S.W. (2001) Identification of animals (pp. 64–69). In: *Introduction to Animal Technology* (2nd edn). Blackwell Science, Oxford.

Gerson, P. (2000) The modification of 'traditional' caging for experimental laboratory rabbits and assessment by behavioural study. *Animal Technology*, 51 (1).

Home Office (1989) *Code of Practice for the Housing and Care of Animals used in Scientific Procedures.* HMSO, London.

Home Office (1995) *Code of Practice for the Housing and Care of Animals in Designated Breeding and Supplying Establishments.* HMSO, London.

Stein, S. and Walshaw, S. (1996) Rabbits. In: K. Laber-Laird, M.M. Swindle and P. Flecknell (Eds) *The Handbook of Rodent and Rabbit Medicine* (Pergamon Veterinary Handbook Series). Butterworth Heinemann Ltd now part of Elsevier.

7

The Ferret

Joanne C. Scott

Introduction

Ferrets are crepuscular and their wild counterparts, polecats, spend much of their time in dark or semi-dark burrows. Table 7.1 lists the classification of ferrets. Albino ferrets have poor eyesight and rely on a keen sense of smell and acute hearing to capture food and communicate with each other. Anal glands are used for scent marking, attracting a mate during the breeding season, and their contents can be expelled as a defence mechanism if they are angry or frightened.

Although polecats are known to live solitary lives in the wild, ferrets do appreciate company of their own kind and live happily together in groups (known as a business). Entire males can be housed together outside the breeding season but may become very aggressive towards each other once the breeding season starts.

Ferrets sleep up to fourteen hours per day but when awake are extremely alert and active. A male ferret is called a hob and a female is a jill. The average lifespan is eight to twelve years.

Ferrets can be restrained by clasping them around the neck ensuring their rear end is supported.

Use in regulated procedures

Ferrets suffer from influenza and the disease will readily be passed between ferrets and man. The ferrets' response to the infection is similar to that of humans, they therefore provide a valuable animal model for research into the influenza virus.

Ferrets are also able to vomit; therefore they can be used in studies where the incidence of vomiting and nausea needs to be recorded. The ferret is used as an alternative animal model to dogs and cats for this type of work.

Table 7.1 Classification of ferret *Mustela putorius furo*.

Kingdom	Animalia
Phylum	Chordata
Sub-phylum	Vertebrata
Class	Mammalia
Order	Carnivora
Family	Mustelidae
Generic and specific names	*Mustela putorius furo*

Environment

The environmental parameters recommended by the Home Office code of practice (1989) and the ferret supplement to the *Code of Practice for Breeding and Supplying Establishments* (www.homeoffice.gov) for ferrets are listed in Table 7.2.

A temperature should be chosen from the range in Table 7.2 and should not vary more than ± 2 °C.

Ferrets have poorly developed sweat glands; temperatures above 30 °C can lead to hyperthermia. Clinical signs of hyperthermia include severe agitation and distress, breathing with a gaping mouth, lethargy, vomiting. If left unattended the ferret will collapse and die. To rectify the condition the animal needs to be cooled down quickly. In mild cases this

Table 7.2 Environmental levels for ferrets (Home Office 1989, 1995).

	Scientific procedure establishments	Breeding and supplying establishments
Temperature	15–21 °C	15–24 °C
Humidity	55% ± 10%	No need to control or record.
Air changes	10–12 per hour	10–12
Photoperiod	12 hours light: 12 hours dark	Not less than 8 hours light daily.
Light intensity	350–400 lux	Sufficient to enable all animals to be inspected.

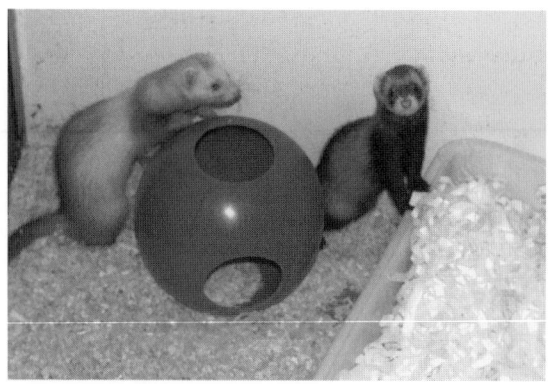

Figure 7.1 Ferrets in floor pen.

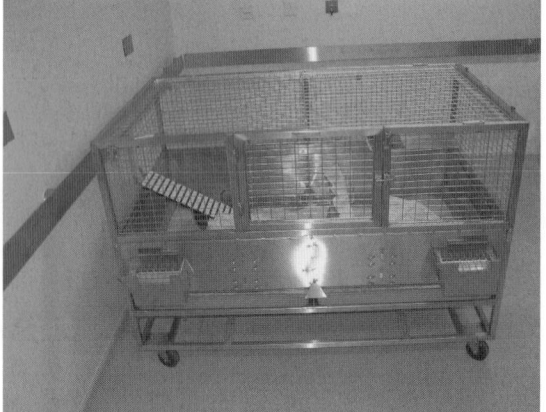

Figure 7.2 Large ferret cage.

can be achieved by placing the ferret in a cool area and spraying it with cold water.

Breeding and supplying establishments are not required to keep records of relative humidity because the welfare of ferrets has not been shown to be compromised if levels fluctuate.

The number of air changes per hour needed to maintain a healthy environment for ferrets is determined by the stocking density. A fully stocked room needs more air changes than one containing few animals.

Housing

Guidance on stocking densities can be found in the current *Codes of Practice for the Care and Housing of Animals used in Scientific Procedures* (Home Office 1989) and the Ferret supplement to the *Code of Practice for Designated Breeding and Supplying Establishments*.

Ferrets are sociable animals and appreciate company of their own kind and should only be housed singly when absolutely necessary. This should be a last resort but may be necessary if the experiment requires it or if the ferret needs to be isolated for health reasons, in these cases the animal must have increased human contact.

It is preferable to house ferrets in social groups in large pens (Figure 7.1) or cages (Figure 7.2). The environment can be enhanced by supplying lengths of drain pipe, boxes, shelves, paper bags, hanging hammocks etc. (Figure 7.3). Deep litter of wood

Figure 7.3 Ferret in cage with paper bag.

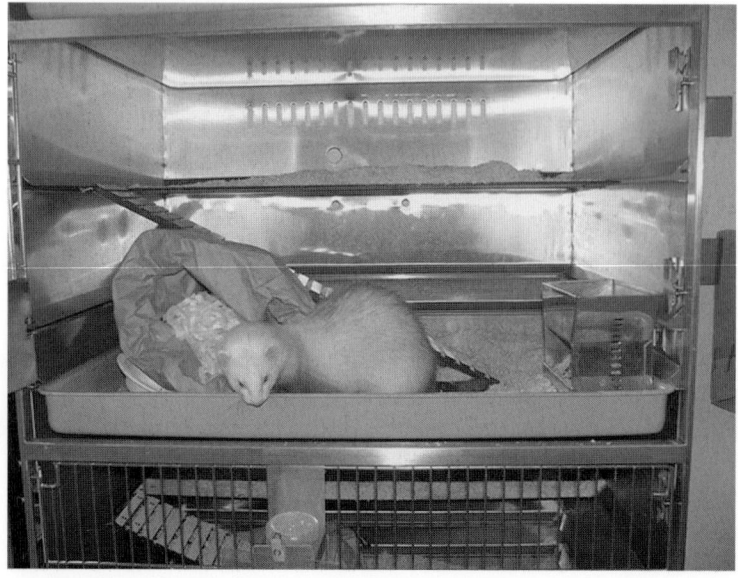

shavings will be greatly appreciated by the ferret and will aid in the removal of faeces and urine.

Breeding females need to be housed singly ten to fourteen days before parturition. They require a supply of nesting material (preferably straw) and a secure darkened area in which to give birth, a large area will be required for the young, known as kits, to play when they leave the nest.

Routines

Ferrets use a selected corner in which to defecate and urinate, they will generally all use the same area and can easily be encouraged to use a litter tray. This must be cleaned at least once a day. The cage or pen needs changing weekly.

Food and water

Ferrets are carnivores. Their natural diet is whole raw carcasses such as rabbit or squirrel. Dry complete ferret diets are suitable and are readily available from commercial suppliers (see Chapter 26) (Figure 7.4). Carnivores have short digestive tracts and a high metabolic rate, their diet needs to contain around 35–40% protein, 20–30% fat/oil, 10% fibre, and vitamins and minerals including A, D, E, B12, Iron, Manganese, Zinc.

Ferrets can suffer from hypoglycaemia if not fed regularly and benefit from being fed small frequent meals. An adult ferret will consume approx 65 g of diet a day.

Vitamin pastes are available from diet manufacturers and prove irresistible to most ferrets, they are therefore invaluable in gaining the ferrets' co-operation for experimental and husbandry procedures, e.g. toe nail clipping, training. The pastes must only be given in moderation as they are a form of supplementary feeding formulated to aid recovery and boost nutritional intake in sick or elderly ferrets. Manufacturers of the pastes provide instructions as to how much to allow each ferret per day.

Ferrets need a continuous supply of fresh drinking water; they drink around 75–100 cm^3 per day. Ferrets fed on dry diets will need greater volumes of water and can be seen to drink quite large quantities at a time. Water can be supplied in drinking bottles, bowls or via an automatic watering system. Ferrets enjoy playing in water so a bowl would need regular cleaning and re-filling.

Breeding

There is significant sexual dimorphism in the ferret, with the hob frequently being twice the size of the jill. The ano–genital distance in the jill is minimal and in the hob is about two to three inches. Both males and

Figure 7.4 Ferret with pelleted diet in hopper.

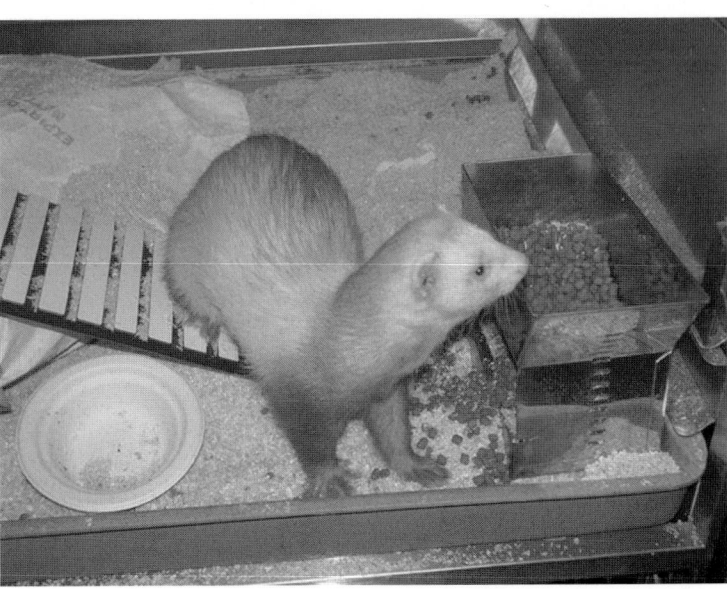

female ferrets have a breeding season. Out of season the vulva of the female has a shrunken appearance; the testes of the male also shrink and move back through the inguinal canal into the body cavity.

Under natural lighting conditions the onset of the breeding season occurs when there is an average of fourteen hours of uninterrupted light per day, usually from March to September. Under these conditions ferrets can have up to two litters per season. By using artificial lighting the breeding season can be manipulated to allow up to four litters per year. This can be achieved by providing non-breeding females with a short day length of eight hours, then by increasing the day length each week by thirty minutes until it reaches between twelve and fourteen hours. At this point the jill will be in oestrus and ready to breed.

Males can be maintained in breeding condition for up to a year if they are kept on a short day (eight hours light) regime (Fox 1998).

All ferrets lose body weight (up to 50% in some cases) and may suffer hair loss during the breeding season so particular care must be taken not to exhaust ferrets involved in intensive breeding programmes.

Oestrus is identified by the swollen appearance of the vulva. The jill will be ready to mate ten to fourteen days after the vulva begins to swell. Jills are induced ovulators; if they are not mated they remain in oestrus long term which can cause health problems (see Health section below, p. 45).

Hobs come into season in early spring, sometimes as early as January. The onset will be evident by the testicles moving into the scrotal sac and a distinctive strong musky scent. The male's strong scent encourages the female to his territory for mating.

Breeding data for ferrets is summarised in Table 7.3, care must be taken when interpreting this data as strain differences exist.

All ferrets will live amicably together during the winter months but at the onset of the breeding season entire hobs housed together will start to fight, possibly causing serious injury. Jills not intended for breeding must be separated from hobs.

Breeding systems

In addition to the enlarged vulva, signs of oestrus in the jill may also include a watery discharge and she will smell a little stronger than usual.

Table 7.3   Summary of breeding data for ferrets.

Age when sexually mature	6–8 months
Age at first mating	9–12 months
Weight at first mating	700–800 g
Breeding season	February–July
Length oestrous cycle	Extensive if not mated
Duration of oestrus	Extensive if not mated
Pseudopregnancy	42 days
Gestation period	42 days
Birth weight:	10 g
Average litter size	8
Return to oestrus post partum	End of lactation or next season
Weaning age	6–8 weeks
Weight at weaning	300–400 g
Adult weight: male	1.5–2.5 kg
Adult weight: female	0.75–1.5 kg
Economic breeding life	6–8 litters over several years

Arranged mating systems are used with ferrets. Oestrus occurs ten to fourteen days after the first signs of the vulva swelling and if the jill is to be bred she should be taken to the hob's enclosure at this time. Mating can appear quite fierce and can last several hours, the hob will grab the jill by the scruff and drag her around before mounting her, and the jill can end up with a sore neck. The jill should be removed from the hob's enclosure after 24–48 hours. Mating induces ovulation.

Implantation occurs around twelve days after copulation. The vulva reduces in size over the next seven to ten days.

Pregnancy and parturition

Gestation lasts from 40–44 days with an average of 42 days. Approximately two weeks before parturition is expected the jill should be moved to a cage in a littering room. The cage should have a nest box with suitable nesting material, e.g. vet bed, shredded paper. The average litter size for ferrets is six to eight but they can give birth to up to fifteen. The kits are born blind, deaf, and naked and rely totally on the mother for the first four to six weeks of life. Stages in the development of ferret kits are given in Table 7.4.

Castration

If male ferrets are not to be used for breeding they may be castrated. A castrated ferret is called a hobble.

Table 7.4 Stages in the development of ferret kits.

5 days old	Fur erupts
10–14 days	Deciduous teeth erupt
14–21 days	Start crawling out of the nest
22–35 days	Ears and eyes open
47–52 days	Canine teeth erupt
42–56 days	Weaning occurs
4–5 months	Adult weight attained
8–12 months	Sexual maturity

Castration is best carried out during the breeding season, when the testicles have exited the body cavity into the scrotal sac. If the procedure is carried out when the hob is not in season the testicles will be retracted into the body cavity and more invasive surgery will be required to complete the procedure.

Health

The general signs of disease outlined in Chapter 2 on the mouse apply to the ferret. Failing to eat and weight loss are early signs of ill health. Ferrets are susceptible to a number of viral diseases, such as distemper. Where appropriate the named veterinary surgeon may advise vaccination to protect from these diseases. The rectal temperature of the ferret ranges from 37.8–40 °C.

Ferrets can contract human influenza virus, so staff suffering from colds should be excluded from ferret units.

After mating, females should be checked to see if they have been damaged by the male's violent mating behaviour. Breeding makes heavy demands on the female and she must be inspected carefully after her young are weaned to ensure she is fit enough to go on breeding.

Effects of prolonged oestrus in jills

When a ferret is in oestrus, the level of the hormone oestrogen rises dramatically. If she is not mated the level remains raised for a prolonged period. The raised level of hormone suppresses production of blood cells in the bone marrow, which in turn causes aplastic anaemia. This condition is almost always fatal if not treated. The reduction of red blood cells causes anaemia, the reduction in white blood cells reduces the immune response and causes the jill to succumb easily to infection, and the reduction of platelets inhibits blood clotting resulting in internal bleeding.

In addition, the female's enlarged vulva can be physically damaged and it also makes her more susceptible to infection. The condition can be controlled in several ways.

- An injection of the hormone proligestone administered subcutaneously at the start of oestrus – this will take the jill out of season. There is a small risk of alopecia at the injection site but this is rare and if it does occur the hair will quickly grow back. The hormone will not affect the productivity of the female for the next breeding season.

- Mating the jill with a vasectomised hob is carried out solely to take the jill out of season by inducing ovulation.

The named veterinary surgeon will advise the most appropriate method of dealing with this condition.

Pseudopregnancy

Using a vasectomised male or the hormone method can stimulate pseudopregnancy. The jill will seem to be pregnant, go through all relevant signs, nest making, milk production, etc. but no young are produced. The pseudopregnancy will last as long as a normal pregnancy.

Ferret diseases are covered in detail in Fox (1998).

Identification

Tattoos in the ear or subcutaneous transponders can be used as permanent methods of identification.

References and further reading

Fox, J.G. (1998) *Biology and Diseases of the Ferret* (2nd edn). Lea and Febiger, Philadelphia.

Home Office (1989) *Code of Practice for the Housing and Care of Animals used in Scientific Procedures*. HMSO, London.

McKay, J. (2000) *Complete Guide to Ferrets*. Swanhill Press, Shropshire, UK.

8

The Laboratory Cat

Brian K. Lowe

Introduction

Cats are sensitive creatures with specific husbandry requirements. When these requirements are not met the cat will become stressed, which is bad for the cat and the experiment. Cats are particularly intolerant of poor handling and are likely to express their unease by scratching and biting. It is important that this is borne in mind when caring for them so the risk of injury to the cat and to laboratory personnel is minimised.

Cats use visual, olfactory and audio cues for communicating between themselves and interacting with their environment. Sound and odour are effective for communication over long distances, which may be significant when housing cats in different parts of the animal unit. The cat is very sensitive to odour having both a large area of sensitive nasal epithelia and a high concentration of nerve endings in the epithelia. The cat also has a vomeronasal organ (Jacobson's organ) which it uses during sexual communication (the Flehmen response). Tom cats (males) in particular will mark their environment with a pungent scent, which they deposit around their environment by spraying urine. Cats have an excellent auditory range, detecting frequencies well, within our range of hearing and into ultrasound frequencies. A cat is able to move its pinna to locate the source of a sound efficiently, and then make visual contact. The feline eye has evolved to detect movement at a distance and to see in poor light. Once an object is close, the cat uses its other senses to investigate the environment. The vibrissae (whiskers) are particularly sensitive to tactile stimuli. The vestibular system is very well developed, and is connected to a large cerebellum where motion control is organised. This means the cat has an excellent spatial awareness and motor

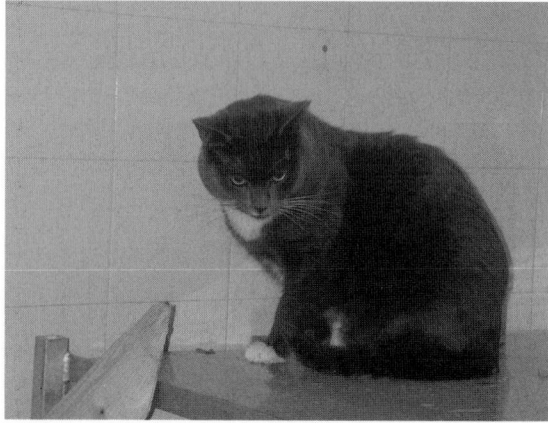

Figure 8.1   Tom cat.

control, resulting in the characteristic feline grace, agility and dexterity. Like many carnivores the cat is naturally lazy, sleeping for around eighteen to twenty hours a day, but when not asleep the cat is alert and eager to seek food or play (Figures 8.1 and 8.2). Classification of the cat is given in Table 8.1.

Cats must be bred and obtained from a designated breeding establishment (see Chapter 36).

Table 8.1   Classification of the cat *Felis silvestris catus*.

Kingdom	Animalia
Phylum	Chordata
Sub-phylum	Vertebrata
Class	Mammalia
Order	Carnivora
Family	Felidae
Generic and specific names	*Felis silvestris catus*

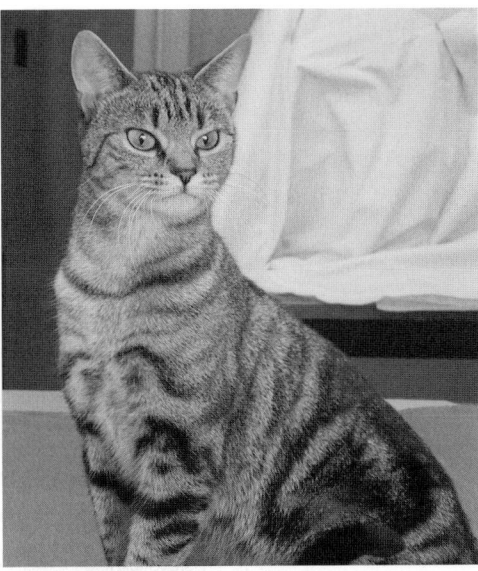

Figure 8.2   Queen cat.

Use in regulated procedures

The domestic cat has been used in many areas of experimental research, including: neurophysiology, neuropharmacology, toxicology, vaccine research and companion animal nutrition.

Environment

The environmental levels recommended by the Home Office codes of practice (1989; 1995) for cats are given in Table 8.2 (see also Chapter 33).

Lighting may be adjusted in breeding units to control the reproductive cycle. Cats appear to be able to tolerate wide fluctuations in humidity, therefore in breeding units it is not considered necessary to control or record relative humidity. Air changes per hour may be reduced from those stated in Table 8.2 if stocking densities are low.

Housing

A reduction in the amount of environmental stimuli is probably more important to the laboratory cat than the limitation on its available space providing the Home Office's code of practice recommendations are met (1989; 1995). Providing a suitable environment is not just about the amount of space, but is more about the animal's ability to make use of the available space, and how this space meets the animal's behavioural and physiological needs. In this instance a crucial, possibly the most crucial welfare issue, is the cat's ability to choose its immediate environment and its immediate activities. For example, in times of stress the cat has three options, to flee the stress, to fight the stressor or to freeze. The ability to choose which response it makes will depend upon the cat's environment. Giving the cat the opportunity to flee and hide when stressed should reduce the risk of it opting for the 'fight' response, which would increase the risk of injury to the handler and the cat. The provision of retreats has been shown to lower the stress response in cats exposed to stressful situations.

Cats can be housed individually or in groups. However, they are social animals and are better housed in stable groups where possible. Where group housing is used it is important to ensure that the animals are checked regularly, including bodyweight, to ensure that they all have access to food and water, and that no cat is being bullied. Cats form relatively stable hierarchies when housed together, but each time new cats are introduced to the group there is likely to be scuffling while a new hierarchy is formed.

Table 8.2   Environmental levels for cats (Home Office 1989, 1995).

	Scientific procedure establishments	Breeding and supplying establishments
Room temperature	15–24 °C	15–24 °C
Relative humidity	55% ± 10%	Not necessary to control or record
Room air changes per hour	15–20	10–12
Photoperiod	12 hours light: 12 hours dark	14 hours light: 10 hours dark
Light intensity	350–400 lux at bench level	Adequate to allow staff to perform husbandry duties safely

If entire males are group housed together they should be housed away from any entire females (queens), as fighting may occur when a female starts an active oestrous cycle. Staff should not go from a room of entire queens to a room containing males as olfactory signals carried on their clothing may be sufficient to unsettle the males.

Stud tom cats are usually housed individually, as they tend to view any company in terms of mating or fighting. Any cats which are housed alone will require special attention to ensure they achieve suitable environmental stimulation. This can be provided by paying attention to the pen design, through human socialisation and specific exercise periods. All singly housed animals should be given access to an exercise area on a regular basis, preferably daily. This may simply be by allowing them to explore the room outside their cage for a period during the day. Most cats, other than stud males, will mix well (providing there is adequate supervision). They can be allowed their exercise period at the same time. Where a cat does not mix with the others it should be exercised away from the other cats. Having a separate room for exercising the stud toms works well. The stud toms are placed in this room while their pens are being cleaned, and again for a period later in the day. The order in which the toms are placed in the cage will vary each day. The room is only cleaned at the end of the day, so the toms have the opportunity to investigate the odours left behind by the other cats. As always care must be taken when handling tom cats as they may become excitable during their exercise periods.

All cat housing must be easy to clean. Singly housed animals or queens in late gestation and with litters can be housed in cages made from fibreglass or other robust plastics. These cages usually have gridded fronts, so there is adequate airflow. Individual pens can be constructed from wire mesh or glass. Groups of cats are housed in rooms. Scratch posts made from softwood should be available at all times. Shelves, especially if hinged and arranged at different heights can be used to vary the environment for the animal and provide areas for rest or retreat (Figure 8.3).

In addition to litter trays and shelving, each room should contain boxes for hiding and playing in and areas for climbing. Cats will enjoy playing with toys, but these need to be small, light and unpredictable in their movements if they are to occupy the cat for long.

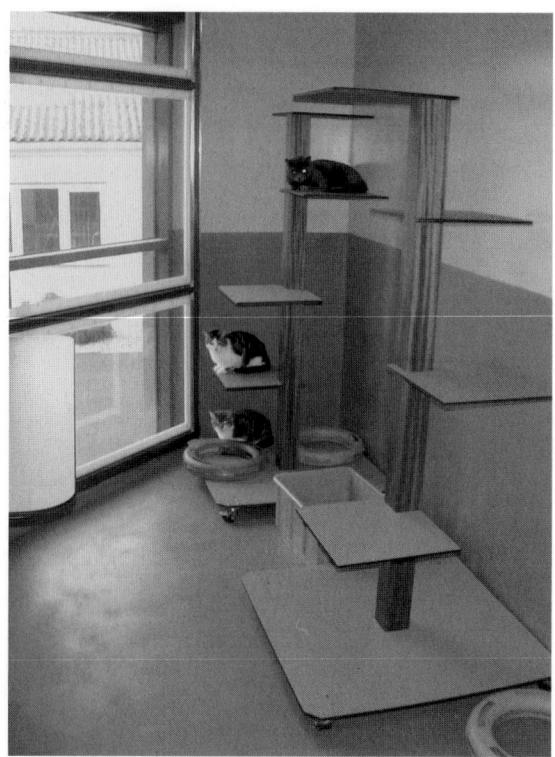

Figure 8.3   Shelf and scratching unit.

Routines

Nesting material can be provided through the use of commercial cat beds or sheets of fleece material such as Vetbed®. Cats learn at an early age to use litter trays. They will not use dirty trays so sufficient clean litter trays must be provided. If there are insufficient clean litter trays, or the litter trays are monopolised by the more dominant cats then soiling of the general environment will occur. Cat litter is generally considered too heavy, expensive and difficult to dispose of to be used as a general bedding material. Cats will readily use softwood sawdust or woodchips. Woodchips being preferable as this material is less likely to get into the eyes or be inhaled.

Cat areas should be cleaned daily. It is insufficient just to remove soiled bedding material. Each litter tray should be emptied, cleaned in a disinfectant solution, well rinsed and dried each day. The living area should be washed out with a suitable disinfectant solution and rinsed each day. Feeding bowls should also be cleaned daily.

Figure 8.4   Cats playing.

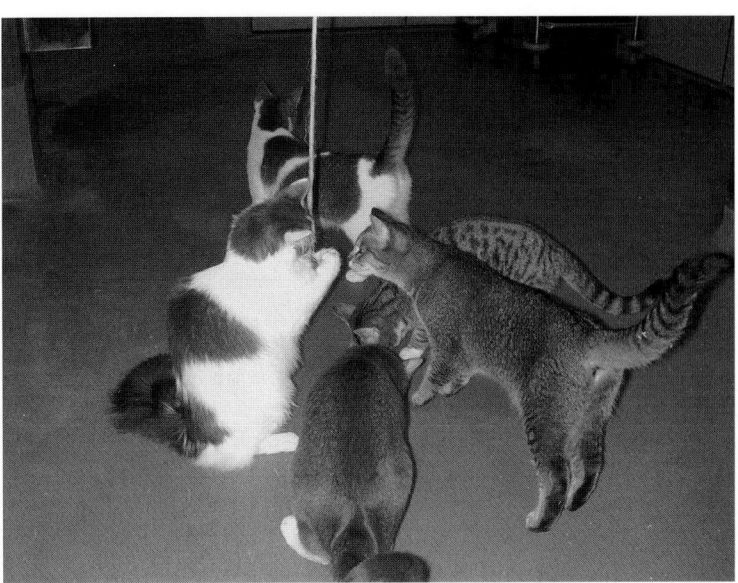

All cats will require regular contact with humans. These periods of contact should be as pleasant for the cat as possible so that it becomes relaxed and confident with human contact. Many cats enjoy being groomed and when working with long-haired cats grooming becomes essential. During these socialisation sessions the animal can be acclimatised to the different handling techniques it is likely to encounter during veterinary, husbandry or experimental procedures, so it becomes accustomed to these procedures and will be relaxed and confident.

In summary, the design of the confinement area should encourage the use of the cat's visual, auditory, olfactory, vestibular and cognitive abilities. In terms of space, quality is more important than quantity. The quality can be improved by including environmental complexity – different textures, toys, adjustable shelves, boxes or other retreat areas as well as access to odours and sounds from outside the room (Figure 8.4). The use of wire mesh allows the passage of air carrying sound and odours to pass in and out of the area.

Food and water

Cats are obligate carnivores, for details see Chapter 26. Adult cats can be fed once a day and the food presented should be consumed within one hour. Kittens, heavily pregnant and lactating females should be offered small regular feeds, e.g. three times a day. Cats can be fed good quality tinned meat (with minimal cereal content), fresh meat or a proprietary dry cat diet (which can also be fed as a mash). In some cases it may be necessary to restrict food intake to control obesity. Sufficient trays must be provided to ensure that all cats have access to the food, and monopolisation by individuals or groups of cats is not possible. The food is usually presented in large shallow trays offering a good surface area for the cats to feed from. Cats are usually fed proprietary dry, wet or a mix of wet and dry foods, fed *ad libitum* and left in overnight or throughout the day. Fresh meat can be offered but care needs to be taken to ensure the cat receives a balanced diet. Unless there are specific reasons for feeding fresh meat it is safer and more controlled to feed diets with a known nutritional profile specifically prepared for laboratory cats.

Water must be available at all times. It is presented in open dishes which are designed so that they cannot be tipped up.

Breeding

Although naturally a seasonal breeder (being sexually active between January and October), in the lab the breeding season can be maintained throughout the year by controlling the photoperiod. Twelve to fourteen hours of light will maintain the queen's period of sexual activity. Oestrus in the queen can be synchronised by reducing the photoperiod to eight hours of light for a few months, until the queen becomes anoestrus. Gradually increasing the light by half an hour a day until it reaches fourteen hours should bring the queens into oestrus together. Synchronisation can be encouraged further by giving the females olfactory access to the sexually mature tom cats.

During pro-oestrus, rising follicle stimulating hormone (FSH) leads to the development of ovarian tissue, which produces oestrogen. The oestrogen leads to profound behavioural changes, which are apparent during late pro-oestrus and oestrus. The queen will show: increased vocalisation (wailing or crying), will become more affectionate (rubbing themselves against people and inanimate objects), will demonstrate lordosis and hind feet treading, and may become anorexic. Some will spray urine. Breeding data is summarised in Table 8.3.

The queen is an induced ovulator. During mating, the penis of the tom cat (which has barbed protrusions) stimulates neurones in the posterior vagina, ultimately leading to the release of luteinising hormone (LH) from the anterior pituitary organ. Providing sufficient LH is released (four matings will normally ensure this, although it may occur with fewer matings) ovulation will occur three days later. Ovulation leads to the production of progesterone

causing the queen to eat more and gain weight, and the mammary glands will start to develop. If the released ova are not fertilised then the cat is said to be pseudopregnant. This normally ends by day 40 post mating, but may continue for 70 days. Once the progesterone level drops to 1 ng/ml a new oestrus cycle will begin. If the ova are fertilised, the queen will become pregnant and will litter down nine weeks after mating.

Breeding systems

Cats can be arranged-mated or mated as harems.

Arranged mating
In the arranged-mating system, the queen is assessed for oestrus through her behaviour. She should show signs of lordosis and hind leg treading; her tail should be deflected to one side to expose the vulva. These signs are usually more apparent if the back is stroked and the scruff gently pulled. It is important to confirm that the female is in oestrus before she is placed in the male's pen. It is a good idea to remove the litter tray and any other furniture from the pen before introducing the female. Initially, the cats investigate each other by sniffing each other and the male may groom the female before he mounts her. Mating is usually rapid, although this varies significantly between pairings. Ejaculation occurs on penetration, the female will 'yowl' and attack the male. An experienced tom will usually jump off the female and retire to a safe distance, where he will groom himself. The female will show a characteristic post-coital behaviour pattern, involving intermittent bouts of licking her vulva, and frenzied rolling across the floor. If the male gets too close she will attack him. The period of post-coital behaviour is variable, but she will usually allow another mating within five to twenty minutes. The cats should be allowed to mate a number of times before the queen is returned to her room and the breeding records are completed.

The harem system

In the harem system the male is placed in a room of sexually mature queens and allowed to mate the females in oestrus. All queens must be weighed regularly – a pregnant queen will start to show a weight gain within two weeks of being mated.

Table 8.3 Summary of breeding data for the cat.

Age at first mating	12 months
Weight at first mating	Minimum of 2.5 kg
Breeding season in nature	January–October
Oestrous cycle	14–21 days
Duration of oestrus	3–10 days
Pseudopregnancy	40–70 days
Gestation	63 weeks
Birth weight	90–120 g
Litter size	3–6
Return to oestrus	Fourth week lactation
Weaning age	6–8 weeks
Weight at weaning	600–1000 g
Adult weight: males	4 kg +
Adult weight: females	3.5 kg +
Economic breeding life	6–8 litters over several years, stop breeding around 6 years of age

Pregnancy can be confirmed and the queens caged before they are likely to litter down.

Systems using more than one male have been described. A mature male is placed in a colony of sexually mature females and one or two sexually immature male(s) (of different ages) are also placed in the colony. As soon as one of the younger males has matured sufficiently to assert himself against the dominance of the eldest male, the eldest male is removed and the younger male takes his place.

Pregnant queens are removed from their room around 55 days after mating and are individually housed in cages for littering and raising their young.

Artificial insemination of cats is possible and can be achieved without the use of drugs or expensive equipment; however it should only be carried out by experienced people.

Pregnancy and parturition

Pregnancy can be confirmed by ultrasound from twenty days post mating, or by radiography from six weeks post mating. Hormone analysis of relaxin from day 20 post partum should also confirm pregnancy. The foetuses can be palpated throughout mid and late pregnancy. The level of circulating progesterone can be used to determine that ovulation has occurred. It should be noted that queens are capable of resorbing or aborting some or all of their litter if a problem develops during gestation, so careful and regular monitoring throughout pregnancy is essential.

A pregnant female should be individually housed about 55 days after mating, so she has time to get used to her new cage and so she can be observed carefully. One week before the expected parturition the queen should be provided with a nesting box containing a suitable litter, e.g. soft shredded paper or Vetbed®. The average gestation period is quoted as 63 days, although the exact period is variable. Any kittens born less than 60 days after mating are premature and have a very poor chance of survival. A veterinary surgeon should check a gestation period in excess of 70 days, or where a queen is showing clear signs of unproductive contractions. Parturition problems are relatively rare in cats, most queens will litter down overnight and the kittens will be clean, dry and feeding by the time you arrive the next day. Queens make excellent mothers and will readily foster kittens from other litters.

Weaning

Weaning should be done gradually. The young are removed from the queen for progressively longer periods over one to two weeks. This gradual weaning process reduces the risk of mastitis and develops the kittens' independence. The young can be fully weaned from six weeks of age, but eight weeks is preferable.

Kittens are born with eyes and ears closed, but have a complete body covering of fur. The ears begin to open around three days of age, and the eyes open around eight to ten days of age, after which they soon begin to eat solids. At around eighteen days teething is usually under way. By eight weeks there is a full set of milk teeth, which are gradually shed from twelve weeks onwards. Kittens are usually born with deep blue eyes, which gradually change in colour as they develop.

Health

Due to the high prevalence of cats outside the laboratory, either as pets or as feral animals, there is a large reservoir of disease which can readily infect the laboratory cat. It is advisable to house cats under full barrier conditions or ensure that cats are routinely vaccinated. High standards of hygiene should be maintained in the facility at all times. Named veterinary surgeons will advise on an appropriate vaccination programme.

As with all laboratory animals, cats must be checked by a competent person at least once every day, better still is a check first thing in the morning and again before leaving at night. In addition to this, the cats should be given a thorough examination and weighed weekly. A record of any abnormalities or causes for concern should be recorded in the appropriate history record for future reference. The rectal temperature of the cat is 38–39.5 °C.

Identification

The Animals (Scientific Procedures) Act 1986 requires cats to have a permanent method of identification. Non-permanent methods can be useful adjuncts for identifying specific groups or individuals (for example different experimental groups) easily. The methods available include:

- tattooing;
- transponders;
- collars and tags;
- coat colour and pattern;
- shaving the fur (this is a temporary system used to mark kittens within a litter).

For further details, see *Introduction to Animal Technology* (Barnett 2001).

References and further reading

Ademic, R.E. and Stark-Ademic, C. (1989) Behavioural inhibitions and anxiety: Dispositional, developmental, and neural aspects of the anxious personality of the domestic cat (pp. 93–124). In: J.S. Reznick (Ed.) *Perspectives on Behavioural Inhibition*. University of Chicago Press.

Barnett, S.W. (2001) Identification of animals (pp. 64–69). In: *Introduction to Animal Technology* (2nd edn). Blackwell Science, Oxford.

Bradshaw, J. (1992) *The Behaviour of the Domestic Cat*. CABI Publishing, Oxfordshire, UK.

Home Office (1989) *Code of Practice for the Housing and Care of Animals used in Scientific Procedures*. HMSO, London.

Home Office (1995) *Code of Practice for the Housing and Care of Animals in Designated Breeding and Supplying Establishments*. HMSO, London.

Robinson, R. (1999) *Genetics for Cat Breeders*. Butterworth Heinemann, Oxford.

Turner, D.C. and Bateson, P. (1989) *The Domestic Cat. The Biology of its Behaviour*. Cambridge University Press.

9
The Dog

Stephen W. Barnett

Introduction

Dogs are one of the species which are given additional protection by the Animals (Scientific Procedures) Act 1986. Project licence applicants must make a special case to justify their use (see Chapter 35). Dogs must be purchased from designated breeders unless a convincing case is made to use a type of dog not bred by a designated breeder and the Home Secretary gives specific permission to obtain them elsewhere.

As most dogs used for research are Beagles this chapter will concentrate on them; a few other breeds or cross breeds are used, mainly for veterinary research. There are different strains of Beagle, largely distinguished by their adult body size.

Dogs are social animals and unless there is a very good reason should be housed in pairs or groups. They communicate with each other and with humans acoustically, visually and through smell.

The sounds dogs make include social (the howl), calls for attention (short sharp barks) and threatening (growling) (Nott 1992). Dogs can hear in a wide frequency range (0.04–46 kHz), both below and above human hearing, but their peak frequency sensitivity is between 0.5–16 kHz (Sales and Milligan 1992).

Visual communication is used when dogs are in close proximity, for instance a dog with hair raised, lips drawn back and tail raised is in an aggressive mood.

The dog produces odours in urine, faeces, vaginal secretions and the anal glands. These odours are used for territory marking and for identifying the sexual status and status in the colony. It is often noticed that when a dog is returned to a newly cleaned cage the first thing it does is spray urine over the walls, remarking its territory. Classification of dogs is given in Table 9.1.

Table 9.1 Classification of dog *Canis familiaris*.

Kingdom	Animalia
Phylum	Chordata
Sub-phylum	Vertebrata
Class	Mammalia
Order	Carnivora
Family	Canidae
Generic and specific names	*Canis familiaris*

Use in regulated procedures

Beagles are good-natured animals, easy to handle and they adapt to laboratory conditions well. There is also a great deal of background biological information available for them. These factors make them an ideal laboratory species.

The major use of dogs is in pharmaceutical safety evaluation. They are also used in respiratory and cardiovascular research, alimentary, skin, genetic and immunological studies.

Environment

Dogs can tolerate a wide range of environmental conditions and can even be kept outside in all but the most extreme temperatures, providing they have access to shelter. Those kept for scientific procedures are housed inside, although some have access to outside runs.

Environmental requirements for the dog are given in Table 9.2. In common with other species, once a suitable temperature has been selected from the range it should not vary more than ± 2 °C. Dogs are less affected by humidity changes than some other

Table 9.2   Environmental levels for dogs (Home Office 1989, 1995).

	Scientific procedure establishments	Breeding and supplying establishments
Temp.: adults	15–24 °C	15–25 °C
Temp.: pups 0–10 days	–	26–28 °C
Relative humidity	55% ± 10%	Not necessary to control or record
Air changes per hour	10–12	10–12
Photoperiod	12 hours light: 12 hours dark	Not less than 12 hours light
Light intensity	350–400 lux	Adequate to allow safe working and inspection of animals

species and it is unnecessary to control or record relative humidity (Home Office 1995), however most facilities do so. Air changes may be decreased if stocking levels are less than those recommended in the codes of practice. Photoperiod is less critical than with other species and they benefit from access to daylight. Figure 9.2 shows how glass bricks can be used to provide day light without diminishing security.

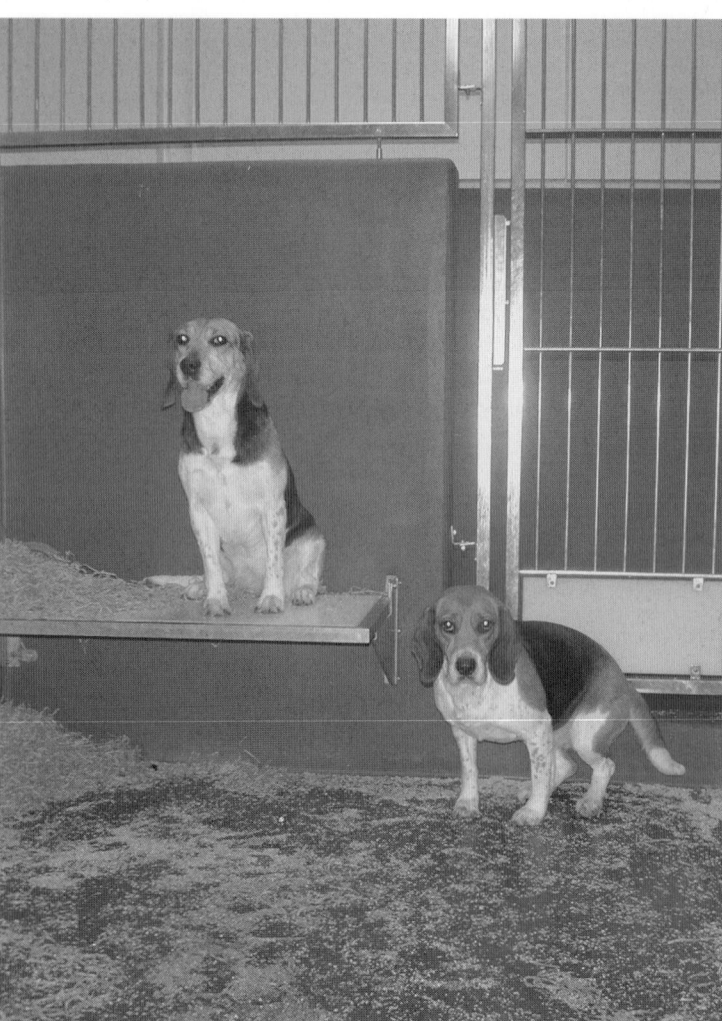

Figure 9.1 Dog pen, with enviro-dry bedding.

Housing

Current stocking levels for dogs used for scientific procedures are stated in the current *Code of Practice for the Housing and Care of Animals used in Scientific Procedures* (Home Office 1989) and those for breeding animals in the *Code of Practice for the Housing and Care of Animals in Designated Breeding and Supplying Establishments* (Home Office 1995).

Dogs should always be pair or group housed. Singly housed animals should only be permitted for established welfare reasons, e.g. separating a late stage pregnant bitch or an injured animal, or where group housing can be shown to be incompatible with particular scientific objectives. In these cases the dogs should be allowed to exercise, wherever possible, with other dogs under staff supervision. Where dogs have to be singly housed, additional welfare resources must be afforded to those animals. They should have visual, auditory and, if possible, tactile contact with other dogs, as well as increased human interaction.

Pens can be manufactured in a number of ways and from a variety of materials; they should be large enough for the defecation area to be kept separate from the living area. Most pens consist of some sort of transparent or bar design to maximise contact between dogs and humans (see Figure 9.2). A variety of additional features can be added to the pen, including heated dog beds and raised platforms. Increasing the complexity of the pen offers the dog choices and somewhere to withdraw from visual contact. Other environmental enrichment, such as toys, can be added to the pens but these can lead to aggression between animals and so must be monitored carefully. Chewing is a natural behaviour in dogs so items allowing this should be provided.

Dogs must have an exercise area within their room. This can be provided by either wide corridors between rows of pens (Figures 9.1 and 9.3) or an attached exercise room.

Dogs can be very noisy particularly at feeding time, consequently soundproofing is necessary. Good soundproofing prevents sounds leaking to neighbouring areas but also reduces the echoing effect within the room. A room of barking dogs can easily exceed the sound levels that damage human hearing (90 dBA); it is essential to wear some form of ear protection when working.

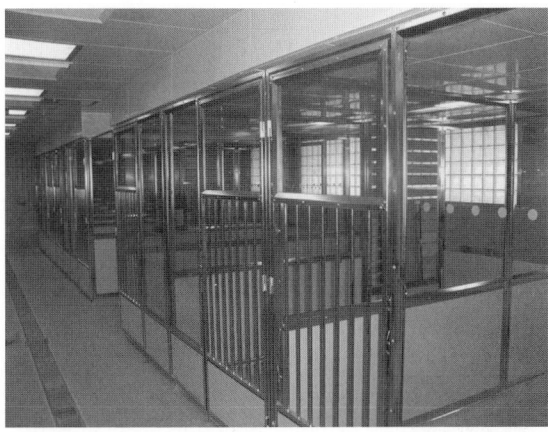

Figure 9.2 Dog room showing toughened glass dividers, glass wall bricks and wide exercise corridors.

Figure 9.3 Dogs exercising in the corridor.

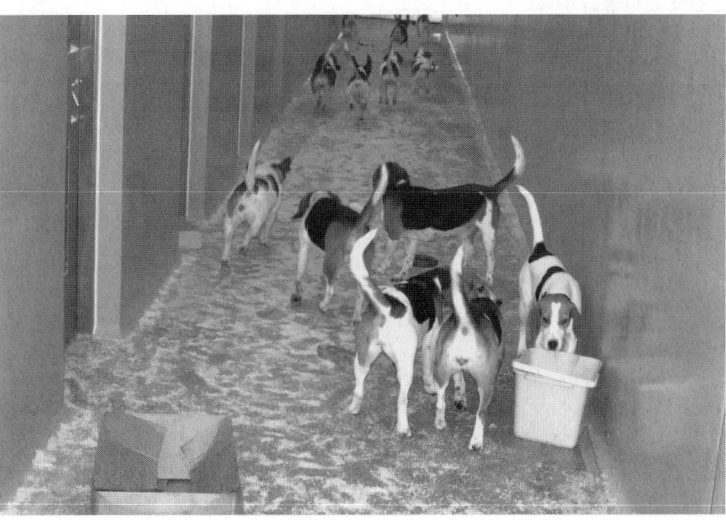

Routine care

Substrate on solid floors is recommended for most dogs. Some may suffer sore hocks on sawdust in which case another bedding such as Envirodry™ (Figure 9.1, see p. 54) can be used instead. Vetbed® can be provided in the sleeping area.

Pens need dry cleaning (removal of soil and replenishing bedding) every day. Once or twice a week the dogs should be removed from the pen so that it can be hosed down and disinfected. The dogs are replaced when the pen is dry.

Regular exercise is essential. A typical regime would be to run dogs in groups with their technician for fifteen minutes, three times a week (Figure 9.3, see p. 55). Novel objects can be added to the run to encourage activity. Dogs should be groomed several times a week. Not only does this ensure good coat condition, it also allows close inspection of the animal and close interaction between handler and animal.

Experimental and stock dogs have to undergo a variety of procedures during their lives; these procedures are much less stressful if time is taken to habituate the animals to them. They can be trained to walk on a lead and obey commands so they can then be walked to where they are needed. This training provides activity (and therefore enrichment) and lessens stress for the dog.

Examples of useful habituation are:

- walking a dog around the procedure rooms on a regular basis so that they get used to the sounds and smells of the room;
- exposing dogs to the sound of hair clippers;
- holding dogs in a position for a procedure (e.g. having an intravenous injection);
- getting dogs used to being in slings or metabolism cages.

Food and water

Dogs are usually fed dry carnivore diet in a bowl or on the floor. Maintenance, breeding and puppy diets are available (see Chapter 26). Wet food in the form of tinned meat may be fed from time to time to provide variety to the diet, to encourage sick dogs to eat or for small dogs needing supplement to their nutrition. Prescription diets can be fed to dogs with special dietary needs.

Adult dogs are fed 300–400 g of maintenance diet a day. This amount can be increased or decreased according to the condition of the dog. The feeding of breeding animals is covered in the breeding section (see below).

Water can be provided in bowls but because the risk of contamination and spillage is high, it is more usual to provide automatic watering devices. An adult dog drinks approximately 1.5 litres of water a day.

Breeding

Breeding data for the dog is summarised in Table 9.3. The oestrous cycle in bitches lasts six to seven months, but can vary by several months. It consists of four stages, pro-oestrus (lasting seven to ten days), oestrus (lasting seven to ten days), metoestrus (lasting one to three months) and anoestrus, which lasts until the next season. Bitches are first used for mating at their second oestrus when they are about a year old. Pro-oestrus is easily identified as the vulva begins to swell and there is a discharge containing blood. At oestrus the discharge becomes straw coloured. During pro-oestrus dogs are attracted to the bitch but bitches are not receptive. In oestrus a bitch will display lordosis by arching her back, lifting her tail to one side and exposing her vulva, she will allow herself to be sniffed and licked and will stand to be mated.

Some bitches exhibit pseudopregnancy – they have signs of pregnancy and will even show nesting behaviour and lactation after the normal gestation

Table 9.3   Summary of breeding data for the dog.

Age when sexually mature	9–12 months
Age at first mating: female	12–15 months
Age at first mating: male	18 months
Weight at first mating	10–12 kg
Time between oestrous cycles	6–7 months
Duration of oestrus	7–10 days
Length of pseudopregnancy	60 days
Length of gestation	63 days
Birth weight:	400 g
Average litter size	6
Return to oestrus post partum	Next season
Weaning age	Eight weeks
Weight at weaning	1–1.5 kg
Adult weight	12–15 kg
Economic breeding life	6–8 litters over several years

Figure 9.4   Dogs in the tied position.

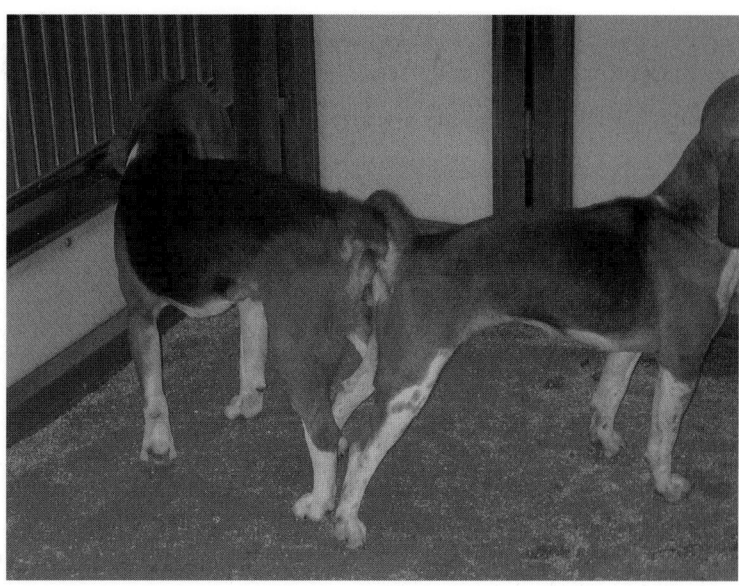

period has elapsed but then produce no young. This can be very disturbing for the animal.

Mating can be prolonged (twenty to thirty minutes) and a large amount of ejaculate is produced. During mating swelling of the bulbourethral gland of the penis in the vagina causes the animals to become locked or tied together. After the initial stages of mating they alter their relative positions so that they end up back to back until mating is finished (Figure 9.4).

Breeding systems

Dogs can be bred by arranged mating or in harems; harems being more common when dogs are bred for scientific procedures.

Arranged mating
In arranged systems the bitch and dog are introduced ten to fourteen days after pro-oestrus is first noted. The animals should be left together for several hours, during which time they will mate repeatedly.

Harem breeding
Harem breeding is usually carried out in closed colonies; detailed breeding records must be kept to ensure only unrelated animals are mated together. Computerised systems are available which make following the family tree of any individual animal a quick

and accurate procedure. These systems, however, are only as good as the information that is logged in.

The animals are grouped in harems of one male to five females. Routine inspections two to three times a week will identify bitches showing signs of oestrus so they can be watched. The male will mate the bitch at the most appropriate time.

Pregnancy and parturition

Twenty-five to twenty-eight days after mating has taken place the bitch can be scanned using ultrasound to confirm pregnancy (Figures 9.5 and 9.6). In experienced hands ultrasound scanning can be used to accurately determine the birth date. If ultrasound is not available trained staff can confirm pregnancy by palpation at about the same time post mating.

If pregnancy is confirmed, the bitch is placed directly into a whelping (birthing) area with another pregnant female, she will remain in this housing until one week before she is due to give birth (whelp). At this stage the bitch should be vaccinated to ensure the antibodies in her colostrum remain high (Table 9.4).

The food ration is increased to 600 g of breeding diet; the condition of the animal must be carefully observed and feeding adjusted by decreasing the amount or supplementing it as required.

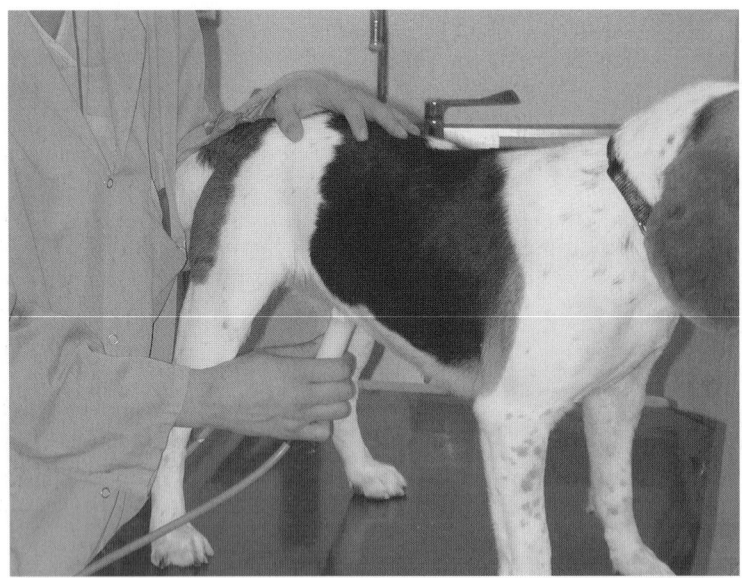

Figure 9.5   Ultrasound pregnancy investigation.

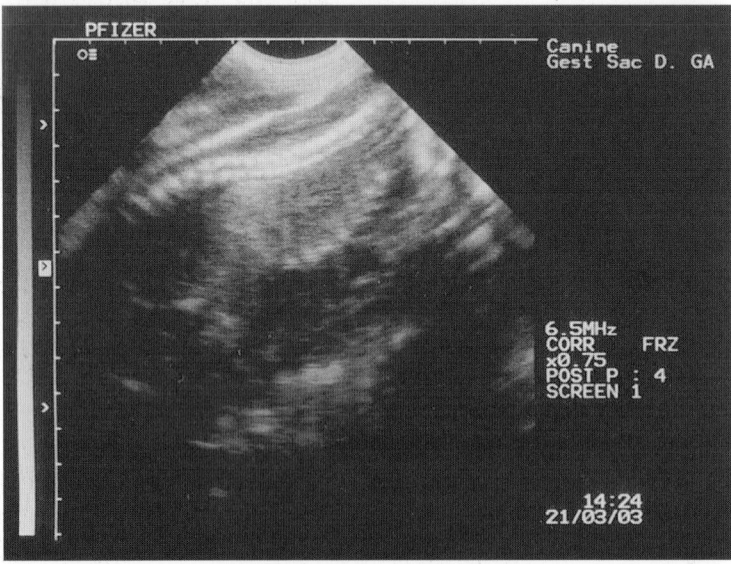

Figure 9.6   Ultrasound scan of fifty-day-old pregnancy.

Table 9.4   Example of vaccination programme.

Time	Animals	Protects against
4 weeks post partum	Bitch and pups	*Bordetella bronchiseptica*
6, 8, 12 weeks	Pups	Combined vaccine covering: Canine distemper virus, Canine hepatitis virus, Canine parvovirus, Canine parainfluenza virus, Canine adenovirus, *Leptospira canicola* and *Leptospira icterohaemorrhagiae.*
Annually	All dogs	Booster for combined vaccine
On confirmation of pregnancy	Bitches	Combined virus
Day following parturition	Bitches	Booster for combined vaccination

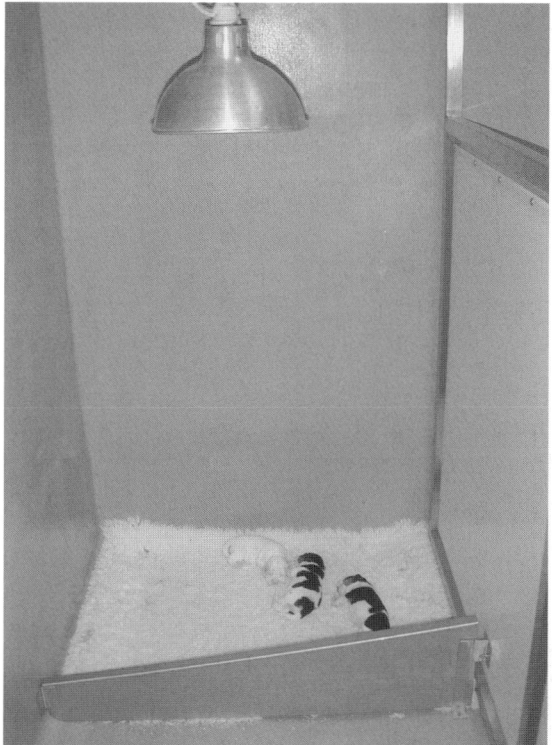

Figure 9.7 Nesting area with heat lamp and vet bed.

One week before the expected birth date the bitch is singly housed in the whelping pen. Within this pen there should be a nesting area fitted with a Vetbed® and a heat lamp to provide supplementary heating (to raise the temperature to 26–28 °C for the pups) (Figure 9.7). Hygiene is essential in the whelping unit and the pen must be thoroughly cleaned and disinfected before the bitch is installed.

The rectal temperature of the bitch can be recorded during this period. It starts to drop from five days before parturition, reaching 4–5 °C lower than normal (38–39 °C) one day before parturition. Bitches must be monitored carefully during parturition but should not be interfered with unless there is an obvious need. Breeding records of established bitches should be consulted so that any previous problems can be watched for. Very close attention must be given to primaparous (first-time) bitches. In some cases parturition may be prolonged, she gets tired and stops pushing and Caesarean section may be necessary, but this can only be judged by an experienced technician or a veterinary surgeon.

The placenta is passed soon after the birth of the pups and the bitch will consume it. On the day after parturition the bitch is given a booster vaccination (Table 9.4, above).

New-born pups are monitored carefully to ensure they are all healthy and are feeding well. Small pups or those not seen consuming enough food may be given supplementary feeding with Lactol. Figures 9.8 and 9.9 illustrate the development of pups in the first few days if life. It is essential to socialise pups between the ages of three to fourteen weeks of age, otherwise they remain wary of humans throughout their lives. In practice they are socialised from day one so that both they and the bitch get used to human interference. Breeding diet is available *ad libitum* for the bitch after parturition, her condition is carefully monitored and supplements given if needed.

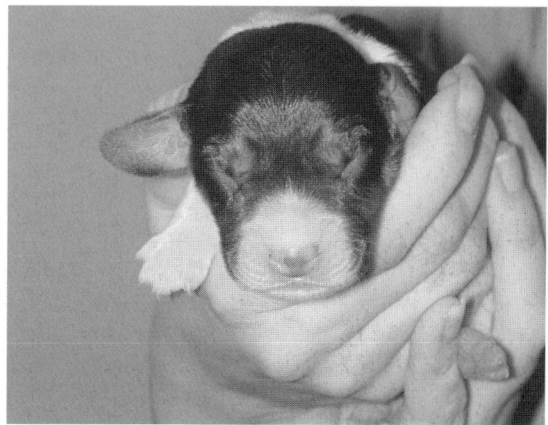

Figure 9.8 Newborn pup.

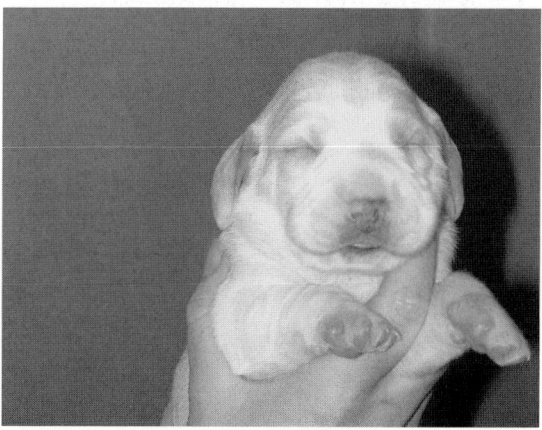

Figure 9.9 Seven-day-old pup.

Human handling can start by the time the pups are three weeks old and they can be identified by microchip at six weeks of age (see section on Identification below).

Weaning is completed by the time the pups are eight weeks old. The bitch should be given a detailed veterinary examination to ensure she is fit to have another litter. If she is, she is housed with other similar bitches for a recovery period of approximately two months. At weaning the pups are housed in a neutral pen with six others of the same size and sex where they remain until they are twenty weeks old. They continue to be fed breeding diet until they are twelve weeks old, then are introduced to maintenance diet over a two-week period until, by fourteen weeks old they are given maintenance diet only.

At twenty weeks the number in each group is reduced to four per pen until they are issued for use.

Health

The normal rectal temperature for a dog is 38–39 °C. Regular health checks should be carried out and dogs showing any signs of ill health should be referred to the named veterinary surgeon. Dogs are susceptible to a number of infectious diseases (see Tables 9.5 and 9.6), fortunately vaccinations are available for the major problems (see Table 9.4, p. 58). Further description of dog diseases can be found in MacArthur (1999).

Identification

The Animals (Scientific Procedures) Act 1986 requires dogs to be individually identified by a method agreed with the Home Office inspector. The method used must be permanent and should be applied before weaning. The law also states that the method chosen should be the least painful possible. As well as identifying the dog, the Act requires all establishments housing dogs to keep records of their identity and place of origin. Good laboratory practice regulations also require dogs to be identified.

The methods which satisfy the legal requirements are tattooing in the ear and microchip. Collars with name tags or coat colour distribution may be used in addition to the more permanent methods.

Table 9.5 Major clinical signs of viral diseases covered by vaccinations.

Disease	Main clinical signs
Canine adenovirus	There are two strains of adenovirus. One also known as infectious canine hepatitis virus, effects can range from subclinical to severe abdominal pain and death. The second strain (also known as infectious canine laryngotracheitis) is a respiratory disease and is one of the causes of kennel cough.
Canine distemper virus	There are widespread clinical signs, which may affect the respiratory, digestive, and/or the nervous systems. Some of the viral strains cause thickening of the skin of the nose and food pads, referred to as hard pad. Young dogs are most susceptible.
Canine parvovirus	In young puppies (3–8 weeks old) infection can lead to heart failure, mortality rate is very high. Older dogs become very ill with vomiting and diarrhoea but the mortality rate is low.
Canine parainfluenza virus	This virus is another one of the agents associated with kennel cough.

Table 9.6 Major clinical signs of bacterial diseases covered by vaccinations.

Disease	Main clinical signs
Bordetella bronchiseptica	This agent is also associated with kennel cough, which is described as a dry, hacking cough.
Leptospira icterohaemorrhagiae	As its name suggests this agent causes jaundice (icterus) and internal bleeding (haemorrhage). In addition there may be vomiting, coughing and diarrhoea. In many cases the disease is fatal unless treated very early. The onset may be so rapid that death occurs without clinical signs.

References and further reading

Home Office (1989) *Code of Practice for the Housing and Care of Animals used in Scientific Procedures.* HMSO, London.

Home Office (1995) *Code of Practice for the Housing and Care of Animals in Designated Breeding and Supplying Establishments.* HMSO, London.

MacArthur Clark, J. (1999) The dog. In: T. Poole (Ed.) *The UFAW Handbook on the Care and Management of Laboratory Animals* (7th edn). Blackwell Science, Oxford.

Nott, H.M.R. (1992) Social behaviour of the dog. In: C. Thorne (Ed.) *The Waltham Book of Dog and Cat Behaviour.* Pergamon Press (part of Butterworth Heinemann, now owned by Elsevier), Oxford.

Prescott, M.J., Morton D.B., Anderson, A. et al. (2004) Refining dog husbandry and care: Eighth report of the BVAAWF/Frame/RSPCA/UFAW Joint Working Group on Refinement. *Laboratory Animals,* **38** (Suppl. 1).

Sales, G.D. and Milligan, S.R. (1992). Ultrasound and laboratory animals. *Animal Technology,* **43** (2).

10

The Common Marmoset

Jeremy N. Smith
© Crown Copyright Dstl, 2004

Marmosets in their natural environment

The ancestors of the Platyrrhini are believed to have evolved from prosimians which entered South America from North America, via a chain of islands around the area now known as Panama. The common marmoset (*Callithrix jacchus*) is indigenous to the Amazon basin in eastern Brazil, its territory stretches from south of the River Amazon to the east of the River Madeira. They live in tropical rainforests, woodland savannah and may often be found in much drier areas. Marmosets are diurnal animals which inhabit the branches of trees in the upper strata of the canopy, but are known to descend to the forest floor to forage for food. Classification of the common marmoset is given in Table 10.1.

Marmosets live in large family groups with one adult male and one dominant female with offspring, which often include older individuals which have become sexually mature. The mother usually produces two young, but occasionally three are born. The dominant female is able to suppress the ovulation of subordinate females within the group, so restricting their ability to reproduce.

Table 10.1 Classification of marmoset *Callithrix jacchus*.

Kingdom	Animalia
Phylum	Chordata
Sub-phylum	Vertebrata
Class	Mammalia
Order	Primate
Infra-order	Platyrrhini
Family	Callitrichidae
Generic and specific names	*Callithrix jacchus*

Groups of marmosets move around the forest at different times of the year to feed on seasonal plants, extracting gum and saps from certain trees between the wet season and the drier months starting in April. They are also known to feed on insects and other animals and are particularly adept at catching large grasshoppers, crickets, cicadas, small lizards and cockroaches. Marmosets are also adept at eating some large fruits while they are still attached to the branches. They achieve this by hanging upside down underneath the fruit with their claws whilst gouging the flesh of the fruit with their teeth.

Use in regulated procedures

Early use within UK biomedical research

Marmosets have been used in biomedical research since the early 1960s, beginning in the USA and later Europe (Rylands 1997). By 1970 breeding groups became established within the United Kingdom providing individuals for studies in virology, metabolic bone disorders, oncology, immunology and toxicology (Grist 1974). Very little was known of marmosets at the time, in comparison to Old World monkeys, which were often used in preference because of the relative ease of looking after them. As knowledge was gathered about the reproductive physiology of marmosets, techniques such as abdominal palpation of pregnant females were established, in addition to the then less favoured vaginal cytology and urinary immunoassay options (Mitchell & Jones 1975).

Use in biomedical research

Marmosets are widely used within research today, including the fields of reproductive medicine, toxicology, pharmacological screening, neurodegenerative disorders and behavioural studies. They are of particular importance to modelling the human response to absorption, distribution, metabolism and excretion (ADME) of compounds.

The recent advances in telemetry technology and remote monitoring over the past fifteen years have enabled extensive studies of the marmoset to be conducted, resulting in a greater understanding of their general physiology. The parameters measured include: blood pressure (BP), heart rate (HR), core temperature (CT), electro cardiogram (ECG), electroencephalogram (EEG) and motor activity (MA).

The long-term collection and analysis of this data has further validated telemetry as a reliable method for gathering information on the cardiovascular system and the effects of related disorders (Schnell 1993, Schnell & Wood 1993). Remote monitoring has also increased our knowledge of environmental and sociological stress within groups of marmosets. The ability to analyse spontaneous cerebral cortical activity via EEG has broadened our knowledge of brain function in both non-human primates and humans (Pearce et al. 1998).

Environment

The environmental levels recommended in the Home Office codes of practice are given in Table 10.2.

Marmosets must be provided with a stable environment. Once a room temperature has been selected from the range given in Table 10.2 it should not vary by more than ± 2 °C (e.g. 24 °C +/− 2 °C). Air changes depend on stocking densities, those quoted in the guidelines can be reduced if the room has low occupancy. Where possible, marmosets benefit from simulated dawn/dusk lighting arrangements.

Housing

Marmosets are housed within cages which allow sufficient vertical flight movement and space for animals to hide from conspecifics (Home Office 1989). Wooden nest boxes serve as excellent places for individuals to take refuge, or sleep at night. Carefully placed wooden perches or sterilised branches are used by animals to climb to different parts of the cage and are often gnawed, as they would in the wild. Link tunnels between cages allow free access to all areas, giving individuals more choice within, and therefore more control over, their environment. Link tunnels may also incorporate forage trays within which an array of different food composites can be mixed with the bedding substrate. Marmosets will then forage for their favourite food at time points of their own choice throughout the day. It has been recorded that, on average, marmosets in the wild spend 35% of their time moving and foraging for food, with only 12% spent on feeding (Stevenson & Rylands 1988). Foraging is a very important behavioural function both to the individual and to the social structure within groups of marmosets, as it promotes cooperation and reduces aggression. Work by Chamove found that allowing groups of marmosets to forage for grain amongst woodchip floor substrate reduced aggressive behaviour by a factor of ten (Chamove et al. 1982).

Cage cleaning and changing routines must take into consideration the importance of scent marking and the messages which may be communicated between individuals. Whilst it is important to keep their environment clean and devoid of a build-up of

Table 10.2 Environmental levels for marmosets (Home Office 1989, 1995).

	Scientific procedure establishments	Breeding and supplying establishments
Room temperature	20–28 °C	20–28 °C
Relative humidity	55% ± 10%	55% ± 15% (higher levels are acceptable)
Room air changes per hour	10–12	10–15
Photoperiod	12 hours light: 12 hours dark	Not less than 12 hours light
Light intensity	350–400 lux at bench level	Sufficient to permit adequate observation of the animals

harmful bacteria, the retention of their own scents is important to the individual and in maintaining the equilibrium of the social structure within the group.

Cages are usually made from stainless steel mesh and are mounted on castors to facilitate their safe movement by the animal technologists. They should incorporate both light and dark areas so that an individual may choose where it would like to be throughout the day. Floor-mounted litter trays filled with sawdust, corn cob or woodchips offer excellent absorption qualities and may also be used to hide food composites within. Breeding cages are generally larger than those used to house smaller groups of experimental animals (Figure 10.1). The structure of a marmoset cage must be such that the animal technologist is able to gain easy access to the inside of it, especially when catching an evasive individual. Marmosets are very adept at hiding in the part of the cage which is most difficult to reach.

Environmental enrichment objects must be safe, easy to clean if they are to be re-cycled and, above all, interesting to the marmoset. It is only by observing how individuals use a particular environmental enrichment device/object that the animal technologist may be able to assess its worth to the animal. Although standing and watching a marmoset use a particular object may give some subjective guidance as to its use, true objective understanding can only be gained via properly designed studies and statistical analysis of the data derived. What seems like a good idea to the human may not be perceived in the same way by the marmoset.

Food and water

Proprietary brands of marmoset diet pellets contain the full range of nutrients required, but should always be supplemented by the addition of a range of natural food composites. Some marmosets do not appear to favour the pellets and will often eat them last, when other food has been eaten. Their diet should include fruit such as apple and banana, boiled egg, raisins, sunflower seeds and millet seeds. High protein porridge-type mix suitable for human babies may be given at a set point throughout the week. This is very

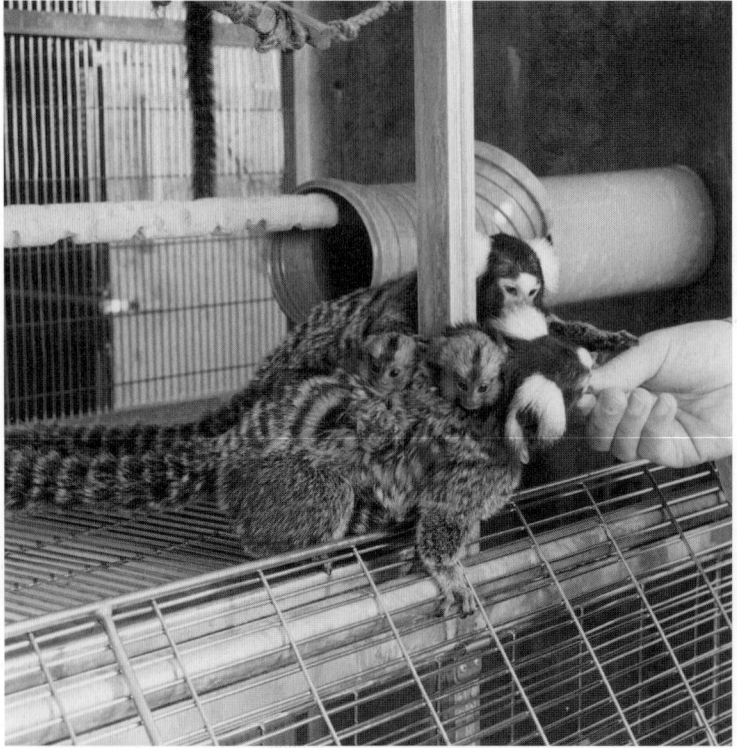

Figure 10.1 Marmoset family group.

palatable to marmosets and allows vitamin D3 drops to be added – essential to their metabolism in the absence of ultraviolet light via sunlight (marmosets must have a source of D3 in the diet rather than D2).

Marmosets are given fresh water via water bottles attached to the cage, which may sometimes be placed at different heights in order to add extra interest.

Breeding and breeding systems

Breeding data is summarised in Table 10.3. Breeding groups of marmosets within the controlled conditions of the animal facility are put together as monogamous pairs at fourteen to eighteen months and will go on to have between one and three young every twenty-two weeks. Figure 10.2 shows a day old marmoset and Figures 10.3 and 10.4 show marmoset growth curves and interbirth intervals. The third young has to be supplementary fed by the keeper if it is to survive, as the mother and father cannot cope very well with looking after any more than two young at a time. The male parent often caries the young around the cage on his back, and siblings from previous births are also known to help out with carrying them. The interaction between siblings of different ages is important for their proper social development, and helps them later when they too may breed.

Marmosets are separated from different family groups at around eight to twelve months of age and are placed together into groups of between twelve and eighteen animals within single-sex gang cages. If the group is made up of individuals from different families then they should be housed together at eight to nine months. Individuals from the same family

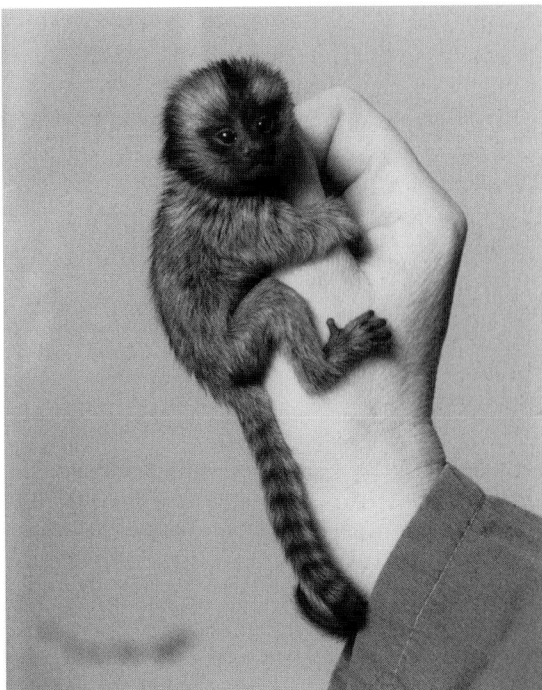

Figure 10.2   Marmoset at one day old.

may be weaned into their gang cage at twelve months of age. It is essential that gang cages of each sex are not kept within the same room, as when the individuals start to approach sexual maturity aggressive interactions within the male gang cage can lead to serious injuries. All newly housed marmosets should be observed for evidence of incompatibility or fighting and some may need to be re-housed in order to maintain the equilibrium within the room.

Training marmosets to co-operate in studies

Marmosets can be caught and held around the waist quite easily, although some individuals do not like this and may attempt to bite. The handler can get adequate protection by wearing flexible leather gloves, thereby allowing the animal to undergo a veterinary inspection or participate in a routine regulated procedure performed by another person. Some marmosets may be handled without wearing gloves

Table 10.3   Summary of breeding data for marmosets.

Age when sexually mature	13–15 months
Age at first mating	14–18 months
Length of oestrous cycle	28 days
Interbirth interval	154 days
Gestation period	144 days
Birth weight	28–38 g
Average litter size	1–3
Weaning age	8–12 months
Adult weight	350–600 g

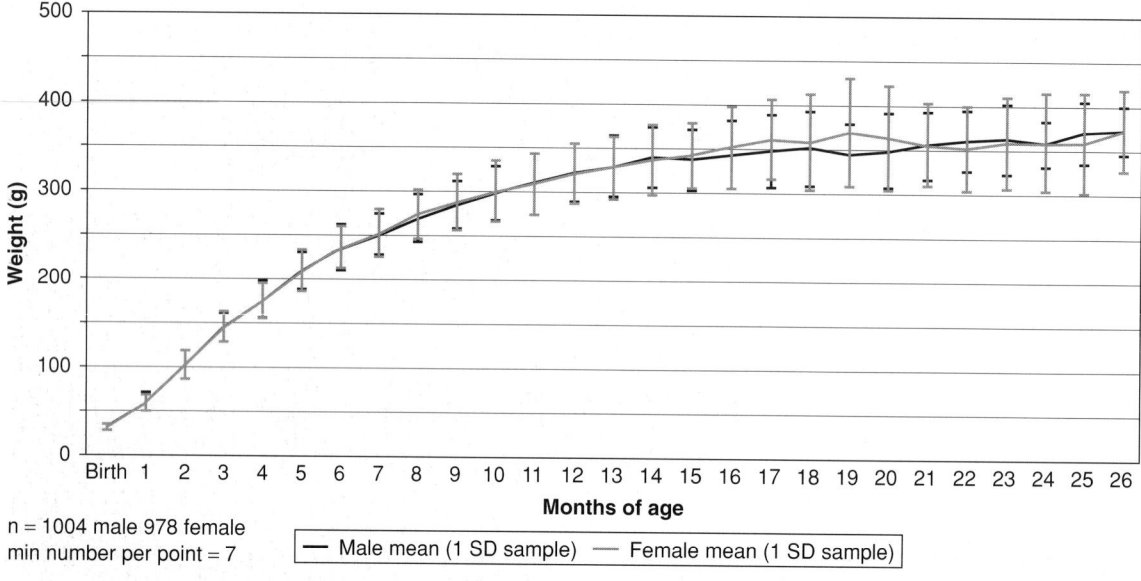

500
400
300
200
100
0
Weight (g)
Birth 1 2 3 4 5 6 7 8 9 10 11 12 13 14 15 16 17 18 19 20 21 22 23 24 25 26
Months of age
n = 1004 male 978 female
min number per point = 7
Male mean (1 SD sample)
Female mean (1 SD sample)

Figure 10.3 Growth curve for marmosets born 1991–1998.

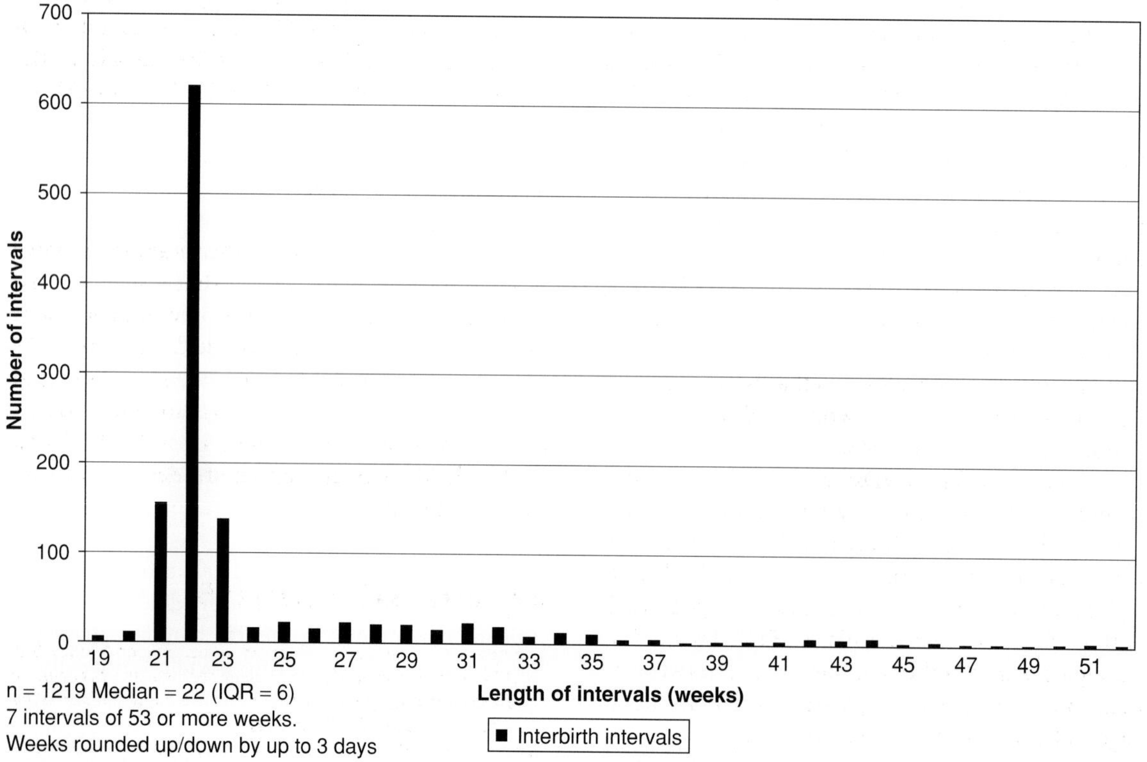

700
600
500
400
300
200
100
0
Number of intervals
19 21 23 25 27 29 31 33 35 37 39 41 43 45 47 49 51
Length of intervals (weeks)
n = 1219 Median = 22 (IQR = 6)
7 intervals of 53 or more weeks.
Weeks rounded up/down by up to 3 days
Interbirth intervals

Figure 10.4 Interbirth intervals for marmosets 1986–2002 (D. Veall, personal communication, 2004).

Figure 10.5   Marmoset at Dstl using the Cambridge Neuropsychological Test Automated Battery ® (CANTAB).

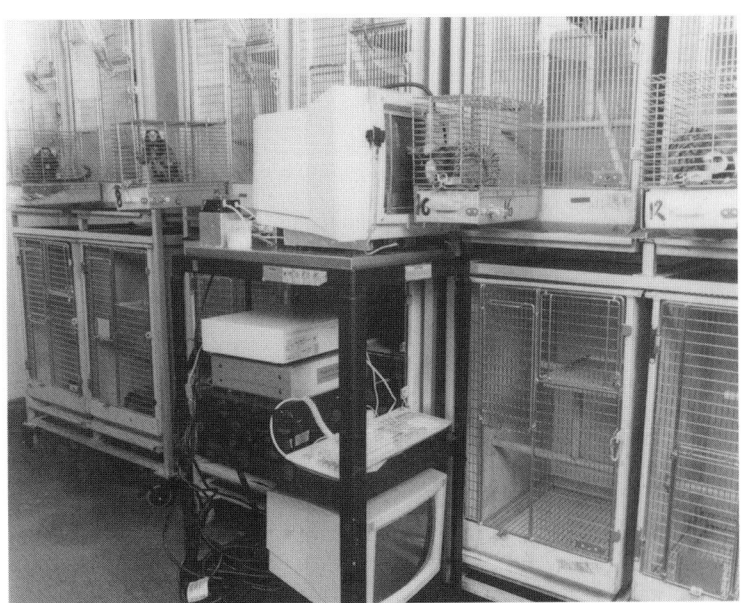

and in all cases the animal should be given a food treat rewarding good behaviour and cooperation.

With careful training marmosets can become very used to cooperating in more complex research programmes. The scientific and welfare benefits achieved with the development of home cage cognitive testing techniques over the past twenty years are many. The use of touch-screen cognitive test equipment at Dstl (the Defence Science and Technology Laboratory) within the marmoset's home environment, removes the need for the animal to habituate to new surroundings (Figure 10.5, above). By using only positive reinforcement via banana-flavoured milkshake, the marmoset is able choose to participate in a particular test or not (Scott et al. 2003). The animal's willingness to participate in such a test programme within the same room as its conspecifics is a further endorsement of its motivation.

Marmosets within the Dstl research facility live as compatible mixed-sex pairs after the male has been vasectomised. They are housed within a bank of four large cages which are linked together with both vertical linkers and horizontal linkers and trays beneath within which forage mix is placed. Prior to and during a particular test the cage linkers are removed and each animal is housed separately within its home cage. All animals are returned to their pair mates at the end of the period of work and the cage linkers are replaced.

Health

Signs of ill health in marmosets are similar to other animals, e.g. anorexia, weight loss, poor coat condition and lethargy. The rectal temperature of a marmoset is 38.5–40 °C. Further details of the health of marmosets can be found in Potkay (1992).

Identification methods

Small coloured discs with either numbers and/or letters may be suspended on short-beaded metal chain and placed around either the animal's neck or waist. The chain must be checked regularly as the animal grows and the disc may require cleaning to remove food deposits. An ID transponder may be installed underneath the loose skin on the back and read by holding an appropriate reader up to 15 cm from the animal.

References and further reading

Chamove, A.S., James, R.A., Morgan-Jones, S.C. and Jones, S.P. (1982) Deep woodchip litter: Hygiene, feeding, and behavioural enhancement in eight primate species. *International Journal for the Study of Animal Problems*, 3 (4).

Grist, S.M. (1974) The common marmoset (*Callithrix jacchus*) – A valuable experimental animal. *Journal of the Institute of Animal Technicians*, 27 (1): 1–7.

Home Office (1989) *Code of Practice for the Housing and Care of Animals used in Scientific Procedures.* HMSO, London.

Home Office (1995) *Code of Practice for the Housing and Care of Animals in Designated Breeding and Supplying Establishments.* HMSO, London.

Mitchell, S.M. and Jones, S.M. (1975) Diagnosis of pregnancy in Marmosets (*Callithrix jacchus*). *Laboratory Animals*, **9**: 49–56.

Pearce, P.C., Crofts, N.G., Muggleton, N.G. and Scott, E.A.M. (1998) Concurrent monitoring of EEG and performance in the Common Marmoset: A methodological approach. *Physiology and Behaviour*, **63** (4): 591–599.

Poole, T., Hubrect, R. and Kirkwood, J.K. (1999) Marmosets and Tamarins. In: T. Poole (Ed.) *The UFAW Handbook on the Care and Management of Laboratory Animals* (7th edn). Blackwell Science, Oxford.

Potkay, S. (1992) Diseases of the Callitrichidae: A review. *Journal of Medical Primatology*, **21**: 189–236.

Rylands, A.B. (1997) The Callitrichidae: A biological overview. In: C. Pryce, E.A.M. Scott and C. Schnell (Eds) *Marmosets and Tamarins in Biological and Biomedical Research.* DSSD Imagery, Salisbury, UK. 1–9. (Private publication.)

Schnell, C.R. (1993) Measurements of blood pressure, heart rate, body temperature, ECG and activity by telemetry in conscious unrestrained marmosets (pp. 107–111). *Proceedings of the Fifth FELASA Symposium, Welfare and Science.* Brighton.

Schnell, C.R. and Wood, J.M. (1993) Measurement of blood pressure and heart rate by telemetry in conscious unrestrained marmosets. *Am. J. Physiol. (Heart & Circ. Physiol.)*, **264** (33): H1509–H1516.

Scott, E.A.M., Pearce, P.C., Fairhall, S. et al. (2003) Training non-human primates to cooperate with scientific procedures in biomedical research. *Journal of Applied Animal Welfare Science*, **6** (3): 199–207. Lawrence Erlbaum Associates, Inc., NJ.

Stevenson, M.F. and Rylands A.B. (1988) The Marmoset, genus *Callithrix* (pp. 131–222). In: R.A. Mittermeier, A.B. Rylands, A. Coimbra-Filtho and G.A.B Fonesca (Eds) *Behaviour and Ecology of Neotropical Primates* (Vol. 2). World Wildlife Fund, Washington DC.

11
Old World Primates

Martin Heath (with additional material from Jeremy N. Smith and Andy Bradwell)

Introduction

The most common species of old world primates used in the United Kingdom for scientific procedures are:

- *Macaca fascicularis*: (Figure 11.1) Crab-eating macaque, usually known as the Cynomolgus.
- *Macaca mulatta*: (Figure 11.2) Rhesus macaque.

This chapter will concentrate on these species. Classification of these primates is given in Table 11.1.

Old World primates account for less than one percent of all animals used in scientific procedures in the United Kingdom. There are many legal and ethical reasons why their use is low, including:

- they require special housing conditions;
- they are expensive to obtain, expensive to maintain; and
- most importantly, their high position in the phylogenic scale requires special justification from the Home Office for use in regulated procedures under the Animals (Scientific Procedures) Act 1986.

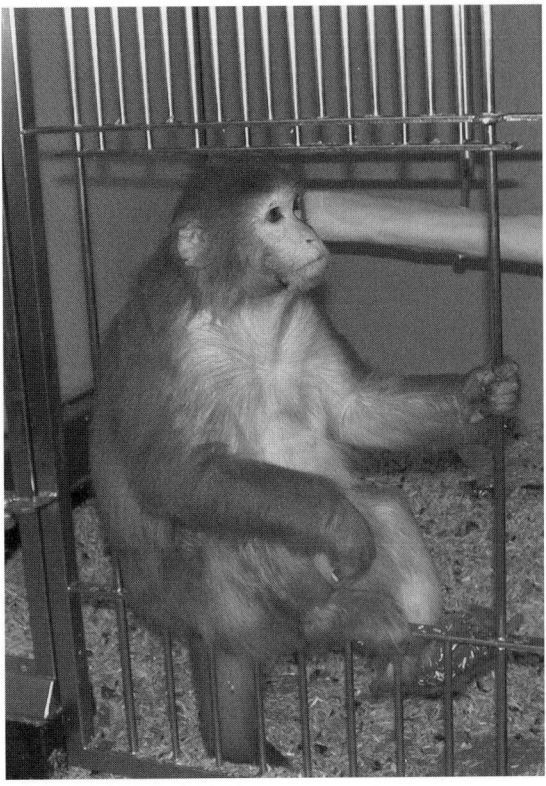

Figure 11.2   Rhesus monkey.

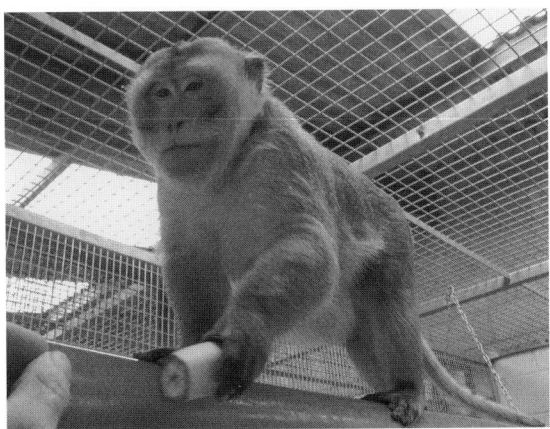

Figure 11.1   Cynomolgus monkey.

Table 11.1 Classification of primates *Macaca fascicularis* and *Macaca mulatta*.

Kingdom	Animalia
Phylum	Chordata
Sub-phylum	Vertebrata
Class	Mammalia
Order	Primate
Family	Cercopithecidae
Genus and species	*Macaca fascicularis*
	Macaca mulatta

Old World primates originate from Africa and countries in Asia such as China, Japan, Indonesia, Malaysia and Philippines. Although they are purpose bred in the UK, imports are currently permitted under strict conditions and with appropriate authority. These conditions include:

- they must come from approved purpose-bred colonies from the country of origin;
- import and export regulations must be strictly observed, i.e. Convention of International Trade in Endangered Species (CITES, 1973);
- transport regulations must be complied with, e.g. Welfare of Animals (Transport) Order 1997 (see Chapter 28).

Primates are given special protection under the Animals (Scientific Procedures) Act 1986 (see Chapter 36), a special case has to be made to be allowed to use any primate and there is a complete ban on the use of any great ape. The Animal Procedures Committee (APC) has a 'Primate subcommittee' which advises the APC on such issues as:

- acquisition of primates;
- housing and care;
- use of wild-caught primates;
- how to minimise or eliminate primate use and suffering;
- primate use in toxicology.

Handling and capture of Old World primates require special skills, as does the execution of regulated procedures. There are special issues of health and safety to consider, especially if the primates are imported. Imported animals must undergo stringent health screening and quarantine procedures. Staff should be aware of the risk of zoonotic diseases such as tuberculosis, Herpes B virus, Shigellosis and Salmonellosis. A routine screening schedule for home-bred primates should also take these diseases into account.

Use in regulated procedures

Old World primates are used in studies involving toxicology, heart disease, infectious diseases and cancer. Increasing human longevity and its associated problems has led to the increasing use of primates in the study of neurodegenerative disorders.

Acclimatisation

Primates, especially those imported, will require a period of acclimatisation after they have arrived in a facility. They are susceptible to stress and on arrival at an alien environment after several hours of travel, they will undoubtedly be stressed. Signs of stress include:

- refusal to eat or drink;
- diarrhoea;
- weight loss;
- loss of condition;
- stereotypies.

It is extremely important to monitor the animals closely and regularly, carry out veterinary health checks and keep detailed health records. In recent years with close association with the end user and with Home Office inspectors, most animals bred abroad are born and raised in facilities which employ such good standards that many of the health problems which existed with imported animals in the past have been eliminated. Acclimatisation both to new facilities and unfamiliar laboratory diets have been reduced in most cases to weeks rather than months. Quarantine under the Rabies Order is still mandatory for laboratory primates bred outside the EU.

Environment

The environmental levels recommended in the codes of practice are given in Table 11.2. (Home Office 1989; 1995).

Cynomolgus macaques originate from tropical climates and may need environmental temperatures at the top end of the scale, whereas Rhesus species come from warm to temperate climates and may be more comfortable at lower temperatures. Indoor housing is usually in the range of 19–23 °C which takes account of staff requirements as well as the animals'. Primates which have the option of outside enclosures should have appropriate heated and ventilated quarters inside (see Figure 11.3) to which they have access at all times.

Housing

Primates exhibit complex social relationships if held in groups and must have housing which is of sufficient

Table 11.2 Environmental levels for primates (Home Office 1989, 1995).

	Scientific procedure establishments	Breeding and supplying establishments
Room temperature	15–24 °C	15–24 °C
Relative humidity	55% ± 10%	55% ± 15%
Air changes per hour	10–12	10–12
Photoperiod	12 hours light: 12 hours dark (preferably with dawn and dusk periods)	–

Figure 11.3 Rhesus in outside pens.

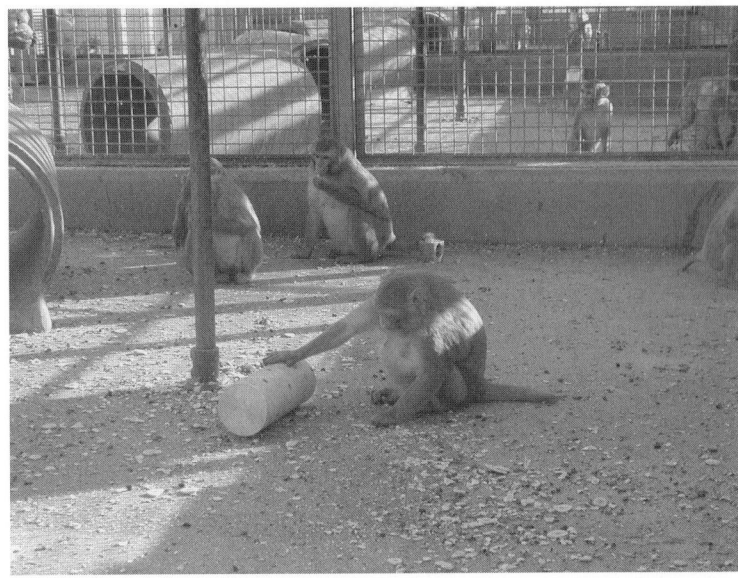

size and complexity to allow these relationships to develop normally. Housing and environment dramatically influence primate welfare, so its design must reflect the needs of the animal. Traditional single housing in metal caging should be avoided wherever possible as this type of caging exacerbates behavioural problems. Pair housing with compatible animals should be a minimum social provision, however it may be necessary to use single cages for experimental or health (e.g. injured or sick animals) reasons, in which case, wherever possible, the cage should be situated where the primate can see other animals. Primates held in this manner should be provided with environmental enrichment in the form of novel play items, food puzzles, etc. It is more important to have a complex cage structure for long-term, singly housed primates to prevent the onset of abnormal behaviour such as stereotypies, self-mutilation and/or aggression due to boredom.

Macaques are mainly arboreal, with complex social structures; this has to be taken into consideration when designing primate group accommodation. They require enough three-dimensional space and pen furniture to be able to express their natural behavioural repertoire. It is preferable to have the height of caging extend above human level so that animals can gain confidence in the presence of humans. Where possible, escape routes or visual barriers should be available for less dominant animals to retreat from dominant cage-mates. Cage and pen design should reflect the complex needs of the animal, whilst at the same time enabling the animals to be captured or restrained safely. All primates benefit from being able to see all parts of the room in which they are held; cages with bow fronts, protruding tunnels or even suspended stainless steel mirrors allow this (Figures 11.4 and 11.5).

The Home Office codes of practice (1989, 1995)

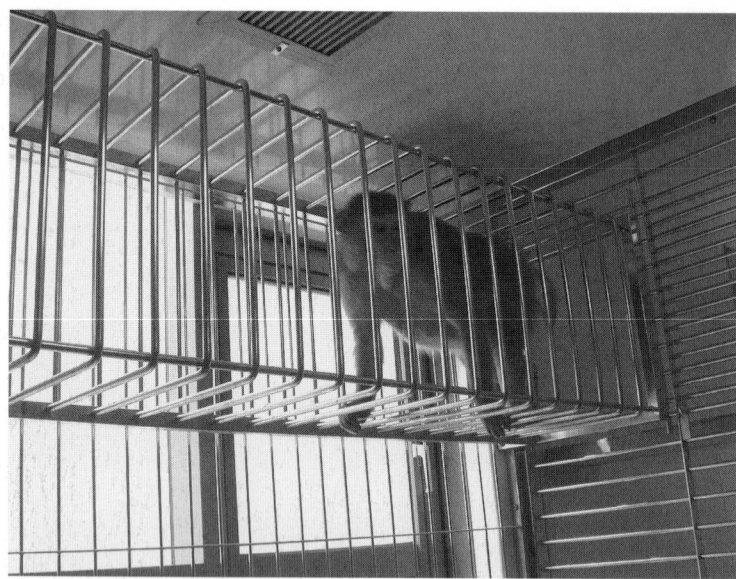

Figure 11.4   High-level protruding tunnel.

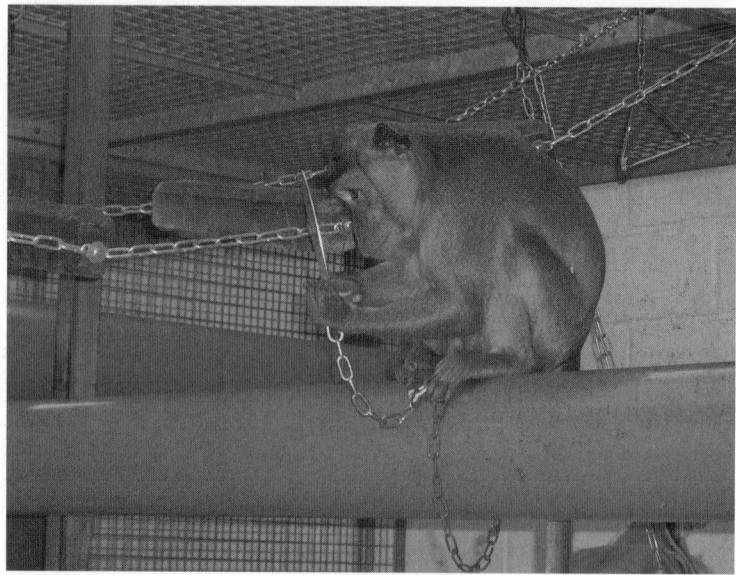

Figure 11.5   Rhesus using a polished metal mirror.

give precise minimum cage dimensions and stocking densities, however, it is important to remember two things:

(1) What is put into a cage in terms of environmental enrichment is more important than the size of the cage alone.
(2) These are minimum size guidelines. The more useable space that can be provided, the better it is for the animal (Figures 11.6 and 11.7).

Primate housing must be strong and escape proof to be able to contain these very strong, manipulative and inquisitive animals. It must be capable of being cleaned regularly and where modular systems are used, flexible enough to join up and enlarge when necessary. If moving parts, such as moveable panels, are used they should be serviced regularly and well maintained. The use of positive reinforcement in training primates to cooperate in routine procedures is hugely advantageous in reducing stress to both

Figure 11.6 Pen with environmental enrichment item.

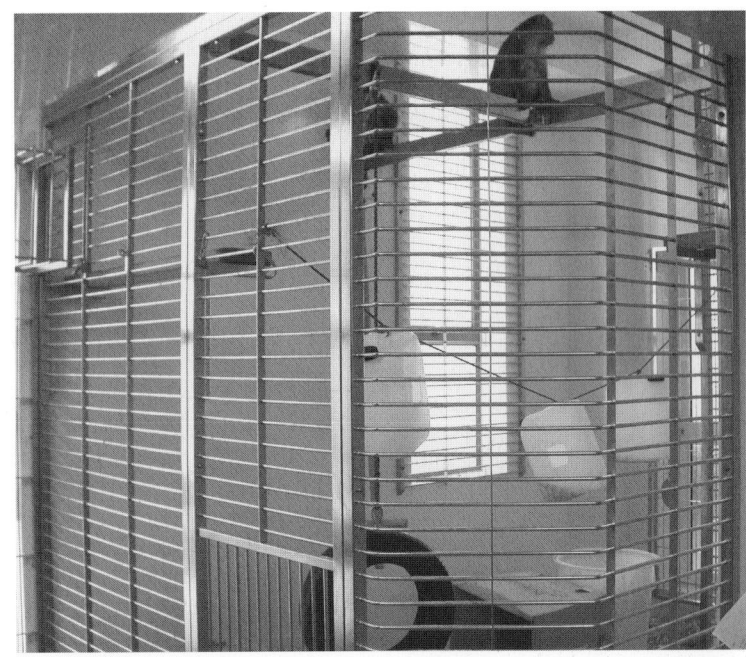

Figure 11.7 Young cynomologus using cage space.

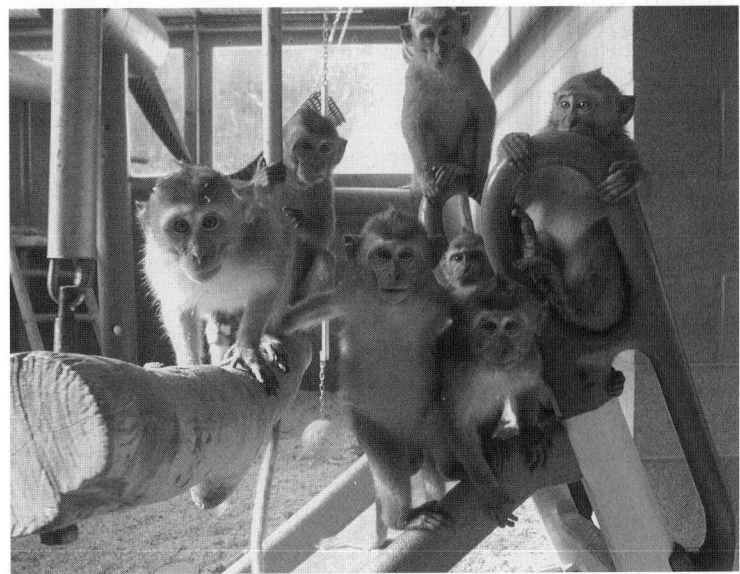

animals and technicians and can reduce or even eliminate the need for crush-back cages and physical restraint methods.

Routines

Traditionally, wire-mesh flooring has been used for primate caging but this is no longer acceptable for welfare reasons and should be replaced by a solid floor with a substrate of woodchips or shredded paper. The only real benefit of mesh flooring is for the convenience of their human carers. In the wild, Old World primates spend the majority of their day foraging for food, so providing a substrate that enables them to carry out this natural behaviour is of great benefit. If mesh floors have to be used, a foraging box should be attached to the cage so that the primate still has an opportunity to carry out this behaviour albeit in a more restricted way.

A typical cleaning regime for Old World primates housed in cages would include changing the cage tray every day, changing the cage contents twice a week and providing a clean cage once a month. Any cleaning regime needs to be adaptable, for instance an animal that is particularly messy will have to be cleaned more often.

Cleaning regimes for group-housed primates are entirely dependent on the size of the caging or pens, the numbers of animals housed and the type and amount of substrate used. Deep litter wood shavings for example will require far less maintenance than a thin layer of sawdust, although either may be appropriate. Good drainage and good drainage protection is a must, as these areas will need to be pressure washed regularly; again depending on size and stocking densities.

Food and water

Primates in the wild spend several hours of daylight looking and foraging for food and sources of water. In the laboratory, food and water is provided for them, usually at the same time of day, therefore the mental stimulation used for searching for food is lost. Making primates look or work for their food is mentally stimulating and fills up several hours of their day, reducing boredom, which otherwise could result in abnormal behavioural patterns.

Primates, like humans, require a daily intake of vitamin C because they are unable to synthesise a supply in their tissues (see Chapter 26). A balanced, as well as a varied, diet is important when primates are kept in captivity. Primates which do not have access to direct sunlight need an increased supplement of vitamin D. Primate diet is usually given in the form of a pre-packaged pellets. Although this type of diet is nutritionally balanced, provided it is used by the prescribed date, it is very dry and uninteresting. Clean fruit and vegetables should be given to supplement the pellet diet to add variety and texture. Animals will undoubtedly prefer fruit and vegetables to pellets and this may result in them consuming insufficient amounts of the pellets for their nutritional needs. This can be prevented if pellets are

provided in the morning and fruit and vegetables later in the day. Fruit given in large amounts, especially oranges, may cause diarrhoea as will any sudden change in diet, so new food must be introduced gradually and the animals carefully monitored.

Water should be provided at all times in water bottles or automatic watering systems. Both have advantages and disadvantages. Bottles for instance only hold a specified amount, but water consumption may be monitored. Automatic watering provides a constant source of water, but is difficult to judge how much is being consumed. During the acclimatisation period, water bottles would be the best choice, as accurate water consumption can be recorded and remedial action taken immediately if the primates fail to drink.

Breeding

Like humans, and unlike other laboratory species, Old World primates have a menstrual cycle characterised by endometrial changes in the uterus resulting in regular menstrual bleeding in the non-pregnant female (see Chapter 15).

Breeding data is listed in Table 11.3. The information contained in the table should be treated as a guide. Individual and strain differences mean that different values may apply.

Rhesus macaques

Rhesus macaques are seasonal breeders, and are in breeding condition from September to January (although variation is seen in animals bred inside under artificial light). During the season, females cycle every twenty-eight days. Readiness to mate in the female is signalled by engorgement of the vulval area making it very red. The face also becomes red and other areas of sexual swelling appear on the legs and face.

Cynomolgus macaques

Cynomolgus macaques breed throughout the year. When they are ready to mate the vulval area becomes pink and there may be evidence of sexual swelling beneath the base of the tail, however there are none of the other dramatic changes seen in the Rhesus.

Table 11.3 Summary of breeding data for *Macaca mulatta* and *Macaca fascicularis*.

	Macaca mulatta	Macaca fascicularis
Age at puberty: female	2–3 years	As for rhesus
Age at puberty: male	3–4 years	As for rhesus
Age at first mating: female	3–5 years	As for rhesus
Age at first mating: male	4–5 years	As for rhesus
Breeding season	September–January	All year
Length of menstrual cycle	28 days	31 ± 1
Gestation	164 ± 5 days	160 ± 7 days
Birth weight	0.5–0.55 kg	0.25–0.45 Kg
Litter size	1	1 (twins exceedingly rare)
Return to oestrus post partum	Normally at the end of lactation	Unknown, many animals return to oestrus during lactation
Weaning age	12 months	10–12 months
Weight at weaning	1.5–1.8 kg	1.2–1.5 kg
Adult weight: female	4–9 kg	3–7 kg
Adult weight: male	6–12 kg	5–10 kg
Economic breeding life	18 years	15 years

Breeding Systems

Old World Primates can be bred by arranged mating systems, or in harems.

Arranged mating

Females are introduced to males when the external signs indicate she is ready to mate. Introducing males and females for the first time can pose problems. If they do not get on they may fight, causing injury to each other and staff who have to separate them. Records of incompatible animals should be kept so that they are not placed together again. Compatible breeding pairs will often mate several times a day, over several days. The female will sometimes reject the advances of the male when ovulation is complete; this can be a good indication of the time to separate the male from the female. The male will take no further part in the procedure.

Harems

Harems are often set up with groups of pre-pubescent animals as these tend to settle down far more quickly and with less aggression than adult groups. Animals are grouped at a ratio of ten to twelve females to one male or two males to twenty females. Such systems require a lot of space and usually include outdoor pens. Several females may be pregnant or have sucking young at any one time and those without young may act as surrogate mothers and occasionally look after another female's baby for short periods. Non-pregnant dominant females may become 'broody' and snatch babies away from their real mothers. This may damage long-term prospects for the infant, and in a minority of cases may even result in fighting between the females.

Such systems are dynamic and can result in hierarchical shifts between females from time to time with some becoming injured. These events may even result in death on rare occasions, usually due to resultant shock rather than the trauma itself. In harems, there will usually be a dominant male, but again fighting between previously settled males is not unknown.

Pregnancy and parturition

Gestation lasts for approximately 160 days $\pm$ 7 days, depending on the species (see Table 11.3). Birth usually occurs at night, the afterbirth or placenta is very often eaten, as this provides the female with beneficial nutrients and hormones required for lactation. A new mother has to learn the complex behaviour of motherhood; she has to understand visual, behavioural and auditory queues from the newborn. Whilst much of this behaviour is innate there is evidence to suggest that chances of successful rearing can be enhanced where the new mother has been present when a sibling has been born, i.e. has not been weaned from her natal colony too soon.

It is important to ensure that the young consumes colostrum shortly after birth. The action of the newborn sucking for the first time will stimulate the mammary glands to let down the milk. Sometimes, either for medical causes or through inexperience, breast milk is not produced. If this happens veterinary advice must be sought.

Weaning

It is important that a young primate learns the art of parenting and socialisation if it is to become a good parent itself in the future, it learns these skills from its mother. Weaning should take place no sooner than eight months old unless there are good veterinary reasons. Most breeders wean at a minimum of ten to twelve months and possibly even longer if they are to be kept for future breeding. It is during this critical period that the infants learn important social skills which enable them to interact successfully with other colony residents and hopefully form stable bonds. Infants weaned earlier than six months may be deprived of these experiences and may exhibit unsociable and/or abnormal behaviour later in life.

Weaned animals should be kept in same-sex groups to maintain their social behaviour. Status within a colony is important for the structure of the groups' stability and survival and a hierarchy will become established. Alpha males and Alpha females will dominate the groups; they will have preference over less dominant animals for things like natural mating selection, food, water, and choice of position within the corral or pen. Food and water should therefore be located in several parts of the pen, allowing access for less dominant animals to eat and drink in peace. There should also be several escape routes allowing less dominant animals to avoid confrontation with Alpha males or Alpha females. If less dominant animals are constantly bullied, stress and ill health will become evident, e.g. weight loss, loss of condition, depression, loss of appetite.

Human contact

Human contact is extremely important from an early age. Trust between primates and their carers creates an environment of harmony, minimising stress. Animal technicians, who have the responsibility of the primate health and welfare on a daily basis, should build up a human–animal relationship beneficial to both (Heath 1989). Primates in captivity need to be kept mentally stimulated as well as physically healthy through environmental enrichment and positive reinforcement.

Health

Signs of ill health in the primates are similar to other animals, they include separation from cage mates, ignoring food, poor coat condition and a hunched appearance. They are susceptible to a variety of infectious organisms, some of which can be introduced into the colony by man and some of which are zoonoses. The named veterinary surgeon will advise on the most appropriate health screening programme to protect both animals and the staff working with them. The rectal temperature of a Rhesus monkey is 38.4–39.6 °C and it is 37–40 °C for the Cynomolgus.

Identification

Micro-chip implants have the advantage of allowing identification to be made without disturbing or stressing the animal if they can be read remotely. They may contain additional information such as the project licence number, date of birth, study number and animal identification number (although if extra information is included the implantation of the chip becomes a regulated procedure). Tattoos have the advantage that they can be seen without the need of a reader. They can be applied to the inside of the leg in the region of the quadriceps muscle; alternatively they may be applied on the chest if visibility from a distance is important, i.e. for animals held in groups. Tattooing should be done under anaesthetic and must be done by a competent person.

The Home Office requires that primates are individually identified using a permanent method, therefore a cage label alone will not be suitable. The addition of the cage label is also required by the Home Office, it should be placed out of the reach of the primate who would otherwise destroy it.

References and further reading

Baskerville, M. (1999) Old World monkeys. In: T. Poole (Ed.) *The UFAW Handbook on the Care and Management of Laboratory Animals* (7th edn). Blackwell Science, Oxford.

Heath, M. (1989) The training of cynomolgus monkeys and how the human/animal relationship improves with environmental and mental enrichment. *Animal Technology*, **40** (1): 11–22.

Home Office (1989) *Code of Practice for the Housing and Care of Animals used in Scientific Procedures.* HMSO, London.

Home Office (1995) *Code of Practice for the Housing and Care of Animals in Designated Breeding and Supplying Establishments.* HMSO, London.

Wolfensohn, S. and Lloyd, M. (1998) Primates. In: S. Wolfensohn and M. Lloyd (Eds) *Handbook of Laboratory Animal Management and Welfare* (2nd edn). Blackwell Science, Oxford.

12
Zebrafish

Neil A. Vargesson

Introduction

Zebrafish (*Danio rerio*) are found indigenously in India, Pakistan, Bangladesh, Nepal and Myanmar, where they populate slow moving to stagnant standing water bodies particularly rice fields, streams, canals, ditches and ponds. They commonly feed on small crustaceans, insect larvae and algae. Zebrafish are popular in home aquariums as they are easy to keep and maintain. The male is thin, torpedo shaped and has a purple tinge to the skin, whereas a female has a white belly and is usually larger than the male. The zebrafish is the latest organism to have its genome sequenced (approximately 1.7 gigabases on 25 chromosomes) by groups in England, Germany and Holland. The full sequence should be available in 2006 (for more information see www.sanger.ac.uk/Projects/D_rerio). Classification of zebrafish is given in Table 12.1.

Advantages of the zebrafish as a model system

A pair of adult zebrafish under the right conditions (see below) can produce up to 200 embryos per day. Embryos develop very quickly; going from a single fertilised cell to a fully patterned embryo in just 24 hours. They can swim by the time they are 48 hours old and are feeding independently by five days. They are sexually mature between two and three months old. Embryos are optically transparent, large and can be observed live, making them ideal for the study of development and molecular genetics. Moreover, zebrafish are easy and cheap to keep and breed. For all these reasons the zebrafish is now a well-established model system (= organism) for scientists studying developmental biology and clinical/translational research (Nusslein & Dahm 2002; Westerfield 2000).

Perhaps the biggest advantages of the zebrafish are:

(1) Its genetic tractability, for example, to enable global or even tissue-specific mis-expression of a gene (i.e. via heat-shock promoters (Halloran et al. 2000)) or to be able to knock down gene expression using morpholinos (which prevent translation of mRNA into proteins).

(2) Mutagenesis screens, where application of a mutagenic chemical to zebrafish can produce hundreds of viable mutant fish lines in order to identify important genes. In fact, mutagenesis screens have led to a database containing hundreds of viable fish lines containing mutations in every body system and bodily process, some of the genes and processes involved in causing these mutations have since been identified (Nusslein & Dahm 2002; Westerfield 2000) (see also www.zfin.org/; www.zfin.org/zirc/home/guide.php and www.eb.tuebingen.mpg.de/services/stockcenter/home.html).

Table 12.1 Classification of zebrafish *Danio rerio*.

Kingdom	Animalia
Sub-kingdom	Vertebrata
Phylum	Actinopterygii
Order	Teleostei
Family	Cyprinidae
Genus and species	*Danio rerio*

Use in regulated procedures

Zebrafish are mainly used to study developmental biology. The transparency of the embryo, *ex-vivo* development, high fecundity and fast development times make the zebrafish ideal to study vascular development (Shawber & Kitajewski 2004), neural development (Nusslein-Volhard & Dahm 2002; Moens & Prince 2002), regeneration (Akimenko et al. 2003), wound healing (Redd et al. 2004), organogenesis (Crosnier et al. 2005), etc. The zebrafish is also used as a model for testing drug action (Zon & Peterson 2005) in order to understand the mechanism of action of the drug as well as test for potential side-effects which may affect humans. In addition, many viable mutant fish lines exist which show characteristics which are similar to human diseases/conditions, allowing the zebrafish to be used to understand more about human disease and cure human conditions (Ackerman & Paw 2003).

Environmental conditions

In order to breed zebrafish successfully in a laboratory two essential requirements must be satisfied.

(1) Temperature – a temperature range of 27–28.5 °C is necessary for optimum breeding conditions. Temperatures below 25 °C and above 30 °C reduce the breeding capability of the fish and consequently the numbers of embryos produced.

(2) Photoperiod – a computer- or timer-controlled light/dark cycle of fourteen hours of light and ten hours of darkness is necessary. The darkness allows the zebrafish to rest and the light returning will trigger fish to breed (see section on Breeding p. 81).

Other important parameters which need to be addressed are water quality, water aeration and removal of waste products. Waste products from fish, including ammonia, are toxic in high concentrations, and therefore need to be removed on a regular basis (see section on Water quality p. 80).

A number of systems can be used to keep zebrafish in the laboratory, the system used depends on the needs of the research. The simplest system consists of a series of tanks on table-top surfaces with a low density of fish per tank and one or two water exchanges per week – to remove waste-product build up.

More commonly in laboratories where large numbers of fish are kept for transgenic studies or mutation analysis, fish are kept in custom-made all-in-one systems. These house multiple tanks, with water-flow controls, and an automatic water recirculation system which filters, UV sterilises and aerates the water. Such systems contain biological filters where bacteria (e.g. *Nitrosomas* and *Nitrobacter*) break down fish waste products into harmless components, preventing toxic waste products building up.

The system operated at Imperial College London (Stand Alone System from Aquatic Habitats, Florida, USA; Figure 12.1) houses 48 transparent plastic tanks, of varying capacities. Each tank has a lid, to prevent

Figure 12.1 Stand-alone aquarium system (Aquatic Habitats, USA).

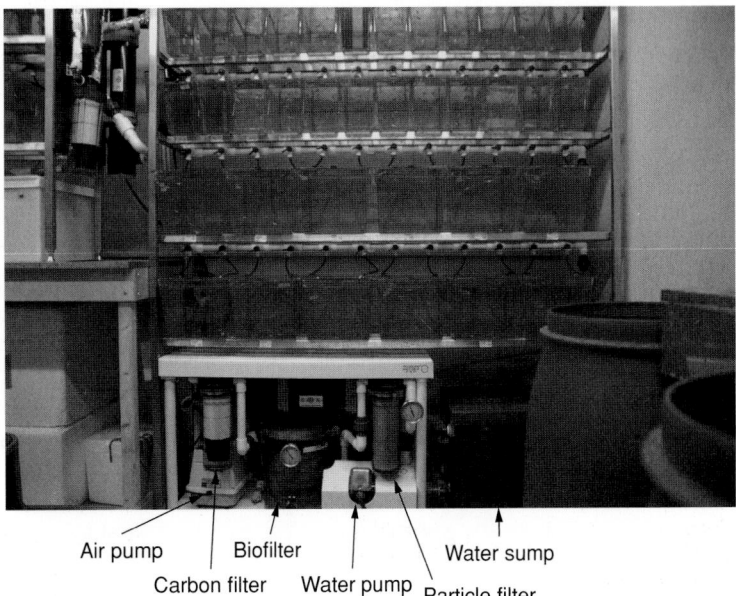

Air pump   Biofilter   Water sump
Carbon filter   Water pump   Particle filter

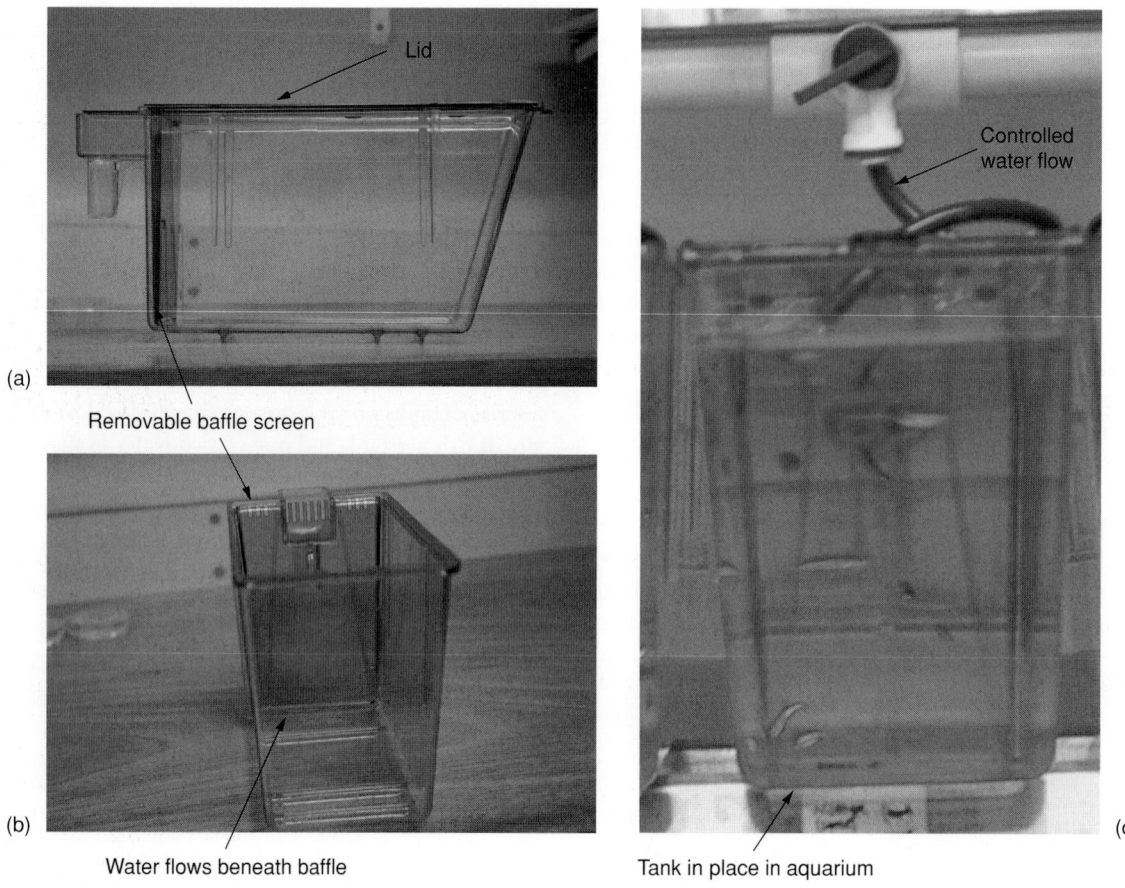

Figure 12.2   A Three Litre Tank Set up.

fish from jumping out and a screen (also known as a baffle) at the back, this has a gap at its base allowing water to pass underneath. This gap also allows waste material and food stuffs to pass through but not fish (Figure 12.2 (a), (b) and (c)). There are different types of screen or baffle to suit the age/size of the fish in the tank to so that young fish cannot escape from the tank. Such a system allows a large number of fish to be looked after at any one time and is time saving, efficient, requires little maintenance and easy is to operate.

Numbers and ratios of fish per tank

In systems possessing filters and a biofilter it is common to find up to five fish per litre, as long as there is good water exchange, a good feeding regime and good water quality. For breeding purposes it is best to have fewer fish per tank (two to three fish per litre). Males and females are kept in separate tanks (which gives good results when crossing pairs of fish, see below). Alternatively, an equal ratio of males to females or, preferably, a ratio of two females to one male are kept. This system is used if a whole tank of fish is to be crossed. To keep fish in good condition and keep waste product build up to a minimum, the maximum number in a tank which does not have filters or a biofilter should be one or two fish per litre. For further information on crossing see the section on Breeding below.

Water quality

Nitrite, nitrate, ammonia and pH levels in water should be monitored on a regular basis. Ammonia is the primary waste material produced by fish. It is

Table 12.2   Safe ranges of water contaminants.

pH	6.5–8.5
Ammonia	0–0.05 g/litre
Nitrite	0 (if using dip-stick test kit)
Nitrate	100–200 mg/litre
Chlorine	0 (if using a dip-stick test kit)

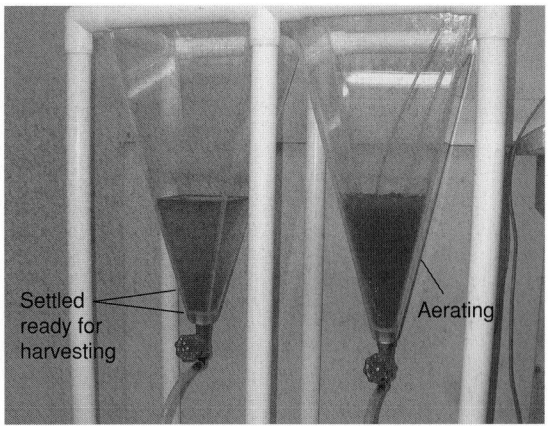

Figure 12.3   Brine shrimp hatcheries.

broken down into nitrite and then later converted into the relatively harmless nitrate. This is all taken care of by means of a biofilter in all-in-one systems, but levels must still be monitored.

Ammonia and nitrite levels are the most important ones to monitor. If these are high (i.e. above the levels indicated in Table 12.2), damage to the fish can occur. For example, nitrite is absorbed through the gills and interferes with the fish's ability to absorb oxygen, resulting in death. High levels of contaminants can be prevented if there is good water exchange, excess food is removed from the tanks, the tanks and system are clean and the biofilter is healthy. If a large increase in ammonia or nitrite is detected, a large water exchange must be carried out immediately.

Ten per cent of the water should be exchanged every day. De-chlorinated tap water must be used, as the chlorine will harm fish. If the tap water normally contains a high base-line of nitrite, pH or calcium carbonate it is a good idea to add some distilled water to the tap water in a ratio of 5 parts tap to 2 parts distilled. One hundred per cent distilled water cannot be used as many nutrients and essential ions required by the fish will have been removed. These nutrients and ions can be replaced by adding supplements which can be obtained from local pet shops stocking fish.

Further information on other systems which can be used to keep zebrafish, as well as further information on environmental conditions and in particular water quality control, etc. is available online (www.zfin.org). This is a wonderful resource full of useful information on zebrafish husbandry.

Food

Zebrafish prefer live food added directly to the tank water. Brine shrimp is commonly used, although paramecium is also suitable. Flake food can be fed when the fish reach adulthood. It is beneficial to the fish to alternate their diet. In general they should be fed twice a day – once in the morning and once in the early evening.

Brine shrimp are reasonably cheap to buy and easy to store in the fridge (ZM Ltd, UK). They are purchased as dried egg cysts which are placed in commercially available brine shrimp hatcheries (ZM Ltd, UK; AHAB, USA; Figure 12.3) in salt water (50 cm^3 of salt in 2.5 litres of tap water) at a temperature of around 28 °C and agitated with an air diffuser. After 24–48 hours the brine shrimp will have hatched and after filtering, to remove the cyst shells and rinsing in tap water, will be ready to feed to the zebrafish. The shrimp should not be kept growing for longer than 48 hours as they will lose their nutritional value.

Although flake food is suitable for zebrafish it is not recommended to feed this alone as it will reduce their breeding efficiency. However, it is a good idea to alternate feeding between brine shrimp and flake. Fish cannot eat large pieces of flake so they must be crushed, through a metal mesh or between two fingers, into a fine powder before lightly sprinkling the food over the surface of the water.

The water flow to the tanks must be turned off or the flow reduced for ten to fifteen minutes while feeding. This allows the fish sufficient time to feed before the food is lost from the tanks since all the food should be consumed within ten to fifteen minutes of being fed. It is important not to overfeed the fish as this will cause them to become fat, reduce breeding, will lead to poor water quality and will increase the chance of disease.

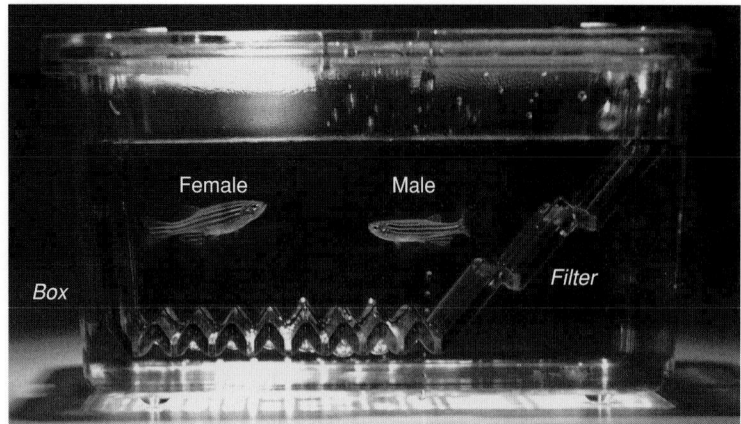

Figure 12.4   Female and male zebra fish in a breeder box (divider removed).

Breeding

Zebrafish will breed in the morning when the aquarium lights come on if environmental conditions are suitable. Approximately one hour after the lights come on the fish will have produced a large number of embryos.

The highest number of embryos can be obtained from fish between the ages of six to eighteen months old. Fish from each tank should only be bred once or twice a week.

High embryo production also requires the fish to be well fed. Extra feeding can be provided by adding highly nutritious bloodworms (bought in frozen form and added to fish tanks after defrosting with a pair of forceps) or flake in addition to their two normal, daily feeds.

There are several ways to breed fish in order to obtain embryos. Two of the most popular are as follows:

(1) Using a breeder box (Aquatic Habitats, USA) to cross a pair of fish (Figure 12.4). This is a transparent, plastic box which contains an insert with small holes in the bottom, a divider to keep the male and female fish separate overnight, a lid to prevent fish from jumping out of the box and a piece of plastic or false seaweed. This method allows the researcher to cross fish of different or the same genotypes with each other to obtain a large number of embryos (up to 200 per cross per day) to found a new line or to use for experiments.

   The procedure is as follows; in the morning when the light has come on, and the divider has been removed from the box, the fish will spawn. The false seaweed aids the spawning as the fish like to rub against it. The eggs/embryos will fall through the holes of the insert so that the fish cannot eat them. When the fish are returned to their original tank/s and the plastic insert is removed, the water can be filtered to harvest the embryos.

(2) The second method uses a one-litre or two-litre breeder box (without the plastic divider or lid) which can be placed directly into the aquarium tanks (either a three-litre or ten-litre tank) containing many fish. This allows the researcher to obtain a good number of embryos from the entire population of fish in the tank (i.e. same genotype). The fish must be over three months of age and must be able to be sexed. A female to male ratio of 2:1 is best for 'tank' breeding. During the process water flow in the tank must be reduced to a minimum.

   Preparation and setting up the breeder boxes should be done one hour after the early evening feed in order to ensure no food is left over to distract the fish and prevent them from breeding. The fish can then be left overnight.

   When the lights come on in the morning the fish will be stimulated to spawn. They are left for 1–1.5 hours before stopping the process and collecting the embryos. Embryos can be placed in aquarium water in Petri dishes, labelled with the date, genotype/name of the embryos and the tank/parents the embryos originated from.

   After six to seven hours the embryos are inspected and infertile or dead embryos are removed otherwise they will rot and kill the remaining embryos.

Fish will not spawn if there is food in the tank, if it is too noisy or there is too much movement/activity around them. Therefore work in the aquarium must be stopped or spawning fish should be placed in parts of the aquarium where the least noise and disturbance occurs. In addition they should be left in a quiet area for at least an hour before obtaining the embryos and feeding the fish.

Husbandry

Growing on fish embryos

Zebrafish embryos can be kept initially in Petri dishes. The embryos contain a yolk sac which provides food for five days, so they do not need feeding for the first five days of life. After two days of development the embryos should have 'hatched' from their protective chorion membrane (which can be removed from the water). By five to six days the larvae should all be swimming on the surface of the water – this shows they have developed a swim bladder, and they can easily be seen with the naked eye.

At five to six days the larvae are placed into a small tank that is a quarter full of water. They are fed with a small amount (i.e. a pinch between forefinger and thumb) of baby/larvae powder (from ZM Ltd, UK; Aquatic Habitats, USA) – gently sprinkled over the water surface. This is done twice a day on weekdays and once on weekends. The water will become cloudy and a 'scum' may form on the surface preventing the larvae reaching food, this can be removed using a brush. The addition of some extra water to the tank will reduce the concentration of waste products.

At nine to ten days the larvae require water exchange and oxygenated water. They are gently poured into a small, clean tank, containing a baby baffle grid/screen. The tank is placed onto the aquarium system and a minimal amount of water is allowed to flow into the tank. This will allow replacement of the water but will not prevent the larvae from swimming or reaching the water surface. Alternatively, they can be given a regular, daily water exchange. They continue to be fed with baby/larvae powder.

At sixteen days a small amount of brine shrimp can be fed to the larvae, i.e. 1–2 ml in a small tank. The brine shrimp must be fresh and moving around in the tank (the larvae will not eat dead brine shrimp). Well-fed larvae have rounded, orange coloured bellies after each meal. A larger size baby baffle grid/screen is inserted to aid water flow and the removal of excess/uneaten food.

At 24–25 days the larvae can be fed just brine shrimp and can also be fed ground-up flake food.

Zebrafish reach sexual maturity at around three months of age by which time they should be fed five to six times the amount of brine shrimp they were initially fed with at sixteen days, depending on fish numbers and tank size. Males and females can easily be distinguished (Figure 12.4).

Fish stocking densities

Up to 50 embryos/larvae can be grown per Petri dish or plastic tank. After one month of development the size/volume of the tank should be increased to allow good, normal growth, as fish growth can be stunted if they are kept in a high density in a small volume. At around two months of development the density should be reduced to two to three fish per litre. For example, at Imperial College a three-litre tank is used for ten to twelve fish and a ten-litre tank for twenty to twenty-five fish. Fish at low densities grow faster, and it is possible to shorten the generation time by raising fish at low densities. However, densities also influence male:female ratios e.g. low fish densities favour female development. Moreover the extra food in tanks needed to support increased/faster development can lead to poor water quality and the rotting food can lead to disease.

Maintaining stocks

Inbreeding is not desirable as it can lead to increased mutation rates and reduced fecundity. Mixing offspring of the same strain but from different parents gets around this problem. Any abnormal or odd-looking embryos should be discarded between day 2 and 5 of development and the remaining larvae mixed together to grow.

Some mutant fish lines require special conditions, indeed some mutant strains are homozygous lethal and can only be kept in the heterozygous state. Therefore, identifying heterozygous mutant carriers requires inbreeding of siblings, raising resulting embryos to adulthood and then identifying the adult heterozygous mutant carriers (either by further intercrossing and identifying those fish which give rise to homozygous embryos which must both be heterozygote carriers, or by PCR (polymerase chain reaction) genome analysis).

Diseases

Zebrafish are hardy fish. Fish diseases can be avoided by ensuring that simple hygiene measures are followed, e.g.:

- fish from a foreign aquarium must be quarantined (i.e. the fish are kept out of the main aquarium) until it can be shown they exhibit no signs of illness (approximately two weeks);
- embryos from foreign aquariums should be gently 'bleached' in 10% NaOCl (Sigma-Aldrich Co. USA) for ten minutes – this reduces the chance of pathogens entering the system (Nusslein-Volhard & Dahm 2002; Westerfield 2000);
- sick fish should be discarded as quickly as possible;
- all equipment should be kept clean and dry (this prevents parasites/organisms living on the equipment);
- water quality must be good and monitored regularly, especially for ammonia and nitrite levels.

One of the most common diseases to affect zebrafish, but not the only one by any means, is fish tuberculosis. This appears to exist in the background of the aquaria and there is no really successful treatment for it. Stressed, injured and genetically inbred fish are at risk. The bacteria *Mycobacteria* causes the fish to look unwell, i.e. be lethargic, have raised scales and waste away. Affected fish should be discarded immediately as there is a high chance of infection to other fish in the system.

All tanks, nets, equipment which came into contact with the affected fish should be cleaned, disinfected and dried. In addition, there is some evidence that fish tuberculosis can be spread to humans so, if dealing with an infected fish, gloves must be worn to avoid any chance of cross contamination. Tanks with a large number of sick fish must be cleaned thoroughly with 5% acetic acid or warm bleach solution, followed by rinsing with cold water and air drying. By maintaining a clean, well-watered system and keeping the fish healthy, this infection should not pose a problem.

For more detailed information on fish diseases, as well as other diseases/problems and suggested treatments please refer to www.zfin.org and Nusslein-Volhard & Dahm (2002) and Westerfield (2000).

Euthanasia

Fish which look ill or are surplus to requirements can be placed in a solution of Tricaine (MS222; Sigma A-5040) (400 mg tricaine powder, 97.9 ml distilled water, 2.1 ml 1 M Tris (pH 9), with a final pH of 7 – which can be stored in 4 ml aliquots at −20 °C in a freezer. A 4 ml aliquot is dissolved in 100 ml water). The fish are left in the Tricaine solution for ten to fifteen minutes, after which their heads are cut off or a slice is made across the brain. Dead fish bodies should be placed into tissue paper and then into an autoclave bag for disposal. Record must be kept of any fish euthanisations and any dead fish found in any of the tanks each day.

References and further reading

Ackermann, F. and Paw, B. (2003) Zebrafish: a genetic model for vertebrate organogenesis and human disorders. *Front. Biosci.*, **8**: 1227–1253.

Akimenko, M., Mari-Beffa, M., Becerra, J. and Geraudie, J. (2003) Old questions, new tools, and some answers to the mystery of fin regeneration. *Developmental Dynamics*, **226**: 190–201.

Crosnier, C., Vargesson, N., Gschmeissner, S. et al. (2005) Delta-notch signalling controls commitment to a secretory fate in the zebrafish intestine. *Development*, **132**: 1093–1104.

Halloran, M., Sato-Maeda, M., Warren, J. et al. (2000) Laser-induced gene expression in specific cells of transgenic zebrafish. *Development*, **127**: 1953–1960.

Moens, C. and Prince, V. (2002) Constructing the hindbrain: insights from the zebrafish. *Developmental Dynamics*, **224**: 1–17.

Nusslein-Volhard, C. and Dahm, R. (Eds) (2002) *Zebrafish: A practical approach.* Oxford University Press.

Redd, M., Cooper, L., Wood, W. et al. (2004) Wound healing and inflammation: embryos reveal the perfect way to repair. *Phils. Trans. R. Soc. Lond.*, *B* **359**: 777–784.

Shawber, C. and Kitajewski, J. (2004) Notch function in the vasculature: insights from zebrafish, mouse and man. *BioEssays*, **26**: 225–234.

Westerfield, M. (2000) *The Zebrafish Book. A Guide for the Laboratory Use of Zebrafish (Danio rerio)* (4th edn), University of Oregon Press. (Available from University of Oregon, Institute of Neuro Science.)

Zebrafish Issue (1996) *Development*, **123**.

Zon, L. and Peterson, R. (2005) *In-vivo* drug discovery in the zebrafish. *Nat. Rev. Drug Discovery*, **4**: 35–44.

Webliography

www.zfin.org
www.zfin.org/zirc/home/guide.php
www.eb.tuebingen.mpg.de/services/stockcenter/home.html
Aquatic Habitats – www.aquatichabitats.com
ZM Ltd – www.zmsystems.co.uk

13
African Clawed Frog – *Xenopus laevis*

Barney Reed

Introduction

Nearly all the *Xenopus laevis* frogs used in research in the UK originate from the Cape of South Africa or are probably the descendants of such individuals. These frogs can typically be found in the stagnant water of pools, ponds, lakes or ditches, usually based on a substrate of deep mud. Under normal circumstances they are totally aquatic. Females are larger than males, growing up to 15 cm from snout to vent compared with 10 cm in the male (Figure 13.1). They can survive for up to twenty-five years in the laboratory (Wolfensohn and Lloyd, 2003). Table 13.1 lists the classification of *Xenopus*.

The front limbs are used to direct food towards the mouth, while the hind legs are larger and primarily used to propel the frog powerfully through the water, to dig out insects and other food items from the mud, and for shredding larger prey into more manageable-sized portions.

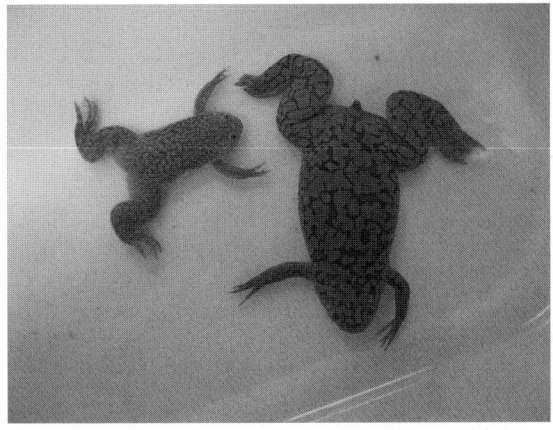

Figure 13.1   Adult xenopus, male on the left, female on the right.

Table 13.1   Classification for frog *Xenopus laevis*.

Kingdom	Animalia
Phylum	Chordata
Sub-phylum	Vertebrata
Class	Amphibia
Order	Anura
Family	Pipidae
Genus and species	*Xenopus laevis*

The skin is damp and slippery. Mucous glands secrete a slimy protective layer, which helps prevent mechanical damage to the skin and provides a barrier against pathogens.

Like fish, these frogs have a lateral line of specialised sensory organs used to locate prey and disturbances in the environment via the perception of water movement and velocity. The lateral line is visible with the naked eye and is seen as a symmetrical pattern of elongated greyish dots or white lines, each 2–3 mm in length which run in a circle around the back of the body, the head and around the eyes.

These animals have a highly developed auditory system facilitating complex underwater acoustic communication between individuals. Studies are now revealing that interactions within populations include the maintenance of territories in underwater habitats (Elepfandt 1996).

Their normal behaviour is to spend most of their time lying motionless below the surface of the water with outstretched arms, waiting for food to pass by.

Recent anatomic, physiological, and biochemical studies, suggests pain perception in amphibians is likely to be analogous to that in mammals (CCAC 2004; Green 2003). Invasive, potentially painful procedures (such as surgical collection of oocytes) should therefore be subject to appropriate ethical review, and accompanied by both anaesthesia and post-operative care including appropriate analgesia.

Use in regulated procedures

Xenopus laevis is the most widely used amphibian research animal. It was the first vertebrate animal to be cloned (Gurdon et al. 1975), and recent years have seen their continued use with the advent of further developments in genetic technologies. They are now one of the most widely used vertebrate species in developmental, cell and molecular biology research (Gurdon 1996).

Developmental biologists, embryologists or geneticists use *Xenopus laevis* because the eggs and early embryos (oocytes) of this animal are large and experimental manipulations are therefore relatively easy (Woodland 2003). Their growth outside the uterus means that embryos can be observed throughout development, which is extremely rapid. Manipulations of the cells within fertilised developing eggs, or of the environment in which the eggs are maintained are often undertaken to discover how subsequent growth and development is affected.

Supply

For many years, large numbers of *Xenopus laevis* frogs have been taken directly from the wild in southern Africa for the purposes of breeding and/or supply to research and testing establishments around the world. More recently, as *Xenopus laevis* can be bred and reared easily under laboratory conditions, an increasing number of captive frogs have been purpose bred for this use. *Xenopus laevis* frogs of either sex and at any stage of development can usually be readily obtained from commercial suppliers.

For animal health and welfare, scientific reliability, and consequently ethical reasons, it is better that animals obtained are from captive colonies bred specifically for the purpose. A researcher must be able to provide compelling scientific justification for using wild-caught individuals.

Transport

The biggest problem for *Xenopus laevis* frogs in transit is exposure to excessive heat. Even a few hours at temperatures above 25 °C can damage egg quality in the females (Sive et al. 2000) though the frogs themselves may *appear* unharmed. Steps must be taken to reduce this risk (see Reed 2005).

Frogs being transported together in the same box should be at a similar stage of development, size and weight, and should not be overcrowded.

Ideally, frogs should be bred at the establishment where they will be used. This will help avoid any potential risks to health or welfare associated with their transport.

Quarantine

A minimum quarantine period of thirty days is advised for all new animals entering an establishment with strong consideration given to extending this period to ninety days for those animals obtained directly from the wild.

Environmental conditions

Lighting

Xenopus laevis are naturally nocturnal animals (Elepfandt 1996). Exposure to continuous light, light deprivation, and inappropriate photoperiods can cause varying clinical symptoms ranging from lethargy to sterility and even death in amphibians (Hayes et al. 1998).

Frogs appear to respond well to lighting regimes of between twelve and fourteen hours of light and twelve to ten hours of dark (Sive et al. 2000). Gradual dimming/brightening of the lights is more akin to natural conditions and allows animals to adapt to the change.

When frogs are exposed to sunlight-equivalent light levels proper vitamin D levels and correct calcium/phosphorous balance can be maintained (University of Arizona 2001) and many researchers believe egg quality improves (Sive et al. 2000). It is therefore important to consider providing full spectrum lighting, including ultraviolet (UV) range, particularly for animals kept over a long period such as six months or more.

Frogs should not be subjected to bright light, though illumination in the animal house must be of an adequate level to allow observation of the animals and for routine housing and husbandry procedures to be carried out. Frogs should have access to places where they can avoid light.

Humidity

Under normal circumstances *Xenopus laevis* frogs are totally aquatic (i.e. equivalent of 100% humidity).

Temperature

If water temperature is sub-optimal, frogs will not eat and their metabolism and immune systems will be depressed. The *Xenopus* immune system operates best above 21 °C (Tinsley & Kobel 1996) and is depressed at low temperatures. Keeping them in laboratories at unsuitable temperatures, such as 15 °C or lower, may be the reason for pathogenic infection occurring (Tinsley & Kobel 1996). Water temperatures of 30 °C can be lethal (Green 2002).

Water temperature should not be maintained below 16 °C or above 24 °C, with strong consideration given to providing a relatively controlled temperature at a point between 18 and 22 °C.

It is also important to minimise significant fluctuations of either room or water temperature. Frogs may be susceptible to thermal shock and suffer mortality if they are abruptly exposed to variation in temperature of 2 °C to 5 °C (Green 2003).

Water

Quantity

Water which is too shallow can increase stress, startle and escape responses in these wholly aquatic frogs. Insufficient water levels can also cause ovary regression in females (Alexander & Bellerby 1938).

The dimensions of the tank and the volume of water must be great enough to allow frogs to move or swim around; to lie fully submerged well away from the surface of the water; to avoid contact with other animals if desired; to turn fully in any direction without impediment either from tank walls or other animals. There should also be sufficient space within the tank to allow the addition of suitable environmental enrichment.

A water depth of *at least* 21 cm is recommended for housing adult *Xenopus laevis* frogs. This is based on

current evidence and knowledge, and should allow them to perform most normal behaviours.

Population density is also important. Under natural conditions, *Xenopus* do not live in direct contact with each other (Council of Europe 2003). *Xenopus laevis* with more area available per animal grow significantly faster than animals kept in a tank with a higher population density (Hilken et al. 1995). It has been suggested that 6–10 litres of water per animal should be provided (Wolfensohn & Lloyd 2003).

Quality

Water should be completely de-chlorinated before use as chlorine attacks the protective mucous layer over the skin and can predispose frogs to infections (Wolfensohn & Lloyd 2003). If local water authorities add chlorine agents to the water this can be removed by running the water through a carbon filter (Sive et al. 2000). In addition, water used directly out of the tap is saturated with dissolved gases and will cause bubbles under the skin and in the toe webs of frogs known as 'gas bubble disease' leading to possible emboli, emphysema, and even death. Therefore, incoming water should be left for twenty-four hours prior to use to equilibrate with the surrounding environment. Incoming water can also be passed through a de-gassing device (vertical packed column) to speed up the process of equilibration of the water (Sanders 2004). The pipes used for transporting water into and around the aquatic system should not be galvanised or copper, since heavy metals can leach from such pipes and may be toxic (Wolfensohn & Lloyd 2003).

Table 13.2 gives one example of typical water quality standards which have been proposed and successfully implemented for *Xenopus laevis* (Sanders 2004). (Note: these are not the only recommendations for good practice and variation exists across establishments.)

Table 13.2   Water quality standards for *Xenopus laevis*.

Alkalinity	> 50 mg/litre $CaCO_3$
Hardness	= 75–150 mg/litre
pH	= 6.5–8.5
Salinity	= 0.4 mg/litre (ppt)
Conductivity	= 50–2000 µS
Un-ionised ammonia (NH_3)	< 0.02 mg/litre
Nitrite (NO_2)	< 1 mg/litre
Nitrate (NO_3)	< 50 mg/litre
Chlorine	= 0 mg/litre
Dissolved oxygen content	> 80% saturation
CO_2	< 5 mg/litre

Group housing

Grouping is advisable as efficient group feeding in this species involves feeding frenzies which are not as prevalent when only very small numbers of animals are kept together (Council of Europe 2004). Grouping animals can also help reduce fear responses.

However, in overcrowded conditions frenzied responses to feeding can lead to traumatic injury of tank mates (DeNardo 1995). The group should be small enough to allow the formation of a stable hierarchy yet large enough to promote feeding frenzies.

It is probable that once the number of animals conducive to encouraging feeding behaviours has been exceeded, *area per frog* is more important than the *actual number of frogs* in the tank. Animal carers commonly consider a minimum of five or six animals per standard tank to be advisable. It is important that animals kept together in the same tank are of similar size.

Cleaning

Frogs are naturally found in murky water, which provides a visual barrier to potential predators (Schultz & Dawson 2003). However, there is a difference between murky, and dirty. Decaying food particles foul the water and frogs routinely shed skin particles and release ammonia and faeces into the surroundings. Cleaning strategies should be designed to minimise disturbance and distress to the frogs.

Xenopus laevis are routinely housed either in tanks of standing water (periodically 'dumped and refilled' every day or few days), or in tanks where a drip-through system continuously and slowly changes the water. In drip-through systems the water coming in may be new, or to reduce overall water use, may be treated and cleaned re-circulating water. Static systems require frequent cleaning of tanks but have the benefit of enabling disease outbreaks to be more easily controlled. This can be harder in re-circulating systems (Sanders 2004). Recommendations for cleaning practices will be influenced not only by the tank or system design in place but also by the feeding regime and quality of water entering the system. There is no current universally applicable regime, but there are many suggestions for suitable general practice. Disinfectants should be used with extreme caution.

Standing water tanks

Water in standing tanks is often changed at least three times a week. However, it has been discovered that frogs disturbed daily for water changes have a slower growth rate and this might negate any improvement gained by better water quality (Hilken et al. 1995). Indeed, frogs were observed to grow better in a tank where water was replaced only once a week.

If complete water changes are undertaken, then this should be done at around the same time of day, preferably post feeding since this is when the water quality is at its worst (DeNardo 1995).

Drip-through water systems

The advantage of drip-through systems is that levels of toxic waste are kept low and solid waste (in suspension) can be drained continuously (Sive et al. 2000). However, they use a lot of water (if not re-circulating) and the quality of the input water must be monitored constantly. In addition, these animals would naturally favour still, stagnant areas of water or, at most, slight and slow-moving waters, so a strong water inflow may cause them stress. Frogs sense water movement through a highly developed lateral line system, the position of in- and out-flowing taps in the tanks and the rate of water flow should be set so water turbulence or motion is minimised.

Tanks

Tanks should have smooth sides, be impervious, easy to clean and be without sharp edges. Tanks for *Xenopus laevis* have traditionally been constructed from fibreglass, stainless steel, glass or polycarbonate. Containers must prevent escape and should allow space for sufficient volume and depth of water and for enrichment such as refuges to be added (Figure 13.2).

Tanks with darkened or opaque sides better approximate pond conditions (Sive et al. 2000) and are also likely to be less stressful for the frogs. Both young and adult frogs may have a preference for dark background colouring (Goldin 1992) and a black background colouring may be better for the frogs' wellbeing than a grey or white one (Hilken et al. 1995). A dark floor may enhance these animals' sense of security (Council of Europe 2004) thereby improving their wellbeing.

Figure 13.2   Multi-tiered *Xenopus* tanks.

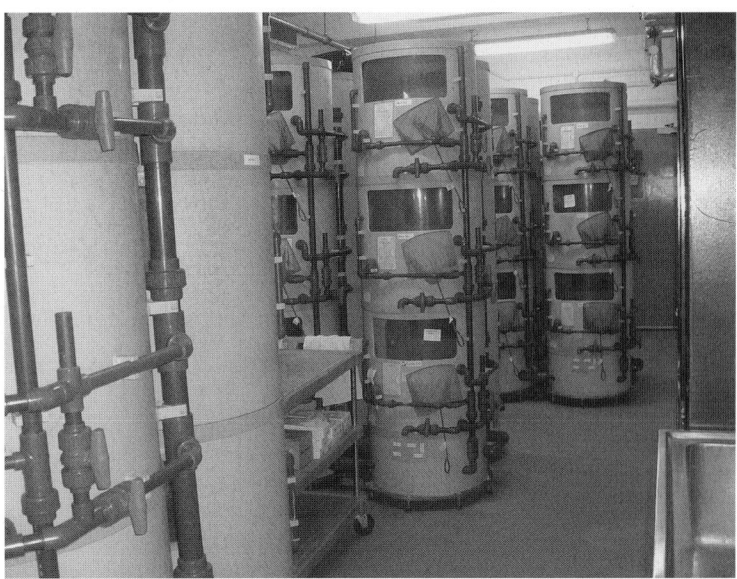

Long, narrow tank designs should be avoided as they restrict locomotor activity and social behaviour such as feeding frenzies (Council of Europe 2004).

Environmental enrichment

It has been shown that these frogs prefer an enriched environment to a barren tank, and that enrichment can be provided without any detrimental effect on egg production or quality (Brown & Nixon 2004).

Frogs are a prey species, therefore it is highly important to provide them with a form of shelter to hide in or under. Enrichment structures should have smooth surfaces and rounded edges to reduce the risk of injury to the animals. Plastic pipes used commercially to safely deliver water to point of use for human drinking can be easily obtained and adapted, and appear to be frequently used by the animals (Brown & Nixon 2004).

Providing cover from above and additional hiding places can also be achieved by placing floating objects in the water (Brown & Nixon 2004). These vary from commercially available plastic 'lily pads' to black bin liners cut into various floating shapes. Surface objects however, must still allow frogs to easily access the surface of the water to breathe (Figure 13.3).

A substrate of small stones should not be used as these can be accidentally ingested and may also be impractical for regular cleaning. Furthermore, it is clear from 'choice tests' that frogs do *not* prefer gravel flooring (Brown & Nixon 2004).

Identification and marking techniques

Marking can have an effect on an animal and its wellbeing through the physical act of marking itself, through the wearing of the mark and/or through the procedures required for observing the mark (Mellor et al. 2004).

Careful consideration should therefore be given to whether identification of individual animals is necessary, and if so, to the method of identification used, particularly where the methods are invasive and likely to cause a degree of trauma.

Non-invasive methods of identification such as group cards or photographs of the dorsal markings of the frogs are the methods of choice.

Handling

Amphibians may be easily disturbed and do not like to be handled, so capture and handling should be minimised, only being undertaken where absolutely necessary and with every precaution taken to avoid stressing or injuring the animals.

The skin of amphibians is more delicate and

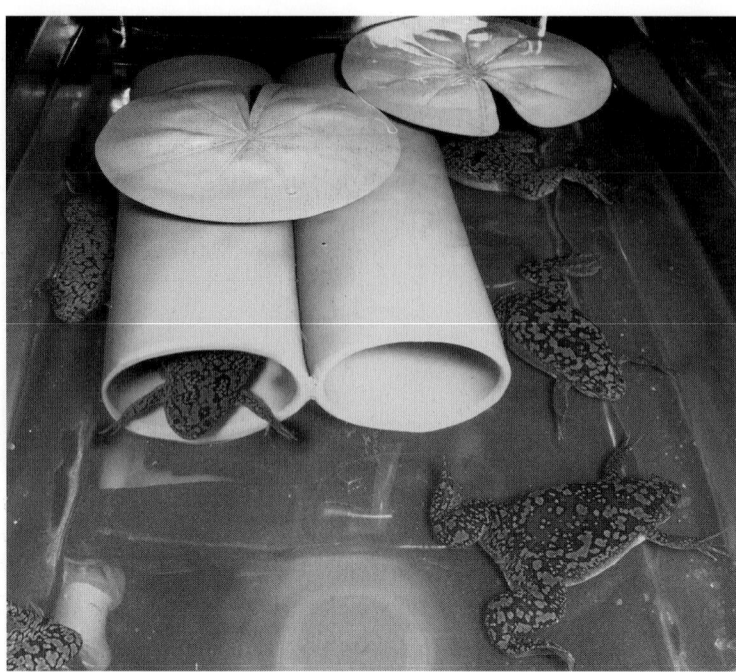

Figure 13.3 Tank enriched with pipes and plastic leaves.

sensitive than that of any other vertebrate (Halliday 1999). Traces of hand lotion, colognes or medicated ointments may harm and even have the potential to kill them. It is also believed that the thin epidermis of the frog's skin could be abraded by the ridges and callosities of the restrainer's hand (Wright & Whitaker 2001). Personnel should consider taking a precautionary approach, wear gloves (non-powdered) and remove frogs from the water with soft-mesh non-abrasive nets.

Unnecessary movements of objects or hands over the tank should be avoided.

Food type and feeding regime

Xenopus laevis frogs are carnivorous by nature and although they will scavenge the carcasses of dead animals, they prefer live food (Green 2002). They are aroused by the odour of food nearby and swim around in search of it until they touch it, often only making a decision about its palatability after the object reaches their mouth (Elepfandt 1996). Examination of the stomach contents of wild *Xenopus laevis* have found the remains of fish, birds, and other amphibians, but it is small insects, slugs, worms and other aquatic invertebrates which predominate (Green 2002).

A number of commercially prepared diets for captive frogs are available. For example, NASCO produce Frog Brittle®, which contains fish meal, meat meal, soybean meal, corn meal, wheat flour, dried yeast, distiller's solubles, whey, wheat germ meal, salt, vitamin supplements and calcium phosphate.

Beef liver is another item commonly provided but when given on its own has been implicated as a cause of vitamin A toxicity, metabolic bone disease and other amphibian diseases (Wright & Whitaker 2001). Meat (such as liver or heart) should therefore be mixed with vitamins (Mrozek et al. 1995).

Maggots and crickets are also provided by some establishments and appear to provide welcome stimulation and enrichment for the frogs.

Frogs are generally fed to satiation (as much as can be consumed in one hour) about three times a week.

Uneaten particles of food may foul the water and so many establishments remove such debris after feeding has taken place. Care should be taken to leave a sufficient time interval (of three to five hours) between feeding and cleaning as frogs may regurgitate food if startled, disturbed, or handled shortly afterwards.

Assessment of health and disease prevention

It is easier to prevent than treat disease in *Xenopus* (DeNardo 1995). They may carry a range of pathogens without the development of disease, unless there is physiological upset caused by additional environmental stressors (Tinsley & Kobel 1996). This can occur as a result of stress through overcrowding, improper handling, over-use or poor water quality.

Diagnosis of disease and assessment of wellbeing can be difficult as *Xenopus* have little ability to express their state of welfare. *Xenopus laevis* is a potential 'prey' species and therefore may well have evolved adaptively to hide overt signs of distress or injury. This means that disease may become established, and pathogenesis may develop to an extreme degree before the frog shows obvious ill effects (Tinsley & Kobel 1996).

Healthy frogs should be placid, with moderately slimy skin and a nice pear shape (Sive et al. 2000). Indicators of poor health include:

- dull skin with subcutaneous haemorrhaging (particularly petechial or 'pinpoint' haemorrhages on the ventral surfaces of the legs);
- failure to feed properly or weight loss;
- erosion or tremors at the animal's extremities (e.g. legs and feet);
- open cuts, lesions or abrasions of the skin or ulcerations;
- excessive coelomic cavity distension/swelling ('bloating');
- changes in activity level, e.g. lethargy;
- postural changes;
- skin discoloration or flaking;
- diminished avoidance response and righting reflexes.

Jumpy frogs, frogs with dry or excessively slimy skin, bloated frogs, and frogs which look grey and thin or reddish are not healthy and should not be used in experimental procedures as this would lead to further deterioration of the animals' condition. Additionally, eggs collected at this time, would be generally unsuitable for experimental purposes (Sive et al. 2000).

The behaviour of the frog can also indicate where an animal is finding a procedure noxious or painful. Behavioural responses of *Xenopus laevis* frogs to aversive stimuli may include startle reactions (sudden movements); activity to physically avoid the stimuli (including 'escape' behaviours); wiping or rubbing of the irritated area (Green 2003).

The potential of laboratory equipment and human activity to disturb or cause stress to these animals must also be considered, as they are sensitive to surrounding vibrations. Steps should be taken to limit the disturbance caused by air-conditioning systems, industrial vacuum cleaners or radios, for example.

Breeding

Field studies in South Africa suggest that breeding is seasonal, notably early spring to late summer (Tinsley, pers. comm.). Seasonal effects impact on breeding frequency and success and in addition, for over five months of the year, no breeding usually takes place in wild individuals.

When a female is receptive, she shows little preference for individuals and instead will be attracted towards any advertising male (Tobias et al. 1998). Cloacal flaps are only visible in the females, while the males develop darkened nuptial pads on inner forearms and fingers to hold on to the females during mating. Amplexus occurs where the male and female frogs clasp together and perform a series of somersaults in the water. Amplexus can last for twelve hours or longer, with the male releasing sperm as the female lays her eggs (usually between 500 and 1000 (Deuchar 1975)). The eggs are scattered over the area and, as there is no further parental investment, they are left unprotected. Environmental conditions experienced by the adult female prior to egg laying, and subsequently by the fertilised eggs, will largely dictate the ratio developing successfully into tadpoles. Oogenesis (the formation, development and maturation of eggs) is a continuous process under favourable environmental conditions and, given suitable temperatures, ovary production is determined primarily by food supply (Tinsley & Kobel 1996). In the wild, females will produce multiple clutches in a season (Measey 2004).

Hatching occurs two to three days after eggs have been fertilised when the transparent, filter-feeding tadpoles measure around 4 mm in length. The tadpoles, which have two long tentacles on their heads and are quite large, hang in the water, head down at a

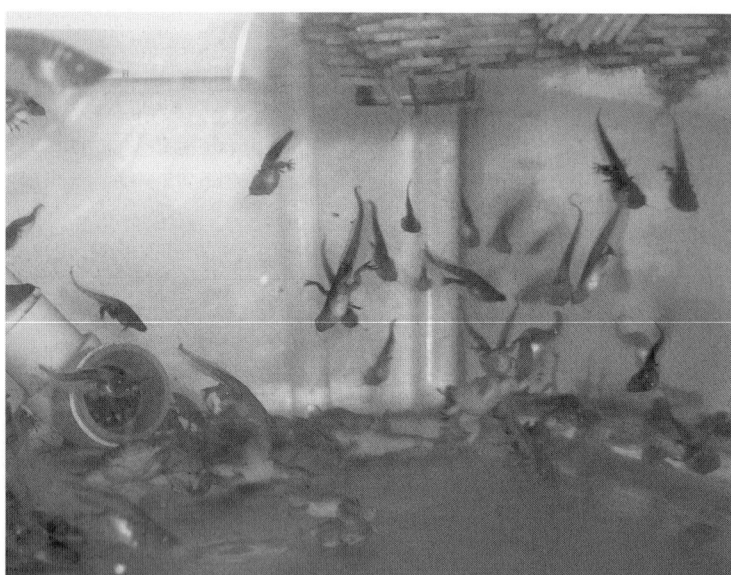

Figure 13.4   Developing frogs.

45° angle, using their tails to produce a current to bring microscopic food to them (Wolfensohn & Lloyd 2003). Tadpoles are herbivorous (eating very small plant particles in the wild, or liquefied fish food or commercial tadpole food in the laboratory) and adopt a carnivorous diet after metamorphosis into a froglet, which may take between two and four months (Figure 13.4). Male frogs typically reach sexual maturity in around ten to twelve months, while females can, depending on environmental conditions, take up to two years. Optimal laboratory rearing conditions can shorten this time to one year for females (Gurdon 1996) or even eight months (Tinsley & Kobel 1996) (although initial batches of eggs from young females under eighteen to twenty-four months may not be suitable for use in scientific manipulation). Females are typically used for egg production from two years of age. As long as the animal remains healthy and egg quality is high, frogs can continue to be used for breeding.

Induction of ovulation and mating behaviour

Leaving reproduction to occur naturally in the laboratory affects both when, and how many, eggs are produced. However, the hormone human chorionic gonadotrophin (hCG) has been used to overcome this, enabling laboratories to have access to a near constant supply of eggs all year. Female *Xenopus laevis* frogs can be induced to ovulate by injecting them with hCG (usually at a level of 500 IU). Ovulation generally occurs within thirty-six hours following injection (NASCO 2003). Males too can be stimulated to perform mating behaviour by injecting 50 units of hCG into the dorsal sac a few days before being placed with a female. Readiness for mating in males is indicated by the production of advertisement calls (in the form of a rapid series of 'clicks') and the appearance of a dark pigment on the front legs.

There is less potential for frogs to suffer when eggs are obtained as a result of natural ovulation, egg laying and mating, the requirement for 'inducing' these behaviours must be justified on scientific grounds. Where undertaken, a minimum interval of eight to ten weeks is recommended between episodes of induced egg laying.

Euthanasia

Immersion in an overdose of buffered MS 222 solution (followed by pithing to ensure death) appears to be one of the least stressful methods to the animals involved (Wright & Whitaker 2001). There must be exceptional justification given for using any other method. A concentration of 0.2% solution should be used for at least three hours (Halliday 1999;

LASA 2001). The agent is absorbed into the animal through the skin. To prevent the frog suffering pain or irritation from this agent (which is low in pH), MS 222 should be buffered to near pH 7 with sodium bicarbonate.

References

Alexander, S.S. and Bellerby, C.W. (1938) Experimental studies on the sexual cycle of the South African clawed toad (*Xenopus laevis*). I. *Journal of Experimental Biology* **15**: 74–81.

Brown, M. and Nixon, R.M. (2004) Enrichment for the captive environment – The *Xenopus laevis*.' *Animal Technology and Welfare* **3** (2): 87–95.

Canadian Council for Animal Care – CCAC (2004) *Species-specific Recommendations – Amphibians and Reptiles*.

Council of Europe (2003) *Revision of Appendix A of the Convention ETS123 – Species-specific provisions for amphibians: Background information for the proposals presented by the group of experts on amphibians and reptiles (Part B)*, (Draft – 7th Meeting of the Working Party). Council of Europe, Strasbourg.

Council of Europe (2004) *Draft Appendix A of the European Convention for the Protection of Vertebrate Animals used for experimental and other Scientific Purposes (ETS No.123)* (8th Meeting of the Working Party). Council of Europe, Strasbourg.

Dawson, D.A., Schultz, T.W. and Shroeder, E.C. (1992) Laboratory care and breeding of the African Clawed Frog. *Lab Animal* **21** (4): 31–36.

DeNardo, D. (1995) Amphibians as laboratory animals. *ILAR Journal* **37** (4).

Elepfandt, A. (1996) Sensory perception and the lateral line system in the clawed frog pp. 97–120. In: R.C. Tinsley and H.R. Kobel (Eds) *The Biology of Xenopus.* Oxford University Press, Oxford.

Goldin, A.L. (1992) Maintenance of *Xenopus laevis* and oocyte injection. *Methods in Enzymology* **207**: 266–279.

Green, S.L. (2002) Factors affecting oogenesis in the South African Clawed Frog (*Xenopus laevis*). *Comparative Medicine* **52** (4): 307–312.

Green, S.L. (2003) Are post-operative analgesics needed for South African Clawed Frogs *(Xenopus laevis)* after surgical harvest of oocytes? *Comparative Medicine* **53** (3): 12–15.

Gurdon, J.B., Laskey, R.A. and Reeves, O.R. (1975) The developmental capacity of nuclei transplanted from keratinized skin cells of adult frogs. *Journal of Embryology and Experimental Morphology* **34**: 93–112.

Gurdon, J.B. (1996) Introductory comments – *Xenopus* as a laboratory animal (pp. 3–6). In: R.C. Tinsley and H.R. Kobel (Eds) *The Biology of Xenopus.* Oxford University Press, Oxford.

Halliday, T. (1999) Amphibians (pp. 90–102). In: T. Poole and P. English (Eds) *The UFAW Handbook on the Care and Management of Laboratory Animals* (Vol. 2: *Amphibious and Aquatic Vertebrates and Advanced Invertebrates*). Blackwell Science, Oxford.

Hayes, M.P., Jennings, M.R. and Mellen, J.D. (1998) Enrichment for amphibians and reptiles (pp. 205–235). In: D.J. Shepherdson, J.D. Mellen and M. Hutchins (Eds) *Second Nature – Environmental Enrichment for Captive Animals.* Smithsonian Books, Washington DC.

Hilken, G., Dimigen, J. and Iglauer, F. (1995) Growth of *Xenopus laevis* under different laboratory rearing conditions. *Laboratory Animals* **29**: 152–162.

Laboratory Animal Science Association (LASA) (2001) *Good Practice Guidelines – Xenopus Husbandry.* (John Cadera) LASA, Staffordshire.

Mattison, C. (1998) *Frogs and Toads of the World.* Blandford Press, London.

Measey, J. (2004) *Xenopus laevis.* Global Invasive Species Database http://www.issg.org/database/welcome/ *(accessed 02/07/2004)*.

Mellor, D.J., Beausoleil, N.J. and Stafford, K.J. (2004) *Marking amphibians, reptiles and marine mammals: Animal welfare, practicalities and public perceptions in New Zealand.* Department of Conservation, Massey University, New Zealand.

Mrozek, M., Fischer, R., Trendelenburg, M. and Zillmann, U. (1995) Microchip implant system used for animal identification in laboratory rabbits, guinea pigs, woodchucks and in amphibians. *Laboratory Animals* **29**: 339–344.

NASCO (2003) NASCO on-line catalogues: http://www.enasco.com/prod/Static?page=xenopus *(accessed 20/07/2004)*

Sanders, G. (2004) (Oral presentation) Water quality for *Xenopus*: Assessment and significance. At Best Practice in *Xenopus* Care meeting: 11 February 2004, University of Sheffield, UK. (Joint meeting by the UK Medical Research Council's Centre for Best Practice for Animals in Research (CBPAR) and the Laboratory Animal Science Association (LASA)).

Schultz, T.W. and Dawson, D.A. (2003) Housing and husbandry of *Xenopus* for oocyte production. *Lab. Animal* **32** (2): 34–39.

Sive, H.L., Grainger, R.M. and Harland, R.M. (2000) *Early Development of Xenopus laevis – A Laboratory Manual.* Cold Spring Harbor Laboratory Press, New York.

Tinsley, R.C. and Kobel, H.R. (1996) *The Biology of Xenopus.* Oxford University Press, Oxford.

Tinsley, R. (2005, pers. comm.) Correspondence between B. Reed and R. Tinsley, Feb 2005.

Tobias, M.L., Viswanathan, S. and Kelley, D.B. (1998) Rapping, a female receptive call, initiates male–female duets in the South African clawed frog. *Proceedings of the National Academy of Sciences*, USA, **95**: 1870–1875.

University of Arizona (2001) Institutional Animal Care and Use Committees (IACUC) guidelines on 'Care and handling of *Xenopus laevis*' http://www.ahsc.arizona.edu/uac/iacuc/xenopus/xenopus.shtml *(accessed 04/06/2003)*

Wolfensohn, S. and Lloyd, M. (2003) *Handbook of Laboratory Animal Management and Welfare* (3rd edn). Blackwell Science, Oxford.

Woodland, H.R. (2003) *Xenopus* Early Development Group. http://www.bio.warwick.ac.uk/res/frame.asp?ID=51 *(accessed 20/07/2004)*

Wright, K. and Whitaker, B.R. (2001) *Amphibian Medicine and Captive Husbandry.* Krieger Publishing Company, Florida, USA.

Further reading

Reed, B.T. (2005) *Guidance on the Housing and Care of the African Clawed Frog, Xenopus laevis.* RSPCA, Horsham (UK).

Note: The Royal Society for the Prevention of Cruelty to Animals is opposed to all experiments or procedures which cause pain, suffering, or distress, and works to promote initiatives which lead to greater application of the 3Rs.

14

Genetically Altered Animals

Roger J. Francis

Introduction

Genetically altered (GA) animals are animals whose genetic make up has been changed by the use of genetic engineering techniques. The change can be an addition (knock-in) or deletion (knock-out) of genes. If added genes originate in a different species the resulting offspring are called transgenics. The term genetically altered animal has replaced the former term genetically modified animal, although genetically modified is still used in some places.

The use of genetically altered animals in scientific procedures has increased greatly since they were first recorded in 1995. Home Office statistics for 2003 (Home Office 2004) show that the numbers used in scientific procedures have more than trebled since that time, now accounting for more than a quarter of all scientific procedures carried out in that year. There are now GA strains of many species of animals including sheep, pigs, rabbits, rodents, poultry, fish, and amphibians, however mice make up 97% of all GA animals used in scientific procedures.

The first genetically altered animals were produced in the early 1970s. Brinster (1974) produced chimeras (organisms composed of cells from two different individuals) by taking cells from one strain of mice and implanting them into an embryo of another strain of mice at the blastocyst stage of development.

The next stage in the development of genetically altered animals involved the use of retroviruses (a family of viruses whose DNA become incorporated into the DNA of the host and can therefore be passed from generation to generation). Stuhlmann et al. (1984) incorporated a specific DNA sequence into a retroviral genome and then used those viruses to pass it on to the cells of an embryo.

At around the same time Gordon et al. (1980) were carrying out the first successful production of GA mice using the pro-nuclear injection technique and this was followed by the development of the stem cell techniques (Gossler et al. 1986).

GA technology is considered of great importance to biomedical science because it enables specific disease mechanisms to be studied in small animals, for instance genes which are known to predispose humans to Alzheimers disease can be introduced into mice and studied in detail.

In addition the specific function of genes can be studied by knocking out genes and by observing the result their actions can be determined.

Legal considerations

A project licence and a personal licence under the Animals (Scientific Procedures) Act 1986 (ASPA) is required to carry out vasectomies, preparation of superovulated females and implanting genetically altered embryos into recipient females. The breeding of GA animals also requires authorisation under ASPA but the pairing of GA animals may be carried out by non-licensed personnel if delegation has been authorised to an appropriate personal licence.

In addition, this work is covered by the Genetically Modified Organisms Regulations. These regulations are controlled by the Health and Safety Executive (HSE). In outline they require:

- a local genetic modification safety committee to be established at the institute where the work is being done;
- a risk assessment to be completed before the work commences;

- the HSE to be notified at least 90 days before it is intended to begin work;
- level of containment commensurate with the type of organism being worked with (in practice transgenic animals will be kept in full barrier units, filter top cages, etc. which will be acceptable);
- records of the work to be kept;
- a report of the work done to be sent to the HSE at the end of the calendar year.

Production of genetically altered animals

Two main methods are used to produce GA animals – pronuclear injection and embryonic stem cell injection.

Pronuclear injection

Pronuclear injection involves the injection of the desired gene sequence (a strand of DNA) into one of the pronuclei in the ova just before they fuse to complete fertilisation (Figure 14.1). The DNA becomes incorporated into the genome of the embryo at fertilisation and will appear in all of the cells of the animal and will also be passed on to its offspring.

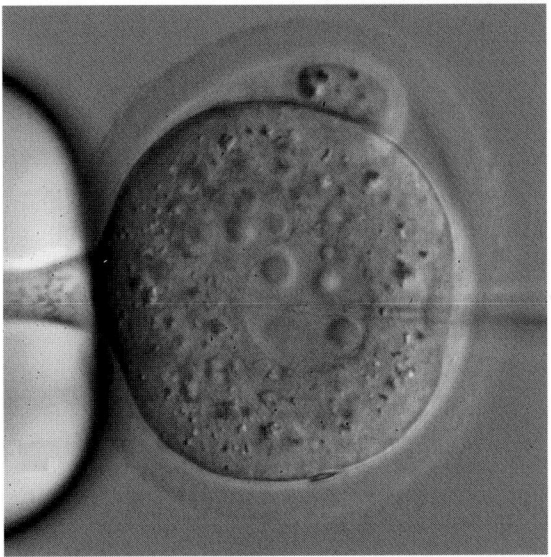

Figure 14.1   Pronuclear injection. Note the fine pipette entering the pronucleus on the right.

Embryonic stem cell injection

Embryonic stem cell injection involves injecting the DNA sequence a little later, after the embryo has developed to reach the blastocyst stage (a hollow ball of cells containing a mass of cells at one end). The cells that make up the ball are called embryonic stem cells because they can give rise to any cell type in the body. These cells are removed from the blastocyst, the DNA sequence is injected into them and they are injected into another blastocyst which is then implanted into another animal. The resulting embryo will be a chimera because there will be two types of cell in their bodies, some from the original mating and some from the engineered stem cells.

Overview

The technique of producing GA animals is similar whether the pronuclear or embryonic stem cell technique is used.

The animals required are:

- vasectomised males;
- stud males;
- superovulated females as donor females;
- recipient females (sometimes referred to as mules).

The procedure starts with the synthesis of the DNA strand in a laboratory. The donor females (females donating the eggs or blastocysts), are treated with hormones to stimulate multiple ovulation. They are mated with stud males and after a suitable time the female is killed by cervical dislocation and the eggs or blastocysts are harvested from the reproductive tract. The DNA is injected using fine glass injection needles under a microscope (Figure 14.2).

Meanwhile a recipient female (mule) is prepared. She will take the engineered embryo to birth. In order to do so she must be in the same hormonal state as a normal female at a similar stage of pregnancy. This is achieved by mating her with a vasectomised male; the mating will induce pseudopregnancy in the female so she will be able to accept the engineered embryo.

The mechanism by which recombinant DNA integrates into the host chromosome is unknown although some information may be inferred from the study by Palmiter (1982) which looks at the organisation of inserts found in GA mice. Because the locus of transgene integration is a random process the effect

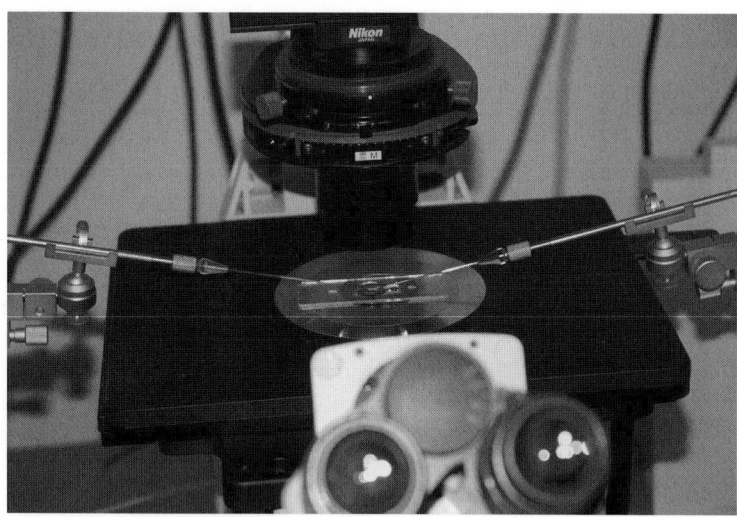

Figure 14.2 The stage of an injection microscope. The pipette holding the cell is on the left and the injection pipette is on the right.

of the insert is unknown. Once expression of a transgene has been successful, this may lead to gain of function (over-expression of the gene, protein or cell), sometimes referred to as 'knock-in', or loss of function or 'knock-out'. Creation of knock-ins and knock-outs allows the study of the function of almost any protein, gene or cell line.

Preparation of animals

Vasectomised males

Vasectomy is carried out under general anaesthesia, it is a relatively simple procedure when performed by skilled personnel, but in an animal the size of the mouse it needs very precise work as the vas deferens is very small. The procedure may be carried out via incision in the scrotal sac (Waynforth 1980) or via a lower abdomen incision. The vas deferens is exposed, ligated and either cut through or cauterised. The muscle wall is then sutured and the skin is clipped (the skin is clipped rather than sutured to prevent the mouse removing the sutures).

Superovulated females

This technique makes use of females between three and twenty-four weeks of age. These animals are injected on day 1 with FSH (50 IU/ml follicle stimulating hormone (Sigma 4877) in sterile water or normal saline) and then 48 hours later with HCG (50 IU/ml human chorionic gonadotrophin (hCG Sigma CG-2) in sterile water or normal saline). These primed females are then placed with stud males to mate overnight, the intention being to produce as many fertilised ova as possible. In addition to the effect on the female of the two injections of hormones, one must also consider the effect on the female of being mated by a male that may be considerably larger than herself, a three week old female mouse weighs 8–9 g and she could be paired to a 30 g plus male. In the case of the rat this situation is far worse when you consider a 40–45 g weaner being paired to a 500 g plus male. Unless absolutely essential older females should be used. The mated superovulated female is killed by cervical dislocation either the following morning for pro-nuclear injection or after two to three days if blastocysts are to be used.

Stud males

The stud male should be of proven ability with a good record of fertilisation. He should be singly housed, preferably in a room without females and, ideally, he should not have been used for breeding for 72 hours to ensure peak breeding efficiency. If he has not been used for longer than several weeks he should be primed by being allowed access to another female.

Recipient females

These animals are prepared by mating with the vasectomised males to cause pseudopregnancy, they will then be implanted with the manipulated embryos harvested from the superovulated females. Implantation, like vasectomy, is a relatively simple procedure in skilled hands. The recipient female is anaesthetised, a single dorsal incision is made, the opening is drawn across to the flank, the ovary and uterine tube can be visualised through the muscle wall, a small incision is made over the uterine tube and the manipulated ova are inserted into the uterine tube, the muscle wall is then sutured, this procedure is repeated on the opposite uterine tube, the wound in the skin is then clipped.

Incubation of eggs

After the fertilised eggs/stem cells have been harvested from the donor female the most important feature of the GA animal must be undertaken – the genetic engineering. The ability to target specific genes has developed considerably since the first genetically altered animal was created, but there is still a high risk of both mechanical damage to the blastocyst and uncertainty regarding the site of insertion of the foreign DNA. Subsequent incubation of the manipulated blastocyst gives the opportunity to operate a degree of selection, discarding any which show signs of damage. Badly damaged embryos will undergo cytoplasmic condensation, causing a change in colour. Care also has to be taken not to incubate embryos for too long a period because this too can have deleterious effects.

Care should be taken with the timing of gestation periods of recipient females to ensure that they give birth at the appropriate time and to ensure that they do not have problems around the time of expected parturition. Consideration must be given to selecting the correct strain to act as recipients, animals with good mothering ability and preferably a phenotype which would show any incorrect generation of offspring, i.e. any pups born as a result of natural mating. Recipient females should be handled carefully as often as possible to habituate them, thus reducing the likelihood of the female killing any of the pups when they are checked at birth.

Monitoring genetically altered animals

Newly born GA animals should be checked as soon as possible to ensure they have no harmful defects, detailed records of any defect and numbers born

should be kept. Many scientists will want to sample the pups' DNA as early as possible, this is frequently by tail tipping. Tail tipping is a very misleading term, Osman (1997) talks of the removal of 0.6 cm of tail from a two-week-old animal. This represents approximately a quarter of its tail. In fact the amount of tissue required for DNA analysis is very small, it can be achieved by harvesting the small piece of ear removed when earmarking, however in practice this is very difficult to find and collect. Other methods are being developed such as analysis by blood, saliva or hair samples. Tail tipping using a local anaesthetic prior to removal of the tip only approximately 5 mm from a three- to four-week-old animal, appears to cause only minimal disturbance to the animal.

One area for concern is the matching of DNA samples to the individual animal. Many people have opted to identify each animal with an electronic transponder at the same time as the sample for DNA is collected. The transponder is a very simple system to use; an electronic transponder is inserted subcutaneously. The transponder emits a precoded number when the animal is scanned with an appropriate reader. Whatever system is used for matching the animal to its sample, it needs to be simple to use, simple to read, permanent and well tolerated by the animal. Electronic transponders appear to satisfy all of these criteria they also have the added advantage that the data can be preserved electronically and can be downloaded onto computers reducing the risk of operator error. It is essential that DNA samples taken for analysis by such methods as Southern Blotting or PCR (see Chapter 17) can be accurately related to the animal from which they originated.

Breeding genetically altered animals

The production of large numbers of genetically altered animals requires very accurate record keeping.

Once DNA analysis has been carried out, future breeding stock can be selected and it is here that a basic understanding of Mendelian inheritance is required to enable the creation of the new lines of GA animals. To create lines of new constructs each animal shown by DNA analysis to express copies of the new construct will be paired to an appropriate inbred animal (called 'wild type'). GA males have the advantage

Table 14.1   Backcrossing onto a selected inbred strain.

Pairing	Genotype
Pair 1	+/− × +/+
Pair 2	+/− × +/−
Pair 3	+/− × −/−
Pair 4	−/− × −/−

that they can be mated to numerous females and create lines faster than their female sibling.

In the initial mating the new line will be in the hemizygous (same as heterozygous but with integrated exogenous DNA) state, it will normally be mated to a wild type (pair 1), this will result in two genotypes of offspring, hemizygous (+/−) GA and homozygous (+/+) for wild type offspring. These offspring will be DNA sampled and hemizygous animals will be retained for further breeding. Selected hemizygous animals may be paired to each other or paired back to their hemizygous parent (pair 2). This pairing will result in three genotypes of offspring, homozygous (−/−) GA, hemizygous (+/−) GA and wild type (+/+). The generation of homozygous (−/−) animals allows the pairing of homozygous to hemizygous animals (pair 3), or the pairing of two homozygous GA animals (pair 4). Each new line should be gradually backcrossed (Festing 1979) onto a selected inbred strain (see Table 14.1).

In the hemizygous animal the effect of the alteration may be regulated by endogenous genetic material of the allelomorph at the site of insertion (in general the hemizygous animal rarely shows any effect, the single normal allele allows the body to function, when both alleles at a given locus are affected. For example if deleted (knocked out), the animal or a major organ etc. may have an inability to function normally. In the knock-in there may be an excess of function which again may lead to a welfare problem). Only when an animal is homozygous −/−, with GA structures on both alleles, will the effect of the genetic alteration be seen. There may be over expression, or negative expression etc. and these may have insignificant or extreme effect upon the animal and may or may not have serious implications for the animal's wellbeing.

Depending on the result of the genetic alteration a decision will have to be made as to how the new line

will be produced in the future. It may be that in the homozygous −/− GA state that the animal cannot reproduce successfully, if this is the case then the line may have to be maintained by heterozygous +/− pairings. Some lines may be able to reproduce in the homozygous state but may be unable to rear their offspring, for instance some lines of females cannot lactate, such lines would require fostering to rear their young.

From time to time lines may no longer be required and the question arises of how long to maintain them, how many pairs are needed to successfully keep the line ticking over and how long will it be before they are required again. It is at this time that the scientist should consider whether or not to preserve the lines no longer in use. Various systems have evolved for the preservation of embryos the most common being that of cryo-preservation – the freezing of embryos at very early stages of development. These embryos can be thawed and then relocated by embryo transfer into a recipient female to resurrect the line of animals.

Cryo-preservation offers several advantages: it prevents waste of animals and resources, loss of valuable GA lines and it is a valuable insurance against genetic contamination and disease. N.B. the current legislation in the UK (ASPA) does not cover the cryo-preservation of embryos frozen before the half-way stage of development, it does however cover the regeneration of the GA lines, this regeneration must be covered by a project licence.

Health considerations

GA animals are far from being of the highest health status (Costa 1997). The movement of GA animals between designated premises within the UK and import and export world wide represents a considerable challenge. Many of the animals in circulation are carriers of diseases such as mouse hepatitis virus and *Syphacia obvelata* to name but two. This leads to recipients of these 'dirty' animals having to decide to maintain an infected colony or to re-derive and clean them up. Restriction of access of a scientist to his animals often leads to conflict, with many scientists being unwilling to be subject to the higher level of containment involved with the higher health status animals.

General care

The general routine care and husbandry is no different from the care of normal stocks of animals. However if specific welfare problems are identified they may require modification of normal husbandry e.g.:

- animals shown to be diabetic may need more frequent cleaning than normal animals due to the volume of urine they produce;
- animals which are ataxic may require special food hoppers to give them access to the food;
- nude animals may need to be kept at slightly higher room temperatures than normal;
- immune-compromised animals will need housing systems which offer special protection, such as individually ventilated cages, filter cabinets or isolators.

Welfare

There has been a considerable amount of concern expressed about the welfare of GA animals. Many new lines appear to have no problems, but a survey of papers published in *Nature* shows that many lines reveal major welfare problems. At what stage are these welfare problems occurring? The first indication of welfare problems may be when there is disruption to the expected genotype ratio. This could indicate embryonic lethality. If sufficient offspring are produced using the pairings in Table 14.1 (see p. 98), the expected ratios of offspring produced should be similar to the expected percentage indicated in Table 14.2.

Table 14.2 Expected ratios of offspring expressed as a percentage using the pairings indicated in Table 14.1 (see p. 98).

Pairing	Genotype	Expected genotype of offspring (%)
Pair 1	+/− × +/+	50% +/+
		50% −/−
Pair 2	+/− × +/−	25% +/+
		50% +/−
		25% −/−
Pair 3	+/− × −/−	50% +/−
		50% −/−
Pair 4	−/− × −/−	100% −/−

Deformity or malfunction could lead to an animal's inability to survive in a litter containing normal siblings and this could lead to a high pre-weaning mortality. If offspring with deformity or malfunction survive beyond weaning their entire life may be compromised. Animals surviving may be infertile or have low fertility, there may be premature ageing or late-life problems.

One of the areas which can be difficult to assess is an inability to adapt to environmental changes, i.e. animals may have an inability to thermoregulate. This would only become apparent if there was a problem with the environmental conditions in which the animal was housed. Any adverse effect seen should be recorded. If the effect is not one that was expected, then it is necessary to report it to the Home Office and to take steps to minimise the effect on the animal.

GA animals should be offered the same sorts of environmental enrichment as their normal siblings but care must be taken to ensure that compromised animals are not further impeded by the materials used to enrich their environment.

References and further reading

Brinster, R. (1974) The effect of cells transferred into the mouse blastocyst on subsequent development. *J. Exp. Med.*, **140**: 1049–1056.

Costa, P. (1997) Welfare aspects of transgenic animals. *Proceedings EC Workshop*, October 1995: 68–77.

Festing, M.F.W. (1979) *Inbred Strains in Biomedical Research* (1st edn). Macmillan, London.

Gordon, J.W. et al. (1980) Genetic transformation of mouse embryos by microinjection of purified DNA. *Proc. Natl. Acad. Sci. USA*, **77**: 7380–7384.

Gossler, A. et al. (1986) Transgenesis by means of blastocyst-derived embryonic stem cell lines. *Proc. Nat. Acad. Sci. USA*, **83**: 9065–9069.

Home Office (2004) *Statistics of Scientific Procedures on Living Animals Great Britain 2003*. Cm 6291 2004.

Osman, G.E. et al. (1997) SWR: An inbred strain suitable for generating transgenic mice. *American Association Laboratory Animal Science* (2): 167–171.

Palmiter, R.D., Brinster, R.L., Hammer, R.E. et al. (1982) *Nature*, **300** (611).

Richa, J. and Lo, C.W. (1989) Introduction of human DNA into mouse eggs by injection of dissected chromosome fragments. *Science*, **245**: 175–177.

Stuhlmann, H. et al. (1984) Introduction of a selectable gene into different animal tissue by a retrovirus recombinant vector. *Proc. Natl. Acad. Sci. USA*, **81**: 7151–7155.

Waynforth, H.B. (1980) *Experimental and Surgical Technique in the Rat*. Academic Press Inc., London.

15
Reproductive Physiology

Janice Lobb

Every new animal develops from a zygote – the result of fertilisation, which is the fusing of a male gamete (spermatozoon) with a female gamete (egg or ovum). The problems involved with breeding laboratory animals are those of ensuring that the necessary gametes come together at the right time.

The male gametes do not usually present a problem. During the time the males are used for breeding, male hormone levels are constant, so their testes maintain a continuous production of spermatozoa and the males are willing to mate at any opportunity. Not so females! Ova are bigger than spermatozoa. More biological material, effort and time goes into their production and they can only be released from the ovary at intervals. This release is called ovulation, and this is the best time for fertilisation. For reproductive success the female needs to mate close to the time of ovulation.

Neither the production of ova nor the urge to mate are under the conscious control of the female. They are under the control and coordination of hormones produced by the unconscious part of the brain and by the ovaries. The body's master clock is in the hypothalamus. It determines the onset of sexual maturity and, thereafter, the overall level of sexual activity.

The hypothalamus is influenced by external stimuli, such as day length, so that some animals, e.g. ferrets and hamsters, are seasonal breeders if they are kept in 'natural' lighting. Out of the breeding season the reproductive tracts of both sexes are shrunken and inactive, and neither sex shows any inclination to mate. This is why controlled lighting cycles are important if you need to breed animals all the year round.

In many types of female mammal, either during the breeding season or throughout the whole year, the hypothalamus orchestrates a reproductive cycle known as the oestrous cycle. Releasing factors, produced by the hypothalamus, control the secretion of gonadotrophic hormones from the anterior pituitary gland, an endocrine gland closely associated with the hypothalamus at the base of the brain. These gonadotrophic hormones, in their turn, control the activities of the ovaries.

During the first half of the ovarian cycle, stimulated by follicle-stimulating hormone (FSH), some developing eggs mature and their surrounding follicular cells multiply and secrete steroid hormones called oestrogens. The larger the follicle, the higher the level of oestrogens produced. The effects of oestrogens on the female body prepare it for ovulation and mating. The endometrium, lining the uterus, thickens. The cells of the vaginal epithelium proliferate and then become keratinised. A vaginal smear first (at pro-oestrus) shows nucleated epithelial cells and then (at oestrus) cornified cells. For timed matings, males and females should be put together at pro-oestrus.

As oestrogen levels rise, the female's general level of activity increases. When they reach a peak, at the stage known as oestrus, the female is ready to mate. This is the stage which gives the oestrous cycle its name. Different mammals display oestrus in different ways. Although the males and females of some species, such as rats and mice, can be housed together permanently, oestrus may be the only time that the males and females of other species, such as adult hamsters, can safely be put together. When the female is not in oestrus she may be very aggressive towards the male.

Most small laboratory mammals, such as rats and mice, are spontaneous ovulators. Their ovaries release eggs, at the right stage of maturation, to coincide with oestrus and the act of mating. This is not accidental but due to hormonal control. The oestrogens produced by the follicular cells act back on the hypothalamus and anterior pituitary. Owing to negative feedback, by the time the eggs are mature, the production of FSH has ceased. Instead, positive feedback causes a new hormone, luteinising hormone (LH), to build up. When the level of LH reaches an ovulatory peak, mature follicles (Graafian follicles) shed their eggs into the uterine ducts. They are fertilised by spermatozoa deposited by the male during mating.

In induced ovulators, such as rabbits, cats and ferrets, ovulation is the result of mating. The oestrogens produced by the Graafian follicles are at a high enough level to put the female into a state of continuous oestrus, so that she will mate at any time, but not quite adequate to produce an ovulatory peak of LH. An extra stimulus, provided by mating, is needed to give a boost to LH. Sensory impulses to the brain alert the hypothalamus, and the pituitary is stimulated to release the extra LH necessary to induce ovulation. An unmated female may lose condition by being in oestrus too long.

In the second part of the ovarian cycle, after ovulation, LH (and, in some species, luteotrophic hormone) converts the remains of the follicles into new endocrine glands, called corpora lutea. Progesterone (and more oestrogens) produced by the corpora lutea prepare the female's body for pregnancy. In particular, the glands in the thickened endometrium become secretory, ready for implantation of the embryos. Progesterone is vital for the survival of the embryos. If eggs have been fertilised, they undergo the first stages of embryonic development as they make their way to the uterus. They soon start to produce their own hormone (chorionic gonadotrophin) which ensures the continued growth of the corpora lutea and the secretion of progesterone. The corpora lutea remain important until placental progesterone production takes over.

If eggs are released without being fertilised, progesterone has a negative feedback effect on the hypothalamus and pituitary, which reduces LH secretion. Eventually lack of LH causes the corpus luteum to shrink and become inactive. The reduction in hormone levels causes a decrease in activity in the reproductive tract. In primates, the top layer of endometrium is shed, resulting in menstrual bleeding. Resorption occurs in other animals; white blood cells invade the endometrium and the vaginal epithelium to remove dead and unwanted cells. A vaginal smear at metoestrus shows many of these leukocytes. The reduction in steroid hormones also means that secretion of FSH can start again, and a new cycle begins.

16

Genetic Monitoring of Inbred Strains

Adrian A. Deeny

Introduction

The last twenty-five years have seen a dramatic increase in the use of specialised inbred strains in biomedical research. Today, well over 1000 different inbred strains and outbred stocks of mice are used in biomedical research. In addition, genetically altered animals (transgenic, knock-out and knock-in) have profoundly changed the way animals are used in research, so that models can be exquisitely tailored, in terms of their genetics, to specific areas of research.

The need for genetic control of inbred animals is well established. There have been several occurrences of non-authentic or genetically contaminated laboratory rats being used in research. Kahan et al. (1982) found genetic contamination in 'BALB/c' mice supplied from a commercial breeder. Lovell et al. (1984) found two 'inbred' strains, which should have been homozygous and congenic with C57BL/6 and DBA/2, which were genetically segregating at several loci. Gubbels et al. (1985) found nude mice, supposed to be on an inbred BALB/c genetic background, which were not fixed for BALB/c markers. Kurtz et al. (1989), using DNA fingerprinting, found WKY rats from different sources which were genetically different. A similar study by Nabika et al. (1991) suggested that there are substantial genetic differences in SHR rats between two major sources of this strain. A survey of genetic markers in 93 colonies found approximately 4% with apparent genetic contamination and several other cases where nominally identical inbred strains differed to a slight extent.

Genetic monitoring of genetically altered animals is also important. Authenticity of the background strain is critical to ensure that unknown or unanticipated variables are excluded from the investigation. Additionally, the genetically altered animal itself must be monitored to ensure the presence or absence of the relevant genetic modification, and to ensure that other genetically altered mice sharing the same room have not contaminated the line. Therefore, it is clear that a programme of genetic quality control is imperative.

Methods used in genetic monitoring

Coat colour

Phenotypic traits, such as coat colour, are useful in confirming the genetic authenticity of an inbred strain. In general, the housing of stocks and strains of the same coat colour within the same room should be avoided. If an accidental mating has occurred between strains of differing coat colour, this may be evident in unexpected appearance in the resultant offspring.

Of course, many strains share the same coat colour. For this reason, animals which have escaped from their cages and are freely roaming the animal room should be culled immediately. Genetic contamination can occur through animal care staff assuming the strain identity of escaped animals and replacing animals into a cage. This should be avoided.

Breeding records

In general, the reproductive performance of inbred strains is lower than for outbred stocks. This is a result of 'inbreeding depression', a general decline in reproductive fitness associated with increased homozygosity. A sudden and dramatic increase in reproductive performance (e.g. litter size) should be investigated immediately, as it may be a result of 'hybrid vigour', a phenomenon which occurs when individuals of different strains are crossed. It is well known that F1 hybrids usually breed substantially better than either of their individual parental lines. Therefore, large litters should be regarded as suspicious.

Behaviour

Observation of behavioural changes are very much the domain of the animal technician and, by their nature, are subjective. For example, many strains have a docile temperament, the hybrids tend to be more active and nervous. Thus any change in temperament should be investigated.

Skin grafting

Skin grafting monitors major, as well as minor, histocompatibility loci. These are distributed over a wide range of the mouse genome. Individuals within an inbred strain should be homozygous at all genetic loci – this can be confirmed by skin grafting. Any individual within a particular inbred strain should accept a skin graft from any other individual within that strain. However, skin grafting has the disadvantage of being slow; it may take several weeks to obtain a result. It may also be practically difficult and animals may appear to reject a graft, although this apparent rejection may be due only to a lack of healing.

Biochemical markers

Genetic monitoring is frequently carried out using groups of enzymes and proteins. These biochemical markers show allelic variations; i.e. they migrate across a gel during electrophoresis at different rates when subjected to an electric charge. As inbred strains are homozygous, any particular inbred strain should show only one type of variant for any one marker. These variations (alleles) are usually designated by a letter, e.g. a, b, c.

Usually, a group of biochemical markers is used. The group can be devised to differentiate a number of strains within the same animal room, or in the same facility. Such a group of (e.g. 7) discriminatory markers is known as a critical subset. The alleles obtained for each strain using the critical subset forms a profile, which is unique to that strain. An example is given in Table 16.1.

Table 16.1   Allelic profiles obtained using biochemical markers.

Strains	Idh–1	Pep–3	Gpd–1	Pgm–1	Gpi–1	Hbb	Car–2
BALB/c	a	a	b	a	a	d	b
C3H/He	a	b	b	b	b	d	b
C57BL/6	a	a	a	a	b	s	a
DBA/2	b	b	b	b	a	d	b
NZW	b	b	b	b	a	d	a

A disadvantage of this system is the relatively small number of markers available. Additionally, the use of these markers requires the use of a number of laborious techniques. A further major disadvantage is that, as tissue samples need to be used for some of the markers, the animal must be killed.

DNA fingerprinting

Over recent years, the use of molecular biological techniques has increased. One such technique is DNA fingerprinting. This involves detection of polymorphisms at multiple loci.

DNA is obtained from tissue (e.g. tail or liver) and is cleaved at particular restriction sites using a restriction enzyme. This results in many fragments of DNA of differing lengths. These fragments are separated on an agarose gel by electrophoresis, blotted (by Southern blotting) on to a nylon membrane. The pattern of bands obtained is visualised using a single multilocus probe, resulting in a strain-specific fingerprint.

DNA fingerprinting involves the use of minisatellites. A minisatellite, also known as a hypervariable region or variable number tandem repeat, is a DNA sequence consisting of multiple copies of a short sequence, typically of fewer than 65 base pairs. These minisatellites occur throughout the mammalian genome. Specific minisatellites can be used as probes, simultaneously detecting hypervariable regions at many separate loci and producing distinct fingerprints on agarose gels.

DNA fingerprinting patterns should be identical for individuals within the same inbred strain. However, the technique can detect hypermutable regions where subtle band differences between individuals within the same strain make interpretation very difficult.

DNA fingerprinting is technically demanding and costly. It has now been superseded by the Polymerase Chain Reaction (PCR).

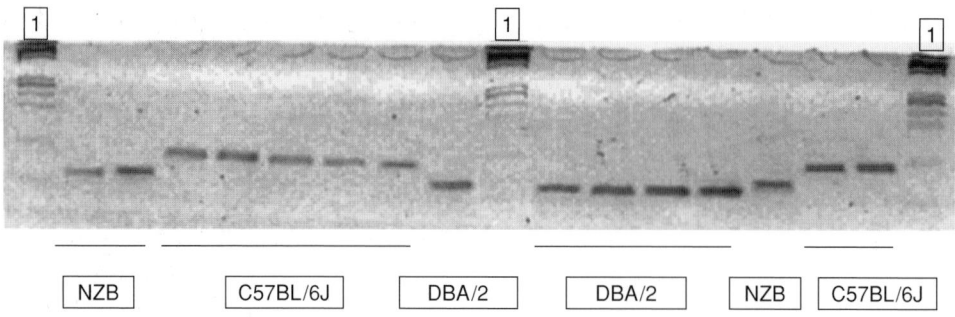

Figure 16.1 Example of a PCR gel showing variation in band sizes between several inbred mouse strains. The marker used in this example is D11Mit236. Lanes marked 'I' are molecular weight markers.

Polymerase chain reaction (PCR)

PCR has provided molecular biology laboratories with a flexible and sensitive method of authenticating inbred strains. PCR is a method for amplifying lengths of DNA defined in terms of a unique DNA base sequence of oligonucleotide primers flanking the stretch of DNA to be amplified. Microsatellites are relatively short, simple sequence repeats, which occur several thousand times in the genome and are often polymorphic in the number of repeats.

They are sufficiently stable to be used as genetic markers, and several thousand of them have been found and mapped in rats and mice.

The advantage of these microsatellites used for genetic quality control is that they are relatively easy to use. DNA is extracted from a small sample of tissue and a PCR reaction is made up with a pair of primers which define the particular locus. After twenty to thirty cycles of amplification, the reaction mixture is run on an agarose gel and visualised after staining with ethidium bromide or using a radioactive tag. So

many microsatellite markers are available that for routine work it is possible to choose a set which can be identified using identical protocols, only varying the primers. In most cases the interpretation of results is relatively easy (Figure 16.1).

PCR does not require the animal to be killed; tail clips, ear snips and other samples (blood, saliva) can be used with relative ease. When using tail clips or ear snips, it should be remembered that the sample needs to be snap frozen, i.e. frozen immediately on dry ice or liquid nitrogen. It is then maintained frozen at −70 °C until processed.

As with biochemical markers, critical subsets can be used. There are literally thousands of primers which have been developed in rats and mice. Their use as markers, however, depends upon whether or not they are discriminatory between the strains to be tested. Critical subsets typically vary between five and thirty markers (Table 16.2).

PCR is such a sensitive technique that it is possible to pool samples from the same strain. Non-authenticity of a strain is recognised as an unexpected band

Table 16.2 Example of a PCR critical subset for mice.

Strain	D1Mit308	D5Mit79	D6Mit102	D9Mit18	D11Mit236
BALB/cOlaHsd	b	b	b	d	c
NZB/OlaHsd	c	a	c	a	c
C57BL/6JOlaHsd	a	a	c	a	b
DBA/2OlaHsd	c	c	d	b	a

Key: DlMit308   a = 150bp; b = 160bp; c = 172bp
  D5Mit79 a = 106bp; b = 136bp; c = 144bp
  D6Mitl02 a = 126bp; b = 140bp; c = 146bp; d = l72bp
  D9Mit18 a = 180bp; b = 204bp; c = 210bp; d = 213bp
  DllMit236 a = 84bp; b = l06bp; c = l08bp; d = 118bp; e = 95bp

appearing on the electrophoresis gel following PCR. To identify the 'rogue' sample(s) the individual samples which make up the pool can be tested separately.

PCR is used extensively in monitoring other specialised strains of, in particular, laboratory mice, e.g. genetically altered and mutant lines. Several mutant strains of rats and mice exist where identification of the heterozygote would provide advantages for the producer and the researcher.

It has been particularly useful in testing for the Lep^{ob} mutation, where the wild type and heterozygote are identical. The ability to test for this gene has resulted in a reduction in the number of test matings required to distinguish the two genotypes.

Genetic monitoring protocols

As mentioned above, critical subsets typically vary between five and thirty markers. Such subsets should be constructed, the profiles and markers used determined by the number and identity of the strains held within the room or facility. Monitoring these markers is key to a successful programme. However, it must be remembered that a colony is based on a foundation colony (FC), from which a production expansion colony (PEC) and a production colony (PC) are derived. It is therefore important to monitor each colony for the occurrence of variation.

Genetically altered animals are backcrossed onto inbred strains in order to minimise variation between individuals. Monitoring of the 'background' strain is important to ensure that variables have not been introduced through accidental outcrossing.

Genetically altered lines are frequently maintained in facilities in open cages, or in individually ventilated cages (IVCs). In such cases, there is a small, but nevertheless ever present, risk that valuable animals will be mixed. Depending upon the strain used in the backcross, the outcrossing may not be apparent by observation of the phenotype, or even through testing. However, a transgene may have inadvertently been introduced into another line. It has been suggested that monitoring lines for the transgene present in other lines in the same room may be recommended.

While there exist many laboratory protocols for genetic monitoring of colonies, observation of colony abnormalities by animal care staff remains integral and fundamental to a genetic monitoring programme.

References and further reading

Kahan, B., Auerbach, R., Alter, B.J. and Bach, F.H. (1982) Histocompatibility and isoenzyme differences in commercially supplied 'BALB/c' mice. *Science*, **217**: 379–381.

Lovell, D.P., Totman, P., Bigelow, S.W. et al. (1984) An investigation of genetic variation within a series of congenic strains of mice. *Lab. Anim.*, **18**: 291–297.

Gubbels, E. and Poort-Keesom, R.J. (1985) Genetically contaminated 'BALB/c' nude mice. *Curr. Top. Microbiol. Immunol.*, **122**: 86–88.

Kurtz, T.W., Montano, M., Chan, L. and Kabra, P. (1989) Molecular evidence of genetic heterogeneity in Wistar-Kyoto rats: Implications for research with spontaneously hypertensive rats. *Hypertension*, **13**: 188–192.

Nabika, T., Nara, Y., Ikeda, K. et al. (1991) Genetic heterogeneity of the spontaneously hypertensive rat. *Hypertension*, **18**: 12–16.

17

Microbiological Control of Laboratory Animals

Adrian A. Deeny

Introduction

The disease status of laboratory animals has improved significantly over the last twenty years. This has resulted in the increased availability of animals free from the major pathogens, which are robust under experimental procedures and do not represent a hazard to other animals in the facility.

At the same time, the increase in the use of transgenic animals and their movement from diverse sources throughout the world has presented a serious threat to animal health and has resulted in the breakdown of some animal facilities with serious infections.

The maintenance of health status of the animals within the facility, whilst fulfilling a research requirement for specialised laboratory animals, presents a difficult challenge. Therefore a programme of health monitoring is essential providing managers and researchers with the assurance that the standard of animal health within the facility has been maintained and that experiments will not be compromised by unexpected infections.

Why do health monitoring?

Infections may be important in laboratory animals for three major reasons:

- They may cause disease in humans, i.e. they may be transmitted from animals to humans and may cause disease (zoonoses). Examples are:

  — *Salmonella* spp.;
  — lymphocytic choriomeningitis;

  — *Streptobacillus moniliformis*;
  — Hantaan virus.

- They may cause disease in animals. Examples are:

  — *Mycoplasma pulmonis*;
  — mouse hepatitis virus;
  — ectromelia;
  — Tyzzer's disease (*Clostridium piliforme*).

- They may alter biological parameters and animal responses. Examples are:

  — mouse hepatitis virus;
  — *Spironucleus muris*;
  — Sendai virus.

Many infections are inapparent; that is, they are not made apparent by gross and obvious lesions. Indeed, many infections only cause disease if the animal is stressed in some way, such as in an experimental procedure or during transport. Therefore, given the human and animal welfare aspects, and the necessity of generating reliable and reproducible research data from experimental animals, a health monitoring programme is essential.

Which organisms should be included in a health monitoring programme?

It has to be accepted that any health monitoring programme is a compromise between what is practicable and affordable to achieve on the one hand, and the significance of the results on the other.

The Federation of European Laboratory Animal Science Associations (FELASA) has published recommendations for the health monitoring of rat, mouse, guinea pig, hamster and rabbit breeding colonies (Nicklas et al. 2002). These are now widely used worldwide.

The organisms listed in the various screening profiles have been included mainly based on the following criteria:

- Are they zoonotic?
- Do they cause clinical disease in animals?
- Are they known to affect physiological and biochemical parameters in animals?

In general, those organisms and agents which should be monitored most frequently are those which are most prevalent within laboratory animal populations and which may have the most profound effects on health and experiments.

However, it is also important to include those organisms which may present a significant risk in specific circumstances. For example, if there are animals within the facility that are known to be positive to rotavirus, but are housed separately from the main population, then this agent may put animals in the general population at risk. Rotavirus would clearly be included in the health monitoring programme for that facility.

It is important to be aware of new/emerging organisms and agents. Two examples of such agents that have become prominent since the publication of the FELASA recommendations are parvoviruses and *Helicobacter* spp.

Parvoviruses

In recent years, evidence has emerged indicating that more parvoviruses exist than the prototypic (KRV, Toolan's H-1, MVM) parvoviruses previously recognised. These newly recognised parvoviruses are now called mouse parvovirus (MPV), rat parvovirus (RPV) and hamster parvovirus (HPV). They have been found throughout numerous tissues and organs and have been shown to have been associated with some effects on research (accelerate tumour graft rejection, perturb the immune response). Identifying their presence is difficult and relies on serology using the appropriate antigen, usually a recombinant VP-2 or NS-1 antigen, combined with confirmation using a polymerase chain reaction (PCR) test on mesenteric lymph nodes or spleen (Livingston et al. 2002; Ball-Goodrich & Johnson 1994).

Helicobacter *spp.*

Various *Helicobacter* spp. have been identified (Fox & Lee 1997). *H. hepaticus* has been demonstrated to cause hepatic disease and lesions in immunodeficient and aged immunocompetent mice (Ward et al. 1994). *H. bilis*-associated typhlitis has been observed in immunodeficient mice. *H. muridarum* colonises the gastric mucosa and intestine of mice but is not associated with intestinal or hepatic disease. *H. rodentium*, also found in mice, causes lesions when associated with *H. bilis* in immunocompromised mice but is not associated with any lesions in immunocompetent mice.

In rats, *H. hepaticus* and *H. bilis* are not associated with clinical or histologic disease, but may have some effects on research such as tumour induction, induction of hepatitis and typhlocolitis, and alteration of hepatic and intestinal function (Livingston et al. 1998; Whary et al. 2000).

Frequency and sample size

It must be true that the more frequent the sampling and the bigger the sample size, the greater the confidence in the information obtained from the health monitoring programme. However, sampling frequency and sample size must be balanced against economic constraints and the availability of animals. The following factors will influence:

- **Microbiological status of the animals and the type of housing**

It could be argued that the stricter the barrier, the less the opportunity for ingress of pathogens. Therefore, it might be concluded that animals housed in such conditions could be screened less frequently than pathogen-free animals housed in non-barrier conditions.

- **The level of risk of contamination from other nearby populations**

Facilities where staff move freely between animal areas of varying health status, and where there is no clear delineation between clean and dirty areas, have a greater chance of disease transmission. They therefore need to be screened more frequently than facilities where the movement of staff and equipment is strictly controlled.

• **Facility environment**

Environmental factors such as temperature and humidity can alter an animal's susceptibility to infectious agents and have an impact on how they respond to the agent.

• **Frequency of animal and personnel population changes**

As the human and animal population dynamics change within a facility, the potential for changes in animal health status increases. Clearly, new animals can introduce new infections, and new personnel may make husbandry errors which increase the chance of new infection.

• **Confidence in the testing methodology**

The sensitivity and the specificity of testing techniques vary with the agent to be tested. As the confidence in the test decreases, so the frequency of testing for that agent increases.

• **Importance of a pathogen or other contaminant to the use of the population**

The work carried out by the research groups at the institution may dictate the frequency with which particular organisms/agents are sought.

• **Economic considerations**

Increased frequency of sampling inevitably leads to increased costs of screening. Thus, economic constraints need to be balanced against maintenance of a statistically significant programme.

• **Sample size**

The purpose of a health monitoring programme is to detect at least one animal in the sample with each of the infections or diseases present in the population. The number of animals to be tested (sample size) is of critical importance and can be determined mathematically with two important assumptions:

(1) rate of infection > 25%;
(2) that the infection is randomly distributed.

As shown in Table 17.1, if one assumes that 40% of the animals in a population are infected with an agent, there is a 99% probability that one infected animal will be detected in a randomly selected sample of ten animals. At a 50% infection rate, a sample size of only five animals is required for a 97% probability of detecting infection in at least one animal.

It should be recognised that although the sample size required to detect a single agent can be determined with reasonable precision, it is virtually impossible to maintain the same degree of precision for all agents to be included in a large test battery. Different agents have typically different infection rates within animal colonies. For example, typical rates for established infections in mouse colonies are greater than 90% for Sendai virus, 25% for PVM and less than 5% for *Salmonella enteriditis*. If screening for these three agents, the lowest assumed rate would be required to be considered, i.e. 5%: a 95% confidence limit would require a sample size of at least sixty animals. This is entirely appropriate in circumstances where *S. enteriditis* infection is suspected.

However, for routine health monitoring programmes, sample sizes are usually based on assumed infection rates of 40–50%, in order to keep sample sizes reasonable.

• **Random sampling**

Correct sampling also requires random sampling of the entire population. This means taking animals from different cages, shelves and racks. Attention should also be given to sampling animals of both sexes and of different ages. Young animals tend to have greater parasite burdens, whereas older animals (adults and retired breeders) are recommended for serological testing. Young adults are preferred for detecting recent viral infections and retired breeders give an indication of the infection history of the colony.

However, the assumption that infections are randomly distributed is not generally true in animal facilities. Infections usually are initiated from an infection focal point. Thus, avoidance of sampling from small, limited areas in the room gives a greater opportunity of finding an infected animal from a 'focal' point of infection, should it be present.

It should be remembered that detection of an infection is always retrospective. Early infections may go undetected, and will not be detected until established in the animal unit. Therefore, health monitoring should not be limited to the laboratory, but must also include:

Table 17.1   Confidence limits for detecting infection using different sample sizes and assumed rates of infection[a].

Sample size (N)[b]	Assumed infection rate (%)											
	1	2	3	4	5	10	15	20	25	30	40	50
5	0.05	0.10	0.14	0.18	0.23	0.41	0.56	0.67	0.76	0.83	0.92	0.97
10	0.10	0.18	0.26	0.34	0.40	0.65	0.80	0.89	0.94	0.97	0.99	–
15	0.14	0.26	0.37	0.46	0.54	0.79	0.91	0.95	0.99	–	–	–
20	0.18	0.33	0.46	0.56	0.64	0.88	0.95	0.99	–	–	–	–
25	0.22	0.40	0.53	0.64	0.72	0.93	0.98	–	–	–	–	–
30	0.25	0.45	0.60	0.71	0.79	0.96	0.99	–	–	–	–	–
35	0.30	0.51	0.66	0.76	0.83	0.97	–	–	–	–	–	–
40	0.33	0.55	0.70	0.80	0.87	0.99	–	–	–	–	–	–
45	0.36	0.69	0.75	0.84	0.90	0.99	–	–	–	–	–	–
50	0.39	0.64	0.78	0.87	0.92	0.99	–	–	–	–	–	–
60	0.45	0.70	0.84	0.91	0.95	–	–	–	–	–	–	–
70	0.51	0.76	0.88	0.94	0.97	–	–	–	–	–	–	–
80	0.55	0.80	0.91	0.96	0.98	–	–	–	–	–	–	–
90	0.60	0.84	0.94	0.97	0.99	–	–	–	–	–	–	–
100	0.63	0.87	0.95	0.98	0.99	–	–	–	–	–	–	–
120	0.70	0.91	0.97	0.99	–	–	–	–	–	–	–	–
140	0.76	0.94	0.99	–	–	–	–	–	–	–	–	–
160	0.80	0.96	0.99	–	–	–	–	–	–	–	–	–
180	0.84	0.97	–	–	–	–	–	–	–	–	–	–
200	0.87	0.98	–	–	–	–	–	–	–	–	–	–

[a] ILAR, 1976

[b] $N = \dfrac{\log\,(1 - \text{probability of detecting infection})}{\log\,(1 - \text{assumed infection rate})}$

- observations from animal technicians;
- observations from veterinary staff;
- observations from research staff.

Methods used in health monitoring

Bacteria

In general, apart from those bacteria detected using serological techniques, bacteria are cultured from specific sites from the animal. For example, a routine microbiological analysis might consist of taking swabs from the nasopharynx and caecum of the animal in order to isolate respiratory and enteric pathogens respectively.

The swabs are plated onto various media. Media may be selective or non-selective. Selective media are used where the organisms to be sought are fastidious in their growth requirements or may easily be overgrown and therefore hidden by other bacterial colonies if another type of medium were used. *Salmonella* spp.

are often grown initially in selenite broth, which is an enrichment medium for this genus, before being subcultured from this medium to another such as DCLS. The latter medium is a solid medium on which salmonellae may grow and be more easily identified than on a non-selective medium.

An example of a commonly used non-selective medium is blood agar. This medium is commonly included in the microbiologist's battery of media as most animal bacteria will readily grow on it.

Once a primary culture has been obtained, the various colony types obtained are subcultured onto individual plates of medium in order to obtain pure cultures, which can be identified. The methods for identification largely rely on their ability to detect products of bacterial metabolism. Several kits are now commercially available for this purpose.

Parasites

The animal, once euthanised, is examined for parasites. Ectoparasites are those parasites that live in, or on, the skin of the animal. They can usually be readily detected behind the ears, around the nose and eyes of the animal, or behind the neck.

Endoparasites, or those parasites whose habitat is within the animal, are best detected by examining wet preparations of the large and small intestines, whilst taking account of any lesions which may be apparent in other tissues and organs, e.g. the liver, which may signal infestation by parasites. Examinations are made using a microscope for trophozoites (the free-living forms of protozoa), worms, cysts, eggs and oocysts (of coccidia) (see Chapter 34).

Viruses (and some bacteria and parasites)

It is a very difficult and expensive procedure to isolate viruses. Therefore, most of the important viruses are detected using an indirect serological test. This test relies on the ability of the animal to produce antibodies in response to an infection by an antigen. Thus, serological tests detect the antibody produced specifically against particular agents.

Clearly, the disadvantage of such testing is that a positive serological test may mean that the animal has at some time in its life been infected with the agent being sought; the agent may no longer be present in the animal.

The most common serological tests used are enzyme-linked immunosorbent assay (ELISA) and indirect immunofluorescence assay (IFA).

As these are antibody detection tests, it follows that the animal must be capable of producing antibody if the test is to be valid. Therefore, such serology tests are not recommended for immunodeficient or immuno-compromised animals. Furthermore, it is advised that animals tested by serology are sufficiently old to produce an adequate immune response (e.g. ≥ 8 weeks).

A common mistake when using serology to determine the causative agent of a disease outbreak is to test animals which are exhibiting symptoms of the disease. Such tests will frequently give false-negative results, as the animal may not yet have had an opportunity to mount an effective immune response. It is better to test healthy cohorts or, even better, animals which have shown symptoms and then recovered.

Even when a good positive result is obtained in, for example, an ELISA test, the result should initially be viewed with calculated scepticism. Because a serology test is far less definitive in diagnostic value than the result of a direct test such as isolation and identification of the agent, it should be supported by one or more secondary tests to confirm the positive result. In many cases, particularly for viruses, a second test such as IFA or hemagglutination inhibition assay (HAI) may well be sufficient. In others, more investigation may be required.

Serological tests for bacterial and parasitic agents, for example, are more prone to false-positive results. Such organisms may appear to be positive by more than one serological test. Another test, such as histopathology, should be used for further elucidation. In some cases, e.g. for *Clostridium piliforme* (Tyzzer's disease) stress testing of the animals may be appropriate and the organism may be observed in histological sections of target tissues and organs.

Molecular biological techniques

In recent years, molecular biological tests have played an increasing role in the detection of infectious agents. The polymerase chain reaction (PCR) has been used to detect almost all of the common viral agents known to infect rats and mice. It has also been used successfully to detect many of the new and emerging agents mentioned above. PCR is a test which detects specific parts of DNA in the genome of the agent under investigation. As its name suggests, PCR can generate relatively large amounts of DNA from a small amount present in a sample.

The availability of oligonucleotide primers is the key to the amplification process. One primer is annealed to the flanking end of each DNA target sequence complementary strand; thermal stable Taq polymerase is added to mediate the extension, as temperatures of up to 95 °C are used in the reaction.

The main components of a PCR reaction are the DNA template, oligonucleotide primers and a DNA polymerase. The PCR cycle comprises denaturation of the template DNA, annealing of the primers and extension of the region between the primers. Synthesis proceeds across the target sequences flanked by the primers with the extension products of one primer acting as a template for the other primer. The amount of DNA synthesised in each successive cycle is doubled, resulting in an exponential accumulation (2^n where n = number of cycles).

This test is now a useful inclusion in the battery of tests available to the health monitoring laboratory.

Health monitoring is not only laboratory based

Health monitoring should not be considered to be the domain of the micro- or molecular biologist. Health monitoring starts in the animal facility with good observation. Animals which are behaving abnormally, i.e. are lethargic, are of hunched appearance, show signs of diarrhoea or exhibit respiratory distress should be reported immediately to managers who can then take appropriate action, such as arranging for diagnostic testing.

Changes in colony parameters may also be a sign of ill health. For example, a rise in pre-wean deaths or a fall in the number of young born may signal a disease outbreak.

The use of sentinel animals

There are some instances when the use of sentinel animals is recommended. Sentinel animals are those that are introduced to the main population specifically for the purposes of health monitoring, when it is difficult or inappropriate to sample animals from the main population.

One example of such a case is when using racks of individually ventilated cages (IVCs), where it may not be practicable to screen the animals in every cage on the rack. Another example is monitoring immunodeficient or immunocompromised animals, where serology is inappropriate.

When using sentinels it is important to remember that the main intention must be to maximise the exposure of the sentinels to any infectious agents which may be present in the main population. To this end, it is recommended to place dirty bedding from cages cleaned from the main population into the sentinel cage(s). However, while the inclusion of dirty bedding in sentinel cages is an important strategy, not all infectious agents are easily transmitted in this way. For example, CAR bacillus, Sendai virus and parvovirus are among the agents which are not satisfactorily transmitted using this technique (Artwohl et al. 1994).

Therefore, if possible, animals from the main population should be included in the sentinel cages to augment direct transmission of infectious agents.

Conclusion

An important consideration is the establishment of a policy agreed by all the relevant parties in an institution which directs what action will be taken in the event of positive results being obtained at health monitoring. In addition, there should also be a documented policy for the criteria for acceptance of animals into the facility from other institutions or commercial breeders.

Health monitoring programmes can contribute to the successful maintenance of high quality animals. However, strict management of the barrier and excellent communication between animal care personnel, veterinarians and researchers achieves the greatest success.

References and further reading

Artwohl, J.E., Cera, L.M., Wright, M.F. et al. (1994) The efficacy of a dirty bedding technique for detecting Sendai virus infection in mice: A comparison of clinical signs and seroconversion. *Lab. Anim. Sci.*, **44**: 73–75.

Ball-Goodrich, L.J. and Johnson, E. (1994) Molecular characterisation of a newly recognised mouse parvovirus. *J. Virol.*, **68**: 6476–86.

Fox, J.G. and Lee, A. (1997) The role of *Helicobacter* species in newly recognised gastrointestinal tract diseases of animals. *Lab. Anim. Sci.* X: 222–255.

ILAR (1976) Long-term holding of laboratory rodents. *ILAR News*, **19**: L1–L25.

Livingston, R.S., Besselsen, D.G., Steffen E.K. et al. (2002) Serodiagnosis of mice minute virus and mouse parvovirus infections in mice by enzyme-linked immunosorbent assay with baculovirus-expressed recombinant VP2 proteins. *Clin. Diagn. Lab. Immunol.*, **9**: 1025–1031.

Livingston, R.S., Riley, L.K., Besch-Williford, C.I. et al. (1998) Transmission of *Helicobacter hepaticus* infection to sentinel mice by contaminated bedding. *Lab. Anim. Sci.*, **48**: 291–293.

Nicklas, W., Baneux, P., Boot, R. et al. (2002) Recommendations for the health monitoring of rodent and rabbit colonies in breeding and experimental units. Recommendations of the FELASA working group on health monitoring of rodent and rabbit colonies. *Lab. Animals*, **36**: 20–42.

Ward, J.M., Anver, M.R., Haines, D.C. et al. (1994) Chronic active hepatitis in mice caused by *Helicobacter hepaticus*. *Amer. J. Pathol.*, **145**: 959–968.

Whary, M.T., Cline, J.H., King, A.E. et al. (2000) Monitoring sentinel mice for *Helicobacter hepaticus, H. rodentium* and *H. bilis* infection by use of polymerase chain reaction analysis and serologic testing. *Comparative Medicine*, **50**: 436–443.

18

Introduction to Farm Animals

Stephen W. Barnett

Introduction

The farm species covered in the next few chapters are cattle, sheep, goats, horses and pigs. These form a small proportion of animals used in scientific procedures (in 2003 2.7% of regulated procedures were performed on these animals).

The care of farm animals differs from most other experimental animals in the following ways:

- they may be kept outdoors in fields;
- indoor accommodation has to be larger than that provided for other species;
- areas for unloading and storing food and bedding have to be able to cope with large volumes;
- waste material is bulky;
- machinery such as tractors may be needed to deal with some of the handling problems;
- specialised animal handling and restraint equipment may be needed;
- the risk of injury to staff is greater than with most other animals.

Any farm animal which is undergoing regulated procedures is subject to the Animals (Scientific Procedures) Act 1986 and must be kept in accordance with the requirements of the *Code of Practice for the Care and Housing of Animals used in Scientific Procedures* (Home Office 1989). If they are not protected by the 1986 Act they are subject to other animal welfare legislation, e.g. the Agriculture (Miscellaneous Provisions) Act 1968; the Welfare of Farmed Animals Regulations 2000 (2001 in Wales) and the Welfare of Farmed Animals (England) (Amendment) Regulations 2003. Under the 1968 Act the Secretary of State at the Department of the Environment, Food and Rural Affairs and relevant ministers in the National Assembly for Wales and the Scottish Parliament are authorised to produce codes of recommendations for the welfare of livestock. These codes contain the minimum standards required for keeping farm animals. Failing to follow the standards laid out in the codes is not illegal but it can be brought as evidence against anyone prosecuted for animal welfare offences. As well as stating husbandry standards the codes contain information about the legislation mentioned above. Anybody working with farm animals must be familiar with the codes which are available free of charge on the DEFRA website (http://www.defra.gov.uk).

Farm animals housed outdoors

All farm animals benefit from being housed outdoors. They are exposed to fresh air, have the opportunity to exercise as much as they want and, if the grass is well managed, they have access to a fresh, nutritious food source. However there are hazards in keeping animals outdoors and, to minimise these, the animals and pasture must be kept under regular observation.

Outdoor housing must provide many of the characteristics we expect to find in cages or pens, e.g.:

- it must contain the animals;
- it must provide for the animals' needs e.g. space, protection from harm and access to food and water;
- there must be protection from draughts.

Containment is provided by hedges and fences, these can be constructed from a variety of materials, e.g. wood, wire, or electric fences (Figure 18.1).

Before animals are placed in outdoor accommodation the fences must be checked to ensure there are no gaps or weak areas where they can push through. Escaped animals can injure themselves, cause injury to people or do damage to property. Apart from the

Figure 18.1 Wire mesh fence.

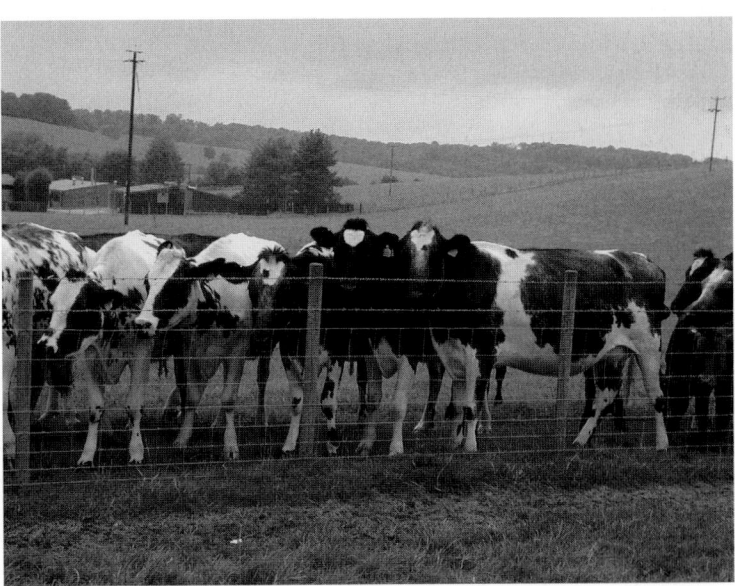

distress caused to the escaped animal, owners are legally responsible for the damage their animals do, so a programme of fence inspection and repair must be instituted.

All animals require some sort of shelter if they are to be kept outdoors in winter. Farm animals can withstand very cold weather but need protection from winds, rain and snow. They also need protection from the sun, some animals are at risk from sunburn and all are at risk of heat stroke.

Protecting animals from harm when housed outdoors is more of a problem. Many of the hazards associated with outdoor housing are connected with the public. The public may leave gates open and may let untrained dogs chase animals. They discard waste in fields which can cause severe injury or even death to animals. Bottles and tin cans can lead to foot damage and plastic bags may be ingested causing blockages in the digestive system. A less common but nevertheless real problem is theft of animals. The only defence against these hazards is continual inspections.

Poisonous plants

Poisonous plants present a risk when animals are at pasture; they are more likely to eat these plants when other food is in short supply, for instance in drought conditions, as many poisonous plants are more likely to survive than grass. When found they must be removed or if this is not possible they must be fenced off to prevent access to the animals. Examples of commonly found poisonous plants are bracken, laburnum, yew and ragwort.

Bracken (*Pteridium aquilinum*)
Bracken is widely seen along minor roads throughout the country (Figure 18.2). It begins to grow in the spring and dies back in autumn. The plant contains a number of toxic agents which affect different species in different ways. These toxic agents remain potent after the plant is dried.

In cattle and sheep these toxic agents cause acute haemorrhagic syndrome resulting in a rapid death from internal bleeding. There is also a chronic form of haemorrhagic disease where small amounts of bracken are eaten over a long period. Long term ingestion causes retinal degeneration in sheep. Horses and pigs are at risk of suffering thiamine deficiency due the presence of thiaminase in the plant. Bracken also contains a number of carcinogens responsible for causing tumours in farm animals.

Laburnum (*Laburnum anagyroides*)
Laburnum is grown as a tree in gardens and is only a problem to animals if they have access over a hedge or if it spreads to grazing areas. The clinical signs it produces are nervous excitement, convulsions and eventually death. All parts of the plant are toxic but the bark and seeds are most dangerous.

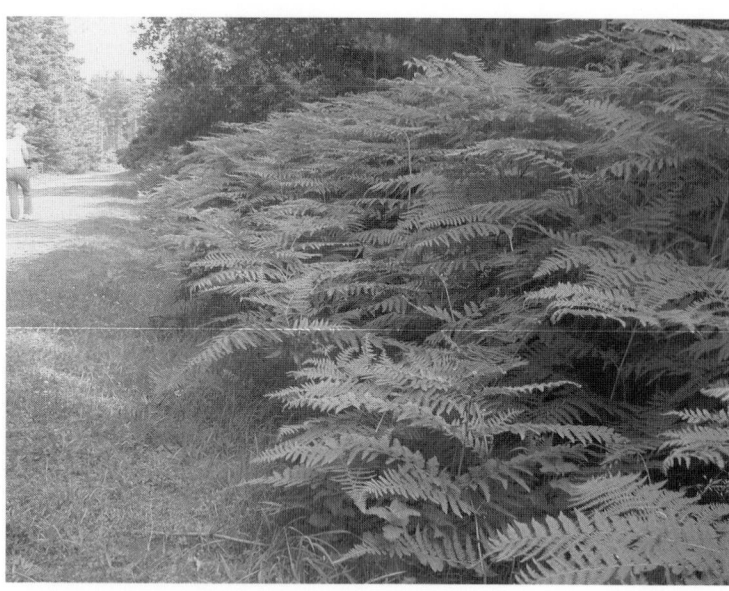

Figure 18.2   Bracken.

Yew (*Taxus baccata*)

Yew trees are found in many churchyards as they have religious significance, in more modern times they have been used for hedging. There are a number of toxic agents in yew, the most important being taxine which interferes with cardiac function. All species can be affected but cases involving cattle and horses are most often reported. Clinical signs include muscular trembling, ataxia, rapid weak pulse and collapse. Sometimes the first sign seen is death.

Ragwort (*Senecio jacobaea*)

Ragwort is a widely distributed weed. It mainly affects cattle and horses but has also been seen to affect sheep and pigs. Deer and rabbits appear to be able to eat it without being harmed.

The poisonous agent in ragwort damages the liver and digestive tract, causing pain, diarrhoea or constipation, straining and rectal prolapse. There may be neurological signs before death.

Further information on poisonous plants can be seen in Cooper and Johnson (1984).

Water

Water can be supplied by piping water to tanks in fields, usually through constant level devices but it can also be provided from natural sources (e.g. streams or ponds). Natural sources must be easily accessible to the animals. In the summer there may be a risk of sources drying up and in hot summers dangerous levels of toxic blue–green algae may build up, these must be treated in the same way as poisonous plants. After heavy storms animals have been known to drown where rivers flow through their fields. Piped water sources must be inspected to ensure the supply remains constant, pipes may rupture or become blocked and constant level devices (e.g. ballcocks) may become blocked. In winter pipes may become frozen.

Grassland management

Grass forms the bulk of the food fed to cattle, sheep, goats and horses. It can withstand repeated cutting and grazing without sustaining permanent damage because its meristem (the region where cell division takes place) is situated at ground level and is not damaged when the plant is grazed or cut. This allows rapid regrowth. In other plants the meristem is situated at the growing tip and is removed when grazed, leading to a very slow recovery period or even death of the plant.

A typical grass crop starts to grow in early spring. Leaves appear first, followed later by stems which bear flowers and seeds after pollination. Stems are reinforced with indigestible lignin and the production of stems, flowers and seeds divert nutrients away from leaf production. So, as the season progresses, the overall digestibility of the crop decreases although the bulk increases. Grazing or cutting grass in the early season delays flowering and therefore lengthens the period of maximum digestibility.

Pasture can be left undisturbed for long periods or it may be regularly reploughed and resown. The former is called permanent pasture and the latter temporary pasture. The choice between the two will depend on local conditions and the productivity required from the land.

Pasture rarely consists of one type of grass. Species with different characteristics are mixed so that the productivity of the land as a whole can be maximised e.g. some species may grow in the early season, others later. Some may be drought resistant others may be tolerant of cold weather.

Clover is a useful addition to grassland particularly where regular applications of fertilisers are unwanted or difficult. Not only does clover contain high levels of nutrients but it is a leguminous plant, having nodules on its roots containing bacteria which can fix atmospheric nitrogen making it available to the plant. However there must be a balance between clover and grass and care must be taken with some species of clover as they produce oestrogenic substances which can interfere with the reproductive cycles of ewes and cows.

Fertiliser application

When grass is cut or grazed nutrients in the soil are lost, some are returned to the land in the urine and faeces produced by animals grazing the land. Where animals are housed indoors their waste is collected as slurry or manure which can be sprayed on to land.

Chemical fertilisers (nitrogen, potassium and phosphates) can also be added. The quantities and timing of the application of these is critical and depends on a number of factors, including: time of the year, stocking levels, grazing system and economic considerations.

In addition to the major elements considered above, other nutrients may be missing from the soil and therefore from the grass. Although they have little effect on the crop they can lead to nutritional deficiencies in animals fed on them. Two common examples are cobalt and copper. Cobalt is required by bacteria in the digestive tract to make vitamin B_{12}. Its absence causes a condition known as cobalt pine typified by poor growth, anaemia and decreased resistance to infection. Copper deficiency also leads to anaemia in many animals and to a condition known as 'swayback' in new-born lambs. In both the above cases the soil deficiency can be rectified by adding the missing element to the soil but because of cost, and in the case of copper, the risk of the toxic effects of overdose, it is more usual to administer them directly to animals either orally or by parenteral administration.

Parasites

Endoparasite build up is a problem when animals are housed on grassland. This can be prevented in several ways. The cheapest is to leave the land idle for nine months to a year or to graze another species on it. Alternatively, the land can be ploughed up and resown. Regular prophylactic treatment of the animals blocks the life cycle of the parasite protecting both the animal and the land (see Chapter 35).

Hay and silage

Grasses have to be preserved in their growing season to provide a source of food in the winter. There are two major ways of doing this, hay and silage production.

Hay

Hay is naturally dried grass. The crop is cut, left in the field and turned periodically until it is completely dry. Three to four days of fine weather is required for the process. It is then collected and baled in either traditional rectangular bails or in big, circular bales.

Grass can be dried artificially in barns and the resultant product has a higher nutrient content than hay but the process uses large amounts of energy and is very expensive. Grass preserved in this way is called dried grass.

Silage

Grass is cut into short lengths and is left in the field to wilt for about twelve hours. It is collected and packed in containers so that as much air as possible is excluded. The containers come in various designs e.g. silage clamps, towers or large plastic bags. Once packed the crop heats up for a while as it is still respiring. This warmth, together with the exclusion of air and the presence of carbohydrate in the crop, provides ideal conditions for anaerobic bacteria (e.g. lactobacilli) to become active. An organic acid (e.g. lactic acid) is produced as a by-product of bacterial activity. Eventually the acid reaches a level which kills the bacteria and prevents other organisms from spoiling the crop. The crop is preserved indefinitely.

In order to ensure good preservation and palatability the crop must be balanced and contain little moisture at the start of the ensiling process. If there are low levels of carbohydrate in the crop (as would be the case if clover content was too high) the bacteria will produce acid too slowly and other organisms, which may spoil the silage, get an opportunity to become established. Additives are available which help to ensure good quality silage is produced. The process is not limited to grass, any green plant can be ensiled.

Haylage

Grass for haylage is cut a little earlier than hay. It is left to wilt until its moisture content is about 45% then it is packed into polythene bags where it ferments. The products of fermentation preserve the nutrients and prevent mould growing. Haylage will keep for up to eighteen months in unopened bags but must be consumed within five days once it is opened because mould grows when it is exposed to air.

Grazing systems

Three main systems of grazing management are commonly employed.

Strip grazing

Animals are allowed access to a portion of a field at any one time. Electric fencing is used to confine animals to one strip of a field. The period of time allowed for grazing the strip depends on the amount of grass growth and the stocking density, but is usually between half a day and two days. At the end of the period the fences and animals are moved to the next strip.

A variation of this system uses permanent fences to divide a field into paddocks, animals are moved from paddock to paddock. This is most often used with sheep. There are several benefits of strip grazing:

- it allows the maximum time for grass to recover from grazing;
- it ensures the animals eat all of the grass plant, not just the more palatable parts;
- it helps to minimise the build up of some parasites.

However strip grazing does have disadvantages:

- it is a labour intensive system;
- if the ground is wet trampling can damage the crop (known as poaching);
- water must be provided in the strip being grazed.

Extensive grazing

Extensive grazing systems allow animals free range over a field. It is also called set stocking. Animals graze for an indefinite period, the stocking density being adjusted (by bringing more fields into the system) as the grass growth rate alters.

An extreme version of extensive grazing is seen with mountain sheep where flocks may wander over many miles to find sufficient grazing.

Zero grazing

Zero grazing is not common in the UK but is used extensively in other countries. As its name implies animals do not graze at all, they remain in barns and the grass is cut every day and is carried to them. It allows maximum utilisation of the grass crop and fences and water sources are not required. It does require a great deal of labour and machinery. Disposal of animal waste products from the barns can be a problem.

Registering premises keeping farm animals

Detailed regulations cover the keeping, identification, recording and movement of all farm animals. The reason for these regulations is to ensure animal disease and human disease originating in animals can be traced and controlled. The regulations used in the UK comply with those in the rest of the European Union.

Registering animals

Before animals are moved onto any premises in the UK for the first time, the premises must be registered and issued with a county parish holding number (CPH). This must be done irrespective of the purpose for keeping the animals and the number kept e.g. one minipig kept as a pet or a commercial herd of 500 milking cows or 2000 breeding ewes.

Application for the CPH has to go to the Rural Payment Agency. They will issue a nine digit number, the first two digits relate to the county and the next three to the parish in which the animals will be kept. The last digits identify the keeper of the animals.

When a CPH has been issued animals can be moved onto the premises. The local Animal Health Divisional Office must then be notified and they will record the CPH and issue a six digit herd/flock mark.

Transport of animals

Control of the movement of animals forms an important part of animal disease surveillance regulations and is detailed in the Welfare of Animals Transport Order 1997 (WATO). As its name implies this order is also concerned with the well being of animals while they are being moved. Further details on the movement of animals are given in Chapter 28 and Chapters 19–23.

References and further reading

Cooper, M.R. and Johnson, A.W. (1984) *Poisonous Plants in Britain and their Effects on Animals and Man*. HMSO, London.

DEFRA website (http://www.defra.gov.uk)

Home Office (1989) *Code of Practice for the Care and Housing of Animals used in Scientific Procedures*. HMSO, London.

Spedding, C. (Ed.) (1983) *Fream's Agriculture* (16th edn). John Murray, London.

19
Cattle

Stephen W. Barnett

Introduction

Cattle are ruminants and so have a four-chambered stomach, which enables them to gain maximum benefit from their herbivorous diet. Their scientific classification is shown in Table 19.1.

Commercially they are bred for their meat, milk and skin. In some countries they are still valuable as beasts of burden. Selective breeding over many years has resulted in cows which are easy to handle despite their large size and obvious strength. Bulls may not be as amenable, dairy bulls can be very dangerous, although beef bulls are often good natured.

Although cows are handled regularly in commercial farming they are usually driven from place to place guided by races. In research organisations it may be necessary to lead them in which case they should be broken in to a head collar as early in their lives as possible.

Terms used in relation to cattle are listed in Table 19.2.

Many different breeds of cattle have been developed to satisfy specific demands of commercial users. They fall into three main types: dairy, beef and dual purpose.

Table 19.1 Classification of cattle *Bos taurus*.

Kingdom	Animalia
Phylum	Chordata
Sub-phylum	Vertebrata
Class	Mammalia
Order	Artiodactyla
Family	Bovidae
Genus and species	*Bos taurus*

Table 19.2 Cattle terms.

Calf	Animal younger than 180 days
	Could be bull calf or heifer calf
Heifer	Female over 180 days can be:
	Maiden heifer (not mated)
	In-calf heifer (confirmed pregnant)
Cow	Female after the start of her first lactation
Bull	Entire male
Steer or bullock	Castrated male

Dairy breeds

Dairy breeds convert food intake into large milk yields, they are strong enough to withstand the heavy physiological demands of long term lactation. Examples of dairy breeds are Holstein Friesian and Jersey.

Holstein Friesian

This breed supplies over 90% of all milk consumed in the United Kingdom. They are large animals, with an adult cow weighing approximately 590 kg. The milk yield per lactation averages 8000 litres. This breed is easily recognised by its familiar black and white colouring (Figure 19.1).

Jersey

An adult Jersey cow weighs about 380 kg. Her milk yield of approximately 3800 litres per lactation is lower than the Holstein Friesian but it is much richer due to a higher fat content. The colour of Jerseys can range from almost black to almost white but is usually golden brown. They have a dish-shaped forehead and a light-brown ring around the mouth (Figure 19.2).

Figure 19.1   Holstein Friesian cows.

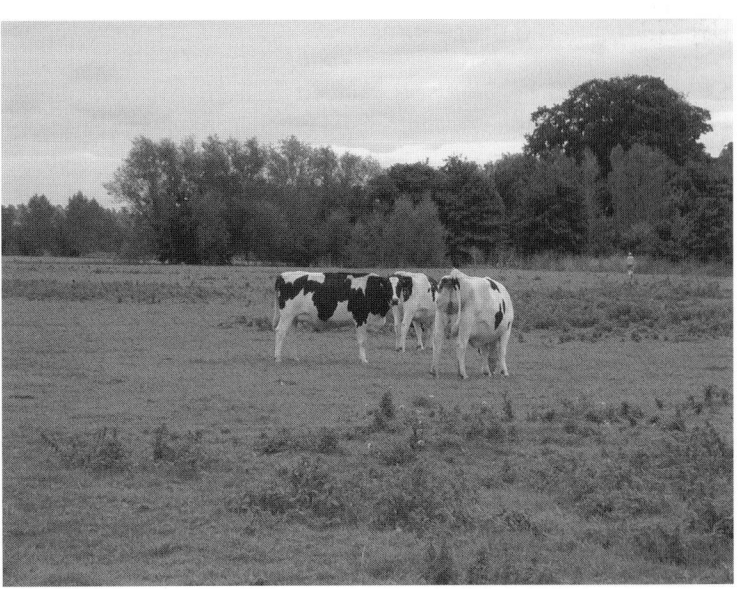

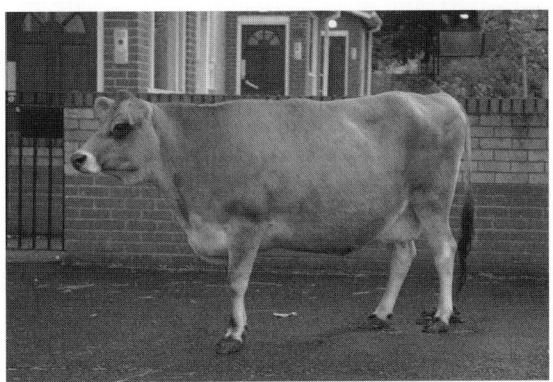

Figure 19.2   Jersey cow.

Beef breeds

Beef breeds are efficient at converting food intake into body mass with a high flesh to bone ratio. Their calves mature rapidly to killing weight. An example of a beef breed is the Hereford.

Hereford

Herefords are very adaptable; they do well in a wide range of environments and are to be found from the warmest to the coldest areas of the world. They are recognised by their white face, belly and feet and red bodies. Bulls average at 850 kg and cows 500 kg.

Dual-purpose breeds

Dual-purpose breeds have some of the characteristics of both the specialists breeds mentioned above. Modern specialised farming practices have made these breeds less popular than they once were but many still survive. An example of a dual-purpose breed is the Dairy Shorthorn.

Dairy Shorthorn

The usual colour of this breed is roan but it can vary from white to red. They produce up to 4700 litres of milk per lactation and good quality calves. A cow averages 500 kg in weight.

Cross-bred animals

In order to maintain economic milk yields dairy cows have to produce one calf a year. If dairy farmers need to breed replacement heifers for their milking herds they will mate their cows with a bull of the same breed, but if they do not need more milkers they often use a beef bull. The calf produced will be larger and mature more rapidly than a pure bred dairy calf.

An example would be using a Hereford bull on a Holstein cow. The resulting calf in this cross will always have a white face and a black body but with varying degrees of white.

Uses in regulated procedures

Extensive research has been carried out on the nutrition, reproduction, disease control and the housing requirements of cattle. Work on their reproductive physiology, artificial insemination, embryo transfer and lactation has been extensively applied to other species. In addition, cattle are used in toxicology studies. Dairy calves have been used in experimental thoracic surgery.

Environment

Cattle undergoing scientific procedures must be kept in accordance with the standards laid down in the Home Office codes of practice (Home Office 1989). If they are not part of a procedure they should be kept in accordance with the DEFRA *Code of Recommendations for the Welfare of Livestock – Cattle* (DEFRA 2003). Both codes describe minimum standards. The environmental levels for scientific procedure establishments are listed in Table 19.3.

The Home Office code states that farm animals can be kept in outdoor accommodation (paddocks, yards, etc.) which have been designated for the purpose. If housed outdoors ambient conditions apply. Cattle can withstand low temperatures very well but they must be protected from drafts and wind.

When housed indoors air changes must be sufficient to provide clean air, free from odours and relative humidity in the range of 55% ± 10%. Cattle produce large amounts of urine and vapours and gases from the digestive system, air changes may need to be high to achieve the desired standards.

The DEFRA Welfare code has less prescribed environmental levels. Ventilation must ensure air circulation, dust levels and temperature are kept within limits that are not harmful to animals. Light levels

Table 19.3 Environmental levels for cattle housed in scientific procedure establishments (Home Office 1989).

Temperature	10–24 °C
Relative humidity	55% ± 10%
Light intensity	350–400 lux
Photoperiod	Natural light periods
Air changes per hour	Sufficient to provide fresh air and prevent a build up of noxious odours

must be sufficient to be able to see all the animals in a unit and to allow the animals to behave and feed normally. Additional lighting must be available to inspect animals.

Housing

The space that should be provided for cattle of different weights, undergoing scientific procedures, can be found in the Home Office code of practice (1989). Space allowance for other cattle can be found in the DEFRA welfare code.

Indoor housing

The *Code of Practice for the Housing and Care of Animals used in Scientific Procedures* states that:

- Pens for cattle should be rectangular and the minimum width should be not less than the length of the animal from its nose to the root of its tail.
- Horned cattle must not be mixed with polled cattle.
- Groups of horned cattle will need more space than groups of polled cattle.
- If slatted floors are used, cattle must have a separate, solid-floored area covered with bedding material.

Loose boxes

Loose boxes are suitable for housing small numbers of calves or cows, for isolating sick animals or cows about to calve. These boxes are usually fitted with stable doors which open in two halves (Figures 23.2 and 23.3, see pp. 158 and 160). All doors on farm animal accommodation should open outwards in case animals fall down behind doors. Hay is presented in racks and concentrate rations in mangers fixed to the wall. Water can be provided by means of constant level devices. Food and water should be available on separate sides of the box to avoid contamination of one with the other. Concrete makes suitable flooring with straw or wood chips as bedding. The floor should slope to a drain.

Cow cubicles

On a larger scale, dairy herds housed indoors are kept in cow cubicles. These consist of rows of compartments separated by wood or tubular metal partitions installed in barns.

Cubicles are designed to fit the size of the cows that will use them. The width is adjusted to prevent injuries caused by knocks against the partition, the minimum width recommended is 1.2 m. The length is adjusted to ensure the cow defecates and urinates into the gully behind the cubicle thus keeping the bedding clean and dry. Tractors with scrapers fitted are used to keep the gullies clean. Cleaning is carried out regularly to ensure good hygiene and to prevent the surface becoming slippery.

Regular cleaning of the lying area is also important to limit the incidence of mastitis in milking cows. Bedding soiled with faeces, urine or milk, all of which encourage bacterial growth, should be removed and replaced with fresh bedding at least three times a week.

Various bedding materials are used in these systems. Straw or sawdust to a depth of 50 mm can be used. Rubber or polyester cow mats covered with either straw or sawdust to a depth of 10 mm are also suitable.

Straw yards

Areas in barns can be sectioned with either permanent or adjustable tubular steel dividers. Adjustable dividers are very useful for experimental animals as they can be altered to take one or several animals depending on the demands of the project. The straw is topped up every day and completely changed every four to six weeks.

If cows are housed singly they should be within sight and sound of other animals. They should be given items of environmental enrichment and extra human contact.

Bull housing

Adult bulls are housed singly. They are potentially dangerous animals so in addition to providing adequate space and comfort for the animals, the pens must ensure they can be cleaned and handled without risk to staff. A number of safety features are incorporated into the design of the pen, for instance barriers are placed across corners so staff can run behind them if the bull gets free while they are in the pen.

Bulls are more tractable if they can see what is going on about them so it is better to situate pens in a busy part of the farm and have walls topped with tubular metal so the bull can see over them.

Feeding adult cattle

Feeding practice varies according to the condition cattle are kept in and the purpose for which they are being kept. In any system the exact amount given must be adapted to the needs of the individual animal. Careful monitoring of body condition is necessary to ensure food intake is adequate. There must be a balance between roughage (hay, straw, grass) and concentrates (e.g. oats, maize, pellets) to reduce the risk of inducing bloat (production of gas in the rumen at a faster rate than the animal can get rid of it).

All rations are divided into the proportion required to maintain body condition in a steady state (maintenance ration) and that required to support growth, pregnancy and lactation (production ration).

Dairy cows

Dairy cows spend ten months of the year lactating and for about six months of this time they are also pregnant. Calving is timed so that they have two months rest from lactation before the birth of the next calf. During this time food rations are carefully managed to build up to support the expected lactation level without causing the animal to get fat.

In the winter, the bulk of a cow's food intake will be hay or silage. There is a great variation in the nutritional quality of these bulk feeds. The variation arises for a number of reasons, such as the time of year the grass was cut, the quality of the land on which it was grown, and the storage conditions. The hay quality is measured in terms of its digestibility (D) and metabolisable energy (ME) content, good quality hay has a digestibility of above 60 and an ME of 9 Mj/kg. Hay of this quality will satisfy the maintenance rations of a cow but hay below this quality will have to be supplemented with concentrate rations.

Silage quality is also stated in terms of its digestibility (D) and ME. Good silage has a D value in excess of 68 and an ME of 10.5–11.00 Mj/kg. If silage is used instead of hay, roughly three times the amount must be fed.

Without expensive nutritional analysis there is no way to be certain of the quality of hay or silage but as a rule good quality hay will be:

- leafy without woody stems or weeds;
- dust free;
- without any sign of mould.

Good hay should also smell sweet but the old practice of holding a sample near to the nose and sniffing must be avoided as inhaling dust or mould spores can lead to serious respiratory disease.

Good silage is leafy, smells sweet and should just produce liquid when a handful is squeezed.

In the summer, grass is available for cows to graze, it is most nutritious in spring and early summer and during this time it will provide for the cow's maintenance and a proportion of its production needs.

Concentrate rations are generally fed in the form of dairy cake, made in a similar way to small animal pellets. These cakes are available with a range of ME and protein levels suitable for different stages in the cow's pregnancy and lactation. Mineral supplements may be needed to make up for deficiencies in the roughage, these can be added to the food or mineral licks can be provided.

Example of a feeding regimen for a dairy cow

Maintenance ration

| Good quality hay | 0.9 kg per 50 kg body weight |
| Good quality silage | 2.7 kg per 50 kg body weight |

Feeding during dry period (when cow is pregnant but not lactating)

Hay for maintenance, plus concentrate ration to give a body weight gain of 0.7 kg/day from six to seven months post partum until birth of next calf.

Feeding for lactation

Mixtures of hay or silage and concentrates are fed depending on milk yield. As a guide, 50 kg of good quality silage with 0.35–0.4 kg of cattle cake can be fed per litre of milk produced.

Concentrate feeding usually takes place in the milking parlour, but where large amounts have to be fed in early lactation there is not enough time to consume it. Some of the ration has to be given outside the parlour.

Feeding beef cattle

Feeding beef animals depends on the age at which it is intended that they are sent to market. This can be from ten months to two years. The aim is to achieve a target daily body weight gain (e.g. 0.8 kg/day). Rations will consist of concentrates, hay and grazing in the spring and summer.

Feeding bulls

| Maintenance | 1.5–2 kg hay per 70 kg body weight |
| Semen production | hay as above + 1.8–2.7 kg concentrates |

Semen quality will fall if bulls are not well fed. However, it is important that they do not become overweight, as this may lead to a drop in ability to perform.

Water consumption

Water should be provided *ad libitum* for all animals. The consumption varies with the type of food supplied and the milk yield. As a rough guide calves require one litre per 10 kg body weight. Adult cows can drink up to 80 litres per day. Consumption is not evenly spread across the day. They drink little in the morning, there is a peak in early afternoon and a much larger peak in the early evening (these peaks are related to morning and afternoon milking). Fifty per cent of the total intake occurs in the evening. Cows can drink up to 14 litres a minute so water containers and constant level devices must be able to cope with very large supply rates.

Water and feeding equipment must be placed where the risk of contamination is low. There should be sufficient of both to ensure easy access to all animals and to prevent a dominant animal stopping others gaining access to food and water.

Reproduction

The age at which heifers become sexually active depends on the breed and level of nutrition they have received. On average it is nine months, a little earlier in small breeds and later in larger breeds. Although the animals reach puberty at this age they are not mated until they are between fifteen and twenty-one months old.

Cattle are polyoestrous. On average the oestrous cycle lasts twenty days in heifers and twenty-one days in cows. Oestrus averages fifteen hours but ranges from two to thirty hours and tends to be shorter in winter than in summer. Ovulation occurs approximately

Table 19.4   Summary of breeding data for cattle.

Average age at sexual maturity: female	9 months
Average age at sexual maturity: male	10 months
Age at first use	15–21 months
Average oestrous cycle (heifers)	20 days
Average oestrous cycle (cows)	21 days
Average length of oestrus	15 hours
Range of oestrus length	2–30 hours
Ovulation	spontaneous
Gestation	283 days
Litter size	1
Birth weight: Jersey	23 kg
Birth weight: Holstein	38 kg
Return to oestrus post partum	3–6 weeks
Economic breeding life	4 lactations

twenty-eight hours after the onset of oestrus. After calving the animals start cycling again within three to six weeks.

The onset of sexual maturity in bulls is also dependent on breed and nutritional state but they are usually sexually active by the age of ten months. Breeding data is summarised in Table 19.4 (there is considerable breed variation in cattle so this table should be interpreted with care).

Mating

In beef herds it is common to run a bull with cows, when they are in oestrus the bull mates them. Raddles (head collars which hold markers under the chin) can be fitted to the bull so that a mark is made on the back of the cow indicating a mating when the bull dismounts.

In dairy herds, and for most experimental purposes, it is necessary to know exactly when the female is mated. So the female is taken to the bull, or is artificially inseminated, when she is observed to be in oestrus. This means that accurate observations must be made and records must be kept to ensure that oestrus is not missed.

Indications of oestrus

Impending oestrus can be identified by changes in behaviour. A cow in pro-oestrus will become restless and will bellow, she will rest her head on the flanks of other cows and may lick them, she will sniff the vulva and urine of other cows and other cows will do the same to her. They may engage in head butting and other cows may attempt to mount the animal coming into oestrus, at first she will walk away but when she is in standing heat (that is when she is in oestrus and is ready to mate) she remains still when mounted. At standing heat the oestrous cow will attempt to mount other cows but at the head end. There are also observable changes in the vulva; it becomes swollen and slack and there is often a clear discharge.

Since in some animals the duration of oestrus is very short and 50% of cattle exhibit oestrus at night, it is easy to miss the signs that an animal is ready for service. The herd should therefore be observed for thirty minutes three times a day (early morning, afternoon and evening) to maximise the possibility of detecting oestrus. Even so, some animals will be missed. Several techniques have been developed to assist in spotting oestrus. Paints are available which can be applied to a cow's tail and which will be removed when she is mounted by another cow (these are similar to the ones illustrated in Chapter 20 on sheep). The Kamar® Heatmount™ detector consists of an inner capsule containing a red dye within an outer clear capsule. It is stuck onto the root of the tail. Pressure from a cow mounting the one in oestrus causes the inner capsule to rupture and releases a red dye which becomes visible in the outer capsule.

Vaginal smears can also be used to determine oestrus and can be useful if single cows are kept.

Artificial insemination

Insemination of cattle is regulated by law which requires commercial AI centres to be licensed. Insemination can only be carried out by a veterinary surgeon, a competent employee from a licensed centre or, in the case of their own cows, an owner or one of their employees who have been adequately trained.

The advantage of using specialist insemination centres is that they have access to a large number of bulls. The bulls are bred from parents who are known to produce good quality offspring and have undergone a rigorous process of testing (see Chapter 1).

AI technique

Bull semen is collected by means of an artificial vagina (AV). A teaser animal (usually a steer) is placed in stocks, the bull is then led to it and mounts. The erect penis is directed into the AV and an ejaculate of a few cm^3 is deposited into the collecting cone of the AV.

The advantages of AI are as follows:

- it obviates the need to keep potentially dangerous bulls on the premises;
- the semen comes from bulls of proven quality;
- semen from one ejaculate can be used to inseminate many cows.

The theoretical risk of inbreeding due to fewer bulls being used is minimised because large-scale AI agencies are constantly replacing their stud bulls with animals from breeding lines not previously used.

Semen can be obtained from the AI centre when a cow in oestrus is identified. A catheter is used to introduce it into the cervix of the cow.

Embryo transfer

A relatively recently introduced method of producing cattle of superior quality is embryo transfer. A cow which has an outstanding performance (in terms of lactation quality and quantity) is chosen as a donor. She is treated with follicle stimulating hormone to induce multiple ovulations. These are fertilised by AI with semen from a superior bull. After six days the embryos are flushed out of her uterus and are implanted into the uteri of recipient cows (hormonally prepared to receive the embryo) who will bring the calves to term.

Unless it is part of a project authorised by the Animals (Scientific Procedures) Act 1986 embryo transfer in cattle is controlled by the Bovine Embryo (Collection, Production and Transfer) Regulations 1995. These require the process to be carried out by or under the direction of a veterinary surgeon.

Pregnancy

The average gestation period of cattle is 283 days but there is variation between breeds (Friesian 283; South Devon 290; Jersey 279). The breed of bull used to service the cow also influences the gestation period. Veterinary surgeons can provide a sure pregnancy diagnosis at six weeks in heifers and nine weeks in cows by assessing changes in the uterus using rectal palpation (inserting the arm into the rectum and feeling the uterus through the rectal wall).

In lactating animals pregnancy can be diagnosed by measuring levels of progesterone in milk twenty-four days after mating.

Pregnancy can also be diagnosed with ultrasound; a rectal probe is used and experienced operators can detect pregnancy at six weeks post mating. Rectal ultrasound scans must be carried out by a veterinary surgeon or by operators who have passed a DEFRA-approved training course (the Veterinary Surgery (Rectal Ultrasound Scanning of Bovines Order 2000)).

Parturition

Calving should take place in a clean, well-bedded box which is disinfected between each calving. The onset of parturition is signalled by structural and behavioural signs. In the month preceding parturition the udder increases in size (known as 'bagging up').

The first stage of labour starts about three to four days before the eventual birth, although timings are not certain and tend to decrease with successive calvings. The behaviour of the cow alters; she becomes restless, repeatedly lying down and getting up again. She also seeks to get away from the rest of the herd.

About twenty-four hours pre-parturition the pelvic ligaments become slack, the vulva increases in size and thick mucous is discharged from it. Throughout the first stage of labour uterine contractions become progressively stronger and these continue into the second stage of labour. The uterine contractions continue to increase in intensity and are joined by more powerful abdominal contractions, the effect of which is to cause the allantoic embryonic sac to protrude from the vulva and rupture. The feet and head of the calf follow, still enveloped in the amniotic sac, but this too is soon ruptured. Up to this point cows generally remain standing but at this stage they often lie down and thus make more room for the calf to pass through the pelvis. The calf is born soon after; the umbilical cord usually breaks when the cow stands up. She licks the calf and so stimulates breathing.

The whole process through to the second stage of labour in normal births may take up to twelve hours.

The third stage of labour results in the expulsion of the placenta and should be complete in six to twelve hours. If it is not expelled within a few days it may be retained and the female may need cleansing (i.e. the removal of the retained placenta) by a veterinary surgeon.

A variety of abnormal presentations may occur in parturition and these need experienced people to rectify them. If cows appear to be in difficulty, veterinary assistance should be sought immediately.

The mouth and nose of the calf should be checked to ensure they are clear of membranes and the navel of the calf must be disinfected as soon as possible to prevent infection.

Calving interval

Farmers aim to produce one calf per cow a year. Lactations are generally terminated after 305 days (ten months) and cows are rested from lactation for two months between the end of lactation and the birth of the next calf. With a gestation period of 283 days this means that cows must be mated at the oestrus nearest to 82 days after the birth of the previous calf.

Milking

Dairy cows must be milked. This is usually done twice a day and cows should not be kept waiting to be milked. The equipment must be properly maintained to avoid damaging the udder. Hygiene measures have to be enforced to prevent contamination of the milk and to minimise the risk of mastitis (inflammation of the udder).

Calves

National statistics show that 6% of calves die in the first six months of life. Careful management is vitally important if they are to live through these early months. Animals with a high birth weight appear to have the best chance of survival. Birth weight depends on genetic factors and on the nutritional state of the dam during pregnancy. An example of a good birth weight for Jerseys is 23 kg and for Friesians 38 kg.

Feeding

As well as a high birth weight, an early and adequate supply of colostrum is essential if calves are to grow into healthy animals.

Colostrum is the milk produced by cows in the first few days of each lactation. It is thicker than later milk because it contains more solid matter. It is important for several reasons:

(1) Some of the solid matter is protein in the form of antibodies produced by the cow in response to pathogenic organisms in her environment. Calves are born with few antibodies and colostrum is their major disease protection until they can manufacture their own. Since antibodies will only be present for organisms to which the cow has been exposed, calves moved away from the birth environment may be subjected to pathogenic organisms to which they lack immunity.

(2) Colostrum has a laxative effect and clears intestines of faeces built up in foetal life (foetal faeces are called meconium).

(3) The high solid content in colostrum consists of a concentrated supply of the nutrients necessary to support rapid growth in the early days of life.

Colostrum is best provided by the cow when she suckles the calf. If the dam dies or calves have to be removed from dams for some other reason, colostrum can be drawn from other newly calved cows. Colostrum can be frozen (at −18 °C for six months) to provide an emergency source. Calves should consume 5% of their body weight of colostrum within six hours of birth (1 kg colostrum = approx. 1 litre). In the twenty-four hours following the first feed three more feeds of the same quantity are given. In the next three to four days twice daily feeds are recommended, still at a rate equivalent to 5% of body weight. This means the amount will increase as the body weight increases.

Post-colostrum feeding of calves

Several different feeding systems are employed to feed calves after the in-take of colostrum.

Suckler systems

Some calves, usually beef animals, are reared by their own dams or with up to three others by a suckler cow. Suckler cows are females with a good milk yield and good mothering qualities who rear a number of calves at a time. Calves have to be introduced with care to ensure they are not rejected or attacked. Weaning practice varies with this system; for instance calves can remain with the cow for six months and then removed for slaughter without weaning (although milk will be an increasingly minor part of their diet). Others are weaned at ten weeks and are then replaced

Table 19.5   Calf feeding.

Day 1	0.75 litres standard mixture after calves have settled into their new environment.
Days 2–3	1 litre, twice daily
Days 4–5	1.5 litres, twice daily
Days 6–7	2 litres, twice daily
Day 8 – weaning	2.25 litres, twice daily

by another set of calves. Good quality hay, calf pellets and plenty of fresh water are available throughout the suckling period.

Artificial rearing

Dairy calves are removed from their dams at an early age so that milking can commence; they are reared artificially on milk substitute. Table 19.5 gives a feeding regimen suitable for home-bred calves being transferred to milk substitute (milk powder), following four days of colostrum feeding. The change to milk needs to be gradual if digestive problems are to be avoided.

Some calves are slow to take to artificial feeding and may need less food more frequently until they are used to it. It is important to note that, apart from poor hygiene, the greatest risk to calf welfare at this stage comes from overfeeding.

Bought-in calves

Calves selected for experimental use should be at least one week old before being moved from their place of birth, be of average weight for their age and breed and be free from overt signs of disease. In particular, the coat should be supple and glossy, the calves should be free from scours, have a clean, damp nose, bright eyes and have a clean, dry umbilicus. If several calves are to be brought in at the same time they should all come directly from the same place of birth; passing through dealers or markets, or mixing animals from different sources increases the risk of cross infection. Stress is minimised if routine procedures, such as disbudding and castration, are carried out at the place of birth. Bought-in calves should be quarantined to ensure they pass no disease to other animals.

Travel is stressful to young calves and can result in digestive upset. This is less likely if the calves are

allowed to settle for at least four to eight hours before food is offered to them, although fresh water must be available at all times. After the settling-in period a warm glucose solution (100 g glucose in 2 litres of water at 38 °C) can be given. Vaccinations and multi-vitamin injections may be given on veterinary advice. Subsequently, milk substitutes are fed at increasing concentration until, after forty-eight hours they are assimilated to the appropriate point on Table 19.5, above.

For example, a seven-day-old calf would enter the unit, be rested for about six hours then would be fed the glucose solution. This would be followed at the next feed by diluted milk after which the concentration of milk is increased until after forty-eight hours it would be fed 2.25 litres of full strength milk substitute twice per day.

Milk presentation

Milk can be presented in several ways:

(1) Bottle feeding is probably the best method from the point of view of calf welfare. It simulates the natural feeding position of calves and allows the feeder to spend time in direct contact with the animal. However, it is so time consuming that it is not a practical method if more than a few calves are being kept.

(2) Bucket feeding is a common way of presenting milk. Calves can readily be taught to feed from a bucket by allowing them to suck on freshly washed fingers which are then lowered into the bucket of milk. A disadvantage of this method is that it forces the calf into an unnatural feeding posture which can lead to digestive problems.

(3) A compromise between bucket and bottle feeding is available which consists of plastic containers with teats at the base.

(4) Automatic feeding systems are available but are only of use where large numbers of animals are kept. There are two main types of automatic feeding. The first one provides cold acidified milk. The second method automatically mixes warm milk on demand. Both provide milk *ad libitum*. Calves on these systems initially grow faster than calves on restricted systems because the milk is always available. Teats should be provided at a

rate of six calves for each teat. If concentrate rations are placed near to the teats the calves will eat them while they are waiting to drink.

Whichever system of calf feeding is used, good hygiene is of the utmost importance. Each calf should have its own bucket or teat and these must be thoroughly washed after use. Automatic feeders must be regularly stripped down and disinfected.

Solid food

In all systems of feeding, solid food in the form of good quality hay and calf nuts (18% crude protein) should be available on the first day. At first the calves will not eat much, so small quantities, changed daily, should be offered. The amount should be increased as the animals get older. Fresh water must be available at all times.

Weaning

Commercial weaning practice varies depending on management systems, the availability of milk and the fate of the calves. As we have seen in suckler systems the calves may stay with the cow for as long as six months. In artificial systems five-week weaning is aimed for. In these systems two factors can indicate the exact time to stop milk feeding, one is when an acceptable weight gain has been achieved (Friesians should weight about 60 kg or have gained 14 kg since birth). The second factor is when the calf is eating sufficient amounts of weaner compounds (750 g consumed on three consecutive days).

Calf housing

Calves are best housed in pens of two or more as this provides companionship. Individual pens may be used for calves up to the age of eight weeks but the walls of the pens must be perforated to allow the animals to see and touch each other. Group housing can produce some management problems, for instance young calves have a strong desire to suck and will suck one another's ears, scrotum, umbilicus and other areas leading to painful and possibly infected areas.

All housing should be constructed of smooth, impervious materials to allow easy cleaning and disinfection.

Where group housing is practised, the group must be made up of animals of a similar age and weight. Once established, animals should not be added to or taken from the group or fighting and bullying may occur.

Weaning to breeding

A week after weaning has been completed but before eight weeks of age, calves of a similar weight and age can be housed in groups of about twelve. Some fighting may occur when they are first put together as the group dominance hierarchy becomes established, but provided adequate space is available to allow submissive animals to escape, this should be short lived and no injury should occur. However, close watch should be maintained in case the fighting becomes too violent. Sufficient food trough space must be provided so that dominant animals cannot prevent weaker ones getting access to food. Good quality hay should be available *ad libitum*, together with pre-weaning concentrates. These should be fed at a maximum rate of 2.3 kg per animal per day.

When the animals are three months old, the concentrates should be gradually replaced for ones with a crude protein content of 16%.

At six months old the animals are fed hay or silage *ad libitum* and concentrates up to 2.7 kg per day. A body weight gain of 0.7–0.9 kg per day is aimed for. A Friesian cow should weigh between 350–400 kg at mating.

In the spring, calves can be housed on clean grass, that is grass that has not been grazed by cattle for the previous nine months. They are put out in the day and brought in at night until they become acclimatised to the conditions. Shelters must be provided in the fields. In summer they are given a parasite treatment and put on fresh grass. Concentrates and mineral supplements will need to be provided at a rate depending on the quality of the pasture. The same body weight gains need to be achieved as those housed indoors.

Handling

Cows are generally good natured animals but may be wary of man, particularly if they are not used to being handled. They may become more difficult when they

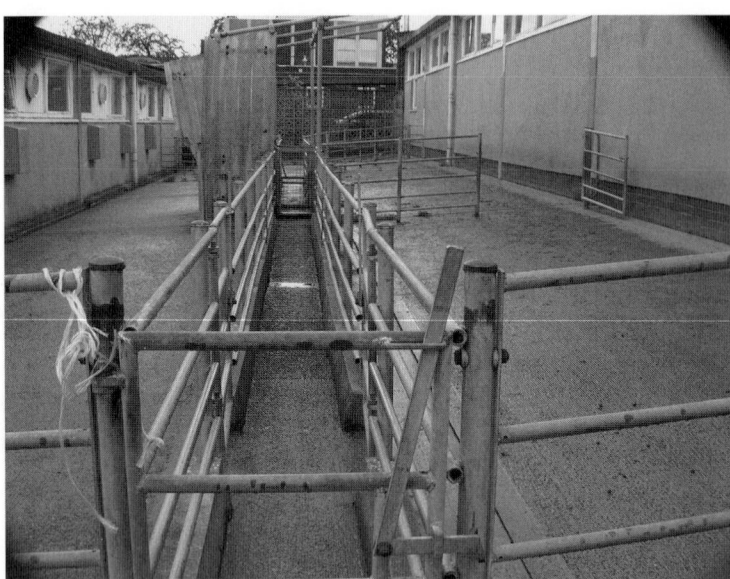

Figure 19.3   Cattle race.

are in oestrus. Gentle, quiet but firm handling gets the best results with these animals. It is easier to drive them from place to place rather than to lead them. However, if they are to be handled regularly they should be broken into a head collar/halter; the earlier this is done the quicker the animal will take to it.

Although it is possible to restrain adult cows manually for procedures such as blood collection or dosing it is better to use proper handling equipment consisting of a race, directing animals into a cattle crush (Figure 19.3).

Procedures

A number of procedures which are carried out on young calves are described below, the DEFRA welfare codes state that they should only be performed after careful consideration of there being necessity for each procedure in each case and not as a routine for every animal.

Castration

Three methods are commonly used to castrate males not required for breeding:

(1) Rubber-ring method. This method is only permitted in the first week of life. The animal is restrained in a sitting position. A rubber ring is placed over the neck of the scrotum using an applicator. When the applicator is removed the ring tightens and cuts off the blood supply to the tissues below it. Within three weeks the scrotal sac and its contents fall off. It is important to ensure both testes are in the scrotum before applying the ring. This method can only be carried out by a trained and competent person.

(2) Bloodless castrators. Bloodless castrators or Burdizzo forceps are used to crush the spermatic cord without breaking the skin, hence the name bloodless castrators. The castrators have to be adjusted properly or they will crush the skin as well. The calf is restrained in the standing position and the procedure is carried out from behind. Again it is essential to ensure both testes are in the scrotum. Each cord is crushed twice and the castrators must be kept closed for five seconds each time. The constrictions on each side should be at different levels.

(3) Surgical castration. Local anaesthetic is injected into the body of the testis. The site is disinfected and an incision is made through the wall of the scrotum, the testis is withdrawn and is gently pulled out. The pull causes the spermatic cord to separate and blood the blood vessels to seal. The operation continues on the other side. It is important to carry out the procedure in clean conditions using no-touch techniques.

Various Acts of Parliament control castrations. The Protection of Animals Act 1911 and the Protection of Animals (Scotland) Act 1912 require operations on animals to be carried out with due care and humanity. The Protection of Animals (Anaesthetics) Acts 1954 make it an offence to use methods which constrict the flow of blood to the scrotum (e.g. rubber-ring method) after an animal is one week old. These acts also make it an offence to castrate a bull over the age of two months without anaesthesia.

The Veterinary Surgeons Act 1966 makes it an offence for anyone other than a veterinary surgeon to castrate a bull over two months of age.

Disbudding

Horns on cattle can cause damage to other animals and to their handlers, it is therefore common practice to remove the horn buds in young animals in order to prevent the horns developing. It is possible to do this by applying a chemical cauterising agent if this is applied in the first week of life, but the welfare codes strongly recommend that it is not used.

A more widely used method of bud removal is to burn out the tissue which gives rise to the horn with a hot iron. The area around the horn bud is rendered insensitive by administering a local anaesthetic to the nerve which supplies the area. A hot iron is then used to burn into the tissue surrounding the horn bud. The tissue must be burned to a depth of about 2.5 mm and usually the bud is removed. The iron used resembles a soldering iron but has a ring bit; it can be heated by gas or electricity. After the removal of the bud the area is dressed with an antibiotic and may need analgesic when the local anaesthetic wears off. This technique should only be used by a trained and competent person.

Foot care

Cattle damage their feet in a variety of ways. They may slip in sheds or milking parlours, they may tread on sharp objects, or they may spend too long in wet fields causing the horn to macerate. The hoof may overgrow forcing the animal to walk in an abnormal manner.

Once the foot is damaged the animal not only has the pain of the injury but also has difficulty in moving about to find food. Minor foot problems which are not noticed may develop into major conditions which result in the animal having to be slaughtered.

The most important element in foot care is regular cleaning and trimming of feet. Cattle rarely allow their feet to be lifted up so to do the job efficiently a cattle crush is required which will enable the feet to be tied up for attention.

Feet should be trimmed so that the weight is evenly distributed on the whole of the sole. Hoof knives and hoof clippers can be used to carry out foot trimming. It is a skill that can be readily acquired but the risks of causing serious lameness if it is done incorrectly are great so it is essential that the skill is gained under supervision.

Identification, records and movement

Recent catastrophic health and welfare issues relating to farm animals (e.g. BSE and Foot and Mouth disease), have led to a tightening of farm animal health control legislation. A cattle tracing system is now operated by a section of DEFRA, the British Cattle Movement Service (BCMS). The system allows government to:

- check which animals are present on any holding;
- check where an animal has been during its life;
- trace animals exposed to a disease risk;
- give assurances to buyers about an animal's life history.

Several elements go together to make the system work – tagging, farm records, cattle passports and notification of movements.

Tagging

Each animal must be identified with two ear tags, one in each ear. One of these tags, the primary tag, must be of a prescribed size and must bear a crown, the letter UK and a unique identification number. The other tag, the secondary tag, must contain the same information but may also contain additional information required by the owner. Since 1998 the tags must be yellow (Figure 19.4).

Tags can only be purchased from manufacturers approved by DEFRA. The owner of the cattle orders the tags. The manufacturers notify the government's

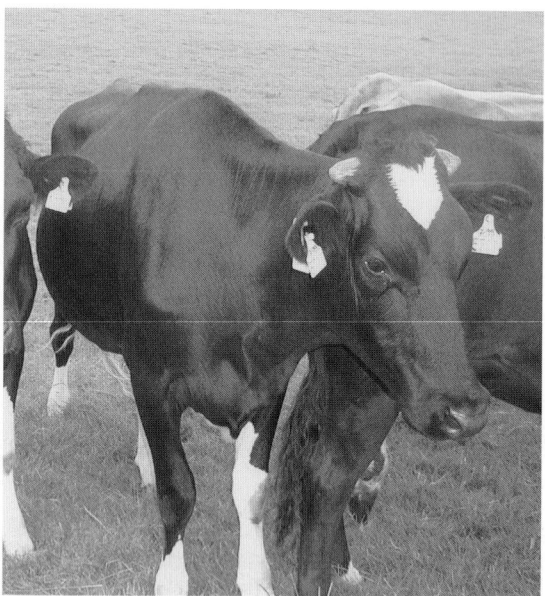

Figure 19.4   Cow with yellow ear tags.

ear tag allocation system who allocate unique numbers crossed-referenced with the farm address. Only one year's supply of tags can be purchased at any one time.

Dairy cattle must have at least one tag fitted within thirty-six hours of being born and all cattle must have both fitted within twenty days of birth.

Passports

All cattle must have a passport which records where they have been throughout their lives.

Herd register

All keepers of cattle must record every birth, every movement on or off their premises and every death of their animals.

Notification of movement

Keepers of cattle must notify BCMS of all movements of their animals, e.g. on and off the premises, to and from markets and to slaughterhouses.

Movement of cattle has to be done under a licence from DEFRA. There are two types of licence, a general licence and an individual licence. The general licence allows movement without applying for permission every time an animal is moved. DEFRA inspectors visit premises on a random basis to ensure the rules of the licence are being obeyed. If they are not then the general licence can be revoked. In this case individual movement licences must be applied for every time an animal is moved anywhere.

One of the important rules under the licence is that six days must elapse from one animal arriving at a premises to any other animal leaving (referred to as a six-day standstill). More details can be obtained from the DEFRA website (www.defra.gov.uk).

Health

Signs of ill health in cattle are similar to any animals, e.g. abnormal gait, isolation from other herd members, unexpected aggression, poor coat condition, discharges. The normal rectal temperature of a cow is 38.5 °C.

Dairy cows are at risk of certain diseases connected to high milk yield e.g. mastitis (inflammation of the udder) and milk fever (hypocalcaemia – lowered blood calcium levels around the time of calving leading to a lack of muscle function). All cattle are at risk of a range of infectious and non-infectious diseases. A veterinary surgeon can advise on an appropriate vaccination programme to protect animals against those diseases prevalent in the geographical area. They will also advise on appropriate protection against internal and external parasites. Further consideration of cattle diseases goes beyond the scope of this book; for further information see Blowey (1999).

References and further reading

Blowey, R.W. (1999) *A Veterinary Book for Dairy Farmers* (3rd edn). Farming Press, Ipswich, UK.

DEFRA (2003) *Code of Recommendations for the Welfare of Livestock, Cattle.* DEFRA Publications, London.

Home Office (1989) *Code of Practice for the Housing and Care of Animals used in Scientific Procedures.* HMSO, London.

Spedding, C. (Ed.) (1983) *Fream's Agriculture.* John Murray, London.

20
Sheep

Sarah Lane

Introduction

Sheep, like goats and cattle, are ruminants, they spend a large part of the day eating fodder and chewing the cud. The classification of sheep is given in Table 20.1. Sheep breeds are classified according to the type of land they occupy, that is hill or mountain breeds found on high lands, and lowland breeds which live on the richer lowland pastures. Hill breeds dominate the flock in the UK and it is these ewes that are used as the mothers of the crossbred sheep found mostly on the lowlands and better uplands. This crossbred type combines the mothering and foraging ability of the hill breeds with the greater prolificacy and size of the lowland breed rams such as the Blue-faced Leicester or Border Leicester. Cross breeding is unique to the UK and provides sheep which are ideal for heavy stocking on lowland pastures.

Sheep are mainly farmed for their meat and, to a lesser degree, their wool, with some specialised milking units.

Terms specifically used in relation to sheep are given in Table 20.2.

Breeds of sheep

Hill breeds

These are small, hardy, active animals. They are able to withstand the long, cold winters and short summers characteristic of hilly regions. They are slow to mature and produce fewer lambs. Commonly, these animals roam over large areas to obtain their food and are adept at finding shelter. They are usually only brought down to the farm for specific purposes such

Table 20.1 Classification of sheep *Ovis aries*.

Kingdom	Animalia
Phylum	Chordata
Sub-phylum	Vertebrata
Class	Mammalia
Order	Artiodactyla
Family	Ovidae
Genus and species	*Ovis aries*

Table 20. 2 Sheep terms.

Ewe	Adult female sheep
Ram or tup	Entire male sheep
Lamb	Young male or female under 6 months old
Hogg	Male or female between weaning and first shearing
Gimmer	Female between first and second shearing
Wether or wedder	Castrated male
Tupping	Mating
Folding	The use of temporary fencing to give access to small areas of forage crops, e.g. swedes, rape or kale

as lambing and selecting for market. Farmers do not generally supplement their feeding and do not have to spend much time and effort fertilising the land, it is an example of low input, low output farming.

The wool from these breeds is coarse and light and is generally used for carpets and tweeds. The carcass quality is good, as it is leaner than that of lowland breeds.

Examples of hill breeds are:

- Welsh Mountain (Figure 20.1);
- Scottish Blackface;
- Swaledale.

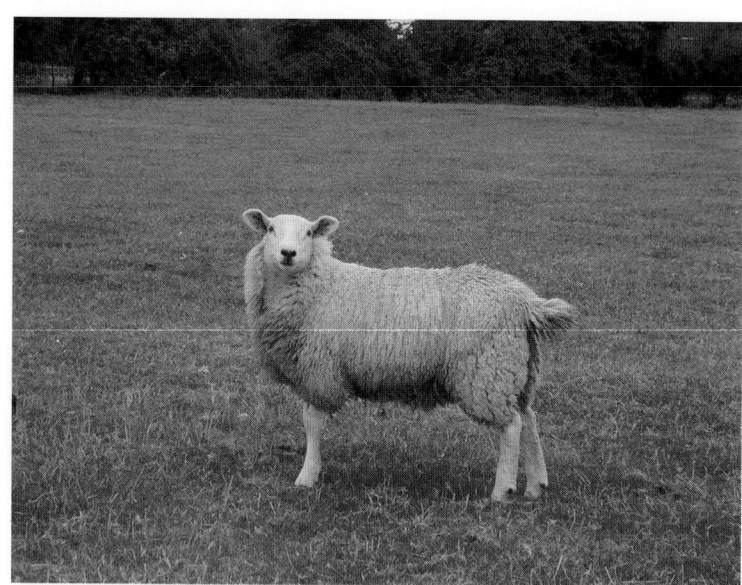

Figure 20.1   Welsh Mountain sheep.

Lowland breeds

These include Longwool and Down breeds. They are kept in more intensive conditions, with good pasture and supplementary concentrate rations available. As a result they produce more lambs which develop faster than hill breeds.

Longwools

These are large with heavy fleeces but their meat is comparatively poor. They are prolific breeders and produce good quantities of milk. The rams are used to cross with other breeds, especially hill breeds, to increase the size and number of lambs they produce. Examples of longwool breeds are:

- Border Leicester;
- Leicester;
- Romney Marsh.

Downs

Downs vary in size and are all polled (hornless). Their meat and wool are of superior quality. The lambs mature early and have good growth rates. Examples of down breeds are:

- Dorset Down;
- Southdown (Figure 20.2);
- Suffolk (Figure 20.2).

Use in regulated procedures

A relatively small number of sheep are used in regulated procedures in the UK, 38 371 in 2003, of which 254 were genetically altered. Genetically altered sheep are listed on Schedule 2 of the Animals (Scientific Procedures) Act 1986 and must be obtained from designated breeders or suppliers. Non-genetically altered sheep can be obtained directly from any sheep breeder. They are used in biomedical research for nutrition and lactation trials, in models of asthma, for foetal medicine research, and for polyclonal antibody production where the antibodies are harvested from the milk. They are also used for experimental surgery because they are a convenient size and their organ size is similar to man.

The various characteristics of the different breeds and crossbreeds available make them especially suited to particular uses in research, for example size and temperament, fleece length or absence of horns.

Environment

Like other farm species, if sheep are part of a scientific procedure they must be kept in accordance with the Home Office codes of practice (Home Office 1989). Otherwise they must be kept in accordance with

Figure 20.2 Southdown ram in front, Suffolk rams with black faces.

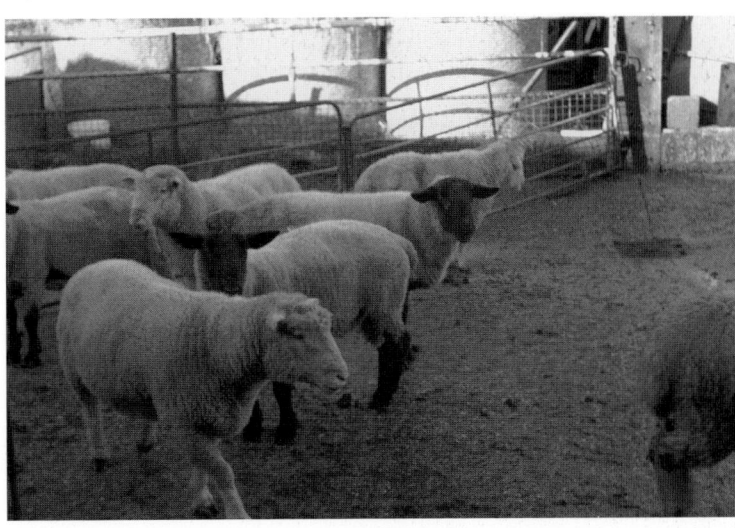

Table 20.3 Environmental levels for sheep housed indoors in scientific procedure establishments (Home Office 1989).

Temperature	10–24 °C depending on fleece length
Relative humidity	55% ± 10%
Photoperiod	Natural light periods
Light intensity	350–400 lux at bench level
Air changes per hour	Sufficient to provide fresh air and prevent build up of noxious odours

agricultural welfare legislation (see Chapter 18) as described in the DEFRA Code of Recommendations for the Welfare of Livestock, Sheep (DEFRA 2003). Environmental levels for sheep housed indoors in scientific procedure establishments are given in Table 20.3.

When housed indoors sheep do not normally require a temperature which is higher than outside. Effective ventilation with good air movement is necessary to prevent a build up of humidity and condensation. Draughts should be avoided, as sheep are particularly susceptible to respiratory diseases. If housed outdoors ambient temperature applies.

The DEFRA welfare codes for sheep on agricultural premises state that air circulation, dust levels, temperature, relative humidity and gas concentrations should be within limits which are not harmful. The ventilation system must permit the free circulation of air above sheep height and avoid drafts at sheep level. In basic farm buildings this can be achieved by building solid walls to a height of about 1.25 m with space boarding above that (Figure 20.3).

There must be sufficient lighting in these buildings to meet the physiological and behavioural needs of the animals. If natural light is insufficient for this, additional artificial lighting must be provided. Enough lighting must be available to enable all animals to be seen and inspected at any time.

Housing

The stocking densities for animals housed in scientific procedure establishments can be found in the current Home Office code of practice (1989). Space allowances for sheep housed on agricultural premises are stated in the DEFRA welfare code (DEFRA 2003a).

Outdoor housing

Permanent fencing, using wire mesh and concrete, metal or wooden posts, can be used to contain sheep. The fence should be a minimum of 1.2 m high and have a mesh size of 0.31 m. Alternatively, electric fencing can be used (except for horned sheep) but must be designed, installed and maintained so that contact with the fence will not cause more than momentary discomfort to the sheep. Animals housed outside must be able to shelter from adverse weather conditions.

Indoor housing

Sheep can be housed in loose boxes, barns or pens constructed so as not to cause any discomfort or injury to the animal. If they have to be housed on their own, e.g. surgically prepared animals, they should

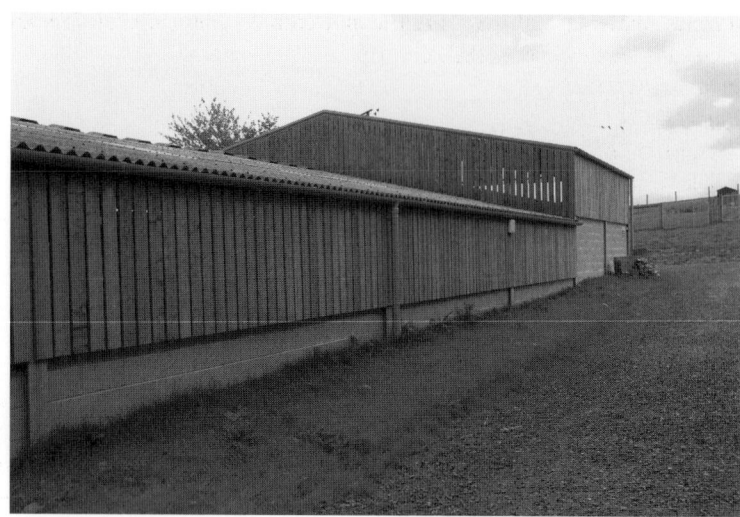

Figure 20.3 Space boarding above solid walls.

be in sight and sound of other sheep. All internal surfaces should be made from materials which can be cleaned easily and disinfected and can be replaced easily if necessary.

Floors can be solid or made from wooden slats. If the floor is slatted the gap between slats should be no more than 16 mm. Slatted floors tend to be less labour intensive as they can be hosed down or mechanically scraped. This type of floor provides no comfort or insulation for the animal and should not be used for newly born or young lambs.

Solid floors must be well drained and the sheep should be provided with some form of dry bedding. It is important to maintain dry, clean, comfortable conditions underfoot as wet and dirty floors may lead to foot-rot. Sawdust or straw can be used as bedding material. Pens bedded with sawdust should be cleaned out every other day and those bedded on straw twice weekly.

Feeding and watering

Sheep should have access to sufficient food and fresh, clean water at all times. Ruminants do well with cellulose, starch or sugar as an energy source, and a nitrogen source, which need not be a protein. The energy source may be calculated in terms of metabolisable energy (ME), digestible energy (DE), starch equivalents (SE) or total digestible nutrients (TDN). The protein is calculated as crude protein or digestible protein (see Chapter 26). Straw has the lowest energy content and grasses the highest.

Hay is still the preferred foodstuff, although grass silage may be fed to sheep housed indoors. An adult sheep will consume approximately 0.9–1 kg/day. This amount will satisfy their maintenance needs and provide some production ration. Growing lambs and pregnant ewes will need extra production rations and these can be provided as cereal-based concentrates, which will contain adequate levels of vitamins, minerals and trace elements.

The use of condition scoring in sheep is a practical method of appraising the fatness or thinness of the animal so that those which require improved nutrition can be housed together. Condition scoring gives a clear indication as to whether ewes, especially those on hill farms, are fit enough to withstand the winter if they are returned to the hill. Body condition is assessed by handling the ewe over and around the backbone, in the area of the loin behind the last rib, and by assessing the amount of fat and muscle under the ends of the bones. The ewes are then scored between 0 and 5, score 1 being when the spine feels sharp, muscle on the back shallow and an absence of fat, and score 5 being where the spine cannot be felt and there is a very thick deposit of fat over the rump and tail.

Feeding is usually increased prior to the breeding season, to improve body condition, increase conception rates and the chance of multiple births. This practice is called 'flushing'.

Clean water should be available at all times. Water troughs and bowls should be constructed and sited so that fouling is avoided and to minimise the risk of freezing in cold weather. Automatic watering should be checked regularly to ensure it is in working order. An adult sheep will drink about 4.5 litres of water a day.

There should be sufficient feeding space to allow group-housed animals to feed together (at least 0.35 m per sheep). Hay racks should be constructed and positioned to avoid the risk of injury.

Sheep kept outside are often 'folded' on root crops in autumn and winter, but they must have a clean area on which to lie down. Sheep will generally do better on legumes than grasses, so a mixture such as rye grass and white clover will achieve the best total production, i.e. body weight and fleece.

Creep or strip-grazing management systems can be used to increase stocking rates. One system is to keep ewes on higher marginal land, leaving the lower, better quality grazing for the growing stock. Bringing the sheep in over winter (in-wintering) is becoming more popular as it prevents wastage of grass by trampling or over grazing.

Breeding

Sheep are seasonal breeders and during the season the ewes are polyoestrous. The season lasts from late summer to early winter in most breeds. One breed, the Dorset Horn, has a season which lasts from July to May and is able to have up to three lambings in two years rather than the one lambing a year of other breeds. Breeding data are given in Table 20.4. All data

in the chart are approximate, there are considerable breed differences.

Mating

Before being put together for mating, the body condition, genitalia, feet and teeth of both ewes and rams must be inspected to ensure they are fit for breeding. Damaged feet and poor dentition reduce the animal's ability to find and eat food and therefore affects its welfare.

Flock mating is the most commonly used method of mating with a ratio of one ram to thirty-five to forty ewes. The ewe will stand close to the ram and will allow herself to be mated and as many as 75% of ewes will seek out the ram. The rams are fitted with a raddle, a harness holding a coloured marker (Figure 20.4), or alternatively a greasy paint applied to the sternum (Figure 20.5) both of which leave a coloured mark on the rump of the ewe when she has been mounted. The colour of the raddle marker or paint is changed every sixteen days so that the oestrus when the ewe was mated can be identified.

Table 20.4 Summary of breeding data for sheep.

Average age at sexual maturity	7–10 months
Age at first use: hill breeds (female)	18 months
Age at first use: lowland breeds (female)	12 months
Age at first use: rams	8–9 months
Average length of oestrous cycle	16–17 days
Average length of oestrus	1–3 days
Mechanism of ovulation	Spontaneous
Gestation period	147 days
Birth weight: lowland twins	3–4 kg
Birth weight: singles	4.5 kg
Litter size: hill breeds	1
Litter size: lowland breeds	2–3
Return to oestrus post partum	Next season

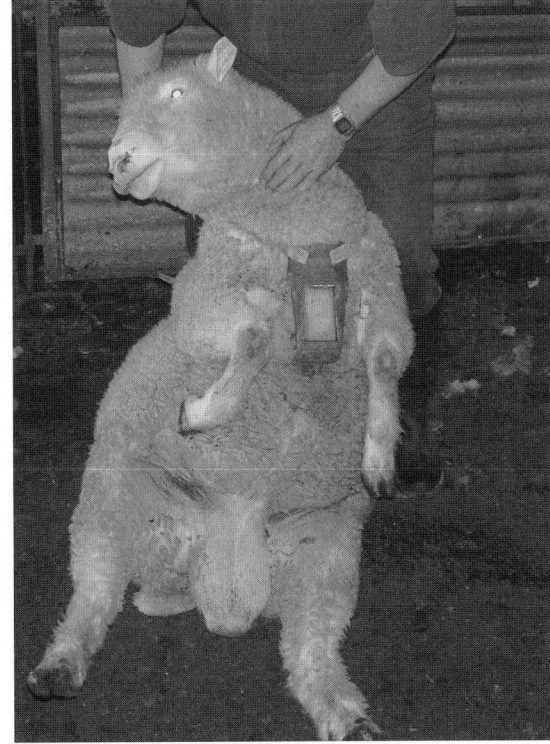

Figure 20.4 Ram fitted with raddle.

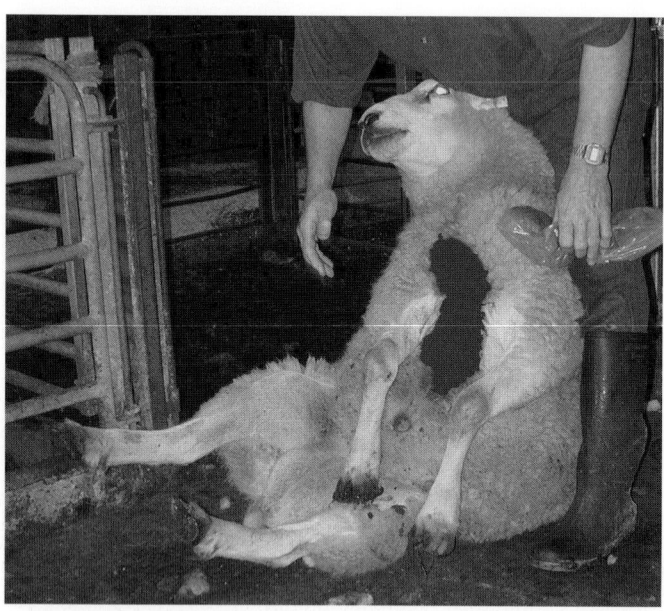

Figure 20.5　Paint applied to the sternum.

Artificial insemination can be used with sheep but is not common because of its cost and because there are no clearly identified external signs of oestrus in the ewe other than a willingness to mate. Oestrus is synchronised so that batches of ewes can be mated within a few days of each other. This can be achieved in the following ways:

- Vasectomised rams: being mounted by a ram tends to stimulate the ewe to come into oestrus. Three weeks before the entire rams are to be introduced, a vasectomised ram is placed with them. His mounting ensures the ewes will be ready for the entire male.

- Hormone sponges: a progesterone-impregnated sponge is placed in the vagina of the ewe. It is left in for fourteen days then removed, oestrus occurs 24–48 hours after its removal. The mating season can be brought forward if the sponge treatment is followed with an intra-muscular injection of luteinising hormone.

Pregnancy and parturition

Non return of oestrus and failure to mate at next oestrus are indicators of pregnancy. Ultrasound, used at twenty-eight days post mating, provides a reliable method of confirming pregnancy. Ultrasound carried out between 80–100 days will show the difference between singles and twins. An indication of the number of lambs being carried by the ewe is important as it enables the shepherd to adjust her food intake.

When parturition is imminent, the ewe will separate herself from the rest of the flock. She will lie down with her head in the air and will begin to strain. The amniotic sac ruptures within one or two hours and the lamb is born soon after. Subsequent lambs are born after the ewe has cleaned the previous one. It is usual to bring the ewes into a barn to give birth.

Lambs

As with all animals, it is essential that the lambs get an early supply of colostrum. Some shepherds will milk colostrum from the ewe and dose the lamb with a stomach tube. The lamb(s) and ewe are housed together so that they can bond. Where possible, lambs should be put onto clean pasture with their ewes.

Orphaned lambs can be fostered onto ewes which have lost their young. This has to be done carefully as ewes will attack lambs other than their own. The skin of the dead lamb can be removed and placed onto the orphan to fool the ewe into thinking it is her own. The skin is left on until the orphan has taken in enough of the ewe's milk to take on her odour.

Artificial rearing

It is possible to rear orphaned lambs by hand using bottles or on automatic feeding devices as described for calves in Chapter 19.

Lambs need ewe milk. Replacer ewe milk has a different composition to cow's milk, therefore cow milk replacer is not nutritionally suitable for lambs.

Milk should be fed at a rate of 0.57 litres per day in four feeds rising to 1.14 litres per day at five weeks of age until weaning. Weaning age varies but is usually complete between twelve and sixteen weeks. Good hay and lamb concentrates should be available from a few days old.

Procedures

Lambs, like most other young farm animals, are subject to a number of procedures early in life.

Castration

The DEFRA welfare code says that castration should only be carried out where absolutely necessary, for instance where problems might arise if entire males are kept after they become sexually mature. There should be no reason to castrate males which will be sent to slaughter before reaching puberty. Lambs, up to three months of age, can be castrated by a trained, competent person, after that time it must be carried out under anaesthesia by a veterinary surgeon. The methods used are the same as those described for calves.

Tail docking

The main reason for tail docking is to help keep the area around the anus free from faeces, and therefore prevent fly strike (see External parasites, p. 138). Again the DEFRA welfare codes say this should only be done if failure to do so would lead to welfare problems. It is rarely done to hill breeds as the risk of fly strike is much lower on high land and a wool-covered tail provides extra protection from the winter weather. Tail docking may be performed by the application of a rubber ring between the coccygeal vertebrae. This cuts off the blood supply to the tail causing it to atrophy and drop off after a few weeks. Enough tail must be left to cover both the anus in the male and the vulva in the female. The rubber ring must be put on in the first week of life.

Surgical methods of tail removal, which may be necessary if the animal is injured, must be carried out by a veterinary surgeon.

Disbudding

Disbudding is not usually considered necessary for lambs. If welfare concerns make it necessary it must be carried out by a veterinary surgeon.

Health

Sheep must be inspected regularly for signs of ill health or injury. Both the Animals (Scientific Procedures) Act 1986 and the Welfare of Farmed Animals (England) Regulations 2000 require health records to be kept. Animals kept outdoors will require frequent observation during lambing, and before and after shearing and dipping. A written health and welfare programme must be established for all animals, covering a whole year. The health programme will detail the timings of health inspections, vaccinations, foot care, parasite treatments etc.

A well-designed set of handling pens will assist the close inspection of the flock and aid routine tasks throughout the year, e.g. vaccinations, worming and foot trimming. Care should be taken to ensure that these routine tasks are performed correctly and the equipment used correctly to limit potential welfare problems, such as abscesses after vaccinations and damage to the feet after trimming. Figure 20.6 shows a handling device which allows sheep to be restrained and moved, to enable access to all parts of the body with minimal disturbance to the animal.

Sheep should never be caught by the fleece alone and should never be lifted by the tail, fleece or horns. Animals should be handled gently and restrained by placing a hand or arm under the neck and holding the neck fleece if necessary, with the other arm placed on or around the rear of the sheep.

Diseases

Sheep are susceptible to a range of diseases; some important examples are mentioned here, others can be found in Fraser & Stamp (1987).

Lameness

This is usually due to foot-rot, an infectious disease

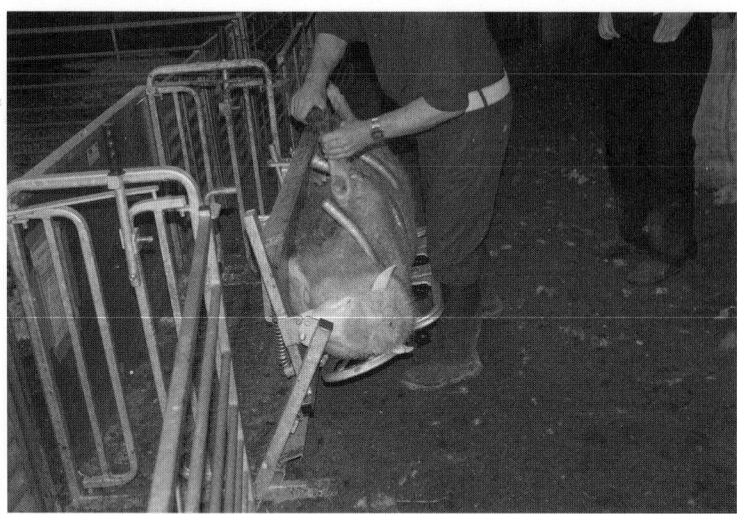

Figure 20.6 Sheep restrained and turned over for feet trimming.

common in poorly drained pastures or damp sheep pens. The organism primarily responsible is *Dichelobacter nodosus*, which is able to get under the hoof if it is damaged or soft due to being kept on wet ground. Foot-rot can be prevented by regular trimming of the feet, once every six to eight weeks or by vaccination.

Clostridial diseases

Sheep may suffer from a number of diseases caused by various species of the bacterial genus *Clostridium*, e.g. tetanus and enterotoxaemia. These diseases can be controlled by vaccination. Veterinary surgeons can advise on the appropriate vaccination programme.

Parasites

Internal parasites

Sheep should be routinely treated for internal parasites by the use of oral or parenteral anthelmintics. Grassland should be rotated to provide clean grazing areas and lambs should be turned out onto these clean areas before the remainder of the flock. Excessive or inappropriate use of anthelmintic drugs may lead to resistance. This can be avoided by alternating types of anthelmintics and by using rotational grazing systems. Veterinary surgeons will advise on the most appropriate treatment.

External parasites

Ectoparasites also present a risk to the health of sheep. Sheep scab (see Chapter 34 on parasitology) and fly strike being the most common.

Fly strike is caused by an infestation by the larvae of blowfly or green-bottles. This normally occurs in the spring when sheep are turned out onto new, lush grass which causes scouring. The flies are attracted to the smell and lay their eggs in the stained wool around the anus. Where there is sufficient moisture, the eggs can hatch within twelve hours and the larvae will burrow into the skin causing raw areas. Clinical signs include tail wagging, withdrawal from the flock and a characteristic odour. Unless the animal is treated death may occur within a week. Sheep can be treated with a dressing, which will kill the larvae. Prevention is by dagging or crutching (removal of the fleece from around the anus) or by spraying or dipping with insecticides.

Dipping consists of putting the sheep into a bath consisting of an insecticide compound. The sheep must be in the dip for a minimum of one minute and the head must be completely immersed at least once. The design of the dip will depend on various factors, including the number of animals, and land and materials available. Generally, the sheep will have a sudden drop into the dip and a steady climb out. Those sheep which have just travelled or have open wounds or sores, or have just been sheared should not be dipped.

Shearing

Shearing is the removal of the fleece, at least once a year, by mechanical or chemical methods. Mechanical shearing either by hand or machine is the most common method used, generally leaving a fleece length of approximately 6 mm. Chemical shearing may well become the preferred and most economical method of the future. Three drugs have been identified, including cyclophosphamide, which causes the wool to loosen so that it can be easily plucked. For those sheep housed outdoors, the usual time of year for shearing is between May and July. Sheep housed indoors can be sheared again in the winter. Care must be taken to avoid nicking or cutting the skin, or nipples, (remember that males also have nipples) and any wounds should receive immediate attention. All shearing equipment should be disinfected between flocks.

Identification, records and movement

All sheep and goats must be identified by the time they are twelve months old or before they are moved to another holding or to slaughter. The identification must be by ear tag, on which will be the letters UK, the herd/flock mark and the animal's unique number.

If sheep and goats are moved onto other premises they must have another tag (called the S tag) which has an 'S' followed by the mark indicating the flock or herd from which it originated.

Further information on identification can be obtained from the DEFRA website (DEFRA 2003b; www.defra.gov.uk). This site should be consulted as the regulations on identification may change.

Ear tags are required for official identification as described above. Care should be taken when fitting the tags to minimise the risk of infection or fly strike. Paints can be used as temporary methods of identification.

Records and movements

By the end of January each year the total number of sheep or goats that were on the premises on the 1st January must be recorded. Records must also be kept of all animals moved onto or off the premises. These movements must be entered within thirty-six hours of them taking place. The person who receives the animals must report the movement to their local authority within three days.

References and further reading

DEFRA (2003a) *Code of Recommendations for the Welfare of Livestock, Sheep.* DEFRA publications, London. www.defra.gov.uk

DEFRA (2003b) *Rules for Livestock Movements.* DEFRA Publications, London. www.defra.gov.uk

Fraser, A. and Stamp, J.T. (1987) *Sheep Husbandry and Diseases.* Blackwell Science, Oxford.

Home Office (1989) *Code of Practice for the Housing and Care of Animals used in Scientific Procedures.* HMSO, London.

21

Goats

Stephen W. Barnett

Introduction

Goats are the third of the ruminant species dealt with in this book. Unlike sheep and cattle in the wild they are browsers not grazers. They use their mobile lips to obtain leaves and shoots from inaccessible places and are able to survive difficult mountainous landscapes and live on poor quality food. Classification for goats is given in Table 21.1.

Although there are breeds of goat which live in extremes of temperatures, some in deserts others in very cold conditions, domestic animals in the UK are likely to be more sensitive to adverse weather conditions and will need to be provided with shelter during the cold weather. They are inquisitive animals (a characteristic that has led to their reputation of trying to eat everything) and readily accept contact with humans.

Commercially, they are farmed for milk, meat and skin. Goat meat has not been widely consumed in the UK but its use is increasing and it is popular with some sections of the population.

Terms used in connection with goat farming are explained in Table 21.2.

Breeds

There are many different breeds of goat. Farmers select the breeds they wish to use on the basis of milk yield, milk quality, size of animal and personal preference. Examples of breeds are:

- Saanen (Figure 21.1);
- Anglo-Nubian (Figure 21.2);
- Toggenburg (Figure 21.3).

Table 21.1 Classification of goats *Capra hircus*.

Kingdom	Animalia
Phylum	Chordata
Sub-phylum	Vertebrata
Class	Mammalia
Order	Artiodactyla
Family	Capridae
Genus and species	*Capra hircus*

Table 21.2 Terms used in goat farming.

Kid	Goat up to 6 months of age
Goatling	Female from 6 months to 2 years of age
Buckling	Male from 6 months to 2 years of age
Nanny	Adult female
Billy	Adult male
Wedder or wether	Castrated male

Use in regulated procedures

Goats are used in respiratory studies and to raise antisera. Some experimental studies seek to improve lactation, reproduction and husbandry of goats.

Environment

The notes and the environmental levels described in Chapter 20 on sheep apply to goats. DEFRA has published a *Code of Recommendations for the Welfare of Livestock, Goats* (DEFRA 1989).

Housing

Space allowance for goats housed in scientific

Figure 21.1   Saanen goat.

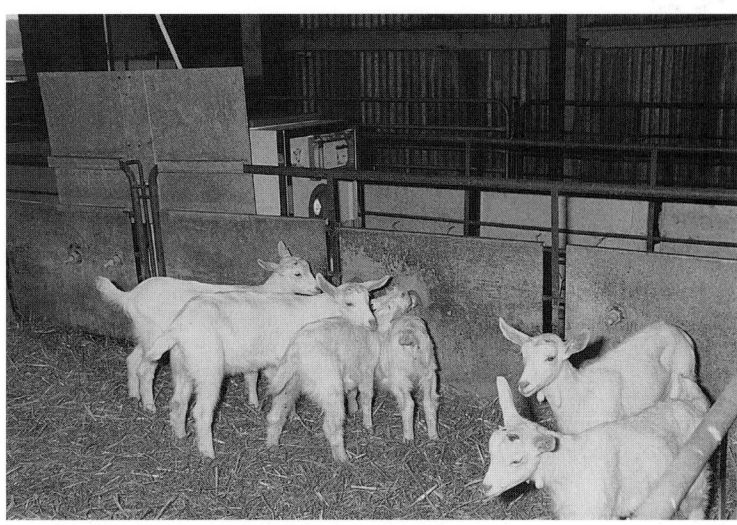

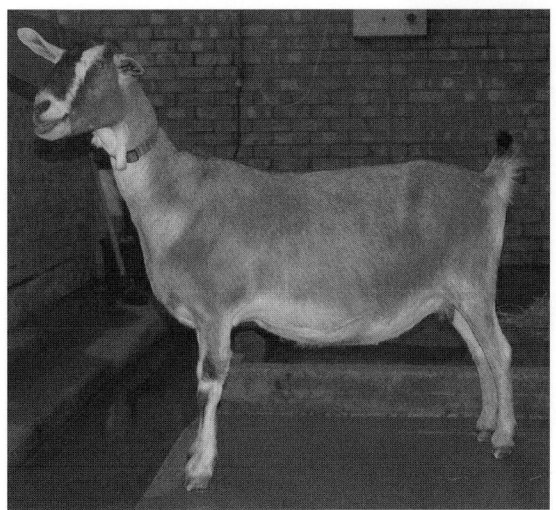

Figure 21.2   Anglo-Nubian goat.

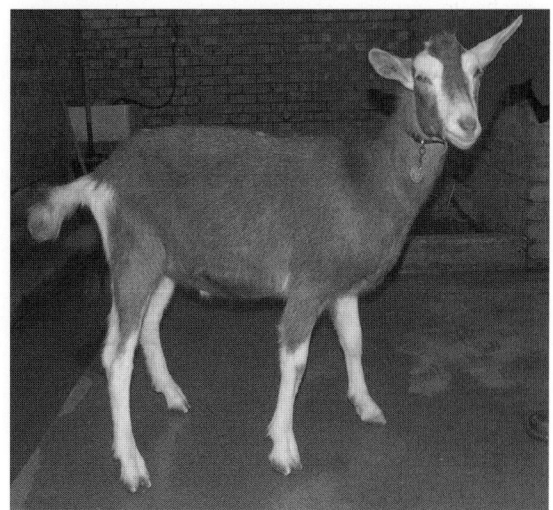

Figure 21.3   Toggenberg goat.

procedure establishments are listed in the current Home Office code of practice (Home Office 1989).

Indoor housing

Goats can be housed in barns, loose boxes and pens (Figure 21.4). Environmental enrichment items can be suspended into the pens; the balls in Figure 21.5 contain food treats. Goats can use their mobile lips to undo door fastenings so these must be placed out of

their reach. They are also able to squeeze through quite small gaps, so if metal bars are used as pen dividers they must be placed close together. Floors should be kept dry, with straw or wood chips for bedding. Normally females and young goats must be housed in groups. If, for experimental reasons, animals have to be housed alone they should be able see other goats and must get extra human contact. Billy goats may be housed alone but these too must be

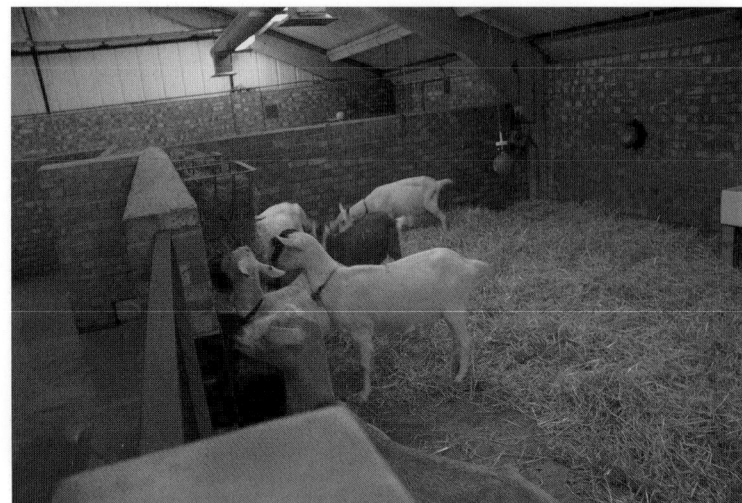

Figure 21.4   Goats in deep litter pens.

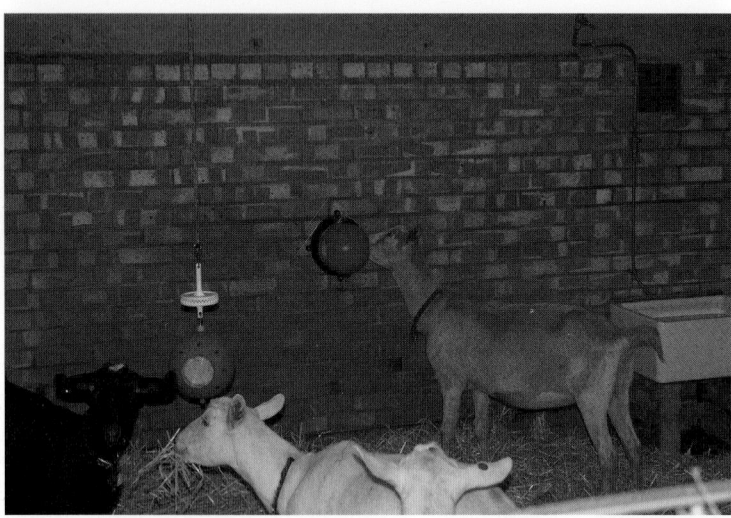

Figure 21.5   Pen with suspended environmental enrichment items.

within sight and sound of other goats. All housed animals should have access to exercise areas. Horned and polled animals should not be housed together unless they have been reared together.

Outside housing

Goats are very agile and are able to climb and jump. Fences should be at least 1.2 m high to prevent them escaping. Troughs and other furniture must be placed away from fences where they could be used to help them clamber over. Climbing frames can be placed in the paddock to add interest for the animals (Figure 21.6). Electric fences can be used but if they are of the mesh type there is a risk of animals getting caught so they should not be used for horned or young animals.

As goats are browsing animals extra care must be taken to ensure poisonous plants, such as yew and laurel (see pp. 113–114), do not overhang the pasture from neighbouring fields.

Feeding and watering

The bulk of feeding is in the form of hay. Good quality hay should provide all the animal's maintenance

Figure 21.6 Climbing frame in goat paddock.

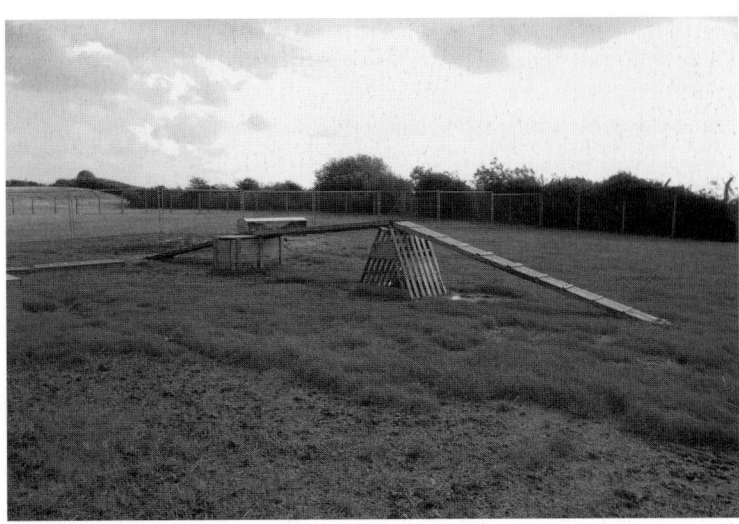

requirements. As a guide, a 45 kg goat will require 1 kg hay per day and a 64 kg goat 1.6 kg of hay. In the spring and summer they can be placed on pasture when grass will provide enough nutrition for their maintenance and part of their production ration. Change from hay feeding to grass feeding needs to done gradually or the animals will suffer digestive upset.

Milking goats will need the addition of concentrate rations, roughly 0.45 kg of concentrates per litre of milk produced should be provided. Pregnant nannies are fed maintenance rations up to eight weeks before kidding, the concentrates are added at a rate of 0.25–0.5 kg per day. All of these quantities are guides only, they are dependent on the size of the goat and the number of young they are carrying. As with all animals the condition of the individual animal must be monitored and the amount of food offered adjusted accordingly.

Hay can be provided in racks and concentrates in troughs, sufficient feeding areas must be provided to ensure all animals get sufficient access; 0.35 m of trough or rack per goat is recommended. Goats will not eat stale or soiled food so old food should be removed.

Water should be provided *ad libitum*, the water troughs should be kept clean and be checked at least once a day to ensure there is sufficient supply. Dry goats need a minimum of 0.61 litres per day and lactating goats between 3.5–6 litres. It has been suggested that food and water should be offered on opposite sides of the housing to reduce the chance of one being contaminated by the other.

Breeding

Goats are seasonal breeders, in temperate zones they come into breeding condition in September and the season ends in February. During this time they continue to cycle every eighteen to twenty-one days if not mated. Breeding data is given in Table 21.3.

Mating

Flock mating can be used where the billy is placed with a herd of nannies and he will mate them when they come into oestrus.

Table 21.3 Summary of breeding data for goats.

Average age at sexual maturity	6 months
Age at first use: female	15–18 months
Age at first use: male	12 months
Average length of oestrous cycle	18–21 days
Average length of oestrus	18–36 hours
Range of oestrus	12–96 hours
Mechanism of ovulation	Spontaneous
Gestation period	150 ± 4 days
Birth weight	3–4 kg
Litter size	2–3
Return to oestrus post partum	Next season
Length of lactation	Variable, 10 months is aimed for

Arranged mating is used when it is necessary to know the exact time of parturition. The female is taken to the male when oestrus is identified. Oestrus is indicated by a red, swollen vulva with a slight, colourless discharge. The nanny is often restless and she bleats and wags her tail. On average, oestrus lasts for eighteen to thirty-six hours but in some animals it can be shorter or much longer (12–96 hours).

When first put together the male and female may mock fight but this is only a form of courtship. When mating takes place it is very quick and is accomplished by a single thrust.

Artificial insemination can also be used.

Pregnancy and parturition

On average, pregnancy lasts 150 days but there are breed differences. Pregnancy can be identified by the use of an ultrasound probe placed against the wall of the abdomen. It can be used at approximately 60 days of pregnancy. In lactating goats, milk samples can be assessed for hormone levels at 50 days post mating. In the later stages of pregnancy the foetus can be palpated through the wall of the abdomen.

Approximately fourteen days before the female is due to kid she should be moved inside in a well bedded pen with room for exercise. Shortly before parturition begins (eighteen to twenty-four hours) the udder fills rapidly with milk and the tissue around the vulva becomes slack. Straining begins and the kids start to be born approximately four hours later. The placenta should be passed between thirty minutes and four hours after the last kid is born. Veterinary help should be called if the nanny has prolonged labour or the placenta is not passed within a reasonable time. Like other animals the nanny licks the kid clean when it is born (Figure 21.7).

Pseudopregnancy

Pseudopregnancy is relatively common in goats. All the normal signs of pregnancy are seen but at the time of the birth only fluid is expelled from the uterus. The condition is commonly called 'cloudburst'. Nannies continue to lactate and achieve a reasonable yield after pseudopregnancy.

Kids

Kids must be seen to consume colostrum within six hours of birth. They may be left with their nannies for the first six weeks of life, she may produce more milk than the kids can consume so the excess must be milked off. From six weeks on the kid can be

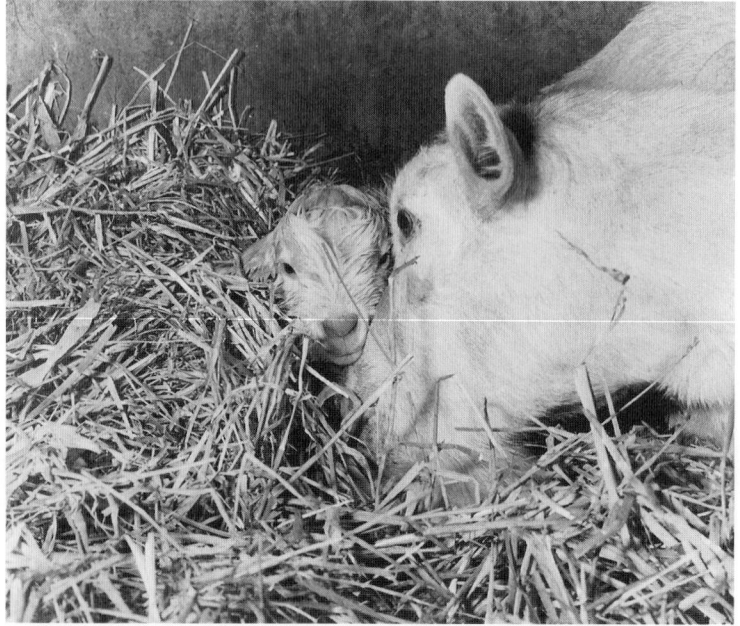

Figure 21.7 Newborn kid.

separated for part of the day from the nanny. The kids should have access to good quality forage and concentrates while separated and the nanny will be partially milked. The amount milked off will increase until weaning is completed at ten weeks of age.

Kids which are to be artificially reared should not be removed from their nanny until they are three to four days old. They can then be fed milk replacers as described for calves (see p. 126).

They are fed at least three times a day. Weaning should be complete at ten weeks of age. Good quality hay and concentrate are offered from two weeks of age.

Procedures

Castration is carried out as described for cattle (see p. 128).

Disbudding, where necessary, must be carried out by a veterinary surgeon.

Health

Signs of ill health in goats include obvious lameness and injury, lethargy, poor appetite, poor coat condition, obvious discharges, diarrhoea or lack of faeces, isolation from other animals. They should be inspected regularly and veterinary help called if there is any cause for concern. The rectal temperature of a goat is 38.5–39.5 °C

They share many diseases with sheep and those mentioned in Chapter 20 on sheep are relevant to goats. Further information on goat diseases can be obtained from Dunn (1987).

Identification, records and movement

The requirements for goats are exactly the same as for sheep (see Chapter 20).

References and further reading

DEFRA (1989) *Code of Recommendations for the Welfare of Livestock, Goats.* DEFRA publications, London. www.defra.gov.uk

Dunn, P. (1987) *The Goatkeeper's Veterinary Book.* Farming Press, Ipswich, UK.

Home Office (1989) *Code of Practice for the Housing and Care of Animals used in Scientific Procedures.* HMSO, London.

22
Pigs

Stephen W. Barnett

Introduction

Pigs are highly intelligent and sensitive creatures. They respond well to human contact, in fact some people keep minipigs as domestic pets. They are omnivorous members of the order Artiodactyla (even-toed hoofed mammals). Their classification is given in Table 22.1.

Commercially, pigs are used for meat production. The skin is also used to make fine quality leather.

As with all farm animals, if pigs are undergoing regulated procedures the work is subject to the Animals (Scientific Procedures) Act 1986 and they must be kept in accordance with the Code of Practice for the Care and Housing of Animals Used in Scientific Procedures (Home Office 1989). If they are not protected by the 1986 Act they are subject to other animal welfare legislation, e.g. the Welfare of Farmed Animals (England) Regulations 2000 and the Welfare of Farmed Animals (England) (Amendment) Regulations 2003. The DEFRA *Code of Recommendations for the Welfare of Livestock, Pigs* (DEFRA 2003) can be downloaded from their website (www.defra.gov.uk). Some terms used in relation to pigs are defined in Table 22.2.

Pig breeds

The most common commercial breeds in the UK are the Large White and the Landrace. Both are general purpose breeds, which means their products are used to produce fresh meat, preserved meat (bacon and ham) and manufactured products (sausages and pies).

Large Whites

Large Whites (Figure 22.1) are prolific breeders. They

Table 22.1 Classification of the pig *Sus scrofa*.

Kingdom	Animalia
Phylum	Chordata
Sub-phylum	Vertebrata
Class	Mammalia
Order	Artiodactyla
Family	Suidae
Generic and specific name	*Sus scrofa*

Table 22.2 Terms used with pigs.

Piglet	Pre-weaner pig
Hog or barrow	Castrated male
Boar	Entire male
Gilt	Young female
Sow	Adult female

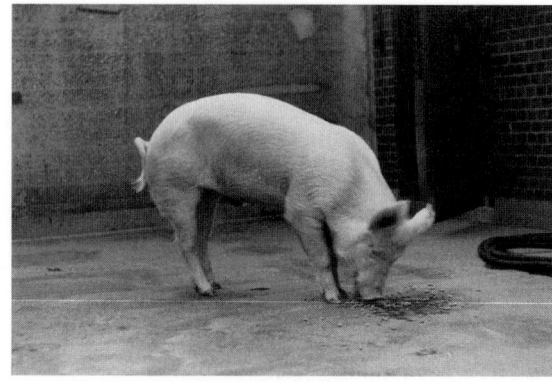

Figure 22.1 Large White boar.

can be recognised by the large head, small ears inclined forward and the sharp right angle between forehead and snout. An adult sow reaches a body mass of approximately 270 kg.

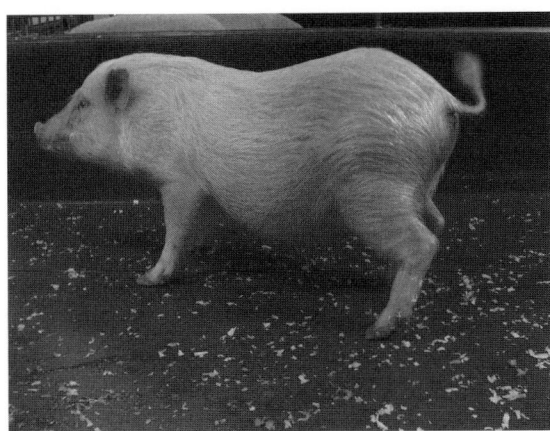

Figure 22.2   Göttingen minipig.

Landrace

The Landrace breed is described as having a small head with ears flopping over the eyes, the back is long and the pelvis well covered. Females reach a body mass of approximately 230 kg.

Minipigs

Although both Large White and Landrace are used for research smaller pigs have been developed specifically for the purpose. Minipigs have the advantage of being easier to handle, require less space and have lower husbandry costs (food, bedding etc.). Several strains of minipig are available; the Göttingen minipig is illustrated in Figure 22.2, an adult female of this breed reaches approximately 40 kg body mass.

Use in regulated procedures

Pigs used for regulated procedures can be purchased from any source unless they are genetically altered, in which case they are listed in Schedule 2 of the Animals (Scientific Procedures) Act (1986) and must be obtained from designated breeders.

Pigs are studied to improve their health and productivity for commercial purposes. They are used extensively in biomedical research because of their anatomical and physiological similarities to humans. Examples of the research areas they are used in are: toxicology, cardiovascular studies, digestion, skin, immunology and transplant surgery.

Table 22.3   Environmental levels for pigs housed indoors (Home Office 1989).

	Scientific procedure establishments
Room temperature	15–24 °C
Relative humidity	55% ± 10%
Photoperiod	Natural light periods
Light intensity	350–400 lux at bench level
Air changes per hour	Sufficient to provide fresh air and prevent a build up of noxious odours

Environment

The environmental levels recommended for pigs housed indoors in the code of practice (Home Office 1989) are given in Table 22.3.

Wide fluctuations in temperature must be avoided, once a temperature from the range is selected it should not vary by more than ± 2 °C. Pigs have few sweat glands and will suffer if exposed to high temperatures for long periods. Newborn animals will need higher temperatures (see section on reproduction, p. 154).

Pigs can be very noisy, reaching levels way beyond those that can cause damage to human hearing (>90 dBA), noise reaches its highest level at feeding time. Ear protection must be worn by staff and care must be taken to ensure other animals are not disturbed by the noise.

If outdoor housing is used, shelter should be provided at all times, in the summer to protect from the sun and in the winter to protect from the cold.

Conditions which should be provided for agricultural pigs are specified in the *Code of Recommendations for the Welfare of Livestock, Pigs* (DEFRA 2003).

Housing

Recommendations for the stocking densities for pigs can be found in the current code of practice (Home Office 1989).

The type of housing used for pigs depends on the type of work being carried out, i.e. in an environmentally controlled laboratory animal facility or in farm conditions. Pigs are strong so whatever the type of housing it must be resilient if it is to contain the animals. Food and water troughs need to be secured to the wall or floor or they will be thrown around

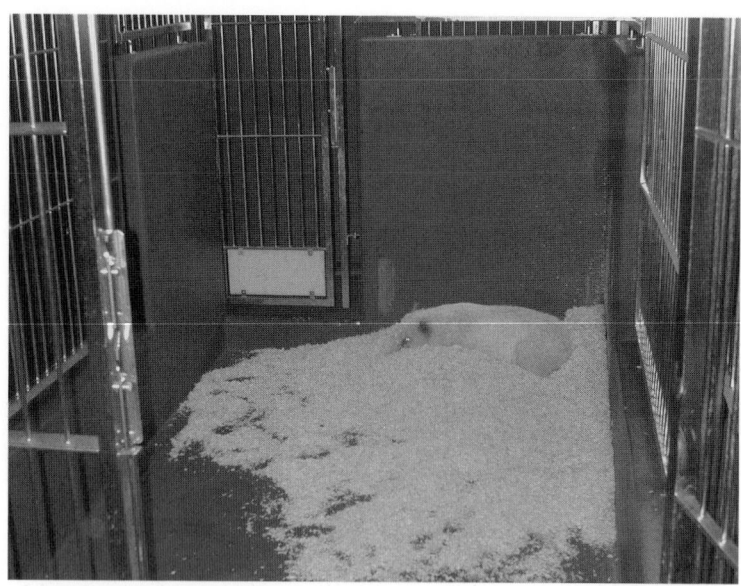

Figure 22.3 Pig pen.

the pen. All surfaces in pens should be smooth; pigs' skin and the soles of their feet are soft and are easily damaged on rough surfaces.

Experimental animal facility

Pens can be constructed of a variety of materials; walls built from brick rendered with a fine grade concrete and sealed with a non-toxic paint is one possibility. Where possible, part of the wall should be constructed of metal bars so that neighbouring animals can see each other (Figure 22.3).

Slatted floors are used in commercial units as they help to deal with large amounts of waste matter produced by adult pigs. Where they are used the gap to slat width must be tailored to the feet size of the pigs housed. Solid floors are more appropriate for experimental pigs; they are more comfortable and the risk of foot damage is less. Floors should slope down to a gully.

A combination of solid and slatted flooring can be used, a slatted area for defecation and a solid area to lie down in. Pigs soon learn to defecate and urinate in the slatted area, particularly if their water drinkers are placed in the slatted area as they tend to soil in wet areas.

Housing young pigs

When weaning is complete, young pigs are grouped with others of similar size, weight and sex in accom-

modation which is new to all of them. Whenever pigs are housed together a dominance hierarchy is established. This will involve some fighting but providing sufficient space is provided and there is plenty of bedding to hide in injuries are usually insignificant and the group settles down within twenty-four hours. In some cases bullying may persist and injuries can be severe, so a close watch has to be kept on newly established groups. No more than twenty to thirty pigs should be grouped together. If large numbers are together, a stable hierarchy is never established and the group never settles down. Once a group has been established, new stock should not be added, the new entrants would be at risk of attack.

Housing boars

Adult boars should be housed singly in pens which have a minimum of 7.5 m³ floor area and have walls of 1.4 m high. This space allows sufficient space for sows to be served.

Young boars housed on their own make poor breeders; they have no opportunity to build up confidence before meeting sows. They should be group housed from weaning until first used for breeding at about thirty weeks of age.

Housing adult females

Dry sows (sows that are not lactating) can be housed

Figure 22.4 Sow house with feeding stalls in front.

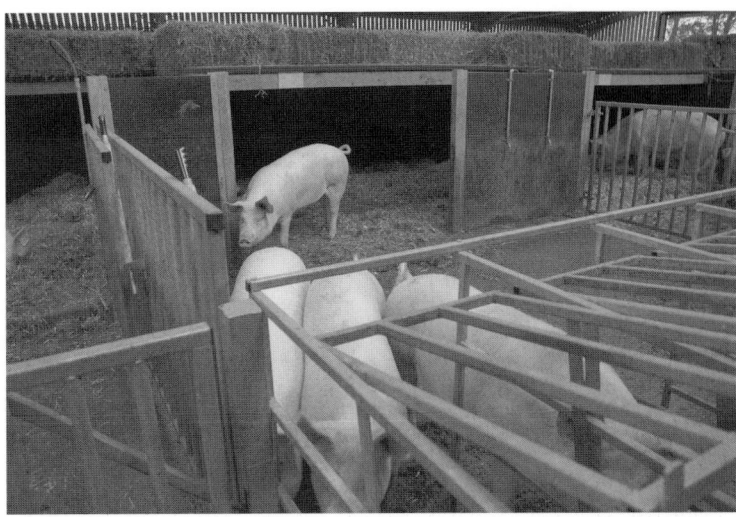

in groups of up to ten in sow houses (Figure 22.4). Food is best supplied individually as this minimises bullying. Feeding stalls can be incorporated into the housing to achieve this, sows enter willingly at feeding time. As well as ensuring each animal gets an appropriate diet this system allows staff to inspect the condition of each animal closely.

Routines

Straw or wood chips make suitable bedding for pigs (Figure 22.3, see p. 148). Contrary to common belief pigs are clean creatures and do not like contact with

their waste. Given adequate space they will often defecate and urinate in one corner of the pen making routine cleaning straight forward. When housed in experimental animal house pens the soil can be easily taken away once a day. Twice a week the pen and corridors should be completely cleaned out and hosed down.

Items such as balls can be placed in the pen to keep the pigs occupied and interested. They will be particularly interested in the items if food is concealed within them, however they soon become bored so the enrichment items should be changed regularly.

Boxes can be placed in pens to act as nests (Figure 22.5). Pigs like to scratch, a brush attached to the

Figure 22.5 Nest box.

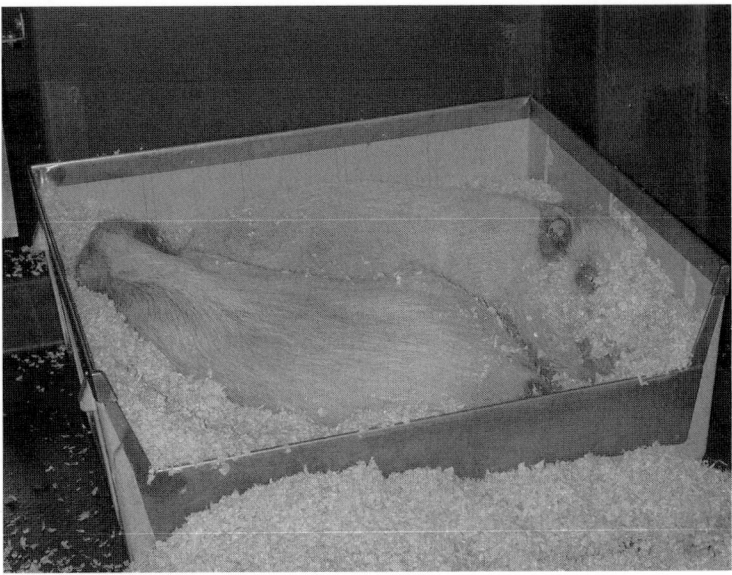

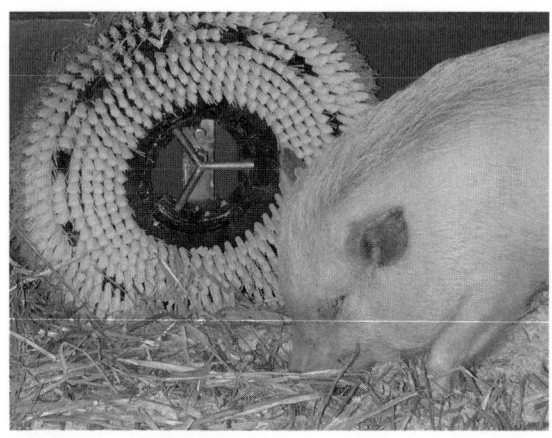

Figure 22.6   Scratching brush.

wall allows them to do this without damaging their skin (Figure 22.6).

Food and water

Conventional pigs

Compounded feeds in the form of mashes, crumbs and pellets are manufactured with nutrient contents to suit pigs in all stages of development and physiological states. Tables 22.4 and 22.5 give typical feeding regimens for commercial pigs at different stages of development (based on ADAS leaflet 104).

A good starting point for newly arrived pigs is to

Table 22.4   Pig feeding chart.

Period	Diet	Presentation/Quantity	Water Consumption	Comments
Young Animals				
Weaning at 5–8 weeks	Creep feed (DE 13.7 Mj/kg; CP18–19%)	*Ad lib*. Animals will eat little at first up to 0.5 kg by 6–8 weeks	5 litres/litter	
Weaning – 65 kg or until selected for breeding at 75 kg	Growers feed (DE13.5 Mj/kg; CP 18%)	*Ad lib* to 35–40 kg then restricted (see Table 22.5)	5 litres/pig	
Breeding Animals				Aim to achieve the following weight gain between weaning of one litter to mating for the next:
Pre-mating				
Gilts 75 kg – 14 days before mating	Medium energy sow breeding diet	2.5 kg/day increase to 3.5–4.0 kg/day	5–10 litres/pig	1st: 20 kg
14 days before mating to mating	(DE 12.5 Mj/kg; CP 16%)			2nd: 15 kg 3rd: 10 kg
Sows – weaning of one litter to remating	Medium energy	4.0–4.5 kg/day		4th +: 5 kg
Pregnancy				Small sows under 180 kg
Gilts and small sows	Medium energy	2.0–2.1 kg/day	5–10 litres	Large sows over 180 kg
Large sows	Medium energy	2.5–2.6 kg/day		The reduction from pre-mating to
Late pregnancy		Bran is sometimes used to replace some concentrates until farrowing.		pregnancy rations should be made gradually. Bran is used to prevent constipation at parturition.
Lactation				Gilts and small sows with large litters may need high energy sow
Small sows	Medium energy	4 kg for sow and 5 piglets + 0.4 kg for each extra piglet	15–30 litres	breeding diets DE 13.5 Mj/kg; CP
Large sows	Medium energy	4.5 kg for sow and 5 piglets + 0.4 kg for each extra piglet		16.5% to ensure they obtain sufficient nutrients.
Boars	Medium energy	2.75–3 kg/day	10 litres	Ration should be adjusted to keep the boar in good, lean condition.
Non-breeding Animals				This average amount should be
Immature	Dry sow feed	See Table 22.5	5–10 litres	adjusted for each pig to maintain
Adults	(DE 12.5 Mj/kg; CP 14%)	2.5 kg/day	10 litres	good, lean body condition.

Table 22.5   Food allowance for growing pigs.

Age (weeks)	Entire males (kg/day)	Gilts/castrates (kg/day)
9	1.00	1.00
11	1.35	1.35
13	1.75	1.6
15	2.05	1.8
17	2.20	1.95
19	2.35	2.05
21	2.45	2.15
23	2.55	2.25*

*should reach approx 75 kg by this age.

Table 22.6   Minimum food trough length (Home Office 1989).

Weight of pig (kg)	Minimum length of food trough (m)
Up to 30	0.2
30–50	0.25
50–100	0.3
100–150	0.35
Over 150	0.40
Adult boar	0.50

find what the suppliers are feeding and to continue with that. The condition of the animal should be monitored and feeding adjusted accordingly.

Adult pigs are normally fed once or twice a day. Food may be placed on the floor or in troughs. If troughs are used they must be long enough to ensure all animals can get access at feeding time, Table 22.6.

Minipigs

Minipigs are fed a low energy diet with a metabolisable energy (ME) value of 10 Mj and a crude protein content of 13.9%. This diet provides for their nutritional needs and should stop them putting on too much weight. Food allowance for minipigs is given in Table 22.7 (see Ellegaard Minipigs, www.minipigs.com).

As with conventional pigs it is essential to monitor minipigs carefully and to adjust feeding according to body condition.

Water

Water should be provided *ad libitum*. Approximate water consumption levels are given in Table 22.4.

Table 22.7   Food allowance for minipigs.

Age (months)	Weight (kg)	Feeds per day	Daily feeding (kg)	
			Males	Females
2–3	5–7	2	0.11	0.11
3–4	7–9	2	0.12	0.11
4–5	9–11	2	0.13	0.12
5–6	11–13	2	0.15	0.14
6–7	13–15	2	0.17	0.16
7–9	15–19	1	0.38	0.36
9–12	19–24	1	0.42	0.40
>12	24–30	1	0.46	0.44
>18	±30	1	0.56	0.54
>24	±35	1	0.56	0.54

Water is usually provided through automatic watering devices. The nipple must be adjusted to suit the size of the animal (Figure 22.7), e.g. adult minipigs drinkers should be no higher than 0.3 m from the floor.

Water drinkers should be placed away from food or lying areas as pigs like to play with water making the area wet. They also tend to urinate and defecate in wet areas.

Reproduction

Breeding data for the pig is summarised in Table 22.8.

Mating in pigs is prolonged, averaging ten minutes, during which an ejaculation of 150–500 cm^3 is produced by the boar. This puts a high physiological demand on the animal, consequently they must not be worked too early in their life or overworked when mature if they are to remain in good condition.

Although boars can be used from six months old it is better to leave them until they are eight months. At this stage they can be allowed a maximum of fifty services evenly spread throughout a year. Adult boars are used for about one hundred services a year. A stocking ratio of one boar to fifteen to twenty-five sows is used.

Gilts (young sows) are first mated at their second or third oestrus, this is when they are six to seven months old. From twenty-four weeks old (when they weigh about 75 kg) the gilts are often housed next to mature boars as this tends to stimulate their reproductive behaviour.

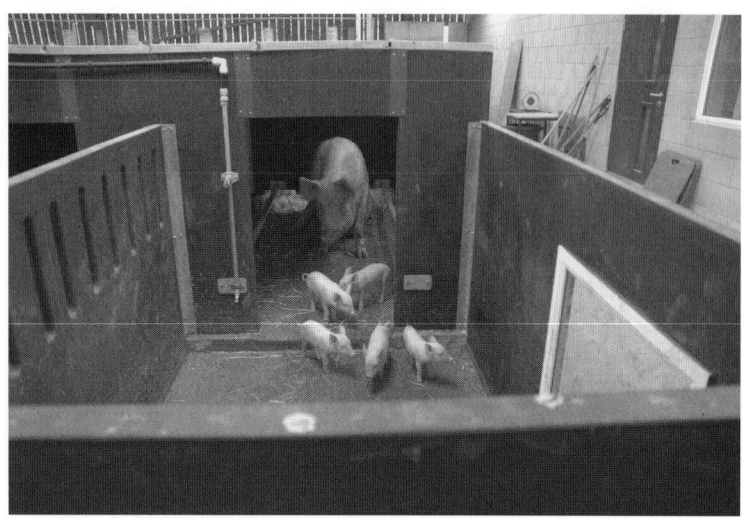

Figure 22.7 Farrowing pen showing two-level nipple drinker – the higher one for the sow, and the lower one for the piglets. The light area at the back of the box is a heated creep area for the piglets.

Table 22.8 Summary of breeding data for traditional pigs and minipigs.

	Traditional pig	Minipig
Average age at sexual maturity: female	5 months	4 months
Average age at sexual maturity: male	6 months	4 months
Age at first use: female	6–7 months	5 months
Age at first use: male	8 months	5 months
Average oestrous cycle	21 days	19.5 days
Average length of oestrus (gilts)	1 day	–
Average length of oestrus (sows)	2–2.5 days	2.9 days
Mechanism of ovulation	Spontaneous	Spontaneous
Gestation	115 days	113–114 days
Birth weight	0.75 – 1.5 kg	0.56 kg
Average litter size	10.5	6.2
Weaning age	3–5 weeks	7 weeks
Weaning weight: 3 week weaning	6 kg	–
Weaning weight: 5 week weaning	10 kg	–
Weaning weight: 7 week weaning	–	1 kg
Return to oestrus post partum: 3 week weaning	10 days	–
Return to oestrus post partum: 5 week weaning	8 days	–

The oestrous cycle takes twenty-one days to complete. Impending oestrus is indicated by changes in behaviour, such as restlessness and drop in food intake. The most convincing sign is a gradual increase in redness and size of the vulva which reaches a maximum some forty-eight hours after it starts. The maximum engorgement indicates the onset of true oestrus or standing heat; from this point and for the next sixty hours the sow will allow herself to be mated.

The willingness of the sow to accept the boar can be confirmed by a test referred to as the 'standing to riding test'. In this test the sow will allow an attendant to apply pressure to her back at the pelvic region (she would be expected to walk away if she was not in oestrus). It is thought the test is more reliable if the sow can smell a boar while the test is being carried out. Where no boar is available, for instance where AI is to be used, an aerosol containing boar odour is sprayed near the snout of the sow before the riding test.

Mating systems

In outdoor systems of management boars can be run with a group of sows, the sows are mated as they come into oestrus. Inexperienced boars and gilts should not be used in this system as they may be bullied by their fellows.

Arranged mating relies on the handler accurately identifying heat. Sows not in standing heat will fight boars who attempt to mount them and this can result in serious injury to both animals and to the handler who has to part them.

Prior to mounting the boar will sniff the vulva of the sow and may put his snout under her belly and lift her hind quarters off the floor, this is normal courtship behaviour. Once mounted, the boar will be restless until ejaculation has started. He then becomes very passive and lies on the sow's back quietly until the ejaculation has finished. Maximum fertility is achieved if mating takes place twelve hours after the onset of standing heat and again about eight to twelve hours later.

Artificial insemination

Artificial insemination in pigs has not yet reached the sophistication of AI in cattle; it is possible to freeze boar semen but when it is thawed for use its fertility rate is very low (about 50%). However, fresh semen diluted with chemicals which maintain normal electrolyte and osmotic balance and stored at temperatures of l8 °C will remain at high fertility for up to four days.

Two methods are used to collect semen from boars. In both cases the boars are trained to mount dummy sows. In one method an artificial vagina filled with water at 50 °C is used. Boar AVs differ in design from the models used for other animals in two ways, first the boar requires pressure to be exerted at the distal end of the penis to stimulate ejaculation so a bulb capable of pumping air into the AV is fitted. Second, the end of the boar penis is spiralled and to accommodate this, the AV is fitted with a wire spiral.

The second method of semen collection needs little equipment, it is called the hand or glove method. When the boar mounts the dummy sow and protrudes its penis the collector, who is wearing a rubber glove, gently holds the free end and tries to push it back into the sheath, when this is no longer possible the boar has achieved full erection and the collector grips the end of the penis firmly. This stimulates the boar to ejaculate.

Once collected the semen is assessed by microscopic examination (see Chapter 1) and is diluted until there is a concentration of 1×10^9 sperm per cm^3. It is packed in plastic bottles of 75 cm^3 capacity.

Insemination

The catheter used to inseminate the sow resembles the boar penis in being spiralled. This is positioned into the vagina of the sow and stimulates contractions. The bottle containing semen is attached to the catheter and, by a combination of uterine contractions, gravity and pressure applied to the bottle the insemination is accomplished. Like natural mating, maximum fertility is reached if the sow is inseminated twelve hours after the onset of standing heat and again some eight to twelve hours later.

Pregnancy and parturition

Gestation in the pig averages 115 days. Pregnancy is indicated by failure to return to oestrus. A more certain diagnosis can be obtained by an ultrasound scan at fifty days post mating. The onset of parturition in sows is indicated by restlessness, nest building (where this is possible), colostrum visible on the end of the teats and sometimes by a clear discharge from an enlarged vulva.

Parturition is usually complete within four hours. The combination of a large mother and small offspring means that problems with parturition are uncommon. Piglets weigh between 0.75 and l.75 kg. Piglets below 1 kg are particularly vulnerable to early death. The average litter size is 10.5. Pre-weaning mortality should be no more than ten per cent.

Death of some piglets due to crushing by sows when they lie down led to very restricted farrowing crates being introduced to protect the piglets. These crates severely compromised the welfare of the sows. Modern farrowing pens provide piglets with warm areas away from the sow (creep areas) while allowing the sow freedom to move (Figure 22.7, see p. 152).

Care must be taken when handling piglets as sows can be very protective and may attack.

The sow is moved into farrowing quarters four to five days before she is expected to give birth. She is usually washed and treated for internal and external parasites.

Pre-weaning care

Warmth is essential to new-born piglets, temperature shock suffered in early life leads to cessation of sucking and increased susceptibility to disease and death. As a guide, areas away from the sow (creep areas) should be kept at a temperature of 30 °C at day one and be reduced to 24 °C by day 17.

Piglets must be seen to suck within the first two hours of birth, if necessary, weak animals can be fed colostrum by stomach tube. If litters are very large, some of the number can be fostered onto a sow with fewer young.

Weaning

In England the law prescribes the age at which piglets are weaned. They must be at least twenty-eight days of age unless their welfare, or the welfare of the sow require it to be done earlier. There is provision for it to be done at twenty-one days providing they would be transferred to a specially designed nursery (WFA Regs 2003). Generally the earlier piglets are weaned the sooner the sow will return to oestrus and therefore the shorter the litter interval. The wellbeing of the animals is more important in experimental animal work so a weaning age of five or even eight weeks is more appropriate.

To minimise weaning stress, the sow is removed from the piglets and they are left for a few days to get used to losing the dam in an environment they are familiar with. After a few days they can be grouped with other animals of similar size and weight in accommodation new to all the animals. The pen should be well bedded with straw and wood chips.

Procedures carried out in first days of life

Several procedures are carried out in the early days of a piglet's life for the welfare of the piglets, the sow or the requirements of the keeper:

- **Umbilicus removal**

The umbilicus is removed and disinfected to prevent infection.

- **Birth weight recording**

Birth weights are useful indicators of animals which are most vulnerable. The earlier these are recorded the better.

- **Iron injection**

Piglets housed indoors, especially those reared in intensive units, are at high risk of suffering from piglet anaemia. This is because little iron is stored in foetal life and sow's milk has a very low iron content. A 200 mg injection of a soluble iron preparation given within three days of birth will normally provide the animal with enough iron to last until it is consuming sufficient creep feed.

- **Teeth filing**

Corner incisor teeth of newborn piglets can be very sharp and may inflict considerable damage to their litter mates and to the teats of their dams. They can be blunted by filing or by removing the tips with bone forceps. However this should not be done as a routine, it should only be done as a last resort and only to individual piglets with problem teeth. In piglets under seven days old the procedure may be carried out by a trained, competent person, it must be done by a veterinary surgeon if the animal is older than seven days.

- **Castration**

Castration should only be done when necessary (not as a routine procedure for all males not intended for breeding). Ideally, it should be carried out at two weeks of age, but should not be performed within one week of weaning or if the animal is sick. Castration plus any other stress will severely risk the life of the young animal. Surgical castration is the only method which is practical for pigs as the anatomy of the scrotum makes it impossible to use bloodless castrators or fit a rubber ring. If the animal is under seven days of age the procedure can be carried out by a trained competent person; over that age it must be performed by a veterinary surgeon.

- **Tail docking**

Tail docking is permitted in herds where there is

evidence of tail or flank biting, but only if other measures such as improving the environment have failed to cure the problem. Veterinary surgeons must remove tails of animals over seven days old.

Handling

Pigs should be walked from place to place. They must not be forced but allowed to walk at their own pace. Food can be used for encouragement but this must be used sparingly. Pig boards can be used to guide animals in the direction they are wanted to go. Flat slap sticks are also used; these are not to hit the animal but to tap it to get it to change direction.

Pigs are difficult to restrain for regulated procedures and may need to be placed in closely confined trollies for this purpose; if these have wheels they can also be used to transport the animal (Figure 22.8).

A twitch can be used to control pigs for some procedures where all else fails and chemical restraint is inappropriate. A twitch is basically a handle through which a stout piece of rope has been threaded. The rope is placed in the mouth and positioned behind the canine teeth. The handle is twisted until the rope tightens around the snout. This method should only be used when other methods do not provide sufficient restraint and only for a very short period.

Health

Signs of ill health in the pig are similar to those described for other animals. They include refusal of food, lethargy, weight loss, lameness, isolation from the rest of the herd, diarrhoea and respiratory distress. They are susceptible to a number of bacterial and viral diseases from which vaccination may protect them. The named veterinary surgeon can advise which vaccinations are appropriate. The rectal temperature of a pig is 39.2 °C. Further information on pig diseases can be found in Taylor (1995).

Records, identification and movement

In order to minimise the spread of serious disease (e.g. Foot and Mouth disease) which could have major welfare and economic effects, it is necessary for DEFRA to be able to track animals and their contacts. In order to be able to do this DEFRA specifies the identification methods which must be used and the records of pigs entering and leaving a unit which have to be kept. They also require movement licences to be obtained before an animal is transported from one keeper to another. These requirements are laid down in the Pigs (Records, Identification and Movement) Order 2003. The main points of the order are:

Figure 22.8   Transport and restraint trolley.

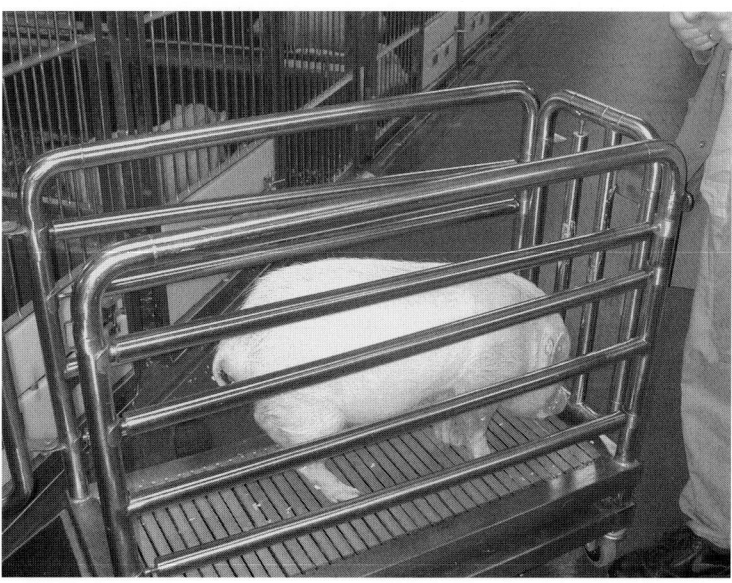

- Keepers of pigs must notify DEFRA (through the Animal Health Divisional Office) within one month of starting to keep them.
- DEFRA will issue a herdmark which must be applied to all pigs.
- Pigs cannot be moved off the premises without being marked with the herdmark unless they are under one year of age and being transferred to another premises. In this case they must be identified with a temporary mark (e.g. paint) which will last until they reach their destination.
- Identification marks must be permanent and must be able to survive the processing that follows slaughter (including singeing). Methods acceptable are:
  — metal eartags;
  — tattoo on the ear;
  — slap mark (a tattoo on the shoulders of the animal).
- Other information, such as the keeper's own individual identification mark of the pig, can be used as long as it does not interfere with the herd mark.
- If the pig is imported into the UK, a letter F must accompany the herdmark.

Movement

The keeper of the pigs being transported must give the transporter a document (form AML2) stating the full source and destination addresses, the date of the movement, the number and identification of the pigs. The keeper at the destination must keep this document for at least six months and give a copy to the local authority within three days.

When a pig moves onto the premises no other pig can move off for twenty days unless it is to go to slaughter (the DEFRA divisional manager may grant exemptions to this under certain circumstances).

References, sources and further reading

DEFRA (2003) *Code of Recommendations for the Welfare of Livestock, Pigs.* DEFRA, London. www.defra.gov.uk

Home Office (1989) *Code of Practice for the Housing and Care of Animals used in Scientific Procedures.* HMSO, London.

Taylor, D. (1995) *Pig Diseases.* Farming Press, Ipswich, UK.

23

Horses

Stephen W. Barnett

Introduction

The horse is a member of the order Perissodactyla, these are hoofed animals with an odd number of toes. Classification of the horse is given in Table 23.1. The equidae bear all their weight on the third toe (the first toe is missing and the other two, commonly called splint bones, are reduced to stunted metacarpals or metatarsals). The teeth continually grow and have a very rough grinding surface to cope with the hard, plant-based diet.

Breeds

Heavy draught

Large breeds have traditionally been used to pull ploughs and heavy carts. Examples include the Shire, which is the largest of the British breeds (measuring 17 hands in height and 1 tonne in weight). Shires are slow but powerful. They have feathers (bunches of long hair) on the legs and are found in all colours except chestnut. Other examples of heavy draught horses are Clydesdale, Suffolk and Percheron.

Light draught

Members of this group of breeds are used to pull carriages and light carts. They also include pacers and trotters which are used for racing. Examples are Cleveland Bay, Yorkshire coach horse and Hackney.

Riding breeds

As their name implies, these animals are used for riding. They include Thoroughbreds, all of which are

Table 23.1 Classification of the horse *Equus equus*.

Kingdom	Animalia
Phylum	Chordata
Sub-phylum	Vertebrata
Class	Mammalia
Order	Perissodactyla
Family	Equidae
Generic and specific names	*Equus equus*

racehorses registered with Weatherby, the Jockey Club agents (the Jockey Club administers horse racing in the UK). To be registered, both parents must have been registered. Thoroughbreds have a wide range of appearances. The average height is 16 hands (Figure 23.1).

Other examples of riding breeds are Arab, Hunter and Polo Pony. With the exception of Arabs these are breed types and not pure bred.

Pony

A pony is an animal whose adult height is under 147 cm. There are many different pony breeds which are usually named after the place they originate from, e.g. Welsh, New Forest, Dartmoor, Shetland.

Some terms specifically used in connection with horses are given in Table 23.2.

Although donkeys and mules are included in equidae, this chapter will concentrate on horses.

Use in regulated procedures

Nearly 9000 procedures were carried out on horses, donkeys and other equids in 2003. An example of their

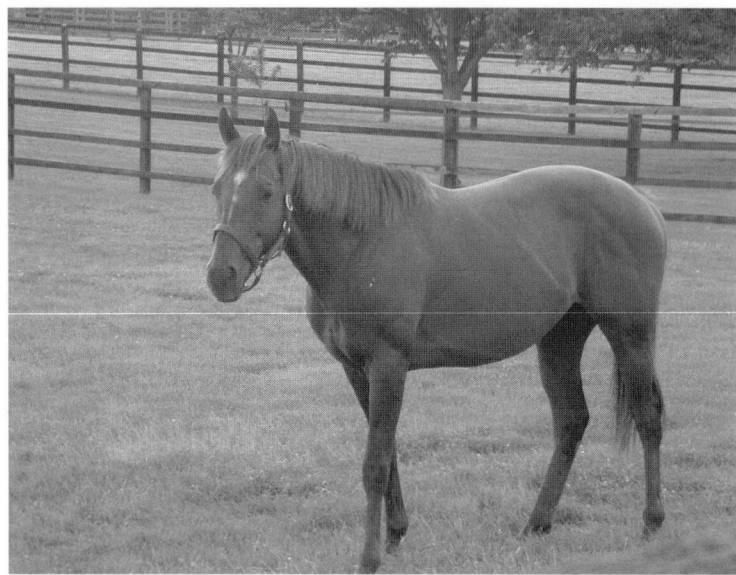

Figure 23.1   Thoroughbred stallion.

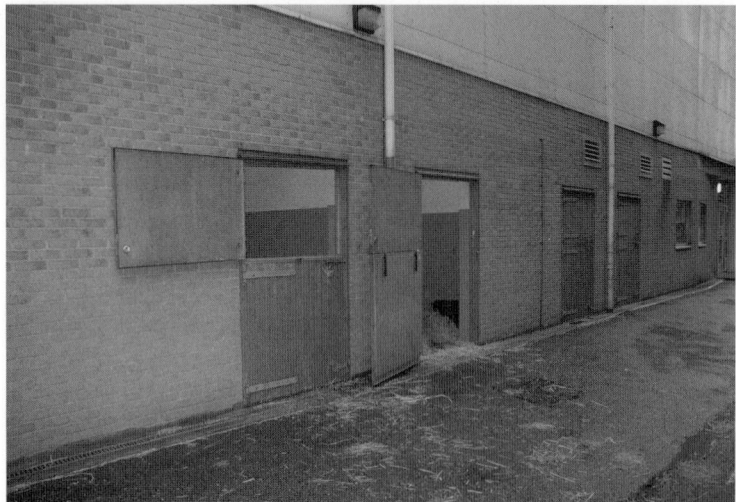

Figure 23.2   A row of loose boxes with doors half closed, open and closed.

use is research connected to advancing veterinary science and raising antisera.

Environment

Table 23.3 lists the environmental levels which should be provided for horses housed indoors in scientific procedure establishments (Home Office 1989). If housed indoors, wide fluctuations in temperature must be avoided. Once a temperature from the range in Table 23.3 is selected, it should not vary by more than ± 2 °C. Forced ventilation systems must provide an even distribution of fresh air without causing any horse to be in a draught. If horses are housed in loose boxes outside (Figure 23.2), open doors and windows may be sufficient to maintain good air quality. Sufficient light must be available to ensure all horses can be seen clearly. Supplementary lighting should be available so that there is enough light for close inspection should it be necessary.

Table 23.2 Terms used in relation to horses.

Foal	A horse from birth to one year old. Can be colt foal (male) or filly foal (female)
Colt	Entire male 1–4 years old
Filly	Female 1–4 years old
Mare	Female over 5 years old
Stallion	Entire male over 5 years old
Gelding	Castrated male
Brood mare	Female kept for breeding
Rig (cryptorchid)	A male whose testicles have been retained in the abdomen. These animals can be difficult to handle
Hand	Horses are traditionally measured in hands and inches or centimeters. One hand is 4 inches or 10 cm.
Pony	An animal 14.2 hands (14 hands 2 inches) or 147 cm
Horse	Animal over 147 cm

Table 23.3 Environmental conditions for horses (Home Office 1989).

	Scientific procedure establishments
Room temperature	10–24 °C
Relative humidity	55% ± 10%
Photoperiod	Natural light periods
Light intensity	350–400 lux at bench level
Air changes per hour	Sufficient to provide fresh air and prevent a build up of heat and noxious odours

Housing

Space allowance for horses in scientific procedure establishments can be found in the Home Office code of practice (1989). Horses are commonly housed in loose boxes, these have doors divided in two halves, the top half is usually left open so the horse can see out and to increase ventilation.

The loose box must have a wide door to prevent the animals knocking themselves as they enter. The height should allow them to stand up straight and to have the full range of head and neck movement. The floor should have good drainage and be non slip. A comfortable covering of straw or wood chip will absorb urine and localise faeces. The bedding also provides a clean, dry surface for the horse to lie down on. Internal materials should be capable of being washed and disinfected.

Horses housed outside must be given shelter from bad weather. They can be fitted with blankets to protect them against the cold and wet but these must be checked regularly to ensure they have not slipped off.

Horses must be inspected at least twice a day while at pasture. Fences must be well maintained and the pasture inspected for poisonous plants and dangerous debris (see Chapter 18). Introduction to new pasture with unfamiliar fences should be done during daylight hours. The position of their eyes, at the sides of the head, mean horses cannot see what is directly in front of them if it is close, and this increases the risk of them running into an unfamiliar fence.

Routines

Soiled bedding should be removed twice a day and the whole bedding replaced once a week. The horse's feet should be picked out regularly so faeces do not become impacted, leading to infection.

Food and water

Horses are herbivores which, in the wild, spend many hours a day grazing. They have a relatively small stomach and are unable to vomit. The very large caecum and colon are populated with micro-organisms which digest the cellulose components of their diet. The horse is able to absorb the products of microbial carbohydrate digestion and microbiologically produced vitamins through the wall of the large intestines. Amino acids, however, are not absorbed very efficiently so the horse has a higher requirement for dietary protein than do ruminants.

An adult horse requires approximately 69 Mj of digestible energy per day for maintenance; in hard work this may well need doubling. Protein should form 8% of the diet for an adult horse. Growing foals require 76 Mj and 16% protein content.

Hay forms the bulk of the food intake for horses housed indoors. This can be provided in hay nets or hay racks (Figure 23.3) and can be available all day. Only good quality hay should be fed to horses, if it is dusty it should be damped down with water before being fed. Haylage may be fed instead of hay, it is said to have a higher nutrient quality but is more expensive. It also has a shorter shelf life (see Chapter 18).

Concentrate rations have traditionally been provided in the form of cereals (oats, corn, barley) and other farm crops and by-products (soybean meal, cane molasses). Pellets are available formulated for

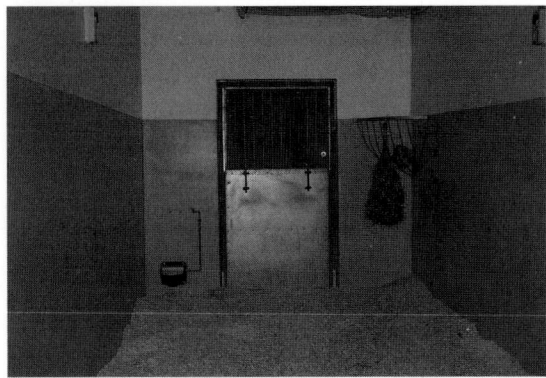

Figure 23.3   Loose box showing hay net and hay rack containing a mineral lick.

horses in various stages of development and physiological condition.

Good quality grass in the summer should provide for their maintenance needs and enough nutrients to support light work (although vitamins and minerals may need to be supplemented).

Feeding regimens for horses should mimic their natural feeding behaviour, basically this is little and often. Hay can be made available all day, but where concentrates are fed they should be divided into three or four feeds spread over the day. Concentrates should not be fed when the horse has recently taken in a large amount of water as they may swell in the stomach causing discomfort.

A rough guide to the amount of food which needs to be provided for horses required to do various amounts of work, and for a pony housed indoors is given in Table 23.4. As with all animals it is the condition of the animal itself which tells if the diet is adequate or too generous. A scoring system is available for horses which can make body condition assessment more accurate (Carroll & Huntingdon 1988). This system has five grades from 0, being very poor (pelvis angular, sunken rump with deep cavity under the tail) to 5, being very fat (both sides of the pelvis so big there is a gutter between them, bone of the pelvis cannot be felt). Score 3 is good, where the pelvis is well rounded but has no gutter and the bones of the pelvis can be easily felt. The system is described in DEFRA (2002).

Horses should not be fed later than ninety minutes before they are be used for vigorous exercise or later than one hour before they are to do light work.

Horses, more than any other species, react very soon after eating if they are fed inappropriately. If they are fed high protein rations when they are not working they will respond by being difficult to handle and with physical signs such as oedematous swellings and stiffness in the legs (a condition called lymphangitis or Monday morning disease).

Water

Fresh, clean water must be available at all times. It can be presented by means of constant-level devices or in a trough. The food trough should be situated away from the water so that one cannot be contaminated by the other. The amount an animal drinks depends on environmental temperature, the type of food available, the amount of work done and the physiological state of the animal (e.g. if a mare is lactating) but is in the region of 19–45 litres per day.

Reproduction

Breeding data for the horse is summarised in Table 23.5. With animals which differ so much in size it is obvious that there will be considerable variation in breeding data for horses.

Before the breeding process begins, mares and stallions must be inspected to ensure they are in

Table 23.4   Food allowance for horses.

	Hay (kg)	Concentrates (kg)
Horse at light work (per 45 kg body weight)	0.6–0.75	0.25
Horse at moderate work (per 45 kg body weight)	0.45–0.6	0.5
Horse at heavy work (per 45 kg body weight)	0.45	0.6–0.75
Pony housed indoors (per 100 kg body weight)	1–2	0.1

Table 23.5 Summary of breeding data for horses.

Breeding season	Spring and summer in the UK. Longer in warmer climates.
Average age at sexual maturity	18 ± 6 months
Age at first use: horse filly	3 years
Age at first use: pony filly	2 years
Age at first use: colt	4 years
Average length of oestrous cycle	21 days
Average length of oestrus	6 ± 4 days
Mechanism of ovulation	Spontaneous
Gestation period	336 ± 5 days
Birth weight (thoroughbred type)	75 kg
Average litter size	1
Weaning age	6 months
Return to oestrus post partum	4–14 days

good body condition. The mare's condition should be monitored continually throughout pregnancy so that any problems can be picked up and dealt with as early as possible. A health programme should be agreed with the veterinary surgeon to cover all possible health problems during the breeding process. Regular exercise must be given to both breeding stallions and mares.

Mating systems

Herd mating is used, where a stallion is run with a number of females and he mates them as they come into oestrus. Generally, arranged mating is a more appropriate method where a mare in heat is taken to the stallion. It is important to identify oestrus accurately as the mare can be very aggressive towards the stallion if he attempts to mount her at any other time.

Indication of oestrus
The mare will stand with her hind legs slightly apart and she will raise her tail to expose her vulva. She opens the vagina to show the mucus lining of the vagina and her clitoris. If a stallion is present she will lean towards him and produce frequent squirts of urine.

Mares and stallions are first introduced with a gate between them to make sure she will accept him. If not it will only be the gate that gets kicked. Arranged mating can be hazardous to handlers as they may get kicked if they are in the wrong place. Training for attendants is essential in order to carry out the procedure with safety.

Artificial insemination can be used with horses but collection of semen and insemination of the mare must be carried out by a veterinary surgeon or by a person trained and approved by the British Equine Veterinary Association.

Identification of pregnancy

Pregnancy can be identified by the following methods:

Rectal palpation by a veterinary surgeon	21 days
Ultrasound probe (per rectum)	21 days
Pregnant mare serum gonadotrophin levels in blood	45–60 days

(this method is not foolproof as levels may remain elevated even if embryo has slipped)

Parturition

Birth usually occurs at night. The mare should be housed in a large, well-bedded box on her own. In specialised studs foaling boxes will be fitted with closed circuit television or with a two-way mirror so the mare can be inspected without disturbing her.

Males disturb mares when foaling so they should be removed from the area (this includes geldings).

Parturition is divided into three stages:

(1) Udder development; wax secretions on teat ends (pre-colostrum); milk may run out of teats. Mare may kick her belly, roll and sweat.

(2) The mare usually lies down and strains, the first membrane (allantochorion) bursts and the foetus is seen at the vulva. One foot is in front of the other with the head resting between them. The mare may rise to eat. The foal is born inside its amniotic membrane. This stage takes about thirty minutes.

  It is best to leave the mare alone as long as everything is progressing normally. Interference may be needed if the amniotic membrane covers the nose of the foal. The umbilicus breaks when the mare moves.

(3) The placenta is expelled (the mare does not eat her placenta) usually within three hours.

Veterinary assistance will be needed if any of the stages takes longer than the expected time or the mare is in obvious distress.

Foals

After birth, the foal must be seen to take colostrum and to be feeding regularly; it usually starts feeding within one to two hours. Newborn foals should consume 250 ml of colostrum per hour for the first twenty-four hours. If the mare dies, frozen or artificial colostrum can be given and the foal can subsequently be reared by hand on foal milk replacer. However the best chance of survival for an orphan foal is to foster it on to a mare which has lost her foal.

Foals have a tendency to suck very enthusiastically when feeding from a bottle. There is a danger of them inhaling milk if they are not watched.

Good hay or grass and foal nuts should be available to all foals by the time they are seven to ten days old.

Foals may have problems passing meconium (faecal material produced during the foetal life). If this does not pass veterinary assistance may be required.

Weaning is completed at six months of age by the foal being removed from the sight and sound of the mare. Both will be upset and a companion should be provided for both. The mare will require reduced food intake for 24–48 hours to dry the milk supply.

Health

Obvious signs of ill health such as abdominal pain, lameness, prolonged sweating etc. should be reported to a veterinary surgeon as soon as possible. Condition scoring can be used to identify long-term problems such as weight loss. When at rest, a horse has a respiration rate of ten to fourteen breaths per minute and this is quite easy to monitor (unlike the much more rapid respiration rate of smaller animals). The normal temperature range of a horse is 37.5–38.5 °C. Horses are at risk from internal parasites. Using grazing management techniques referred to in Chapter 18 and a programme of anthelmintic treatment recommended by the named veterinary surgeon these can be controlled. Ectoparasites must also be treated on veterinary advice.

Vaccinations may be necessary for infectious diseases of horses. Tetanus is a fatal bacterial disease (caused by *Clostridium tetani*) which can affect all horses and for which a vaccination is advised.

Influenza virus is another widespread disease organism causing similar signs in the horse as human influenza does. Vaccination is advised and is compulsory for animals involved in activities under the control of the Jockey Club. Other vaccinations may be advised in certain circumstances, e.g. in breeding animals. Veterinary surgeons will advise on a vaccination programme suitable for specific situations. Further information on horse diseases can be found in Knottenbelt and Pasco (2003).

Horse hooves need to be inspected regularly, apart from the need to clean them out daily, they need to be trimmed. This is a skilled job and should only be carried out by a registered farrier. As a guide this should be done every four to eight weeks.

Because horse teeth are growing continuously and being worn down there is a risk that the wear will be uneven and hooks may appear. These can catch upon the cheek and prevent the animal eating. Teeth must be checked at least annually and more often in animals where uneven wear has occurred before. Where overgrowth has been identified it has to be rasped down. Currently all but the most simple dentistry on horses must be carried out by a veterinary surgeon.

Handling

Horses should be handled gently and quietly. Time must be taken to train them to do what is needed. If they are frightened they may respond by kicking with their back legs or rearing with their front. Sometimes they bite, a rare occurrence but a painful one. In most cases horses used in research will be used to being handled and will respond to human contact. They should be trained to be lead by head collar as early as possible in life (Figure 23.4).

Records, identification and movement

All horses must have a passport. This is issued, on behalf of DEFRA (and the agricultural departments in Scotland, Wales and Northern Ireland) by Weatherby's and recognised breed societies. The passport must be kept by the keeper of the horse (who

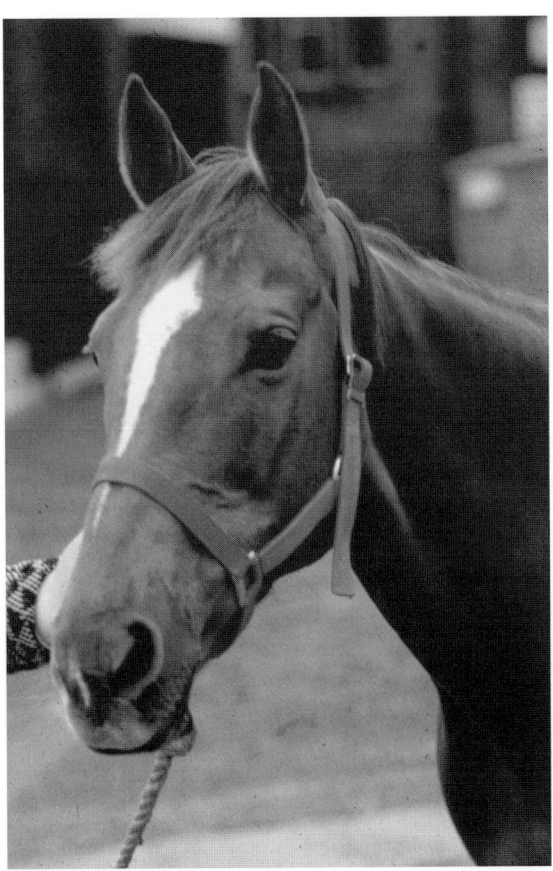

Figure 23.4 Horse in head collar.

may be different to the owner) and must accompany the horse when it is transported. Veterinary surgeons must record when certain types of treatment are given to the horse. If the horse is sold, the seller has to return the passport to the issuing organisation, with details of the new owners, within twenty-eight days.

The passport must record the identity of the horse. Several methods of identification can be used e.g.:

- physical description of the colour markings of the horse, filled in on a silhouette in the passport;
- lip tattooing;
- transponders;
- freeze branding (application of a copper brand cooled to −70 °C and applied to the skin for 27 seconds; the hair is destroyed and when it regrows it is white).

Horses should be transported as described in Chapter 28.

References

Carroll, C.L. and Huntingdon, P.J. (1988) Body condition scoring and weight estimation in horses. *Equine Veterinary Journal*, **20** (1): 42–45.
DEFRA (2002) *Equine Industry Welfare Guidelines Compendium for Horses, Ponies and Donkeys*. ADAS Consulting Ltd. www.defra.gov.uk
Home Office (1989) *The Code of Practice for the Housing and Care of Animals Used in Scientific Procedures*. HMSO, London.
Knottenbelt, D.C. and Pasco, R.R. (2003) *Diseases and Disorders of Horses*. W.B. Saunders Co., Philadelphia.

Further reading

Abbott, E.M. (1999) The Horse. In: T. Poole (Ed.) *The UFAW Handbook on the Care and Management of Laboratory Animals* (7th edn). Blackwell Science, Oxford.

24
Chickens

Roger J. Francis

Introduction

There are three main types of chicken breed which have been developed for meat production (broilers or heavy), specifically for egg production (layers or lights) and dual purpose breeds which are reasonable layers and can be used for meat. In addition there are miniature breeds called bantams.

Modern day broilers such as the Ross 1 have been developed to grow very quickly (reaching a weight of 1.8–2.7 kg by six to eight weeks of age) whereas hybrid laying strains such as Babcock 380 and Warrens (Figure 24.1) have been developed specifically for laying (such strains may lay up to 300 eggs per year without going broody). There are also pure bred strains such as White Leghorn (Figure 24.2), Rhode Island Reds, Light Sussex, Welsummer and Marans to name but a few. The classification of chickens is given in Table 24.1.

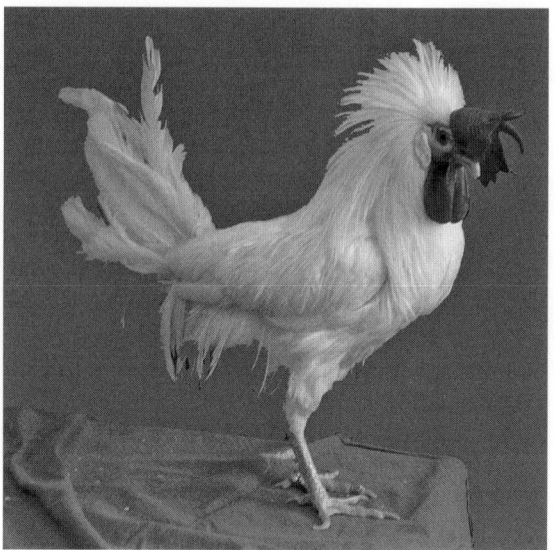

Figure 24.2 White Leghorn cockerel.

Table 24.1 Classification of chickens *Gallus domesticus*.

Kingdom	Animalia
Phylum	Chordata
Sub-phylum	Vertebrata
Class	Aves
Order	Galliformes
Family	Phasianidae
Generic and specific names	*Gallus domesticus*

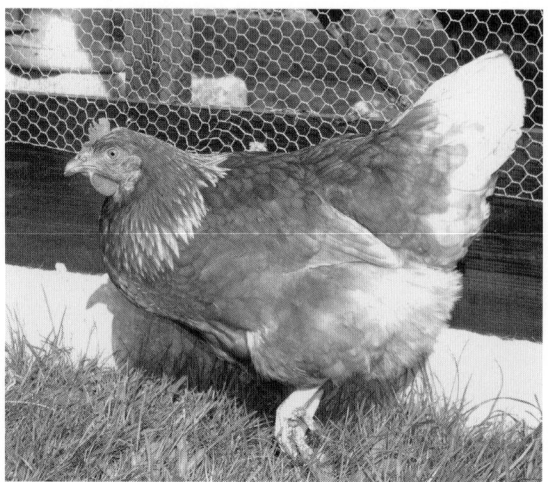

Figure 24.1 Warrener hen.

Given the range of strains available, care must be taken to ensure selection of the appropriate one for a given experimental task. If rapid growth rate is a key factor, for instance in toxicology, then broiler strains should be used but if egg production is required for antibody production then a laying strain or even a bantam strain would be more appropriate.

Table 24.2 Terms used in relation to chickens.

Chick	Bird from hatching to 8 weeks old
Grower	8 weeks to 20 weeks
Pullet	Female in the first year of lay (20 weeks to 18 months)
Cockerel	Male from 20 weeks to 18 months
Hen	Female over 18 months
Cock	Male over 18 months
Capon	Castrated male
Boiler	Laying female at the end of lay
Broiler	Meat bird killed at 9 weeks
Roaster	Meat bird killed at 20 weeks

Both broiler and hybrid laying strains are readily available from commercial hatcheries; pedigree and bantam strains are available from specialist breeders. Terms related to the chicken can be found in Table 24.2.

Use in regulated procedures

Domestic fowl are frequently used as laboratory animals especially in the areas of agricultural research, toxicology, antibody production and behavioural research (124 629 chickens used in 2002). A large number of chicken eggs are also used to culture viruses but as the experiments are often over before the incubation period is halfway through these do not appear in Home Office statistics.

Environment

The environmental conditions for chickens required by the Home Office code of practice (1989) are given in Table 24.3. DEFRA has issued a *Code of Recommendations for the Welfare of Livestock, Laying Hens* (2002) which describes the minimum standard of husbandry required for chickens not protected by the Animals (Scientific Procedures) Act 1986 (DEFRA 2002).

Table 24.3 Environmental conditions for chickens (Home Office 1989).

Temperature	12–24 °C
Relative humidity	30–70%
Air changes per hour	15–20; 10–12 (depending on stocking density)
Photoperiod	See Lighting section p. 000

Chickens can tolerate a wider humidity range than mammals. Once a temperature has been selected from the range it should not vary more than ± 2 °C.

Housing

Current stocking levels for chickens can be found in the code of practice (Home Office 1989). Chickens housed in the laboratory may be kept in large cages or in floor pens with considerably more floor space than is common in agricultural practice. The type of housing used will often depend on the number of birds to be kept. Birds may be housed on grid floors with droppings trays underneath, while others may be kept on solid floors with woodchip substrate allowing far more natural behaviours, such as scratching for food and dust bathing. If grid floors are used the code of practice states that the mesh size must be no greater than 10×10 mm for young chicks and 25×25 mm for growers and adults. Whatever type of housing is used the chickens should be provided with perches.

Lighting

Care must be taken with the lighting levels provided for chickens, especially where they are intensively housed (very bright levels may lead to feather pecking and cannibalism, whereas low levels of lighting may reduce this behaviour); levels as low as 1–2 lux are used for broilers. In commercial broiler stocks the photoperiod may be increased (23 hours light; 1 hour dark) to enable birds to have a greater food intake and enhance growth. Laying strains are frequently maintained at quite short day lengths (six hours light) while immature, with a gradual increase of day length as the pullets (young females) reach 'point of lay' (the stage at which the bird starts to lay eggs) at 18–19 weeks old. Manipulation of the photoperiod may be used to delay point of lay from 18–24 weeks, because birds which start to lay later are likely to produce larger eggs.

Food and water

Chicks should be fed and watered on the perimeter of the heat circle of the brooders. Water should be given *ad libitum* and chicks should be fed chick starter crumbs. Laying strains should be maintained on chick starter crumbs for approximately eight weeks after which point they should be given growers' mash. Broilers are given chick starter crumbs for approximately three weeks. They are then placed onto finisher pellets. Broilers maintained for the meat trade and housed in 23 hours of light outgrow their own skeleton; they put on weight so fast that their skeletons are unable to support their mass. If they are required for breeding their weight may be controlled by housing them in shorter photoperiods and feeding lower protein content foods.

Adult chickens may be fed a variety of commercial foods such as dry mash, wet mash, crumbs or pellets, such diets normally include grit (to help grind down cereals in the gizzard) and calcium to ensure adequate supplies for growth or egg production. Mixed corn (kibbled maize and wheat mixtures) may be fed and this may be scattered onto the substrate to provide the opportunity to forage, if corn is used grit and oyster shell must be provided.

Breeding

Fertile eggs can be obtained from commercial hatcheries. Alternatively a breeding flock can be maintained. Breeding birds will need to be kept at a ratio of one cockerel to approximately twenty hens, groups are established before the birds are fully sexually mature in order to minimise fighting.

Artificial insemination can be used with chickens. Semen collected from cockerels is introduced into the vagina by means of a syringe. This allows maximum use of superior males and makes it easier to produce fertilised eggs using a cage system.

Pullets chosen for egg production usually come from strains which do not go broody, that is they do not stop laying after producing a clutch of eggs to incubate them. Egg laying begins at about twenty weeks of age, a little irregularly at first but they settle down to producing one egg a day for up to seven days then they stop laying for a day before beginning again. They continue to do this for about one year before going into a moult. The moult, where they stop laying and lose feathers and body condition, lasts approximately two months. The first laying season is considered the most efficient period as the birds lay fewer eggs in subsequent seasons.

Collecting eggs

Eggs should not be collected for incubation until five days after mating as it takes that amount of time for the egg to pass down the uterus, gaining its membranes and shell. Eggs intended for incubation should be collected frequently to reduce the risk of premature incubation. Eggs should be of average size (48–65 g for chickens), with good shell quality (no ridges or cracks) and shape (i.e. not misshapen). In pedigree flocks (or flocks maintained for antibody production), where it is necessary to know which hen has laid the egg, trap nest boxes may be used. A trap nests closes when the hen enters and holds her until she is released, it must be checked hourly to minimise the time the bird is shut in the box, each egg must be recorded against the bird that has produced it. When marking fertile eggs, a soft graphite pencil should be used, not a spirit-based pen, as this may damage the embryo.

Storage of eggs

Where small flocks of breeders are maintained, eggs may be collected as soon after laying as possible and can be placed in a cooled store at 12–16 °C and relative humidity (RH) 80–90% until adequate numbers have been collected. Stored eggs will need to be turned at least once per day, storage beyond ten days will lead to a reduction in fertility.

Incubation

Very few establishments use natural incubation (by broody hens) to produce chicks, most use artificial incubation. The type of incubator usually depends on the numbers of eggs to be incubated. Small numbers of eggs are frequently incubated in natural draught incubators which rely on natural convection to distribute the heat. Larger numbers are usually incubated in forced draught incubators where the heat is forced around the incubator by fans or paddles (Figure 24.3).

Whichever form of heating is provided, eggs need to be turned daily. The eggs may be turned manually or automatically, if eggs are turned manually they should be turned at least five times a day. Most incubators, even small ones have automatic turning

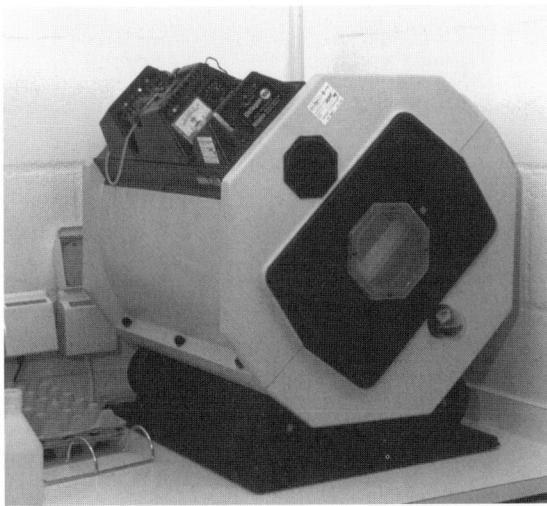

Figure 24.3 Small-scale incubator.

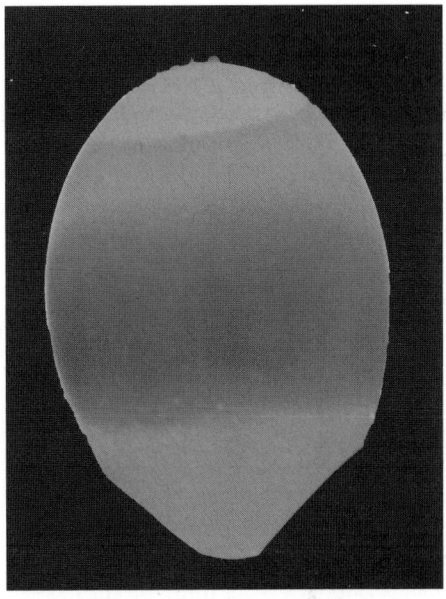

Figure 24.4 Appearance of candled egg. The air sac is clearly visible at the top.

devices. Turning the eggs prevents the developing embryo adhering to the membrane and shell of the egg which may lead to distorted development of the embryo and prevent hatching. Commercial hatcheries use very large incubation rooms which may take thousands of eggs per room.

All types of incubator should be run for 24 hours prior to setting the eggs to ensure the correct temperature is being maintained. Eggs which have been stored at 12 °C should be allowed to warm up before being set (placed) into the incubator. The temperature for incubation should be 37–38 °C for 19 days with an RH of 60%. If a hatching tray or hatcher is available, eggs should be placed in them at 19 days of incubation. The temperature is reduced to 36 °C and the RH increased to 65% for hatching. If RH is too low chick size will be reduced and hatching may be impaired leading to increased numbers of dead in shell, high RH may lead to large wet chicks with reduced survival. Large scale incubators are also able to control oxygen and carbon dioxide levels in which case O_2 levels should be 21–22% and CO_2 levels should be 6%. Chicks which hatch in the hatching tray should remain there until they are fully dry and fluffy (up to twenty-four hours) during which time they will absorb the yolk sac.

The progress of the egg during incubation can be checked by candling. This involves shining a bright light behind the egg so a shadow of the contents can be seen (Figure 24.4).

Rearing (brooding)

Chicks should be reared in specialist cages (called brooders) or restricted areas in a pen (similar to that shown in Figure 25.5, p. 173). The cage or restricted area (in large holding pens, temporary brooders can be made using cardboard or hardboard circles) should be maintained at a temperature of 35 °C for seven days and then reduced by 3–4 °C per week until 21 °C is reached.

The light period will depend on the breed type, broilers may be maintained on 23-hour light period to enhance feeding and growth, whereas layer strains would be placed on a reduced light period (8 hours light) to reduce food intake and control sexual maturity. When maintained in circular pens with a heat lamp suspended over them, if chicks are too hot they will be on the perimeter of the pen trying to escape the heat source, if they are cold they will huddle under the heat source.

Thermostatically controlled brooders are available for large scale chick rearing.

Sexing

Chickens are sexually dimorphic, i.e. males have different plumage and sexual characteristics from the females. Males have larger combs and wattles. They may also have large spurs on the legs. The males also have different feather types, especially the hackles (neck feathers); in the male these are elongated and pointed, in the female short and rounded. Adult males also have elongated curved tail feathers.

Some breeds such as Brockbar and Brussbar are autosexing breeds, i.e. the chicks can be sexed from a day old as they have different plumage.

Some pure breeds may be crossed to produce sex-linked chicks, crossing brown males, such as Rhode Island Red, to white females, such as Light Sussex, produces chicks where the males will have white plumage and the females brown plumage (this sex linkage does not work if the breeds of male and female are switched).

Chicks may also be sexed at a day old by examination of the cloaca but this method demands considerable skill.

Identification

There are a variety of rings which can be placed around the leg of the adult chicken. The rings may be plastic spirals, split plastic rings or metal bands placed around the leg, these rings may be simply different colours or they may be engraved with numbers (Figure 24.5). When rings are applied to young growing stock regular checks must be made to check that it allows room for growth. Wing tags may be placed through the web of skin formed by the wing, these tags must not be put through the muscle. Electronic transponders may be inserted subcutaneously and will provide a safe and efficient method of marking. The application of coloured dyes to the feathers can provide temporary marking, red markers should not be used as this may lead to feather pecking.

Handling

When handling poultry sudden movement should be avoided. The bird should be approach slowly with the

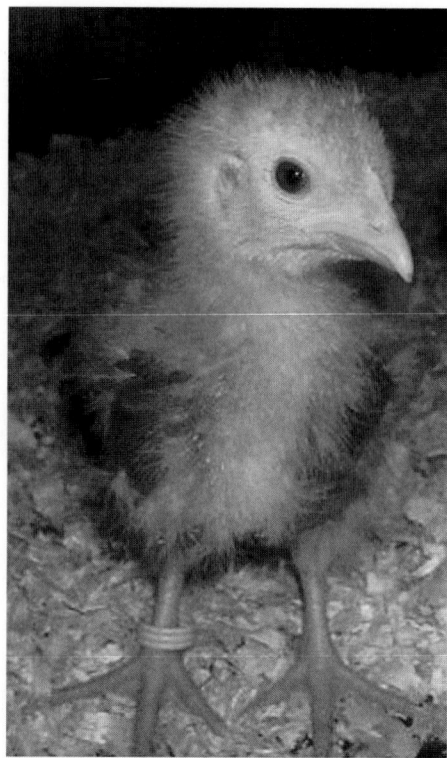

Figure 24.5   Chick with leg ring.

fingers spread so that the bird's wings can be clasped to its body; the wings must be kept close to the body to prevent fluttering. The bird can be conveniently carried with its head pointing behind the handler, its body tucked under the arm and the legs held from underneath.

Health and transportation

Chickens exhibit the same signs of ill health that are seen in mammals – a drop in food intake, weight loss, lethargy. In laying birds there will be a drop in egg laying. The named veterinary surgeon should be consulted whenever there is concern about the condition of a bird. A summary of chicken diseases is given in Duncan (1999). A number of chicken diseases are notifiable (e.g. Newcastle Disease). It is important to be aware if any of these diseases are a problem in the surrounding area as the movement of chickens will be restricted. Information of movement restrictions can be obtained from the local DEFRA divisional manager.

If the establishment holds large flocks of birds veterinary advice should be sought on appropriate vaccinations and health control regimes.

References and further reading

DEFRA (2002) *Code of Recommendation for the Welfare of Livestock, Laying Hens.* DEFRA, London. www.defra.gov.uk

Duncan, I.J.H. (1999) The domestic fowl. In: T. Poole (Ed.) *The UFAW Handbook on the Care and Management of Laboratory Animals* (7th edn). Blackwell Science, Oxford.

Home Office (1989) *The Code of Practice for the Housing and Care of Animals used in Scientific Procedures.* HMSO, London.

25
Quail

Roger J. Francis

Introduction

The Japanese quail (*Coturnix japonica*) (Figure 25.1) is the most common species of quail used in the laboratory. Other species used include the European quail (*Coturnix coturnix*), the Californian (*Lophortyx californica*), the Bobwhite (*Colinus virginianus*) and the Chinese painted quail (*Excalfactoria chinensis*). Both the Japanese and the Chinese painted quail have been bred in many colour mutations. Within the United Kingdom the European quail is a Schedule 2 listed species and may only be obtained from a designated breeder or supplier. The classification of quail is given in Table 25.1.

Use in regulated procedures

In the laboratory, quail are used for studies in the areas of genetics, growth and nutrition, behaviour, physiology, pharmacology and in toxicological testing of agriculture substances and pollutants.

Table 25.1 Classification of quail *Coturnix coturnix* and *Coturnix japonica*.

Kingdom	Animalia
Phylum	Chordata
Sub-phylum	Vertebrata
Class	Aves
Order	Galliformes
Family	Phasianidae
Generic and specific names	*Coturnix coturnix*
	Coturnix japonica

Environment

The environmental levels required by the Home Office codes of practice (1989; 1995) are listed in Table 25.2.

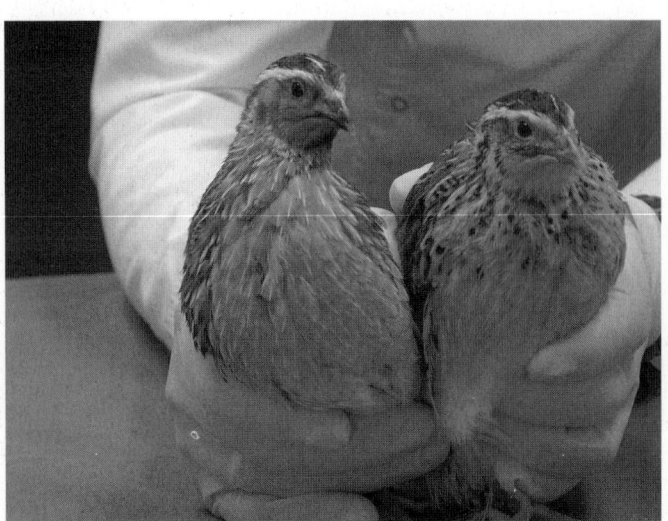

Figure 25.1 Male and female (mottled plumage) quail.

Table 25.2 Environmental levels for quail (Home Office 1989).

	Scientific procedure establishments	Breeding and supplying establishments
Room temperature	16–23 °C	Adults 16–23 °C
Relative humidity	55% ± 10%	30–80%
Room air changes per hour	None stated	Sufficient to provide constant fresh air and extract moisture and waste gases
Photoperiod	12 hours light: 12 hours dark	16–24 hours light
Light intensity	350–400 lux at bench level	None stated

Once a temperature has been selected from the range in Table 25.2 it should not vary more than ± 2 °C. Newly hatched chicks should be kept at 35–37 °C then the temperature should be reduced slowly so that it reaches the adult temperature range by the time the chicks are four weeks of age.

Caging

Recommended stocking densities can be seen in the Home Office codes of practice (1989; 1995). In the laboratory, quail are often maintained in battery-type wire grid cages (wire used for these battery cages should be plastic coated to prevent injury to the bird), but are also housed in larger cages (Figures 25.2 and 25.3), aviaries or pens. Less stereotypic behaviour is seen in floor pens than cages. Quail fly vertically if they are frightened, this must be taken into account

when designing cages for quail to avoid them causing damage to their heads. The suggested cage height is 60 cm and cage tops can be lined with foam padding.

Routine care

Battery-type cages are normally stood over paper tray liners which are changed once or twice per week; this does not entail any handling or disturbance of the birds.

If housed in larger cages, pens or aviaries, birds may be slowly driven to the opposite side of the pen while cleaning out the substrate. In very large aviaries it may be necessary to use nets to catch the birds. A bird can be removed from smaller cages by placing an open hand on each side of it and gently clasping it so that it cannot flap its wings. It can then be held in one hand, with the animal facing the operator, its legs can be placed between the first and second fingers

Figure 25.2 Large tiered cages.

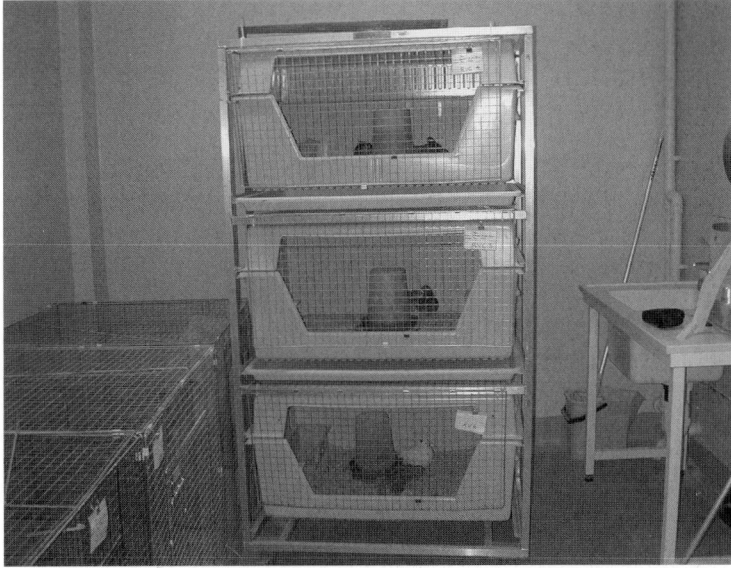

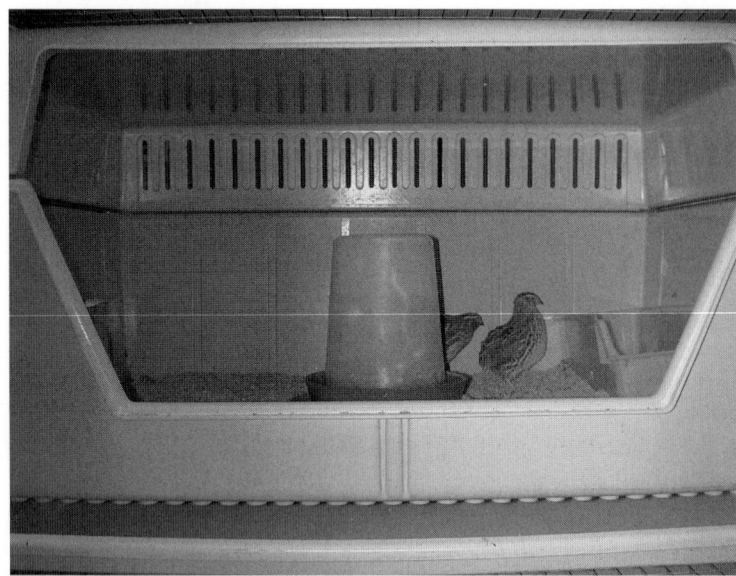

Figure 25.3 Inside large cage, showing water container.

and the wings restrained by enveloping the bird with the palm of the hand and the thumb.

When birds are housed on solid floors with substrate, special attention must be paid to the feet of the birds, as they are prone to build up of faeces and food 'clogs' on their toes and claws. If this does occur, the clogs should not be pulled off as this will damage the toes and risks breaking a claw off. Clogs can be removed by standing the bird in a shallow dish of warm water; this will soften the clogs and allow easy removal without foot damage.

In small battery cages there is not usually room to add any form of environmental enrichment, but in larger cages and pens, with adequate floor space, enrichment is possible. Deep litter substrate and dust baths (Figure 25.4) will allow birds to scratch and bathe, loose hay will allow the birds to hide as will light boards leant against the pen walls, lengths of 4 inch piping can also be used to provide cover.

Small seeds, such as pannicum millet, may be used as a forage food for enrichment.

Feeding and watering

Most laboratory quail are fed high protein diets such as turkey starter crumbs and this is presented *ad libitum*. Fresh water should be available at all times, it is normally offered in open troughs or shallow dishes. Special care should be taken to prevent chicks drowning, this can be done by filling the water dish with marbles or by placing an inverted flower pot into the dish preventing the chicks from getting into the water.

Breeding

Japanese quail are sexually dimorphic as are most species of quail. Both *C. coturnix* and *C. japonica* share the same types of plumage, the males have light brown breast feathers with a lighter central stripe, while the females have light brown breast feathers with a black or dark brown speckle (see Figure 25.1, p. 170).

Aggression can be reduced in breeding groups by establishing them before they are sexually mature. Breeding groups should consist of one male mated with from two to ten females.

Egg laying commences at 6–8 weeks of age in *C. japonica* and 18–20 weeks in *C. coturnix*, the eggs vary in colour from pale blue–green to heavily blotched with brown–black. The eggs weigh 8–10 g and incubation takes 16–17 days at a temperature of 37.5 °C.

C. japonica rarely incubate their own eggs. Eggs should be collected daily and stored at between 12–15 °C until sufficient numbers have been collected

Figure 25.4 Old mouse cage used as a dust bath.

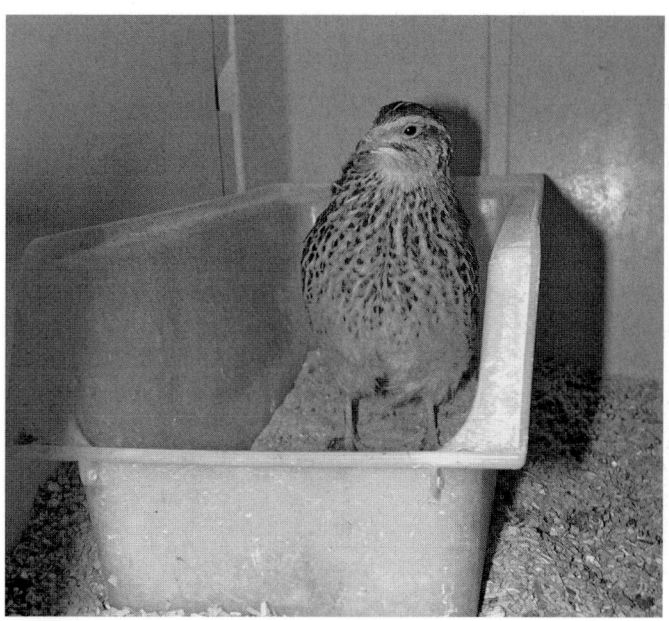

Figure 25.5 Quail brooder.

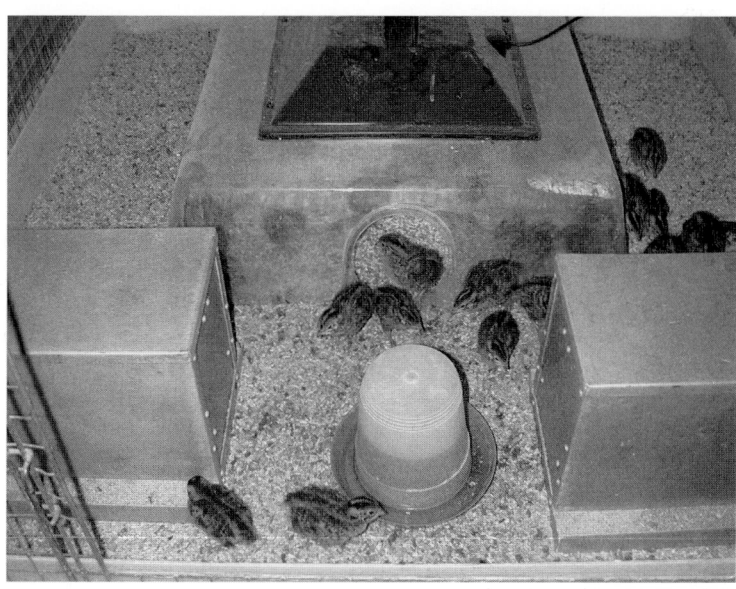

for artificial incubation. Stored eggs must be turned daily. Hatching success reduces the longer the eggs are stored.

Chick hatching weight is approx 8–10 g and growth is rapid, they reach 18–30 g by the time they are seven days old.

Once hatched and dried, chicks are placed in a brooder (Figure 25.5). Quail chicks are precocial, but need to be kept at a temperature of 35–36 °C for the first few days, the temperature can then be reduced by 0.5 °C per day until they are housed at a temperature of 20 °C at three weeks of age.

Health

As chickens, see Chapter 24.

Identification

As chickens, see Chapter 24.

References and further reading

Home Office (1989) *Code of Practice for the Housing and Care of Animals used in Scientific Procedures.* HMSO, London.

Home Office (1995) *Code of Practice for the Housing and Care of Animals in Designated Breeding and Supplying Establishments.* HMSO, London.

Mills, A.D., Faure, J.M. and Rault, P. (1999) The Japanese quail. In: T. Poole (Ed.) *The UFAW Handbook on the Care and Management of Laboratory Animals* (7th edn). Blackwell Science, Oxford.

26

Nutrition – The Basic Nutrients and a Balanced Diet

Brian K. Lowe

Introduction

Seven characteristics distinguish living organisms from non-living objects. These are the ability to:

(1) move;
(2) sense environmental stimuli and make appropriate responses;
(3) grow;
(4) excrete potentially harmful waste products;
(5) reproduce to ensure future generations;
(6) produce energy through respiration;
(7) feed.

Feeding provides the fuel for the living organism, which is 'burnt' to produce energy, and the basic substrates (known as nutrients) which are necessary to support the other characteristics. There is a difference between a diet and a food. A diet is a regime of food provision. This means that a diet is concerned with more than just the type of food eaten, it also includes the amount of food consumed and the frequency of feeding bouts. The amount of food given on a daily basis is often called a ration. A food is a substance which, when ingested, supplies nutrients. A nutrient being a substance which fulfils one or more of the following:

(1) can be used to generate energy;
(2) provides materials which can be used to build new tissue, or repair damaged tissue;
(3) provides materials that are needed for the animal's metabolic processes to continue.

Feeding is a mechanism for ensuring an animal has sufficient raw ingredients to meet its anatomical, physiological and energy requirements. Most nutrients are taken directly from the diet or manufactured within the body from other dietary nutrients. Nutrients which can be synthesised in the body do not require a dietary source, assuming that the animal eats sufficient levels of the precursors required to manufacture enough of the nutrient to meet the animal's needs. For example, most mammals use vitamin A (retinol compounds) from the diet, but are also capable of splitting ingested β-carotenes (which are essentially two units of inactive retinol joined together) into active vitamin A. When there is little vitamin A in the diet, the animals split the precursor β-carotenes into active retinol, and so avoid hypovitaminosis A (vitamin A deficiency). An animal can obtain many nutrients directly from the diet or by synthesising them in the body from dietary precursors.

Nutrients which cannot be synthesised in the body, and therefore have to be supplied in the diet, are termed essential nutrients. Examples of these include essential fatty acids, vitamins, minerals and some amino acids (e.g. methionine and cystine).

While it is true that the majority of nutrients are supplied in the diet, some nutrients can also be obtained via other routes. Vitamin D can be synthesised from the action of the sun on the skin. Gut micro-organisms also produce a number of nutrients (including biotin, vitamin K and volatile fatty acids) as by-products of their metabolism in the hindgut. Although the hindgut is relatively impermeable, some of these may pass into the host's blood stream, even more of these nutrients can be obtained by ingesting the faeces (coprophagy).

Table 26.1 Examples of differences between a generalised herbivore and carnivore. Omnivores are somewhere between these extremes.

	Carnivore	Herbivore
Incisors	Small, used for grooming and manipulating objects.	Large, sharp edges for nibbling vegetation.
Canines	Large, curved and pointed. Used for holding and killing.	Absent, sometimes replaced by a toothless gap (diastema).
Pre-molars Molars	Possess sharp ridges. PM 4 and M1 of lower jaw form enlarged 'carnassials'. The lower jaw bite is inside the upper, and shears slices of flesh and splits bones.	Alternating ridges of hard enamel and furrows of softer dentine. Used to grind food and spilt plant walls to expose contents.
Tooth growth	Closed roots, no growth after milk teeth.	Open roots, continual growth to replace wear after grinding.
Jaw action	Firm jaw articulation. Vertical movements grip and shear flesh. Large temporal muscles.	Loose jaw articulation. Moves in all directions for efficient grinding. Large masseter muscles.
Behaviour	Little chewing, food may be bolted. Many eat large volumes infrequently. Intense activity during hunting is followed by prolonged rest. Felids may rest 18 hours or more a day. Play is important throughout life to hone hunting skills.	Constant or prolonged grazing. Constant alertness for predators. Play less obvious after juvenile phase, but still often present where possible. Play is less important in developing a feeding strategy.
Gut	Relatively short and simple.	Longer, large specialised appendix and caecum, housing commensal micro-organisms.
Eyes	Forward, good judge of distance.	On side of head, for all round vision.

This chapter is primarily concerned with the commonly kept mammalian laboratory species, which in the wild would exhibit many different feeding strategies to meet their nutritional requirements. These strategies have evolved over thousands of generations and mean that a particular species has developed a characteristic set of behavioural, physiological, anatomical and nutritional needs. Despite domestication, laboratory animals retain many of the feeding drives of their wild ancestors. As feeding takes up a considerable amount of an animal's time in the wild, and forms a significant part of an animal's total behavioural repertoire, feeding will be an important part of meeting a laboratory animal's ethological needs. This should be taken into account when devising a diet for laboratory animals. Table 26.1 highlights a few of the differences between animals with widely differing feeding habits.

The basic nutrients

Nutrients are brought together under six broad headings based on their physical characteristics and chemical structure. A summary of the main nutritional groups is given below. (Fibre, although not a nutrient, is also included below.)

Proteins

Proteins contain the elements carbon, hydrogen, oxygen and nitrogen, and sometimes sulphur. They are large molecules comprised of chains of amino acids. The type of protein depends upon the number and arrangement of the amino acids. It is the joining of the amino acids into characteristic shapes which determines the functional ability of the protein. The amino acids are used as building blocks for the growth of new tissue and the repair of existing tissue. Therefore, protein requirements will increase during growth, reproduction and following trauma or ill health. In addition, enzymes which catalyse the animal's metabolism are all proteins, and proteins act as important carrier molecules and chemical messengers within the body.

There are approximately twenty different amino acids, of which these are required in the diet:

- Arganine
- Histidine
- Isoleucine
- Leucine
- Lysine
- Methionine and Cystine
- Phenylalanine
- Treonine
- Tryptophan
- Tyrosine
- Valine

These are termed essential amino acids. The rest

can be assembled in the body from other amino acids. In practice, this means that the amount of individual amino acids provided in the diet (particularly essential amino acids) are more important than the total amount of protein, as a lack of an essential amino acid will still lead to a deficiency syndrome in spite of an excess of other amino acids. First-class proteins provide all the essential amino acids in appropriate quantities and are usually from animal origin, although soya is an example of a first-class plant protein. Second-class proteins lack one or more essential amino acid. The amino acid which is missing is termed the limiting amino acid.

Proteins can be used to provide energy for the animal, but in comparison to carbohydrates and fats, are relatively expensive dietary ingredients. To reduce the costs when manufacturing diets, other nutrients (usually carbohydrates) are used to supply energy. The use of one nutrient to reduce the need of another is called 'sparing', in this case the carbohydrate is 'protein sparing'. Excess protein is not stored like carbohydrates or fats, but tends to be broken down in the liver and excreted in the urine. Meat, eggs and soya are good sources of good quality protein. Cereals are generally second-class proteins as the lysine, cystine or methionine content is often low.

An imbalance in protein levels will show itself in a number of different ways depending upon the nature of the imbalance. A diet high in good quality protein will be expensive, but will give good reproductive performance, growth rates and body condition (assuming it is otherwise nutritionally balanced). If the high protein levels are not required, some of the protein will be burnt for energy and a lot will be excreted, so too much protein can be an expensive waste. In addition, high protein diets fed for long periods have been associated with behavioural changes, tumour formation and renal and hepatic disease.

There is a minimum amount of protein required in the diet to meet the body's demands (the obligatory protein requirement) for repairing the body and replacing proteins which have been metabolised. If the amount of protein supplied in the diet is less than the animal's minimum requirement there will be signs of protein deficiency, including reduced growth, poor coat condition, muscle wastage, anaemia, hypoproteinaemia (low protein levels in the blood), oedema formation, poor reproductive performance and increased neonatal mortalities. If the diet meets the animal's obligatory protein requirement, but is supplied by poor quality protein then there will also be signs of protein deficiency, as the diet is likely to be deficient in at least one amino acid. The signs of the deficiency may vary depending on which amino acid is absent (due to the role of the particular amino acid in the body's metabolic processes); so tryptophan deficiency may cause cataract formation, corneal vascularisation and alopecia; whereas lysine deficiency is associated with dental caries, impaired bone calcification and blackened teeth; and methionine deficiency may cause a fatty liver.

Carbohydrates

Carbohydrates are comprised of carbon, hydrogen and oxygen. The general formula is $C_x(H_2O)_y$, where x and y are variable. For example glucose has the formula $C_6H_{12}O_6$, and sucrose has the formula $C_{12}H_{22}O_{11}$. Table 26.2 shows a few common sugars. Carbohydrates are used principally to provide energy for the body. Excess carbohydrate is stored as glycogen and fat. In its simplest form carbohydrate exists as simple sugars (monosaccharides), i.e. glucose and fructose. If two simple sugars combine they form disaccharides, i.e. sucrose. Longer, more complex chains are called oligosaccharides (two to ten simple sugar chains) and polysaccharides (greater than ten simple sugar chains), i.e. starch or cellulose. Cereals are a good source of carbohydrates.

As the number of chains increases the carbohydrates become increasingly difficult to digest, become less soluble in water and lose their sweet taste. Complex carbohydrates release glucose at a slower rate, avoiding peaks and troughs in blood sugar levels.

Pasta, rice and raw oats are particularly good at releasing sugars gently. Apart from providing energy,

Table 26.2 Carbohydrates.

Carbohydrate	Examples	Characteristics
Polysaccharide $(C_6H_{10}O_5)n$	Starch Glycogen	Unsweet Insoluble
Disaccharide $C_{12}H_{22}O_{11}$	Maltose Lactose Sucrose	Sweet and soluble
Monosaccharide $C_6H_{12}O_6$	Glucose Fructose Galactose	Sweet and soluble

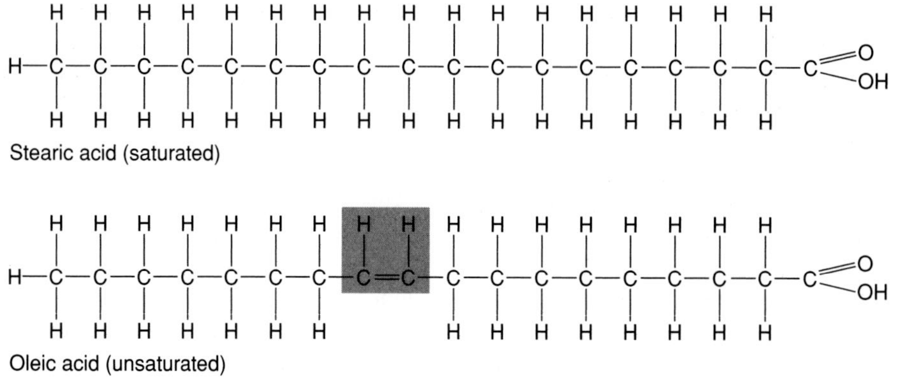

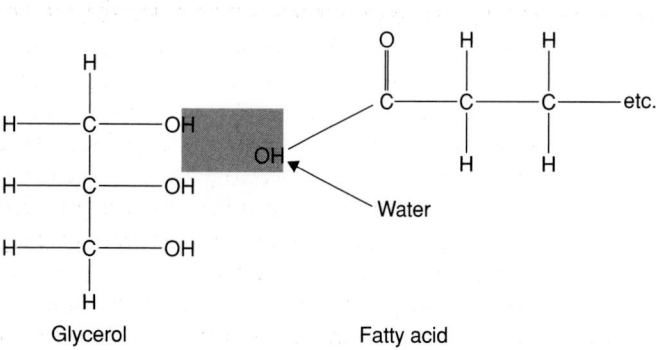

Figure 26.1   Fatty acids.

sugars are important elements in nucleic acids. There is much debate over how essential carbohydrates are in the diet, as some amino acids (gluconeogenic amino acids) can be broken down to supply glucose. In practise, as carbohydrate is readily available and comparatively cheap it will form a significant part of the diet for most laboratory animals, including that of carnivores.

Lipids (fats and oils)

Lipids also consist of hydrogen, oxygen and carbon atoms. The characteristics of lipids are related to the number of carbon atoms forming a chain and the degree to which these carbon atoms are combined with hydrogen atoms. Each carbon atom in the chain can bond with up to three hydrogen atoms if it is at the end of the chain, and two hydrogen atoms if it is in the chain (Figure 26.1). If it binds with the maximum number of hydrogen atoms it is said to be saturated. If a carbon atom is capable of holding more hydrogen atoms due to it being double- or triple-bonded to one or more of the hydrogen atoms, it is

said to be unsaturated. If there is only one carbon atom which is not saturated the lipid is a monosaturate. If more than one of the carbon atoms are not fully bound to hydrogen then the lipid is polyunsaturated. Unsaturated lipids tend to be less solid at room temperature and are more prone to rancidity. An unsaturated lipid can be made more saturated, and therefore more solid and less prone to rancidity, by forcing hydrogen atoms to bind to the double or triple bonded carbon atoms in the chain. This process is called hydrogenation.

An animal's diet must include a supply of the essential fatty acids linolenic and linoleic acids. Linoleic and linolenic acids are parent compounds for the manufacture of longer chain fatty acids, including another essential fatty acid called arachidonic acid. Lipids are relatively insoluble in water but readily soluble in organic solvents. Most dietary lipids are a mixture of three different fatty acids linked to a glycerol molecule (triglycerides) (Figure 26.2). Corn oil, fish oils and tallow are good are examples of lipids.

Each glycerol hydroxyl group (OH) reacts with the carboxyl group (COOH) of the fatty acid. In the

Figure 26.2   Formation of a lipid.

process a molecule of water is formed at each bond. In a triglyceride, three fatty acids are joined to a glycerol molecule, in diglycerides there are two fatty acids and monoglycerides there is just one fatty acid.

Lipids yield twice as much energy as carbohydrates or proteins, around 38 kJ/g compared to only 17 kJ/g from proteins and carbohydrates. They are also used to carry fat-soluble vitamins and essential fatty acids. Intakes of dietary fats and carbohydrates which exceed the animal's immediate metabolic requirements can be stored in the body as glycogen and body fat. Body fat acts as a long-term energy store, forms an insulation layer for cold environments and may offer a degree of protection to some internal organs. Cells rich in fats are called adipocytes and are found in specific regions of the body. The exact position differs between species and sexes.

Neonatal animals have pockets of metabolically active fat, brown fat (due to the rich blood supply) which is used to generate heat and energy immediately after birth and helps to limit the risk of hypothermia. Typically, these pockets are found between the shoulder blades and along the back. The steroid hormones, prostaglandins and leukotrienes are important lipid-based chemical mediators for many physiological processes. Lipids are also important components of cell membranes and the myelin sheath surrounding neurons. A deficiency in essential fatty acids leads to poor growth, dermatitis, fatty liver, impaired reproduction, increased skin permeability and kidney lesions.

Table 26.3 shows the structure and melting point of some common lipids. Lipids are described by the number of carbon atoms and the number of unsaturated bonds, so the C prefix refers to the number of carbon atoms, and the number following the colon refers to the number of unsaturated bonds.

Water

Water is not considered by everyone to be a nutrient as it does not contribute either energy or physical materials for growth and new tissues. However, it is essential to the animal's wellbeing; a lack of water will kill an animal far quicker than a lack of any other nutrient. Water acts as a solvent for dissolving water-soluble molecules, and as a transport medium for moving soluble and insoluble materials around the body. Water is also essential for many metabolic processes (i.e. the hydrolysis of proteins), diluting toxins (urine formation and oedema), heat regulation (sweating/panting) and providing intracellular support. Water can be found in most foods, but the amount varies. In meat the water content can be as high as 70–80%, but in most pelleted diets it is less than 12%. The water content of the food will be inversely proportional to the amount of water an animal needs to drink. A small amount of water is produced by metabolic reactions (condensation reactions, such as the joining of amino acids to make proteins, within the body). The majority of water is supplied in the diet or by drinking. Water is lost in urine, faeces, milk, bleeding, vomiting, sweat/panting or during respiration. An animal must balance its water intake to match any losses if it is to remain healthy.

Water must be clean and fresh when presented to the animal. Domestic mains water is generally sufficiently clean to prevent ill health, although some species may be sensitive to the taste or odour of the chlorine. Chlorination or fluoridation of the mains supply may be a potential problem in some experimental procedures. Water can be treated by ultraviolet irradiation, filtration or acidification to ensure it is not a potential source of infection to animals kept under barriered conditions. Drinking water should never be taken from hot water tanks, as these can be reservoirs for potential pathogens, including *Legionella* sp. Whenever possible, water is provided *ad libitum* to reduce the risk of an insufficient intake, which would lead to the animal dehydrating. Where animals are group housed care must be taken to ensure that all animals have access to the water. If

Table 26.3 The structure and properties of some important lipids. (Adapted from *Animal Nutrition*, P. McDonald, R.A. Edwards, J.F.D. Greenhalgh. Longman Scientific & Technical 1989.)

Lipid	Structure	Melting point (°C)
Butryric	C4:0	−7.9
Caproic	C6:0	−3.2
Capric	C10:0	31.2
Palmitic	C16:0	62.7
Stearic	C18:0	69.6
Palmitoleic	C16:1	0
Oleic	C18:1	13
Linoleic	C18:2	−5
Linolenic	C18:3	−14.5
Arachidonic	C20:4	−49.5

necessary more than one source of water should be provided (see Chapter 27).

Vitamins

Vitamins are organic substances which are required in very small amounts. They are essential for good health. If they are absent in the diet deficiency signs will occur. Some vitamins are unstable and deteriorate in the diet during storage, particularly vitamin C. Vitamins A, D, E and K are fat soluble, while the B vitamins and vitamin C are water soluble. Fat-soluble vitamins are stored in the body, while excess water-soluble vitamins are excreted in the urine. As water-soluble vitamins are not stored, an animal requires a regular supply, but these vitamins are less likely to produce toxicity signs. Excessive intake of the fat-soluble vitamins leads to a build up in the body which interferes with the normal physiological processes and toxicity signs may occur. Table 26.4 shows the main signs associated with a vitamin excess or deficiency, the precise clinical signs will vary between the species.

Some vitamins (i.e. vitamin K and biotin) are synthesised by gut micro-organisms and may be

Table 26.4   Sources, action and deficiency signs of vitamins. Clinical signs may vary with age, species and sex.

Vitamin	Source	Deficiency signs	Toxicity signs	Uses
A (retinol) Carotenes	Milk, fish oils, carrots, green vegetables	Disease susceptibility Xerophalmia Dry scaly skin	Skeletal deformity	Maintains healthy epithelium Forms visual pigments in retina
B_1 Thiamine	Yeast, wheat germ, peas, beans, meat	Nervous disorders Digestive upsets Inappetance Nervous disorder, limb paralysis	–	Needed for carbohydrate metabolism
B_2 Riboflavin	Yeast, liver, milk, green vegetables, cereals	Skin disease, diarrhoea Pellagra	–	Involved in energy formation
Pantothenic acid	Offal, eggs, cereal	Loss of hair colour Inappetance Staining of eyes	–	Growth and skin
B_6 Pyridoxine	Fish, offal, eggs, cereal, yeast	Dermatitis, anaemia Increased activity, convulsions	–	Protein metabolism Blood formation
Folic acid	Offal, yeast	Anaemia, embryonic deformities	–	Blood formation CNS development
Biotin	Microbial synthesis	Dermatitis, paralysis Poor hoof and nail quality	–	Skin and hoof development
Niacin	Offal, eggs, cereal, yeast	Black mouth, salivation, and mouth ulceration. Blood, diarrhoea	–	Can be synthesised from tryptophan
B_{12}	Offal, meat, milk, eggs	Hypochromic anaemia Decreased growth and poor reproduction	–	Formation of glycogen, fats and protein Erythrocyte formation
C (Ascorbic acid)	Citrus fruits, milk, meat, green vegetables, potatoes	Scurvy – bleeding gums, salivation Poor wound healing	–	Antioxidant Wound healing
D Cholecalcipherol and Ergocalciferol	Fish oils, milk, eggs Formed in skin by sunlight	Soft bones	Calcification of soft tissues	Calcium and phosphorous absorption
E (Tocopherol)	Wheat embryo	Muscular dystrophy Poor reproduction including reduced spermatogenesis	–	Antioxidant
K	Green vegetables Synthesised by gut bacteria	Poor blood clotting	–	Antioxidant Blood clotting

absorbed into the animal's blood stream so reducing the animal's dietary requirements for it. Large intakes of these bacterially produced vitamins can be achieved through the practise of coprophagy (faeces eating) which is a natural behaviour of many laboratory species. If an animal has its gut microflora compromised (through ill health, antibiotic therapy, or experimental manipulation, such as gnotobiotic rearing) synthesis of these vitamins may be reduced, and a dietary supplement becomes more important. Animals which are prevented from practising coprophagy, for example if they are housed on grid floors, may also rely more heavily on dietary vitamins.

Vitamin D

Vitamin D occurs in two main forms, D_2 (ergocalciferol) and D_3 (cholecalciferol). Ergocalciferol results from ultraviolet irradiation of ergosterol synthesised by plants (although it is not found in living green tissue as chlorophyll screens the necessary wavelengths for its production). Cholecalciferol results from ultraviolet irradiation of 7-dehydrocholesterol in the skin of mammals. Both can also be digested from dietary sources. Both compounds are hydroxylated in the liver and kidney to form 1,25 dihydroxycholecalciferol that acts on the bone, intestines and the kidney to maintain calcium and phosphate homeostasis. Chickens and New World primates have a limited ability to use ergocalciferol, so require a source of cholecalciferol to remain healthy.

Vitamin C (ascorbic acid)

Primates and guinea pigs are unusual in that they cannot synthesise sufficient vitamin C to meet their daily needs. The inability to manufacture sufficient vitamin C stems from a genetic mutation which results in reduced L-gulonolactone oxidase activity. This has been seen occasionally in other species, including a strain of rat. As vitamin C cannot be stored in the body it must be supplied regularly. Without it the animal will develop scurvy; staring coat, bleeding gums, stiff joints and bone problems. In guinea pigs the teeth may overgrow and there is often increased salivation, leading to a brown staining of the mouth and chest.

Minerals

These are inorganic elements needed for growth, development, and the maintenance of normal metabolic reactions. The macro-minerals – calcium, phosphorous, sodium, potassium, chlorine and magnesium – are needed in comparatively large amounts (although still very small amounts in absolute terms). The rest are known as trace elements due to the minute amounts in which they are required. Table 26.5 shows the main minerals, their importance and deficiency and toxicity signs. The signs may vary between species. Animals may receive additional minerals unintentionally through licking and chewing items in their environment such as galvanised metals and stones; or intentionally through placing mineral licks into their pens.

Fibre

Fibre is not a nutrient, but is included here due to its importance in maintaining the health of an animal. Non-starch polysaccharides (fibre) include cellulose, hemicellulose, lignin and pectin. They are found in whole-grain cereals, oats, nuts, beans, lentils and hay. Fibre cannot be completely digested but does provide bulk to prevent hard masses of food collecting and spreads food out to increase the surface area in contact with digestive enzymes. Fibre may have an important function in stimulating the muscular contractions of the gut. It also delays absorption into the blood stream of glucose from easily digestible sugars and starch, reducing glucose peaks and troughs in the blood. Soluble fibre forms a gelatinous mass creating a physical barrier in the gut to slow fat absorption.

Fibres are fermented in the gut by commensal microbes, a suitable quantity of fibre is necessary to ensure the well being of these commensal gut microbes. Fermentation increases the production of hydrogen, carbon dioxide and methane excreted in the breath and via the rectum. Fibre helps with appetite regulation and satiety, reducing energy intakes which might otherwise lead to weight gain. Fibre helps to fill the stomach and gut, making the animal feel full. This might be important for inactive animals where the volume of food required to keep them healthy is small, and hunger may be a problem due to the reduced food intake. Soluble fibre may be better for satiety. Too high a fibre intake can lead to abdominal pain, flatulence and diarrhoea. The amount of fibre required in the diet will vary between species – dogs, cats and primates require relatively

Table 26.5   Sources, activity, deficiency and toxicity signs of minerals. Clinical signs may vary with age, species and sex.

Mineral	Sources	Deficiency	Toxicity	Use
Calcium and phosphorus	Milk, meat and bone meal	Soft bones, impaired neuro-muscular function, impaired reproduction.	Calcification of soft tissues, poor absorption of other minerals.	Skeletal and teeth development, blood clotting, cardiac function, important blood buffer, energy releasing enzymes, nucleic acid formation.
Potassium and Sodium chloride	Salt, potassium is widespread	Nervous disorders, muscular weakness.	Poor absorption of other minerals, death if insufficient water.	Osmoregulation, nervous function.
Magnesium	Widespread	Neurological conditions, impaired reproduction.	Urinary caliculi formation.	Skeletal development.
Iron	Offal, some green vegetables, wheat and oats	Anaemia.	Poor absorption of other minerals, inappetance.	Red blood cell formation.

Trace elements	Sources	Deficiency	Toxicity	Use
Fluoride	Some domestic water supplies, sea foods (fish)	Increased susceptibility to dental caries.	Possibly implicated in certain cancers at high levels.	Skeletal and teeth development.
Zinc	Meat and diary products	Anaemia, poor skin and coat condition.	Interferes with other mineral absorption.	Skin and coat formation.
Copper	Offal, fish, meat, cereals	Anaemia, poor skin and coat.	Haemolytic anaemia.	Erythrocyte formation, skin and hair formation.
Iodine	Plant tissue, fish, iodised salt, salt	Enlarged thyroid.	Reduced food intake and weight gain.	Production of thyroxin.
Manganese	Cereals, nuts, vegetables	Poor fertility, bone deformities.	Little evidence of toxicity.	Reproduction, bone formation.
Chromium	Widespread	Impaired glucose metabolism.	Liver and kidney damage. Only seen when doses in excess of $500 \times$ normal dose have been fed experimentally.	Glucose metabolism.
Selenium	Quantity in an ingredient depends ultimately on the soil content at source	Poor fertility, muscular dystrophy.	Hair loss, lameness, liver disease.	Antioxidant.

little fibre, but herbivores can handle larger volumes of fibre.

The gut microflora in the large intestine utilise nutrients to reproduce and grow. Most nutrients have already been absorbed before they arrive in the large intestine, but fibre and 'resistant starch' cannot be digested early in the gut and arrive in the large intestine where commensal microbes utilise them to produce fatty acids (butyrates), which have anti-cancer properties, and various other potential nutrients, including biotin and vitamin K. Fibre increases stool weight, dilutes the bowel contents, increases the numbers of gut microbes, speeds up the gut transit time and reduces the risk of constipation. Whole grain cereals are important in large intestine health as the carbohydrate is trapped within the whole grain cereal or seed and cannot be absorbed in the ileum. In addition, starch and oligosaccharides (peas, beans and garlic are good sources) are particularly favoured by beneficial large intestine microbes (i.e. *Lactobacillus* and *Bifidobacteria*).

Lactobacillus and *Bifidobacteria* are also found

in live yoghurts and can be used to help restart the large intestinal colonies after a particularly bad digestive upset. Helping the beneficial bacteria reduces the opportunity of harmful bacteria (including *Salmonella* spp. and *Listeria* spp.) from establishing themselves in the gut, reducing the risk of digestive pathogens establishing themselves.

Energy

Energy is not a nutrient, but is the end product of respiration after the carbohydrate, fat or protein has been broken down in the Krebs cycle. A distinction needs to be made between how the nutrients the animal takes in are used. Nutrients which are used to repair damaged or worn-out tissue, or to manufacture new materials and chemical messengers, or which regulate metabolic processes are known as anabolic or synthetic nutrients. Catabolic nutrients are those which are broken down to produce energy. There is a finite need for anabolic nutrients, after which the remaining nutrients are stored in the body, excreted as waste or used as fuel (becoming catabolic nutrients). An animal needs to meet its nutritional needs in terms of anabolic nutrients to avoid deficiency signs, and must have sufficient catabolic nutrients to meet its energy requirements.

An animal needs to balance its energy intake with its energy expenditure. An animal which is metabolically active will increase its energy requirements. Exercise, low environmental temperatures, growth, pregnancy and lactation all increase the energy demands of the animal. The energy an animal requires is related to the animal's basal metabolic rate. The basal metabolic rate is the metabolic rate of the animal in a resting, fasting condition, within its range of thermoneutrality.

Gross energy (GE) is the energy content of the food, usually calculated by burning the food in a bomb calorimeter. A bomb calorimeter is a closed, metal canister which is filled with oxygen under pressure, and contains a known amount of food. When the food is ignited the food burns completely, giving off heat. The amount of heat given off is measured and used to calculate the gross energy of the food. The digestible energy (DE) is the actual energy available to the animal; it ignores the amount of energy excreted in the faeces. The metabolisable energy (ME) is the amount of useful energy available to the animal; it removes the part lost in the urine. Metabolisable energy is the figure most often quoted when discussing the energy needs of the animal. Net energy is that energy actually used, i.e. metabolisable energy minus energy lost as heat. Figure 26.3 summarises the relationship between these figures.

A diet must be balanced with regard to its energy content. If the diet is high in energy it must also be high in nutrient density as the animal will need very little food to meet its energy demands, but will still need the minimum absolute amount of individual nutrients for anabolic purposes. If the food is too energy dilute, the animal will need to eat a lot of food to meet its energy needs, and consequentially may ingest too high a level of nutrients in order to meet its energy demands, leading to toxicity syndromes. In addition, an active or physiologically stressed animal may be unable to eat sufficient food to meet

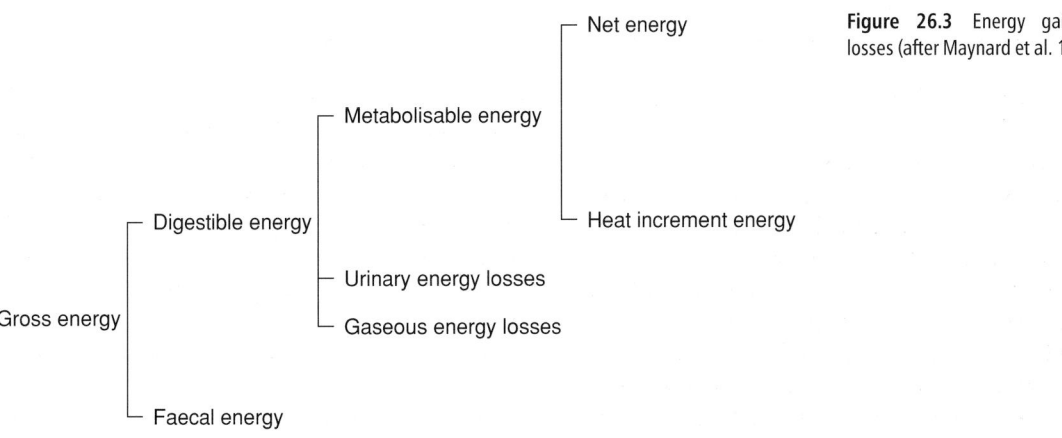

Figure 26.3 Energy gains and losses (after Maynard et al. 1981).

its nutritional or energy demands. This is a particular risk to a heavily pregnant female where the abdominal cavity is full of developing offspring and the stomach has little room to expand.

If the diet is balanced but restricted, the animal will be constantly hungry. If only mildly restricted, the animal will be lean, but healthy and alert. As the restriction increases the animal will become increasingly thin, losing condition, becoming lethargic and miserable. If restricted for long periods the animal will become emaciated and may suffer other nutritional deficiencies as body stores are depleted.

Animals eat to satisfy their energy requirements, but other factors also influence food intake. It is obvious that many animals are not good at regulating their food intake from the high incidence of obesity. The inability to regulate their intakes may be due to an inability to recognise the energy density of the diet, or may be due to other factors. Two factors are particularly obvious, palatability and boredom. A highly palatable food will encourage the animal to eat more. Giving variety to avoid monotony may also increase food intake. Feeding a palatable food is important, as an uneaten diet contains no nutritional value to the animal! Boredom may also lead to an excessive food intake. The animal may have nothing to do but eat, and having restricted space is unable to exercise and use up any excess energy it consumes.

Animals have an absolute minimum requirement for energy – the basal metabolic rate. The energy expenditure is measured by heat loss, which will vary with changes in the surface area of the animal. The larger the surface area of the animal the greater the blood supply near to the environment for heat loss. As an animal grows, the ratio between its surface and body volume decreases. Therefore bodyweight is not necessarily a good predictor of energy requirements. To avoid this, the metabolic bodyweight is used to calculate energy requirements. This figure differs between species but is normally within the range bodyweight$^{0.67-0.75}$. The energy requirements of an animal differ greatly between the species, sexes and physiological state. Table 26.6 lists the energy requirements of animals in various physiological states.

The SI unit for energy is the joule. The joule is a measure of work done when 1 Newton acts through one metre. Another unit you may see is the calorie, which is the amount of heat required to heat 1 g of water by 1 °C. The calorie will therefore vary with

Table 26.6 Physiological status and energy requirements.

Physiological state	Energy requirement	Protein contribution (%)
BMR	0.3 MJ/BWkg$^{0.75}$	–
Maintenance	0.45 MJ/BWkg$^{0.75}$	18
Pregnancy	0.6 MJ/BWkg$^{0.75}$	22–25
Lactation	1.3 MJ/BWkg$^{0.75}$	22–25
Growth	1.2 MJ/BWkg$^{0.75}$	22–25

The figures quoted are an approximation for most laboratory mammalian species, it is intended to indicate how energy requirements change. For specific requirements for particular species the National Research Council's guidelines should be consulted (National Research Council 1995).

pressure, however this variation is so slight as to be insignificant for the purposes of laboratory animal nutrition. As these are small units they are usually expressed as kilojoules or kilocalories (being a factor of a thousand times larger).

A balanced diet

It is important that a diet is balanced. A balanced diet supplies all the nutrients the animal requires in sufficient quantities to avoid deficiency signs, and below the maximum threshold over which toxicity may occur. An animal can usually control the levels of most nutrients within its body by eating more, or excreting or metabolising excess nutrients. However, if a diet is lacking or low in a specific nutrient, it is difficult for the animal to obtain sufficient quantities of that nutrient (without ingesting an excess of other nutrients) to meet its needs. If the diet is very high in a specific nutrient, or the nutrient is stored within the body (such as the fat-soluble vitamins) toxicity can occur. It is not essential that an animal's diet remains perfectly balanced every meal, as the animal is generally able to maintain a good homeostatic control over its nutritional stores. But over time it will become harder for the animal to maintain homeostasis if the diet is unbalanced. Marginal deficiencies or excesses may take a long time to show as body reserves are used up, or excesses gradually accumulate in the body.

Any food must be palatable if it is to have any nutritional value. If the food is not eaten it cannot be digested and the nutrients cannot be absorbed into the animal's body. Palatability is not just about taste;

the odour, texture and size of the pellets or chunks will also help to determine the acceptability of the food to the animal.

Nutrient interactions

Some ingredients or manufacturing processes can interfere with the uptake of other nutrients by:

(1) Competing for binding sites in the small intestine. Zinc, copper, iron and calcium compete for the same binding sites in the small intestine. In practice this means that an excess of one of these minerals will reduce the opportunity for the others to bind and be absorbed.
(2) Binding nutrients, reducing their availability for absorption. Phytates in some cereals can bind zinc and calcium making them unavailable for absorption. Avidin in raw egg whites binds biotin.
(3) Altering their structure, which inactivates them as nutrients. Thiaminases in fresh fish destroy thiamine.

Coprophagy

Many animals practise coprophagy (ingesting their own faeces). Ingested faeces are rich in vitamin B and K, and any other nutritional by-products of microbial fermentation. They also contain a significant population of the microbes which, when swallowed, may help to maintain healthy gut colonies by constantly re-seeding the gut with vigorous robust microbes which have survived their trip through the intestinal tract. A healthy colony of these microbes helps to reduce the risk of pathogenic microbes establishing themselves. Most laboratory species will ingest some of their faeces from time to time, although the rabbit has a particularly well-developed practice. The rabbit produces specific pellets (different from its normal faecal pellets) covered in a thin membrane, these pellets are produced only at night and are ingested directly from the anus without chewing. They are then stored in the stomach where microbial fermentation within the membrane occurs. Eventually the pellets break down and are digested. The ingested pellets from rodents are not as clearly defined as rabbit pellets and are chewed.

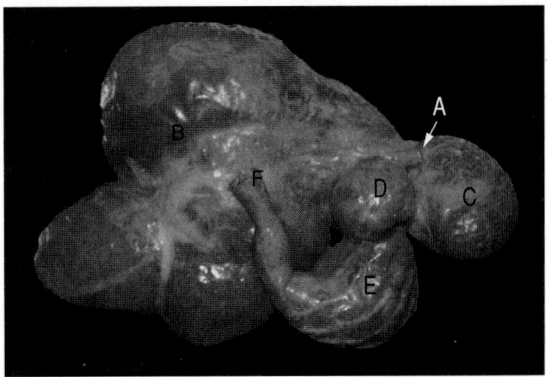

Figure 26.4 Rumen, right side view. A = oesophagus; B = rumen; C = reticulum; D = omasum; E = abomasums; F = duodenum.

Ruminants

Many of the larger herbivores (cows, sheep, goats) are ruminants. These animals have an additional section of gut which greatly increases the breakdown of vegetable matter before it enters the rest of the intestinal tract. Instead of a single stomach, a ruminant has four chambers; rumen, reticulum, omasum and abomasum (Figure 26.4). Food is chewed in the mouth, mixed with copious amounts of saliva and swallowed, where it enters the rumen. The rumen contains a rich community of symbiotic micro-organisms (bacteria, fungi and protozoa). These micro-organisms ferment the food and produce cellulase to break down cellulose. In return for a good food supply and a warm environment in which to live, the micro-organisms produce many nutrients as by-products of their metabolism, including carboxylic acids (ethanoic, propanoic, butyric) and many vitamins. Fermentation also produces methane and carbon dioxide which is excreted by eructation (belching). The micro-organisms can utilise inorganic nitrogen compounds, including urea (which can be included in the diet as a cheap nitrogen source) which is a circulating waste product of nitrogen breakdown from the liver. The partially digested food (cud) passes to the reticulum where it is pelleted and regurgitated for rumination (re-chewing). It is then reswallowed into the omasum for more fermentation. Eventually the processed food passes to the abomasum that is, the true stomach, and then follows the usual mammalian digestive process.

The main advantages of this system include:

- an ability to recycle nitrogen from hepatic urea;
- repeated processing of the food which increases the breakdown of vegetable matter and improves digestive efficiency;
- the products of microbial fermentation are produced anteriorly to the main sites of absorption.

At birth, the rumen and reticulum are underdeveloped so there is little fermentation. The milk bypasses the rumen and reticulum via an oesophageal groove which is stimulated to close (forming a tube) by sucking. Milk enters the abomasum where the milk is clotted and partially digested in the normal mammalian pattern. The eating of solids stops the reflex closure of the oesophageal groove so the rumen fills and becomes functional.

Chickens

The digestion of food by chickens is fundamentally similar to most mammals, however there are significant differences in the organisation of the intestinal tract. Lacking teeth they are relatively inefficient at breaking up large particles. Food which can be picked up easily is swallowed, along with saliva (containing the enzyme amylase), and passes along the oesophagus into the crop (diverticulum). The crop is a pear-shaped extension of the oesophagus which acts as a food reservoir and is a site of microbial activity. These micro-organisms start the digestive processes, and produce useful by-products, including acetic and lactic acids and vitamins. The crop can also secrete milk for nourishing young birds before they are fledged. At the end of the oesophagus is the proventriculus – the true glandular stomach. After the proventriculus is the gizzard which generally contains grit. Birds use insoluble grit (sand, quartz, silica) which is not digested and remains in the gizzard to aid in the mechanical breakdown of food. Soluble grit (oyster shell, cuttlefish, limestone, gypsum) provides minerals. The gizzard is highly contractile and grinds the food into fine particles, aided by the grit. The duodenum and pancreas are similar organs to those found in mammals. In the small intestine are two, paired, blind-ending sacs called caeca. The caeca are absorptive organs which are not essential to the bird's well being. The large intestine is relatively short. Faeces and urine leave the intestinal tract at a common point called the cloaca.

Diet manufacture

The manufacturing process begins with a nutrient specification. This details what constitutes a balanced diet for the particular species to be fed. The nutritional specification is compared with a known nutritional profile of the available ingredients in order to formulate a suitable recipe. Nutritional losses likely to occur during the manufacturing process and any possible nutrient interactions are taken into consideration at this point. Any data on the relative digestibilities of the ingredients also needs to be taken into account. The nutritional profile of some commonly used ingredients are shown in Table 26.7. Modern feed plants are now completely computer controlled. Computers can be programmed to select the raw ingredients from the appropriate store, move these to the processing line and control the whole processing process.

A fixed-formula diet refers to recipes which use the same raw ingredients at the same levels for each batch. Although this helps to maintain a degree of consistency, natural nutrient variations between batches of ingredients will mean that batches of the finished diet will vary in their nutrient content. This variation must be contained within tolerable limits. The price of ingredients will fluctuate with their availability, which can affect the profitability of the diet for the manufacturer, and the cost to the consumer. To control the costs, a variable formula diet can be manufactured. This means that a manufacturer will choose the cheapest ingredients at the time the diet is made to meet the nutritional specifications. There is obviously less consistency between batches of variable formula diets, in particular the digestibility values for different ingredients will vary significantly, affecting the availability of the nutrients to the animal. Fixed formula diets are normally used for laboratory animals.

Ingredients have different physical properties, such as density, particle size, hardness and mixing properties. This means that they are difficult to form into a homogenous pellet without grinding up into a suitable particle size. The main dietary constituents are ground and mixed together, the mixing process

Table 26.7 Nutritional content of some common diet ingredients. Blank spaces indicate that the value is unknown or of no significance. (Adapted from *Basic Animal Nutrition and Feeding* by W.G. Pond, D.C. Church & K.R. Pond, 1995.)

	Moisture (%)	NFE (%)	Crude Lipid (%)	Crude Protein (%)	Fibre (%)
Cereals					
Wheat	11–13	60	2	8–15	2
Oats	11–13	60	5	12	11
Barley	11–13	60	2	10	5
Maize	11–13	65	4	10	2
Bran	11–13	50	4	12–16	8–12
Wheatgerm	11–13	40	9	22–32	low
Straw	15	40	1–2	3	35
Animal products					
Fish meal (Herring)	7	1–2	14	75	Trace
Meat meal	12	4	8	55	2–3
Meat and bone meal	–	1	14	40–70	–
Whole milk powder	–	40	30	25	–
Skimmed milk powder	5–10	50	1	30–35	Trace
Soya oil	–	–	100	–	–
Corn oil	–	–	100	–	–
Vegetation products					
Linseed cakes		20–30	1–6		5–25
Soyabean meal	10	24	1	52	6
Hay	15	40	2–4	5–15	20–30
Grass	75–80	10	<2	3–4	4–8
Silage	75–80	10	1	3	4–8
Roots	80–90	10–20	Trace	1–2	1
Alfalfa	10	40	2–4	15–20	20–25
Grass meal	–	–	–	18	20
Other ingredients					
Yeast	–	40	1	40	–

Ammonium, manganese, potassium, sodium, iron, copper, magnesium, zinc, cobalt, calcium and iodine sulphates, carbonates, phosphates or oxides. Limestone. Individual amino acids and vitamins can be added in their pure chemical state.

Supply supplementary minerals Oystershell.

must be long enough to allow thorough mixing but not too long to allow particles to clump together due to their individual physical properties, such as natural stickiness or electrostatic attraction. Ingredients which contribute less than one per cent of the diet (vitamins and minerals) are mixed separately and added to the main ingredients after mixing. Adding the ingredients in this way will help to ensure an even distribution throughout the diet. It is also generally easier to calculate more accurately the correct amount of vitamins and minerals to add once the bulk ingredients have been ground down to even particle sizes and the bulk volume is known. Sometimes it may be necessary to use a small volume of the main mix to act as a carrier vehicle for the vitamin and mineral mix to ensure it mixes evenly without separating.

The heat used in the pelleting process gelatinises starch which helps to bind the ingredients together.

Extruded pellets are made by mixing ingredients with hot water and forcing them through dies, the temperature at the die face reaches 95 °C. This process forms a lot of heat, killing off most pathogens. Extruded pellets are hard, dense and brittle.

Expanded diets are made by mixing the ingredients with hot water under pressure (so the water is hotter than 100 °C), after mixing, the pressure is reduced to atmospheric pressure causing the water to turn to steam and the mixture is extruded through dies. The temperature at the die face is between 130–180 °C. The steam aerates the mixture causing it to expand as it leaves the die. Expanded diets are lighter, having a texture like biscuits, and are relatively free from pathogens.

After extrusion, the diet is dried on perforated beds through which hot air (95–100 °C) passes. The final pellet has a moisture content of less than twelve percent. After drying, the diet is cooled to prevent condensation. Once cool, the diet passes on to dressing beds. A dressing bed consists of two vibrating screens lying in parallel one above the other. The top screen has perforations which allow pellets of the appropriate size to pass through. The lower perforations are much smaller and retain the pellets but allow dust to fall through. Pellets which are too big can be collected and re-processed.

If a powdered diet is required the pellets are ground up. Grinding at this stage ensures that the powdered diet is exactly the same as the pelleted diet in terms of nutritional value.

This diet will be homogenous, clean and generally more digestible due to the heating during pelleting. The powder or pellets are weighed and packaged into clean multilayered paper sacks. The bags may be lined with heavy gauge, heat-sealed polythene bags for additional protection. Diets designed for irradiation are packed in a lightweight polythene bag, within a heavy-duty polythene bag inside the standard paper sacks. Diet may also be vacuum packed for use in isolators, the diet is contained within a paper inner, inside a heat-sealed, vacuum-packed polythene nylon laminate bag, inside a polythene dust cover in a cardboard box.

Canned diets

Ingredients are chosen to meet the nutritional specification of the diet. Ingredients for canned diets are bought in advance and stored frozen in large weighed bins. It is important that the ingredients are frozen, as they are easier to break into smaller pieces while solid. Thawed meats tend to mush and block up the grinding machinery. The weighed, frozen ingredients are dumped into large grinding receptacles where they are broken down into smaller pieces. Once the bulk ingredients have reached a suitable particle size, the other ingredients (supplements of vitamins, minerals, anti-oxidants etc.) are added. Many commercially manufactured canned foods contain synthetic chunks which represent meat; these are added at this point. The complete diet is thoroughly mixed and poured into cans. The filled cans are then moved to the pressure cooker. The high temperatures used in the cooking sterilise the food (similar to an autoclave). The cans are cooled and labelled before distribution.

Quality control

As a rule, non-nutritive additives (coccidiostats, growth promoters, antioxidants and antibiotics) are not added as they may interfere with any tests to be carried out on the animals. Antibiotics and coccidiostats are sometimes added to control infectious disease. Antioxidants combat free-radical formation. Free radicals are unpaired electrons which damage cell structures (including membranes and DNA) and interfere with chemical reactions within the body. Ascorbic acid and tocopherol are natural antioxidants. Butylated hydroxanisols, butylated hydroxytoluene and benzoic acids are also used as antioxidants.

The Food and Drug Administration of America (FDA) has laid down specifications for diets which are to be fed to animals undergoing trials under their jurisdiction. These set appropriate levels of hygiene, administration and manufacture for laboratory diets. Only specified antioxidants and mould inhibitors may be added to increase the shelf-life of the diet. The nutrient capability and contaminant contents must be known prior to feeding.

Reliable food manufacturers will have their own quality control systems to ensure high quality, standardised diets. These may run along aside FDA regulations, but generally will be less rigorous in order to reduce costs for diets not designed to meet FDA requirements. Procedures should be in place to monitor the quality of the whole process, including the formulation, hygiene, machine functioning, ingredient quality, storage, processing and suitability of the finished product.

It is not practical to test every bag of diet comprehensively. Representative samples are taken from the start, end and middle of each production batch, and from batches of individual ingredients and supplements. The frequency at which ingredients will be tested and the type of tests will depend upon the potential risk to the diet. Animal proteins would require a thorough microbiological screening, while vegetation is more at risk from aflatoxins. All are generally tested for proximate analysis, which gives a crude idea of quality. Reference data has been built up over the years against which each ingredient can be checked to ensure it appears within normal tolerance limits. These tests usually include:

- a proximate analysis;
- minerals;
- vitamins;
- heavy metals and other inorganic contaminants (i.e. lead, arsenic, cadmium, mercury, selenium, fluoride, nitrate and nitrite);
- aflatoxins;
- pesticide residues (i.e. dieldrin, lindane, DDT, PCB);
- microbiology – total viable organisms, mesophilic spores, fungi, salmonellae, *E. coli* count;
- where necessary other tests can be requested.

There will be variations between analytical results, so absolute values are not set as guidelines. Instead reference ranges of tolerable limits are set. The size of the range depends on the natural variation in the ingredients being used (cereals will vary depending upon where they were harvested, the time of year and quality of the soil in which they were grown), and the repeatability of the analytical procedures. The manufacturing process (differences in time, temperature and pressures), sampling methods and type of formula will also influence the variation between batches.

The nutritional profile of each batch should be established, recorded and checked against reference ranges to decrease the risk of malnutrition or contamination and for reference if unexpected experimental results occur.

Measuring nutrient levels

A food can be analysed chemically to define its nutrient content. A crude measure can be obtained by looking at the proximate analysis, which measures the following.

Crude protein

The Kjeldahl method measures the nitrogen content of the food and multiplies this by 6.25. This assumes that all dietary nitrogen comes from protein, and that on average the nitrogen forms 16% of the protein molecule.

Crude fat

This measure is obtained by boiling with hydrochloric acid and extracting with diethyl ether. It will include waxes and resins which have little nutritive value.

Ash

This is the residue left after food is incinerated at 500 °C. Ash is used to calculate the nitrogen-free extract.

Moisture

This is the amount of moisture lost after drying to a constant weight in an oven at 100 °C. Moisture meters measure the electrical conductivity of a sample and can give approximate moisture contents. Freeze-drying methods can also be used.

Nitrogen-free extract (NFE)

Carbohydrate is calculated from adding up the other parameters (as percentage values) and subtracting the total from 100. The NFE will include starches, polysaccharides, simple sugars and some fibre (lignin, hemicellulose).

Further parameters

Other parameters can also be measured. Crude fibre is obtained by boiling the sample in dilute acid and then alkali. It is then washed and dried. After weighing it is burnt and the ash weight is subtracted from the pre-burned weight to give the crude fibre figure.

Using more sophisticated techniques (chromatography, flame spectrometry) the levels of specific nutrients can be determined more accurately. These techniques are expensive so need to be targeted selectively. The results are then compared with published recommendations on nutrient levels, such as those published by the National Research Council, prior to feeding.

The concentration of nutrients

The concentration of nutrients within a food can be described in a number of ways:

(1) 'As is' – the quantity of a nutrient in a given weight of the food (e.g. g/100 g). This takes no account of the moisture concentration of the food, so it is difficult to compare foods varying significantly in moisture content in terms of the nutrients they supply. The figure is often expressed as a percentage, 1.5 g/100 g is the same as 1.5%.

(2) On a dry matter basis. The nutrient concentration is expressed taking into account the moisture content of the food. This allows a comparison between foods of very different moisture concentrations on an equal basis.

(3) On an energy basis (g/unit of energy). This allows an estimation of the concentration of nutrients the animal will eat, as the animal needs to satisfy its energy demands.

Tests for measuring the availability of nutrients

Chemical analysis will tell you precisely what the food contains, but tells you little about the availability of the nutrients to the animal. Although a food may contain a certain amount of nutrients, the process of digestion is not one hundred per cent efficient. If the nutrients cannot be absorbed into the body they can contribute no nutritive value for the animal. The actual availability of the food to the animal needs to be evaluated. This is most commonly done by feeding the diet to the animal and collecting the faeces which the animal produces on that diet. By comparing the nutrient content of the diet and faeces, the actual amount absorbed by the animal can be deduced.

In vitro tests are also available. For example, microbiological tests use micro-organisms (*Tetrahymena pyriformis, Streptococcus zymogenes*) instead of animal models to predict the nutrient availability. These are quicker and cheaper to run. One example is the use of *Streptococcus zymogenes* to predict protein quality. The growth of this organism can be sustained by a supplement of casein. The casein acts as the control. Instead of casein, the growth media is supplemented with the test protein and the growth rates of organisms are compared with the casein control. This gives a relative nutritive value (RNV) which correlates well with *in vivo* methods.

Increasingly sophisticated *in vitro* modelling systems are being developed to mimic specific regions of the intestinal tract, so ingredients or foods can be tested without the use of expensive and lengthy animal tests during diet development.

In vivo tests are also conducted to ensure nutritional adequacy. These tests involve feeding the diet to animals at different lifestages. The health and appropriate physiological parameters are measured throughout the trials to ensure that the diet meets the animal's needs. Health checks are carried out by a veterinarian before, during and after the feeding trial has been conducted. Health checks will include blood biochemistry and haematology measurements, to identify less overt signs of malnutrition. Other measurements will depend upon the lifestage being tested, but will obviously include food consumption. For a diet being fed to young animals growth rates will also be important. For a diet designed for reproducing animals then litter sizes, survival rates and neonatal development will be important. Palatability and digestibility tests will also be conducted to ensure the diet is acceptable to the animal (and will therefore be eaten), and that the nutrients within the diet are available to the animal.

Dietary calculations

Digestibility

Digestibility refers to the amount of the diet which can be digested, and is therefore available to the animal. In simple terms it is expressed as:

apparent digestibility (%)

$$= \frac{(\text{food} - \text{food excreted})}{\text{food eaten}} \times 100$$

true digestibility (%)

$$= \frac{\text{food eaten} - (\text{food excreted} - \text{endogenous losses})}{\text{food eaten}} \times 100$$

Endogenous losses refer to the nutrients which although appearing in the faeces do not come from the food, but from body secretions and sloughed alimentary cells. These are difficult to measure and are largely ignored, so apparent digestibility is the figure normally quoted.

A number of factors will affect the digestibility of a food:

- composition of the food, i.e. individual ingredients will have different digestibility values;
- recipe – some ingredients will interfere with the digestion of another, i.e. iron, calcium and zinc;
- the degree of processing;
- species will vary in their ability to digest certain foods.

Protein usage calculations

The protein efficiency ratio calculates how much weight is gained per unit of protein:

$$\text{protein efficiency ratio} = \frac{\text{weight gained}}{\text{protein intake}}$$

Biological value calculates the proportion of the dietary protein absorbed and retained by the body. It is calculated as follows:

$$\begin{aligned}&\text{biological value (BV)}\\&= \frac{\text{nitrogen intake} - (\text{faecal nitrogen} + \text{urinary nitrogen})}{(\text{nitrogen intake} - \text{faecal intake})} \times 100\end{aligned}$$

Biological value (BV) is obviously related to the digestibility of the dietary protein. It is used to highlight the effects of processing, which may damage some amino acids (methionine, lysine and cystine), and protein metabolism in terms of sparing or catabolism for energy. BV may differ depending on the physiological state of the ingredient. Egg protein (around 95%) is considered to have the highest BV, cereals tend to have low BV (40–60%). Animal proteins are around 70–80%. Where a single protein source has a low BV, providing a mixture of protein sources will raise the overall BV.

Calculation of protein in the diet

The amount of protein present in the diet can be calculated as follows:

(1) list ingredients;
(2) calculate the percentage contribution of each ingredient to the diet;
(3) determine each ingredient's percentage protein content;
(4) calculate the amount of protein contributed by each ingredient by multiplying the percentage contribution of each ingredient and its protein content, then dividing this figure by 100;
(5) the protein content of the diet is the sum of these figures (Table 26.8).

Food intake

The total food intake is a useful calculation for estimating the dietary ordering dates and quantities required, or as a crude estimation of palatability and consumption on a given diet. However, a more meaningful figure is the food intake on a bodyweight basis, as this takes the weight of the animal into account. When growth rates are being compared the food conversion ratio is a useful calculation.

$$\text{food conversion} = \frac{\text{food intake}}{\text{weight gain}}$$

This ratio will change with age, temperature, strain, species and sex.

Table 26.8 Calculation of percentage of protein in diet.

Ingredient	Ingredient in diet (%)	Protein content (%)	Calculation	Protein contribution
Fishmeal	10	65	$10 \times 65/100$	6.5
Soya	7.5	44	$7.5 \times 44/100$	3.3
Wheatfeed	30	15.5	$30 \times 15.5/100$	4.65
Maize	40	8.5	$40 \times 8.5/100$	3.4
Barley	12	10	$12 \times 10/100$	1.2
Minerals and vitamins	0.5	–	–	–

Total protein in the diet = 19.05%

food utilisation

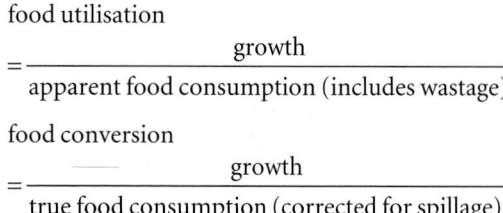

$$= \frac{growth}{apparent\ food\ consumption\ (includes\ wastage)}$$

food conversion

$$= \frac{growth}{true\ food\ consumption\ (corrected\ for\ spillage)}$$

Sterilisation of the diet

Sterilising increases the diet costs and reduces the nutritional value. The processing of laboratory animal diets is carried out to reduce the risk of pathogens being present in the finished diet, and additionally acts as a pasteurising process. Generally, those nutrients most at risk from sterilisation are included at higher levels to allow for losses during processing and sterilisation.

Heat

Pelleting heats the diet up to over 70 °C killing most vegetative organisms. Sterilisation can be achieved by autoclaving the diet but exposure to high temperatures will reduce its nutrient value. Autoclaving should only be used for diets which manufacturers state are suitable and high temperature/short time cycles should be used (e.g. 134 °C for 3–4 minutes). After autoclaving, the diet must be dry, especially hay, to avoid mould growth.

Radiation

Irradiation is another common sterilisation treatment for laboratory animal foods, although it is expensive. One kiloGray kills insects and damages parasite development, five kiloGrays can kill most bacteria, and ten kiloGrays is lethal to spores. Gamma rays from a cobalt[60] source are used to disinfect laboratory animal diets at around 25 kiloGrays (2.5 Mrads) and cause minimal harm to the nutritional profile. Higher doses of 50 kiloGrays (5 Mrads) may be desirable for diets designed to be fed to gnotobiotic animals. Irradiation and heating may increase free-radical formation, which means the level of antioxidants in the diet will be important. Irradiation will also increase the shelf life.

Factors affecting the choice of food

(1) *Microbiological status*. Diets that are not 'clean' are a potential source of pathogenic entry into the colony.
(2) *Palatability*. If the animal does not eat the food it will not receive any nutrition.
(3) *Physical properties*. The hardness, texture, particle size affect how easy it is for the animal to eat the food.
(4) *Volume and availability*. Animals get used to a particular diet, if the diet cannot be obtained when required in appropriate volumes you will need to change the animal's diet frequently. This can lead to digestive upsets and provides another unnecessary experimental variable.
(5) *Reliability of producer*. There must be trust between the manufacturer and the consumer in terms of knowing the quality and consistency of the diet, and the overall service provided. This includes knowing how long it takes from ordering to receiving the diet.
(6) *Cost* in relation to growth rate and productivity. Diets are expensive and need to provide value for money.
(7) *Availability of analytical profile*. It is important that an analytical profile is available for reference if unexpected problems occur with animals being fed the diet.

Feeding

A great deal of research and effort is put into designing and manufacturing laboratory animal diets, all of this is a complete waste of time if the diet is inappropriately stored or presented to the animal. Poor storage leads to deterioration in the quality of the food, which lowers the nutrient content and makes the food unpalatable for the animal. It is worth repeating that any food, no matter how carefully designed and manufactured provides no nutritional value unless it is actually eaten. It is important that the food is presented to the animal in such a way that the animal can get to the food easily and eat it, and that the food is sufficiently palatable to encourage the animal to feed.

The amount of food an animal requires will vary according to:

- species;
- age;
- size;
- sex;
- physiological state;
- environmental conditions.

Storing the diet

The quality of the diet depends upon the:

- quality of the ingredients;
- manufacturing processing;
- delivery and storage;
- presentation methods.

The importance of choosing ingredients which are free from toxins and pathogens, and which reflect a 'normal' nutrient profile for the ingredients has been discussed. However, if the diet is poorly stored, the nutritional value of the diet will deteriorate rapidly. Natural interactions within the diet will lead to a gradual deterioration in diet quality over time, and will increase the risk of contamination from food pests. Although antioxidants are added to a diet, a degree of oxidation will occur over time leading to a general deterioration in the quality of fat, vitamins and minerals. Poor storage increases these losses.

Diet should be stored in cool, clean, dry, dark and well-ventilated storage areas which are dedicated to diet storage. These areas should be vermin proof and protected by insectocutors. The diet should be stored off the floor on pallets or racking. Diet should be used in strict rotation and used by the sell-by date. Dirty or damp food should not be brought into the store. The outer layer of the paper sacking may be removed to limit the risk of bringing disease organisms into the store. Any remaining contents of an opened bag must be stored in airtight sealed containers.

Providing the diet

In a laboratory situation food is normally supplied in specially designed containers. These keep the food clean, reduce wastage and allow accurate recording of food intake. When recording food intake it is essential that the amount of food spilt is taken into account, as diets which crumble may fall through gridded floors and are inaccessible to the animal. If this spillage is not recorded the animal's food intake will be greatly exaggerated.

Where animals are group housed a close eye on the animals' behaviour, condition and bodyweights will be necessary to ensure that all individuals are getting sufficient food, and that no single animal is monopolising the food. It may be necessary to provide more than one feeding point to ensure access for all the individuals within the group.

When checking the animals, the food containers should also be checked to ensure that food is available and that it is within reach of the animal. Small or sick animals may not be able to reach into high-rimmed bowls, or hoppers suspended on cage fronts. Hoppers can get blocked with clumps of pellets, which prevent the food falling into the hopper base where the animals feed.

Food may be offered continually (*ad libitum*) so the animal can eat whenever it wants. This is particularly useful for small species which would naturally eat small amounts frequently. There is a risk that the constant availability of the food may result in over eating and obesity. This risk can be reduced by carefully controlling the amount of food the animal is offered. Food is offered in measured amounts either for a limited period or until the animal has eaten it. This is meal feeding and allows the nutritional intake of the animal to be carefully controlled and measured. Animals soon get used to a routine if the food is offered at the same time each day. The animals become expectant around this time, so care should be taken when planning experimental or other husbandry procedures around this time if they are likely to be hampered by excited animals.

Types of diet

Farm animals, horses and carnivores may be fed 'home-made' diets comprised of natural ingredients. Hay, silage, legumes and root crops can be fed to the herbivores, while cooked meat, offal and bone meals can be fed to the carnivores. It is essential that these diets are tested analytically and supplemented where necessary to ensure a balanced diet is achieved. Care must be taken to avoid microbiological contamination. It is more usual to feed commercially prepared complete foods to laboratory animals.

Antioxidants are added to the diet to prevent oxidisation of the ingredients, which make the diet unpalatable and possibly harmful to the animal. Ascorbic acid, and tocopherol are natural antioxidants, butylated hydroxanisols, butylated hydroxytoluene, ethoxyquin and benzoic acid are other antioxidants. Oxidation leads to the build up of free radicals which can be damaging to the body. Dietary antioxidants are also beneficial in protecting against oxidation within the body.

Antibiotics may still be used in farm-animal diets to increase growth rates and control endemic disease, but are not generally used in laboratory diets. They may influence gut flora, and possibly promote resistant strains of bacteria. Coccidiostats may be used occasionally, but are generally not included in laboratory animal diets.

Natural ingredient diets

These are normal standard diets with limited processing. The diet cannot be completely controlled in terms of nutrient quantity, as there will inevitably be minor batch to batch variations. There may also be a degree of contamination from herbicides and pesticides, although these should be within safe limits. However they may be sufficient to initiate or affect immunological responses.

Canned foods

These are often fed to the carnivore species. They provide a palatable, high-meat diet which is closer to the natural diet that these animals would encounter in the wild. Canned foods can be labour intensive to feed and generally work out more expensive. They are also heavy to transport, but will pass through dunk tanks. It is possible for animals to select items from a canned food, as most of them contain obvious chunks, and this may have a long-term nutritional impact, but this behaviour is unlikely. Canned foods are fed regularly with a limited timed access for the animals, as this type of food will dry out quickly, becoming less palatable. Wet foods left out for long periods are a potential source of infection as they attract insects and other vectors. Feeding bowls will need washing between meals.

Dry diets

Dry diets are normally fed to most of the laboratory species, even the carnivores are increasingly being fed dry foods. As these diets are homogenous, the animals cannot select for particular nutrients. Rodent expanded pellets are about eight to ten millimetres in diameter. Rabbit and guinea pig extruded pellets are about two to four millimetres in diameter. It is important that an appropriate texture is fed to each species. Dry foods, as the name suggests contain very little water (typically less than 12%), so it is important that fresh, clean water is made available at all times. Dry diets are easy to feed, they are less prone to pathogenic gain, and there is minimum wastage. Dry foods generally work out cheaper to buy and feed. However, it is difficult to add medicines/experimental treatments to dry diets unless they are powered. Care must be taken with dry foods during storage to avoid infestation from pests, which apart from causing food spoilage, may act as vectors for disease organisms.

Expanded diets are generally more palatable for dogs, most rodents and primates. This helps to reduce wastage and spoilage of left-over food. The cooking process increases the digestibility of many of the complex ingredients improving the food conversion efficiency, and therefore improving cost efficiencies. The high temperatures used mean the diets, even without further treatments, are clean (less than 1000 micro-organisms per gram). The high temperatures used in expanded diets cause plasticisation of the ingredients leading to a very homogenous pellet, which creates a good powered diet if ground. Standard pellets tend to be less homogenous due to the lower temperatures used.

Mashes

Mashes can be formed by mixing a powered type diet with water. Mashes need to be made up daily as they soon go off and become unpalatable. They also are good breeding grounds for pathogens. The bowls which are used for mash feeding require cleaning before being refilled. Mashes are often used to feed chickens or very young or sick animals as they are easier to eat.

Purified diets

A diet can be manufactured from individual

ingredients whose nutritional content is known and constant. These ingredients are chosen as they provide only one nutritional group. For example casein will provide protein, sugar and starch will provide carbohydrate, vegetable oil will provide lipids and cellulose provides the fibre. Vitamins and minerals are added as required. These diets mean the researcher has better control over any nutritional variation, and reduce the risk of an immune response due to dietary antigens. However, these diets are expensive and generally unpalatable.

Chemically defined diets

These are strictly controlled diets, using purified chemical components to make up the diet, i.e. individual amino acids etc. There is less opportunity for an animal to develop an unexpected immune reaction. They are very expensive and are generally unpalatable.

Liquid diets

Sometimes a liquid form of nutrition is required, especially for very sick animals, neonates or animals whose ability to eat solid foods has been compromised. Liquid diets are formed from soluble ingredients. A good example is the milk replacers used for orphans or to supplement the diet of a neonate whose mother is not producing sufficient milk. If the animal cannot lap the liquid, it can be administered directly into the stomach using a gavage. In extreme situations an animal may be kept alive through the intravenous supply of liquid nutrients.

Special diets

These diets are formulated to provoke certain experimental conditions. The formulation includes specific factors which will predispose an animal to the desired experimental condition. For example, high sugar levels and a sticky texture might be used in studies into dental caries, or high sodium levels might be used for studies into hypertension, or high magnesium and calcium levels used for studies in urolithiasis.

Treats and other dietary provisions

Primates, guinea pigs, rabbits and farm animals may be offered mixed feeding This involves feeding a

nutritionally complete pellet, but the pellets are supplemented with fresh foods, i.e. forages, fruit or vegetables. This system primarily provides enjoyment for the animal as they enjoy these treats. Care must be taken to take in to account any interactions between the treat and the pelleted diet, and to ensure that the animal eats sufficient pellets to obtain all the nutrients it requires. Any treats must be thoroughly cleaned to reduce the risk of introducing pathogenic organisms such as *Yersinia* spp. or *Salmonella* spp.

Treats can be used as rewards to encourage particular desirable behaviours, or as pleasant reinforcers for some experimental procedures. These encourage animals to cooperate with husbandry and experimental procedures, and help bond technicians and animals.

Forages are above-ground herbaceous plants such as pasture, silage and hay. In practice these consist of a mix of perennial and annual plants, so their nutritional contribution is variable. Legumes such as alfalfa and clover are high in protein, vitamins and minerals. Any vegetation must be non toxic and not harmful to the animal, and so should be free from dust, foreign bodies and thistles. Certain plants contain toxins which can poison the animals or interfere with experimental results. Thiaminases and antithiamine agents (i.e. caffeic acid) occur in bracken fern (*Pteridium aquilinum*, Figure 18.2, see p. 113) horsetail (*Equisetum arvense*), yellow star thistle (*Centaurea solstitialis*).

Feeding the young

Neonatal mammals receive all their nutrition from their mother's milk. If the mother cannot produce sufficient milk the neonate will rapidly dehydrate and die. The colostrum (first milk) provides passive immunity from pathogens, so it is important that all neonates are given a source of colostrum. Milk replacers can be used to supplement the neonate's intake. The younger the animal the more frequently it will need feeding.

Rabbits are unusual in that they only suckle their young once a day. Guinea pigs are precocious and can eat solids soon after birth, but do still suckle. As the young develop, they gradually move on to solid foods, this becomes particularly obvious once their eyes open. The change from milk to solids leads to significant changes in the functioning of the digestive system and in the type of micro-organisms living in the gut. The change should be made gradually – sudden changes can lead to digestive upsets. Young can be encouraged to eat solids by offering moistened solid foods, breaking the solids into small pieces and making it available. This may mean sprinkling the food into the substrate where the neonates are living, or offering it in low-rimmed bowls.

Creep feeds are the diets used to wean farm animals off milk and onto solids. For instance lambs start being creep fed ten days after birth, by four to five weeks of age the pellet-fed lambs have a functioning rumen. Development of the rumen depends on gradually weaning onto solid foods, even large lambs only milk fed do not have functional rumen.

Feeding for reproduction

Good quality nutrition is important throughout the reproductive cycle. This begins prior to mating as nutrition may well influence ova maturation and quality. Flushing is a process used in sheep to increase the incidence of twins. Before mating the sheep are moved on to a diet of increased nutrient content. It has been suggested that the change to a high protein diet increases the action of hepatic steroid metabolising enzymes, which may lower steroid levels increasing the secretion of gonadotrophins and improving ovulation efficiency. Ewes on pasture are supplemented with harvested forage, or up to 0.5 kg of grain per ewe per day; the supplement beginning two weeks prior to mating and continuing two to four weeks into the breeding season. The effects are especially good in thin ewes.

During gestation there are two broad phases: an anabolic phase characterised by the laying down of fat and protein which act as nutritional maternal stores, and a catabolic stage during late gestation, where these stores are used to supplement the maternal dietary intake. Initially, due to the increased laying down of fats and protein, and then in late pregnancy by the rapidly growing foetuses, the weight of a pregnant female increases during pregnancy. Her food intake will also increase. In addition to meeting the mother's needs, the developing young also require increasing amounts of nutrients as gestation

continues. These nutrients are used to form new tissue as the young grow and mature. In general, reproductive diets will require increased amounts of energy, protein, vitamins and minerals. The frequency and amounts of feeding may need amending as the abdomen of the pregnant female fills with developing young, which may press on the stomach. Small frequent meals will be better for the female as they do not fill the stomach and are easier to digest.

Inadequate maternal nutrition is associated with poor breeding performance, increased neonatal mortality, deformities and even a long-term predisposition to disease throughout the life of the surviving young, and possibly into future generations.

The energy demands of the lactating female increase further still, as she supplies milk to the rapidly growing young. The nutritional demands upon the mother are usually related to the litter size. Poor nutrition will rapidly compromise the mother's condition, and may even lead to her failing to produce milk. The young will be thin and emaciated and will rapidly dehydrate. Water must be supplied at all times due to the mother's increased demands. As the young reach weaning age, normally from the point at which their eyes open, they will start to eat solids and become less reliant on the mother's milk.

Feeding the sick

Sick animals may well have a reduced appetite and reduced ability to handle large, hard foods. Sick animals are often also dehydrated. Offering moistened, softened foods may improve food acceptability. Any diet fed to these animals must be nutrient dense so only small volumes are required to be eaten. In severe cases, liquid diets can be administered by gavage or drip. Carnivores may appreciate warmed, soft food. All food must be within easy reach of the sick animal.

Feeding specific animals

Table 26.9 lists the typical food and water intake for common laboratory animals. Table 26.10 lists specific nutritional requirements for some laboratory animals.

Table 26.9   A guide to adult food and water intakes (see text for notes on factors affecting food intakes) .

	Food type	Adult weight (kg)	Daily intake (g)	Feeding frequency	Water (ml)
Mouse	Expanded	30	5	*Ad libitum*	6
Rat	Expanded	300	15	*Ad libitum*	35
Syrian hamster	Expanded	100	10	*Ad libitum*	8
Guinea pig	Pellet	600	40	*Ad libitum*	100
Rabbit	Pellet	5	190	*Ad libitum*	500
Cat	Expanded	4.5	70	1–2 times a day	360
	Canned		350		90
Dog	Expanded	10	200	1–2 times day	800
	Canned		600		350

Source: Special Diet Services, Essex, UK.

Table 26.10   Specific nutritional requirements for laboratory animals.

Animal	Nutrient	Reason
Guinea pigs, primates	Ascorbic acid	Lack the enzyme to manufacture suitable amounts
Cat	Food of animal origin to supply vitamin A, arachidonic acid, high levels of protein, taurine	Lack of selective pressure to use non-animal tissue has left it requiring certain nutrients found only in animal tissue.
New World primates, chickens	Dietary vitamin D	Chickens and new world primates require vitamin D_3 as they have a limited ability to use this vitamin.
Gnotobiotic animals, sick animals, animals on antibiotics	Additional B and K vitamins	Altered gut microbe population may reduce production of these nutrients.

References and further reading

Maynard, L.A., Loosli, J.K., Hintz, H.F. and Warner, R.G. (1981) *Animal Nutrition* (7th edn). McGraw-Hill Education, UK.

McDonald, P., Edwards, R.A. and Greenhalgh, J.F.D. (1989) *Animal Nutrition*. Longman Scientific & Technical, London.

Report of the Laboratory Animals Centre Diets Advisory Committee (1977) Dietary standards for laboratory animals. *Lab. Anim.* 11: 1–28.

National Research Council (1995) *Nutrient Requirements of Laboratory Animals* (Nutrient Requirements of Domestic Animals series). National Academy Press, Washington DC.

Taylor, D.J., Green, N.P.O. and Stout, G.W. (1997) *Biological Science* (Vols 1 & 2). Cambridge University Press.

Pond, W.G., Church, D.C. and Pond, K.R. (1995) *Basic Animal Nutrition and Feeding*. John Wiley, New York.

27
Animal Drinking Water

E.K. Edstrom and B. Curran[1]

Introduction

Since humans first domesticated animals, providing water has been a basic, everyday animal husbandry task. In animal research facilities the watering task is extremely important to the well being of the animals and the validity of the research. However, water can carry contaminants harmful to animals and which can introduce variables into research. To protect both the animals and the research, it is important to understand the common water delivery and purification methods used in modern research facilities.

Water delivery

There are several ways in which water is delivered to animals in modern research facilities, including water bottles, plastic bags or pouches, and automated watering systems. The choice depends on the species at the facility, the number of animals, water quality requirements and, of course, budget.

The current trend in animal facilities is towards automation, and there are two driving factors behind this. First, by eliminating routine tasks animal facilities can employ labour resources towards more productive work, saving time and money. Secondly, concerns for worker safety, especially from musculoskeletal injuries due to repetitive motion and heavy lifting, have lead to automating high-risk operations. Animal watering falls into both of these categories and there are a range of systems employed in facilities today which both increase efficiency and protect workers.

Water bottles

The default method of watering animals such as rabbits, rats, mice and most other laboratory animals, is the water bottle. Because open water sources like pans and dishes are easily soiled or spilled, bottles are a simple and effective way to provide clean water to animals. Bottles range in size from 200–500 cm^3 and are most commonly made of plastic. Animals drink from water bottles by way of a metal sipper tube which is fixed to the bottle cap or stopper. When the bottle is inverted with the stopper and sipper tube in place, a vacuum is formed above the water which keeps the water from pouring out. As animals drink, air bubbles are drawn upwards into the bottle, replacing the volume of the water consumed. Some sipper tubes have steel ball bearings at the opening to provide a surer seal against drips.

The water bottle process in the animal facility starts when the bottles are filled. Usually, bottles are kept and transported in wire baskets which hold from twelve to thirty bottles. Specialised bottle fillers are employed to automate the filling. An operator positions a basket of bottles in the filler, which is fitted with a manifold, having outlets above the opening of each bottle in the basket. The operator then presses the fill button and all bottles are filled at once. At that point stoppers and sipper tubes are place on the bottles, and the basket is put on a cart for transport to an animal holding room.

During cage cleaning or cage changes, the water bottle is exchanged for a full, clean one. The soiled bottle is placed into a basket and transported to the cage wash area where it will be dumped, cleaned and

[1] Portions of this chapter first appeared in the Lab. Animals Magazine. Edstrom, E.K. and Curran, B. (2003) Quality assurance of animal watering systems. *Lab Animals*, **32** (5): 32–5.

refilled. The time between changes depends on the volume of the bottle and species being watered. For group-housed mice this is typically seven days and for rats it is every three to four days.

Bottles have been used successfully for decades in research facilities because they are simple to use and cheap to purchase. The disadvantages of bottles are the labour intensity and ergonomic stress it puts on workers. To reduce these issues, automation is available to handle some portions of the process, mainly in the washing and filling. Another concern with water bottles is maintaining water quality. As time passes, the water in the bottle can become contaminated due to the back bubbling phenomenon of bottles. This can carry contaminants from the animal's mouth into the bottle.

Plastic bags or pouches

The use of polyethylene bags for animal drinking water is growing in popularity in animal research facilities housing mice, rats and other rodents. The bags hold 300–500 ml of water. A drinking valve connects to the bag. The bag is placed in the cage in the same location which holds a water bottle. When the animal activates the valve, water is released. When the animal releases the valve, water flow stops.

The process surrounding bags is different from bottles. Empty, sterile bags are brought into the animal holding room. They are held in packs of 100–200 in outer bags to protect them from contamination. These are placed under a change hood or animal transfer station. At the start of each cage change, a bag is placed on a small, special-purpose filler unit. The filler is supplied by water distribution piping installed for that purpose, usually coming from a reverse osmosis purified water source (see Reverse osmosis p. 201). While the bag fills, the worker carries out the activities of moving the animals from the dirty cage to the clean cage. When the worker is ready to place the bag into the cage, a drinking valve is connected to the bag and the bag is placed in the cage. In general, the bag fits in the exact location a water bottle would go.

The empty bag is placed in a disposal cart, which has a perforated waste bin above a water collection tank. This allows any water remaining in a bag to drain out. Bags can then be thrown out and water emptied at a drain.

Water quality in bags is better preserved than in water bottles. Unlike bottles, bags do not operate on the vacuum principle. Because bags are flexible, they collapse as water is consumed; there is no need for air to replace the volume of water consumed. This means there is no back bubbling with bags, which reduces the chances for contamination.

The chief advantage of water bags is that they are disposable. This eliminates all the transportation of empty bottles, cleaning, filling and re-transport of full bottles back to the animal holding rooms. This in turn allows labour resources to be allocated towards more productive and less ergonomically stressful activities.

On the other hand, because the bags are disposable there is a recurring expense each time a bag is changed and it also increases the waste materials generated by the facility.

Automated water systems

Used for watering most mammalian species commonly found in research facilities, automated watering delivers drinking water to each animal cage. Animals access the water through a drinking valve.

Water is usually reverse osmosis purified and flows through piping called room distribution piping. In each animal holding room, the distribution piping is mounted on the wall surface and has outlets called interconnects for each cage rack or pen. Since most caging is mobile, a flexible hose makes the connection between the room distribution piping and the piping on the rack. For most mobile cage racks this hose is called a recoil hose because it recoils itself when disconnected; this causes the hose to lift up and out of the way. For dogs and primates, hoses are usually straight. Non-human primates need special metal guarded hoses to keep them from being destroyed by the animals.

Water enters the manifold at a connection point near the top of the rack and is carried first to the bottom row of cages, then follows the piping through each course of cages back towards the top of the rack. This configuration, called Reverse 'S', assures that all air is bled from the manifold piping. This is very important because entrapped air could form bubbles at a drinking valve outlet, preventing animals from receiving water. By filling from the bottom shelf first, and by having a single, continuous path, all air can be vented from the manifold.

Water quality in automated watering systems is maintained through water purification, treatment and periodic flushing of the piping. Animals consume a relatively low volume of water compared to the volume held in the distribution and manifold piping. To prevent stagnation and proliferation of bacteria, automated watering piping is flushed every day. This is accomplished either with manual valves or with automated, online flush systems controlled by electronics.

Automated watering has several advantages over bottles and bags. First, it reduces the labour needed to water animals. It also eliminates the ergonomic risks associated with bottles. However, it is a mechanical system which needs periodic maintenance and staff must be trained to use it properly.

Watering systems can provide very high quality water. Since the water is replaced in the manifolds daily through flushing, it provides a cleaner, more consistent quality than bottles or bags which are replaced as infrequently as every fourteen days in some applications.

All watering systems, bottles, bags or automated systems, are significant capital investments for animal research facilities. Before choosing a system, careful analysis of the operational processes should be undertaken to determine the labour resources needed and to understand the ergonomic risks of the process. Finally, a water quality standard which meets the needs of the research being conducted must be established, and methodologies and processes must be designed to test the animal drinking water quality periodically against that standard. It is not uncommon for facilities to employ more than one watering method to satisfy the needs of the animals, the research and the animal care staff.

Water quality of animal drinking water

The importance of water quality

Not only is water a key nutrient needed by all living things, but it can also be a significant variable in medical research. High bacterial loads can cause illness and death in animals, and other contaminants in water can introduce uncertainty in research (Sparks et al. 2002). It is important for animal technicians to understand the contaminants in water and how water may be purified and treated.

What constitutes 'good' quality water?

The Home Office *Code of Practice for the Housing and Care of Animals used in Scientific Procedures* (1989) states 'clean drinking water must normally be available to all animals at all times.' It goes on to say, 'water is a vehicle for micro-organisms and the method of supply should minimise this hazard.' The code of practice requires all equipment for supplying water to animals be sterilisable and that 'water should be monitored for quality and purity to avoid bacterial contamination' (Home Office 1989).

In the UK water is supplied by regional water supply companies. The quality of the water they supply is regulated by a government agency, the Drinking Water Inspectorate (DWI). Water quality regulations require the supply companies to carry out continual analysis of their product to ensure permitted levels of over fifty biological, chemical or physical contaminants are not exceeded. Their analysis is checked by the DWI so that throughout the UK it can be safely assumed that water supplied for human consumption is fit for the purpose, it is described as 'wholesome' or 'potable'.

A copy of the full water regulations can be obtained from the DWI web site (www.dwi.gov.uk) and results of local analysis can be obtained from the local water supply company.

Although facility managers can be confident that water reaching experimental animal facilities will be free from contaminants considered harmful to humans it may not necessarily be suitable either for the health of research animals and or for the validity of the research. It is also possible that the water may become contaminated after it reaches the user's premises (e.g. due to old and leaky pipes). Facility managers and the named veterinary surgeon have to make their own decisions about what contaminants to measure, how often to measure them, and what the limits are for each one.

Edstrom Industries (Waterford, WI), a vendor of animal watering systems, recommends the following when setting up an animal drinking water quality control program:

(1) Meet standards set out in UK Water Supply (Water Quality) Regulations (2000).

(2) Set limits and test for contaminants of concern to your facility's research studies. Examples: for

toxicological studies, test for any interfering chemical contaminants in drinking water; for immune-compromised animals, set tighter limits on bacterial contaminants.

(3) Benchmark against other facilities and organisations. Compare your water quality standard with that of a neighboring animal facility. They are likely to be dealing with similar water source issues.

(4) Monitor the purification process if purified water is specified. Water purification (usually by reverse osmosis, see below) will remove contaminants from water and will provide a standardised water quality, safeguarded against seasonal variation in the local tap water supply.

Methods of water purification and treatment

Because incoming water quality will have some degree of variability which could affect animal health and experimental results, it is safest to assume the water provided to the facility is contaminated. Therefore, the first step in any water quality program is to use a water purification process.

Purification processes – particle filters

These filters commonly range from 5 microns to 0.2 microns and are implemented as salutary defense against water-borne contaminants. However, unless filter cartridges are checked and replaced regularly, they can cause more problems than they solve. The contaminants which filters remove are also nutrients for bacteria. If cartridges are not replaced regularly, the bacteria can 'grow through' the filter into the distribution system. Filters should be considered the minimum protection for an animal water system, and they have value in that they can remove large particles which could compromise the function of drinking valves used in automated watering systems.

Activated carbon filters

Carbon filters are used to adsorb organics from water and can also remove chlorine. Carbon filtration is used as a pre-reverse osmosis purification process for

animal drinking water to remove the organics and chlorine which together can form harmful trihalomethanes (THMs) like chloroform. Care must be given to the maintenance of carbon filters because the organics they adsorb provide an excellent nutrient supply for bacteria. Furthermore, the effectiveness of carbon filters goes down over time as the medium reaches its adsorption limits.

Ultraviolet light (UV)

Bacteria can be deactivated when exposed long enough to ultraviolet light (UV), specifically at a wave length of 254 nanometers. UV does not remove the deactivated bacteria from the water, so it increases the pyrogen load sent downstream. In addition, UV does not remove dissolved ions or organics. Furthermore, the United States Food and Drug Administration's *Guide to the Inspections of High Purity Water Systems* (www.fda.gov/ora/inspect_ref/igs/high.html) states, 'It must be remembered that at best UV light will only kill 90% of the organisms entering the unit.' Due to these disadvantages, it is not employed as a sole purification method, but UV can be part of an overall purification process. UV lights require regular maintenance, including periodic bulb replacement. Also, bulbs need regular cleaning to provide an unobstructed light path to the water.

Reverse osmosis (RO)

Reverse osmosis (RO) is a purification process which forces water under high pressure through a semi-permeable membrane, filtering out contaminants as small as atomic radii (see Table 27.1).

Like most water purification processes, the RO membrane collects high densities of nutrients for bacteria. If proper maintenance is not observed, bacteria can grow through the RO membranes and

Table 27.1 Contaminants removed by reverse osmosis (Edstrom Industries, Inc.).

Contaminant	Reverse osmosis removal
Dissolved ions	> 93%
Organics	99% > 200 MW
Particles	> 99%
Bacteria	> 99%
Pyrogens	> 99%

contaminate the water downstream. Modern ROs incorporate a number of self-monitoring and self-cleaning processes to automate this, but RO membranes will need to be replaced every two to five years.

Dealing with bacteria

Of all the contaminants in water, bacteria are the most difficult to control. It would seem that a distribution system containing RO water would be a low nutrient, hostile environment for bacteria. However bacteria do in fact live in and colonise these systems very successfully by attaching to pipe surfaces and forming a biofilm. In fact, bacteria such as *Pseudomonas aeruginosa* can go into starvation mode, and survive quite easily in low nutrient water (Moore 1997).

Enumerating bacteria

Because biofilm can cover a large proportion of the internal surface area of a piping system, there is no definitive way to enumerate the bacteria present in the biofilm. Yet it is important to understand the relationship between the number of bacteria attached to surfaces as biofilm and the number of free-floating, planktonic bacteria in the water. Facilities are mainly concerned with planktonic bacteria, since that is what animals are exposed to when they drink the water. However, biofilm is important because the majority of planktonic bacteria found in water have detached from a biofilm. Biofilm detachment occurs at irregular intervals making it entirely possible for a facility to conduct tests showing low or no bacteria counts and still have bacteria problems resulting in animal health issues. Furthermore, the standard agar used in heterotrophic plate counts may fail to culture bacteria which are in their low-nutrient mode.

An alternative culturing media is R2A. This is a low-nutrient media, and is specially designed for culturing high-purity water samples. It is optimised to give an accurate representation of the nutrient concentrations found in a typical high-purity water system, therefore the bacteria in those samples will thrive, yielding more accurate counts. Those facilities concerned enough about water quality to invest in a high-purity water system, such as an RO, will need the accuracy of the water quality testing gained by using the R2A media. If facilities are using tap water and very accurate bacterial numbers are not a top concern, then the standard total plate count agar is sufficient.

Controlling bacteria

Since bacteria can detach from a biofilm on piping surfaces at any time, it is important to maintain a residual disinfectant like chlorine in the water. When free chlorine is available in the water it can kill detached bacteria before animals consume them.

Treatment processes

Following the purification process, water goes through a treatment process to control bacteria in the distribution system. Most facilities use a residual disinfectant like chlorine or hydrochloric acid, but some also use ultraviolet light when following a 'chemical-free' water policy. The trade-off between maintaining a residual disinfectant versus 'chemical-free' water is increased variability in bacteria levels in the chemical-free water, since no residual disinfectant is available to control biofilm growth or kill bacteria which have detached from biofilm.

Residual disinfectants

Chlorine is the residual disinfectant used in most animal watering systems. Levels of 2–3 ppm are effective in maintaining low bacteria counts. Acidification using HCl has long been used in animal drinking water because low pH water inhibits bacterial reproduction in water bottles. Acid is used in watering systems at 2.6–3.0 pH; pH lower than 2.5, should not be used as this will degrade the stainless steel and silicone rubber components of the watering system. Chlorinated water should not be acidified below pH 5.0. At lower pH, chlorine will be present as dissolved chlorine gas which may cause swelling of the silicone rubber components in the animal drinking valves.

Sanitisation

In addition to acidifying, water bottles are also sometimes autoclaved. This sterilises the bottles and the water by heating it to 121 °C for fifteen to twenty-five minutes. This kills all microbials in the water.

However, bottles are subject to re-contamination once they are placed on the cages and the back-bubbling phenomenon of water bottles can draw debris from the cage environment into the bottle.

Automated watering systems, distribution piping and manifolds may be sanitised periodically using higher levels of chlorine. Special sanitisation equipment pumps water chlorinated to 30 ppm into the system. The system is then allowed to 'soak' for twenty to thirty minutes before being flushed with un-chlorinated water. Because bacteria live in biofilms attached to surfaces, some bacteria can survive chemical sanitisation efforts. Sanitisation can be effective in reducing measurable bacteria counts in the short term. But bacteria will re-colonise a watering system following a sanitisation event in as little as three days, in the absence of a low-level residual disinfectant.

Eliminating dead legs

There is one key principle which must be applied to any water distribution system: eliminate dead legs. Dead legs are problematic because water turnover is low and they become a haven for bacteria.

Modern system design is careful to avoid dead legs whether the piping is supplying water bottle fillers, bag fillers or an automated watering system. However, a dead leg is more than just a length of pipe which terminates with no outlet, a dead leg can also occur at the bottle filler. If the bottle filler is not used for a few days, the whole filler is a dead leg and needs to be flushed prior to filling water bottles. In automated watering systems, if the cage rack manifolds level is not flushed regularly, the whole manifold is essentially a dead leg.

Recoil hoses which connect the distribution lines to the manifolds can also be dead legs when racks are disconnected. Therefore, when a rack is removed from the system, the recoil hose must either be:

- removed and sanitised; or
- connected to the flush line recoil hose in systems which use automated online rack flushing.

Conclusion

The drinking water quality in animal research facilities is influenced by both system design and system maintenance. Animal care staff must understand what water quality standards they are trying to meet and how the equipment is intended to deliver that quality. Therefore, it is especially important to have a good understanding of bacteria and biofilms, how they survive in low-nutrient environments, and how they can be controlled. With that knowledge in place, the equipment can be employed to suit the needs and specific challenges of each facility.

References and further reading

Sparks, L., Lochhead, J., Horstman, D. et al. (2002) Water quality has a pronounced effect on cholesterol-induced accumulation of Alzheimer amyloid g (Ag) in rabbit brain. *Journal of Alzheimer's Disease* 4 (6): 523–529.

Home Office (1989) *Code of Practice for the Housing and Care of Animals used in Scientific Procedures.* HMSO, London.

Food and Drug Administration (25.01.2006) *Guide to Inspection of High Purity Water Systems.* www.fda.gov/ora/inspect_ref/igs/high.html

Moore, D.M. (1997) *Reference Paper: Pseudomonas and the Laboratory Animal.* http://www.criver.com

Mittleman, M.W. (1986) Biological fouling of purified-water systems. *Microcontamination* (1): 30–40.

28

Transport of Animals

Stephen W. Barnett

Introduction

Movement from place to place is an experience that all laboratory animals have in common. The movement may be over a very short distance within a facility, or it may be from one end of the country to the other. It may even be from one continent to another.

Most animals find the experience stressful, the amount of stress suffered is related to the distance moved, the mode of transport, the time spent travelling and the environment through which they travel. Once out of the controlled environment of a laboratory animal facility the possibility of an animal being exposed to infectious organisms increases. It follows that transport is a risk to the health and welfare of animals and consequently it can have an effect on the quality of experimental results.

The major aim of good animal transport must be to minimise disturbance to the animals by ensuring the journey is as short and comfortable as possible and in as stable an environment as possible so they arrive in good health. This means that all aspects of the transport must be well planned. Factors which need to be considered in the planning include:

- legal requirements;
- duration of the journey;
- health and welfare of the animals being transported;
- transport containers;
- feeding and watering;
- mode of transport.

Legal requirements

Transporting animals is a highly regulated activity. Legislation ensures the welfare of animals while they are being transported and seeks to control the spread of disease through the movement of animals. The farm animal chapters of this manual (Chapters 18–25) describe the regulations concerned with registration and identification of animals for disease control. Several pieces of legislation are concerned with animal welfare during transport. The Protection of Animals Act 1911 (1912 in Scotland) makes it an offence to cause unnecessary suffering to any captive or domestic animal. More specific regulation is detailed in the Welfare of Animals (Transport) Order 1997 (WATO). This order covers all vertebrate animals. It prohibits the transport of any animal in a way which causes or is likely to cause injury or unnecessary suffering and details requirements for the design of transporters, space allowances, travelling times and rest periods, training and experience of people moving the animals, feeding and watering and route planning. Specific requirements will be referred to throughout this chapter.

Welfare of Animals (Transport) Order (WATO) (1997)

Detailed consideration of WATO is outside the remit of this chapter but some of the major points are mentioned below and in subsequent sections of the chapter.

Authorisation and documentation

In the UK, all transporters of vertebrate animals must be granted either general or specific authorisation from DEFRA, through the local divisional veterinary office. General authorisation covers many journeys and specific authorisation has to be applied for before each journey.

General authorisation is required for:

- the transport of farm animals and horses for journeys less than eight hours in a road vehicle;
- all other vertebrate animals.

Specific authorisation is needed to transport farm animals and horses:

- for journeys of eight hours or more in road vehicles;
- all journeys by sea, rail or air.

In addition to the authorisation mentioned above, WATO requires route plans and animal transport certificates to be carried by transporters.

Route plans are required when farm animals and horses are to be transported between member countries of the EU or to other countries, except when the journey or travelling time exceeds eight hours. The route must be submitted to the local divisional veterinary office ten days before the journey is due to commence and must provide sufficient information to allow the local divisional veterinary manager to judge whether the requirements of the WATO are met.

Animal transport certificates are required when farm animals or horses are transported over 50 km except when the journey will not take over eight hours and is not to another country. They are also needed for any other vertebrate animal transported over 50 km when the journey will take over eight hours and is to another member state of the EU or to a third country.

An animal transport certificate must contain the following information:

(1) the name and address of the transporter;
(2) the name and address of the owner of the animal(s);
(3) the place where the animal was loaded and the final destination;
(4) the date and time that the first animal was loaded;
(5) the date and time of departure;
(6) details of the animal(s) being transported;
(7) registration number of the vehicle.

Competent persons

A competent attendant must accompany vertebrate animals being transported over 50 km. The attendant must have specific training or have practical experience. If the animals are farm animals or horses on journeys which will take over eight hours by road or any time by sea, air or rail, they must be accompanied by an attendant who has proven competence by qualification or assessment of practical experience.

Animals which are secure in a transport box and have access to food and water sufficient for at least twice the estimated journey time, do not need to be accompanied by a competent attendant. However, a person must be responsible for them at their destination or transfer point.

Feeding, watering and rests

WATO details the maximum length of journeys, rest times during the journey and feeding and watering requirements of animals being transported.

Intervals between feeding and watering of farm animals and horses depends on the species of animals, the stage of development (e.g. pre-weaning or adult), the type of vehicle and the type of journey (e.g. road, sea etc). For example:

- pigs may be transported for a maximum of twenty-four hours providing they have continuous access to liquid;
- cattle, sheep and goats must be given one hour's rest for food and water after a maximum of fourteen hours' travel;
- horses may be transported for a maximum of twenty-four hours but must be given liquid and, if necessary, food every eight hours;
- domestic dogs and cats must be fed at intervals of not more than twenty-four hours and given liquid at intervals of not more twelve hours – detailed instructions of feeding and watering must accompany the animals;
- other mammals must be fed and watered at appropriate intervals during the journey and clear instructions about feeding and watering must accompany them during the journey.

These timings are given for illustration only. Full details are given in the Welfare of Animals (Transport) Order 1997 and Guidance on the Welfare of Animals (Transport) Order 1997 (DEFRA 2004).

Directives from the European Union require all member states to enforce standards similar to UK legislation, although it is always wise to check with the destination country if animals are being sent abroad because further specific regulations may apply. The same is true for non-EU countries, it is always necessary to comply with local legislation. Failure to do so can result in a waste of time and money but more importantly will involve animals being kept waiting in ports of entry and may result in them having to be killed.

International Air Transport Association (IATA) regulations

If animals are being transported by air the containers they are housed in must comply with the regulations of the International Air Transport Association (IATA). These regulations are issued every year so it is important to ensure current ones are consulted. The transport container designs they advocate not only ensure sufficient space is given to the animals but also ensure the containers will fit the holds of the aircraft and its handling equipment. It is a requirement of WATO to comply with IATA regulations. In addition no airline will accept animals in containers which do not comply with the regulations.

Animals (Scientific Procedures) Act 1986

The Home Secretary must give approval before protected animals can be moved between project licences or before animals listed on Schedule 2 of the act are obtained from non-designated sources. This would include animals imported into the UK from abroad (e.g. genetically altered strains). Authority may be given in a project licence or as a condition of a certificate of designation, otherwise it must be applied for by completing an 'application form for authority to transfer protected animals'. The request must be justified and must be sent to the Home Office at least three weeks before the date of the proposed movement.

Importation of animals

In order to import rodents and lagomorphs into the UK it is necessary to obtain an authority to transfer protected animals from the Home Office and an import licence from DEFRA.

The Rabies (Importation of Dogs, Cats and other Mammals) (England) (Amendment) Order 2004 permits the importation of rodents and lagomorphs for research purposes without the need for six months' quarantine, providing certain conditions are satisfied. The conditions require a certificate to accompany the animals, signed by the veterinary surgeon or medical supervisor from the breeding/research unit that the animals come from which states that:

- the animals have been at the establishment for not less than fifteen days;

- the animals have been isolated from new introductions for fifteen days;
- no cases of rabies have been reported in the unit for the previous twelve months;
- no experiments with rabies have been carried out in the unit for the previous twelve months;
- the animals being exported showed no signs of rabies on the day they were shipped.

Cats, dogs and non-human primates for use in research can be imported into the UK from the EU under the Balai Directive (92/65/EEC). Balai is concerned with allowing free trade throughout the EU. In this context it allows importation of animals, under prescribed conditions, without the need for quarantine. However in the case of Balai, the importer has to be registered with DEFRA and the exporter must be registered with the DEFRA equivalent in their country.

Cats, dogs and non-human primates imported from outside the EU need to be placed in DEFRA-approved quarantine facilities for six months.

Export of animals

Before exporting animals it is necessary to be aware of the import regulations of the destination country so that the necessary documentation can accompany the animals. In addition animals will need to be certified as being fit for the journey by a veterinary surgeon and an export licence must be obtained from DEFRA. If the animals are to be transported by air, the transport boxes must comply with IATA regulations.

Duration of the journey

The length of the journey affects a number of the other factors that have to be considered when transporting animals, e.g. mode of transport, type of transport container, food, water and bedding provided, day on which animals are sent.

For short journeys, within a facility or to another one very near, it may be appropriate to move small rodents in their own cages, or in cardboard boxes on a trolley, providing the ground is smooth and the animals are not exposed to vibration. Larger animals may be moved in trolleys such as that shown in Figure 22.8 (p. 155). Barrier-maintained animals can be moved from area to area in a facility in a transport isolator.

Longer journeys will require more substantial containers able to withstand the activities of the animals they hold.

Longer journeys have an increased risk of being delayed. If the journey requires a change of carrier this could have a significant harmful effect on animals, e.g. if it is by air it could involve at least three changes of carrier – road transport to the airport, aeroplane, road transport from the airport to the destination. In long journeys it is not only necessary to consider the type of container, bedding, food and moisture provided for the animals but the timing of the journey. Sending animals on a long journey where there is a risk of delay should not be started at the end of the working week. A small delay could result in animals arriving at the weekend when staff numbers at the port of entry and destination unit may be low, causing further delay.

Long journeys in warm weather or to warmer parts of the world require consideration of lower stocking densities and increased ventilation space to be incorporated in the container. In cold weather extra bedding should be added.

Health and welfare of animals

Animals selected for transport must undergo a health assessment to ensure they are fit to travel. Sick or injured animals must not be transported unless it is for veterinary treatment or to slaughter. If the journey is within the UK, the inspection can be carried out by a competent person. If the journey is international, a veterinary surgeon must inspect the animals and must sign a veterinary certificate. Animals that are undergoing regulated procedures can only be moved if permission has been granted by the Home Secretary, they also require a veterinary surgeon to confirm they are fit to travel.

European transport directives and domestic regulations prohibit the transport of animals during the last tenth of their pregnancy until one week after parturition. The LASA (Laboratory Animal Science Association) Transport Working Group recommends that they should not be moved during the last fifth of gestation. Their recommendations for each species are given in Table 28.1.

Transport of newborn animals before their navel has completely healed is also prohibited.

Table 28.1 Typical gestation periods of common laboratory species and recommended permissible shipping times (Swallow et al. 2005).

Species	Duration of gestation (days)	Can be shipped up to (days)
Rat	21	17
Mouse	21	17
Guinea pig	56–75	45
Rabbit	30–32	22
Dog	61–65	40
Cat	64–67	42
Common marmoset	144	96
Long-tailed macaque	153–167	102

If animals are to travel together they should be selected and grouped the day before they are due to travel so they settle before undergoing the added stress of transport. When grouping animals, their normal behaviour must be considered. Aggressive animals should be transported alone, mothers and litters should be boxed alone, groups should be of the same age, size and sex. Table 28.2 lists the recommended stocking densities in filtered crates, with temperature-controlled vehicles and where controlled temperature is not available.

Once ready to be transported, animals should be handled as little as possible. When the boxes do need handling this should be done with care.

Transport containers

The *Code of Practice for the Housing and Care of Animals in Designated Breeding and Supplying Establishments* (Home Office 1995) states that a transport container should:

- confine the animals in comfortable hygienic conditions;
- contain sufficient food and water or moisture in a suitable form;
- contain sufficient bedding so that animals remain comfortable and in conditions close to their thermo-neutral zone;
- be of such a design and finish that an animal will not damage itself during loading, transport and whilst being removed from the container;
- be escape-proof, leak-proof and capable of being handled without the animals posing a risk to handlers;

Table 28.2   Stocking densities for laboratory animals in transport containers (Swallow et al. 2005).

Species and weight (g)	Minimum floor area cm² per animal. No active temperature control provided during the journey.		Minimum floor area cm² per animal. Active temperature control provided throughout the journey	
	Filtered crates	Unfiltered crates	Filtered crates	Unfiltered crates
Rats	Minimum height 15 cm			
<50	120	60	96	48
51–75	160	80	128	64
76–100	200	100	160	80
101–125	240	120	192	96
126–150	280	140	224	112
151–175	360	180	288	144
176–200	360	180	288	144
201–225	420	220	336	176
226–250	500	253	400	203
>251	600	300	480	240
Mice	Minimum height 10 cm			
10–20	120	60	96	48
21–25	150	75	120	60
26–30	150	75	120	60
>31	180	90	144	72
Hamsters	Minimum Height 15 cm			
30–60	120	60	96	48
61–90	160	80	128	64
91–120	200	100	160	80
>120	240	120	192	96
Guinea pigs	Minimum height 15 cm			
100–150	330	165	264	132
151–250	400	200	320	160
251–350	440	220	352	176
351–450	480	240	384	192
451–550	520	260	416	208
>551	560	280	448	224
Rabbits and ferrets	Minimum height 20 cm			
600–1000	1000	–	800	–
>1000	2000	–	1600	–
600–1000	–	500	–	400
1001–2500	–	762	–	610
>2501	–	1000	–	800

- be designed to limit the entry of micro-organisms;
- be designed so that they can be thoroughly disinfected between shipments, if intended to be reusable;
- allow sufficient ventilation;
- be clearly labelled.

Rodents and other small animals

Most small animal transport containers are made of disposable cardboard or corrugated plastic (trade name Correx®). Whatever material is used, the box must be constructed in way that will resist distortion

Figure 28.1 Reusable transport box. Note spacers which prevent vents being blocked.

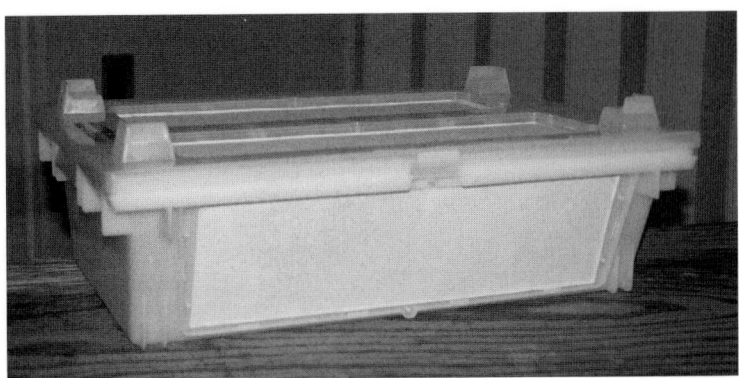

and crushing. Cardboard is only suitable for short journeys, as urine will soften it over time. The resistance of cardboard to damp can be increased if it is coated with an impervious material (thin plastic coat). Correx® is naturally water resistant and is suitable for short and long journeys. Reusable containers made of sterilisable plastics (e.g. polypropylene) are also available; these are often used for international transport (Figure 28.1).

Containers must have smooth inside surfaces so that there is no possibility of animals injuring themselves and to resist animal gnawing. A lining with mesh is often used to further resist damage to the box by the animal. It is recommended that the complete inner surface of hamster transport boxes should be lined with screen wire to prevent escape (Swallow et al. 2005). The container must have sufficient ventilation space to provide adequate air supply. Ventilation space can be provided at the sides of the container and/or on the top. Ventilation on at least two sides is recommended (Swallow et al. 2005). If filters are used they can reduce the ventilation efficiency by up to 70%. Clough and Townsend (1987) recommend suitable vent to surface area ratios for transport boxes (Table 28.3).

Table 28.3 Ratio of vent to surface area (excluding base) of transport boxes.

	Non-filtered vents on side	Filtered vents on side
Mice, hamsters, rats	1:30	1:10
Guinea pigs, rabbits, cats	1:50	1:15
Dogs	1:50	–

The ratios given in Table 28.3 assume the animals are travelling in temperate climates. If they are travelling in a very hot summer, or to warmer parts of the world, the ratio of vent to surface area must be increased and stocking densities decreased.

All ventilation spaces must be protected by mesh so that no part of the animal's body can protrude. Filters need to be protected by mesh on the inside and outside to prevent damage. No vent is effective if air cannot reach it so boxes are designed with sides that slope or with spacers preventing blockage of the vents (see Figure 28.1).

Animals must be able to be inspected on journeys so it is necessary to have a window in the lid of the box. These consist of a cardboard flap which can be lifted to expose a clear, plastic window protected on the inside with mesh. This allows the animals to be viewed without opening the box. This is particularly important for barrier animals where opening the box would make the animals unusable (Figure 28.2).

All rodents should be transported in barrier transport containers to ensure they do not pick up pathogens on the journey (Swallow et al. 2005). This means that in addition to filtered ventilation spaces the lid must be completely sealed, usually with heavy duty tape. It may be appropriate to use a double-box system where the animals are placed in a filtered plastic box within a normal Correx® one for microbiologically clean animals. If animals are transported in isolator transfer or double-box systems, care must be taken to ensure that the inner box is packed in a position that aligns the window in the inner box with the window in the outer box, thereby allowing the inner box to be examined without opening the boxes.

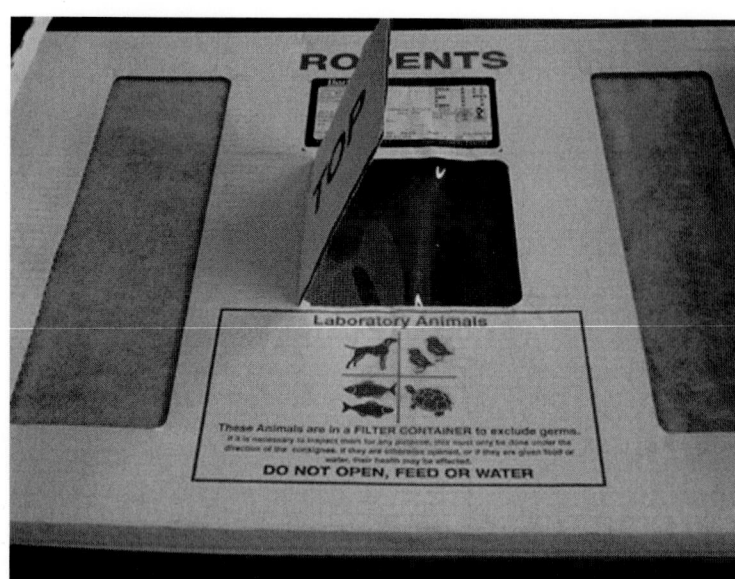

Figure 28.2   Transport box showing viewing window.

Rabbits are transported in boxes made of stronger materials than rodents, e.g. rigid plastic, fibreglass, fibreboard. The LASA Transport Working Group recommends height restrictions in rabbit boxes to prevent the risk of back injuries which might occur if the animals jump when frightened during the journey. LASA also suggests fitting a grid floor above the container floor for long journeys to separate the rabbit from its faeces and urine.

Ferrets are housed in containers similar in size and design and made of the same materials as rabbits.

Cats and dogs

Cats and dogs are moved in containers similar to those used for domestic pets. These must be strong and are constructed of fibreglass or rigid plastic. The door should be constructed of wire mesh so the animals can both be seen and can see out. Doors must be securely fastened so that they cannot be opened by accident. Ventilation holes should be placed on all sides of the container so that a minimum of 16% of the four sides is ventilation space. The animal should not be able to put any part of its body through the door or ventilation spaces. Dogs and cats are often wary of being put into transport containers and the operation can be made less traumatic for them if the container is left in their pens for a while so they become accustomed to it. Dogs may be group-housed

for transport providing they are from an established group and are moved in a purpose-built, double-door vehicle.

Non-human primates

Non-human primates present special problems for transporters. They are sensitive, strong and intelligent, which means they are more likely to be disturbed by abnormal circumstances over which they have no control and they are more likely to be able to work out a way to escape from transport boxes. Small primates such as marmosets can be transported in Correx®, wood or rigid plastic. Larger primates such as macaques are transported in wood, stainless steel or rigid plastic. The containers must be of very strong construction and have locks which the primates cannot break or undo. A slatted floor within the container should be fitted for longer journeys. A minimum of 10% of all sides should be devoted to ventilation space. All openings must be covered with mesh so that no part of the primate can protrude to the outside. Juvenile macaques should be transported in same-sex pairs. Adults should be moved in pairs too unless they are incompatible.

Animals should be provided with bedding and nesting materials to absorb moisture, provide insulation, reduce the effects of vibrations and provide hiding places from aggressive travelling companions.

Wood shavings, wood chips or paper products are suitable for bedding; hay and paper wool are suitable for nesting.

Labelling the container

The LASA Working Group (Swallow 2005) lists the information which should be on each container as follows:

- 'LIVE ANIMALS';
- 'THIS WAY UP' with arrows;
- instructions for handling the crate;
- the type and number of animals in the container;
- the consignor's name, address and a 24-hour telephone contact number;
- the consignee's name, address and a 24-hour telephone contact number;
- feeding and watering instructions, even if these read 'DO NOT FEED'.

Food and water

The Welfare of Animals (Transport) Order (1997) states that enough food and moisture should be provided for twice the expected consumption on the journey. The type of food and the form in which moisture is provided depends on the species being transported.

Rodents and lagomorphs can be fed and watered up to the point they are loaded into the transport container. Food can be provided for the journey by adding their normal pellets to the bedding. Hay can be given for nesting and as an extra food source for rabbits and guinea pigs. Moisture can be provided in the form of gel, mash, fruit and vegetables or in plastic bags with nipple drinkers. If animals are being transported to another country their import regulations must be consulted to ensure they are not breached by plant material added for the animals to eat on the journey. Ensuring that sufficient food and water is available for the journey is particularly important with barrier animals on long journeys as the container cannot be opened up to provide more if the journey is delayed.

Carnivores should not be fed less than four hours before the journey. This is because they may suffer from travel sickness. During the journey they should be inspected every four hours to ensure they are fit and well. During these stops they should be offered a drink of water and then given thirty minutes' rest before commencing the journey. On longer journeys adult carnivores should be fed once a day followed by a rest. Young animals and lactating females need more frequent feeding. The food offered to carnivores on journeys should be the food they have been used to consuming.

Primates can be offered pellets, fruits and vegetables for the journey.

Mode of transport

The type of transport used to move protected animals depends on the distance to be covered on the journey. The fastest and most direct route must be chosen. In practice most deliveries of animals within the UK are made by supplier's own vehicles as these ensure the animals are handled correctly and provide the maximum security. These vehicles should be air conditioned with systems which run independently of the engine (Figure 28.3). There should be warning devices which alert the driver if the ventilation system fails. The vehicles should be insulated and the suspension should minimise vibration and noise. The inside of the vehicle should provide easy loading and unloading of containers and should be able to be disinfected.

Drivers should be experienced in handling the animals and should be trained to deal with problems which may occur on the journey. Methods of communicating with headquarters should be installed so that contact can be made in the event of breakdown or other emergency. Back-up vehicles should be available.

International journeys are usually made by air, mention has already been made about IATA regulations (see p. 206).

Protected animals have been moved by sea on roll-on roll-off ferries. Drivers must ensure that ventilation remains adequate when the vehicle is parked on the ship.

Farm animals are transported in purpose-made vehicles. These must ensure animals can be seen at all times. The inside of the vehicle must be able to be divided so that animals can be separated when necessary. Space provided should be adequate but dividers should prevent them being thrown around when the

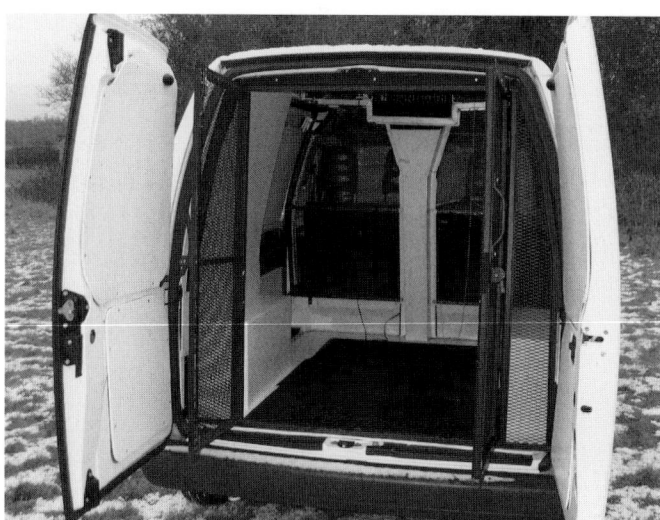

Figure 28.3 Transport van for small animals. Note air-conditioning unit on the roof and the double door security.

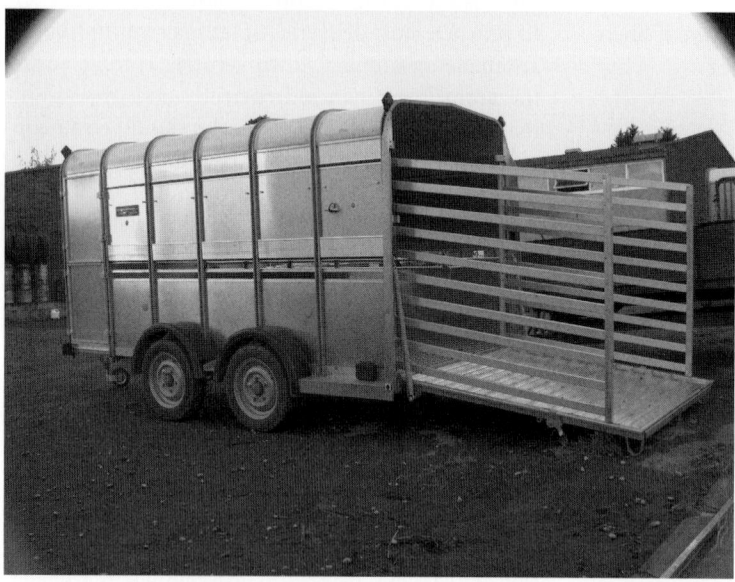

Figure 28.4 Trailer suitable for moving farm animals short distances.

vehicle is in motion. Ventilation must ensure all animals are supplied with fresh air. Loading ramps must enable animals to get on and off the vehicle without risk of injury (Figure 28.4).

WATO describes the design features and the maintenance required for all animal transport vehicles.

Reception of animals

Prior to animals being received into a facility, records should be consulted to establish which animals are

expected and what caging needs to be prepared for their reception. Cages should be prepared with bedding, food and water and be labelled.

When animals are received in a unit they must be unloaded as soon as possible. The boxes should be inspected to ensure they are intact and there have been no escapes. The documentation which arrived with the animals must be inspected, e.g. delivery, health report. The boxes should be opened and the animals inspected to ensure they are all well. The inspection may include weighing a selection of animals as indication of their body condition. The animals which have arrived must be compared with what was ordered. Any sick animals should be dealt with immediately. The animals are then placed in the cages that have been prepared for them. Any problems with the order or the condition of the animals should then be reported to supplier.

Animals may be transferred to a quarantine room or directly to a normal animal room depending on local protocols. Quarantine for animals from within the UK would normally last for twenty-one days, during which time most laboratory animal diseases would become evident. During the quarantine period the animals should be inspected regularly.

References and further reading

DEFRA (2004) *Guidance on 'The Welfare of Animals (Transport) Order' (1997)*. www.defra.gov.uk

Clough, G. and Townsend, G.H. (1987) Transport. In: T. Poole (Ed.) *The UFAW Handbook on the Care and Management of Laboratory Animals* (6th edn). Longman Scientific and Technical.

Home Office (1995) *Code of Practice for the Housing and Care of Animals in Designated Breeding and Supplying Establishments.* HMSO, London.

Swallow, J.J. (1999) Transporting animals. In: T. Poole (Ed.) *The UFAW Handbook on the Care and Management of Laboratory Animals* (7th edn). Blackwell Science, Oxford.

Swallow, J.J. (Chairman) (2005) Guidance on the transport of laboratory animals. *Laboratory Animals*, (1): 1–39.

29
Biodecontamination

Gerald McDonnell

Introduction

The biodecontamination of instruments, equipment and facilities can be achieved using a variety of products and processes, which are described in this chapter. In general, decontamination is a staged process which includes cleaning and then disinfection or sterilisation. The choice and use of these procedures will vary depending on the type and level of contamination, risks associated with contamination, costs, and the safety/efficacy of methods available.

Definitions

Antimicrobial: The ability of a process or product to be effective at killing micro-organisms. This can vary depending on the process/product and the target micro-organism.

Antisepsis: Destruction or inhibition of micro-organisms in or on living tissue, e.g. on the skin.

Biocide: A chemical agent, usually broad spectrum, which inactivates micro-organisms.

-cidal/-static: The suffix '-cidal' refers to lethal activity against a group of micro-organisms (e.g. sporicidal, refers to the ability to kill bacterial spores and bactericidal, refers to the ability to kill bacteria). The suffix '-static' refers only to the ability to inhibit the growth of an organism.

Cleaning: Removal of contamination from a surface to the extent necessary for further processing, or for intended use.

Decontamination: Physical and/or chemical means to render a surface or item safe for handling, use or disposal. The term decontamination can refer to both chemical and biological, but for the purpose of this discussion, biological decontamination only is discussed. It is noted that chemical decontamination may be a concern in some facilities and should be considered separately. Decontamination is generally a combination of cleaning and disinfection/sterilisation.

Disinfection: The antimicrobial reduction of the number of viable micro-organisms/bioburden on a product or surface to a level previously specified as appropriate for its intended further handling or use. In general, disinfection is used to describe a product or process ('disinfectant') which is effective against all pathogens, with the exception of bacterial spores. Bacterial spores are considered to be the most resistant organisms to disinfection/sterilisation.

Fumigation: Delivery of a disinfectant/disinfection process (gas or liquid) indirectly to the internal surface of an isolator/enclosure. Fogging is a form of fumigation, which refers to the indirect application of a liquid product to a given area for the purpose of antimicrobial activity.

Pathogen: Disease-causing micro-organism.

Pasteurisation: Involves heating to a temperature of 70–90 °C followed by rapid cooling.

Preservation: The prevention of multiplication of micro-organisms in products.

Sanitation: A general term for the removal of micro-organisms which pose a threat to public health.

Sterilisation: Validated process used to render a product free from viable organisms, including bacterial spores. When something is sterile it is described as being free from viable organisms.

Washer–disinfector: machine intended to clean and disinfect devices and other articles.

Validation: documented procedure for obtaining, recording and interpreting the results required to establish that a process will consistently yield product, complying with predetermined specifications.

General considerations

Microbiology

Facility concerns: Not all micro-organisms are harmful; many are in fact innocuous and even beneficial. Therefore it is not necessary in all cases to ensure that all surfaces are and are maintained sterile. Facilities are particularly concerned with pathogens and biofouling. Pathogens are disease-causing organisms, and will vary depending on the facility. An understanding of the types and risks associated with the presence of pathogens is important in the choice of biodecontamination process. For example, the environmental control of bacterial pathogens (like *E. coli* and *Salmonella*) can be achieved using a wider range of disinfectants than for certain viral pathogens (like parvoviruses), for reasons described below. Biofouling is a further consideration; for example, water, foodstuff or product contamination, damage over time and unpleasant odour.

Microbial resistance: Micro-organisms can vary from those which are relatively sensitive to decontamination (e.g. lipid-enveloped viruses) to those which are very resistant (e.g. bacterial spores) to it (Figure 29.1).

Resistance is dependant on intrinsic and, to a lesser extent, acquired mechanisms. Intrinsic mechanisms include the external structure of the micro-organism which can be impermeable to a biocide. For example, spore-forming bacteria (including *Bacillus* and *Clostridium* species) are relatively sensitive in their vegetative form, but have the ability to form spores which are resistant to chemical and physical processes. Spores have a unique structure, protected from the environment by multiple external layers. Similar intrinsic mechanisms are responsible for the environmental survival of many parasites, including eggs (*Enterobius*, pinworms) and cysts (*Cryptosporidium*, oocysts). In contrast, lipid-enveloped viruses

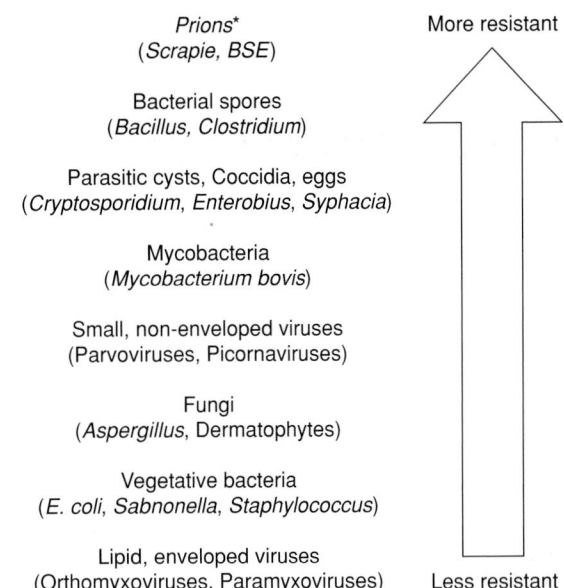

Figure 29.1 Microbial resistance to disinfectants and sterilants. (* Prion resistance remains under debate, but they are generally considered uniquely resistant to physical and chemical antimicrobials.)

(including influenza and Newcastle viruses) are very sensitive to environmental factors and disinfectants. Another example of intrinsic resistance is the ability of organisms to grow in biofilms. Most bacteria and fungi have the ability to attach to surfaces, multiply and produce protective materials (e.g. polysaccharides and proteins) which can protect the microbial community in a biofilm from an antimicrobial. Acquired resistance has been described, in particular in bacteria, for example due to genetic mutations, but in most cases these only partially increase the resistance to a given biocide and remain sensitive under normal product/process treatment.

Product/process application

In the consideration of any cleaning, disinfection or sterilisation product or process the following factors should be considered.

Antimicrobial efficacy

Products/processes should be chosen which have demonstrated broad spectrum efficacy. The required level of antimicrobial activity will vary depending on the risks associated in the use of an area or instrument.

Dirty and/or highly contaminated surfaces will present a greater challenge than clean and/or low bioburden surfaces.

Antimicrobial claims will vary considerably, in particular for liquid disinfectants. Attention should be paid to reviewing product claims, including the test methods used. For example suspension tests (where test organisms are directly inoculated into a test liquid) are only an indication of the efficacy of a product when applied to a contaminated surface. Antimicrobial claims should be supported by standard, recognised test methods. In some cases, efficacy may need to be validated for critical applications in a facility.

As discussed above, the development of intrinsic or acquired resistance should be monitored in a facility. Product or active rotation can be considered.

Process/product variables

- Concentration: in general, as the concentration of the biocide in a given product/dilution increases, there is an increase in the antimicrobial activity.

- Formulation is an important factor when considering liquid-based disinfectants. Formulation effects, including pH, solubility and presence of surfactants, will significantly affect (enhance or restrict) biocidal action.

- Dilution: liquid products should be diluted according to label claims.

- Stability: the stability of an active in a diluted product can vary depending on the biocide and how the product is used. Reuse of the diluted product, where recommended, can dramatically reduce the shelf life of the active.

- Temperature: in general, the higher the temperature the greater the antimicrobial activity, although when used in combination some biocidal products (in particular temperature-sensitive biocides such as oxidising agents) will have a shorter stability time.

- Humidity can be an important consideration for certain fumigation and sterilisation processes. Examples include the use of formaldehyde for area decontamination (>70% humidity) or ethylene oxide for device sterilisation (generally 60%). Both actives are not biocidal unless humidity is controlled during the process contact time.

Presence/absence of soil or inactivating agents

Soils can be organic (e.g. blood, serum, oils, lipids) or inorganic (e.g. heavy metals, water hardness) in nature. Soils inhibit the activity of the antimicrobial process by restricting the contact with the target micro-organisms or reacting with the active, thereby losing activity. Where liquid disinfectants are required to be diluted in water, the quality of the water used can affect the activity of the product. On surfaces, gross soil should be removed by cleaning to ensure the efficacy of subsequent disinfection/sterilisation process.

Materials/surfaces

The efficacy of decontamination will vary depending on the contact surface. Porous surfaces are a particular concern, in comparison to non-porous surfaces such as stainless steel.

Compatibility of contact surfaces should be considered in the choice of decontamination processes. Electrical surfaces are an example, where liquids should not be used. The optimum processes should be non-destructive to surfaces over repeated use.

Safety

Material Safety Data Sheets (MSDS) review and a risk analysis should be considered during the choice of decontamination processes. The optimum processes should be non-toxic, non-allergenic and non-irritant. Special precautions or standard operating procedures should be in place to describe correct handling and use, with provisions for personnel protection and evacuation/clean-up procedures in the case of uncontrolled release/spills.

Many biocides can have serious short- or long-term toxic effects with repeated use. In some cases, reactions of the biocide with certain surfaces or on natural breakdown can produce toxic by-products which should also be considered. Disinfectant residuals may need to be removed from or neutralised on certain surfaces following application.

Care should be taken to consider the compatibility of chemicals/processes which could be used in combination or be mixed inadvertently, in a facility.

Monitoring efficacy

The efficacy of decontamination methods should be routinely monitored. This can be achieved in a variety of ways:

Physical methods

Parametric monitoring of process variables is often considered sufficient for confirming the efficacy of some disinfection/sterilisation processes. This includes measuring temperature, concentration, humidity, air removal and other process variables.

Heat-based systems are widely validated using physical methods which include temperature monitoring at various locations in a vessel to ensure process effectiveness. For steam autoclaves, it is important that correct air removal is confirmed, as well as that the correct temperature and contact time for sterilisation has been achieved.

Gaseous and liquid methods (including cleaning) can also be validated if important variables have been defined and can be monitored.

Chemical methods

Cleaning efficacy is generally monitored by visual inspection. Alternatively, chemical or biochemical methods can be used for sensitive applications. Examples include the use of clean/white cloths which can be wiped over surfaces or swabbing/extraction methods which can be analysed for protein, carbohydrate, lipid or other soil contaminants.

Chemical indicators are used to indicate the qualitative presence of biocide, and can be semi-quantitative. These are usually in the form of small strips with a colour pad which changes on exposure.

Microbiological methods

Direct methods include contact plates and air samplers. Indirect methods use swabs, cloths or surface extractions. There are no universal microbial cultivation methods which can be used for detecting the growth of all micro-organisms. In general, the monitoring of surfaces for aerobic (organisms which grow in the presence of oxygen), mesophilic (organisms which grow at ambient temperatures)

bacterial or fungal contaminants is the most convenient, although specific culture media and incubation conditions may be selected in cases where certain microbial contaminants are suspected or of particular environmental concern.

Biological indicators are also available for monitoring the effectiveness of processes, particularly sterilisation. These are usually in the form of paper or stainless steel coupons which are inoculated with bacterial spores (as the most resistant organism to sterilisation processes), but other test organisms can be used. These are exposed to a process and then cultured to determine the presence or absence of growth.

Cleaning

Cleaning is an essential part of any routine disinfection/sterilisation process, as organic and/or inorganic soils inhibit the activity of any given process. In general, visually clean is regarded as being sufficient for most purposes, although chemical (e.g. protein determination) and microbiological methods (e.g. swabbing) can be used for more sensitive determinations for the presence of soil residues following a cleaning process.

Cleaning can be conducted manually or automatically. Manual methods generally use a cleaning detergent (including alkaline, acid, neutral and enzymatic formulations) in combination with cloths, brushes etc., followed by rinsing and drying. Low-soiled isolators are often cleaned using alcohols, for physical removal and drying. Automated processes include washer/washer—disinfector machines or clean-in-place systems, with or without cleaning detergents. It is recommended that when using any automatic process, equipment is serviced regularly, loads are defined and periodically verified by performing tests which include temperature mapping, probe calibration and cleaning tests.

Disinfection

Although disinfection does not kill all micro-organisms, it is meant to reduce the levels of pathogens to safe levels. Disinfection can be achieved by heat, UV, or chemical means.

Heat

Rapid surface disinfection of materials (or water disinfection) can be achieved by immersion in hot, preferably boiling water or treatment with steam at atmospheric pressure. In general, disinfection time will depend on the temperature, typically > 65 °C. Examples of overkill disinfection cycle times using moist heat (for devices that could be used for invasive procedures):

    100 minutes at 70 °C
    10 minutes at 80 °C
    1 minute at 90 °C
    0.1 minute at 100 °C

Care should be taken to ensure that all surfaces are heat resistant, and exposed for the required disinfection time. Surfaces should be allowed to cool down before use, and should be used immediately. Where surfaces, particularly devices, are not to be used following treatment, they should be dried and should be redisinfected before use.

Pasteurisation is a traditional form of heat disinfection widely used in the food industry, originally introduced to control mycobacteria (tubercle bacilli) in milk. This is achieved by rapidly heating to 65–80 °C, holding for the required disinfection time, and rapid cooling. This method can be used to reduce the load of viable micro-organisms in feeds and liquids.

UV disinfection

UV light is produced from mercury vapour lamps and has maximum antimicrobial efficacy at 240 to 280 nm. Due to a lack of penetration, in comparison to other forms of radiation, the effect of UV is dramatically reduced the further a surface is from the light source, and by shielding and in the presence of soils or other interfering substances. UV is bactericidal, cysticidal and virucidal, but requires longer exposure times or higher radiation levels for fungicidal and sporicidal activity. UV is widely used for water disinfection and small surface-area decontamination (for example, in laminar flow hoods).

Chemical disinfectants

A variety of antimicrobial liquid, foam or impregnated wipe disinfectants are used for localised or area decontamination. It is important that these products are prepared (if provided as concentrates) and used according to manufacturer's labelling (including correct dilution, restrictions on reuse, safety precautions, as described above). In general, all chemical disinfectants have greater efficacy at increased temperatures, where recommended by the product manufacturer. The most widely used biocides are discussed below. It is re-emphasised that the activity of any product will depend on its formulation and use; the discussion below is meant only as a guide for each active.

Alcohols

The most widely used alcohols are ethanol and isopropanol. Both are rapidly bactericidal, fungicidal and virucidal, but have no activity on bacterial spores. Typical used concentrations range from 50–90%, where lower and higher concentrations are significantly less antimicrobial. Alcohols are used for surface disinfection, antisepsis (of the skin) and drying due to their rapid vaporisation. Care should be taken when using high concentrations, due to flammability risks.

Aldehydes

Glutaraldehyde and formaldehyde have broad-spectrum activity, although longer exposure times are required for sporicidal activity. In general, aldehydes are mycobactericidal, but resistant atypical strains to glutaraldehyde have been reported. Glutaraldehyde, usually in liquid formulation at 0.1–2.5%, is widely used as a surface or device disinfectant. Formaldehyde (dilutions of a ~40% aqueous solution) is generally used for fumigation in a gaseous form (<7%). Both actives are particularly sensitive to the presence or organic soils. Due to their cross-linking mode of action, they can fix residual soils onto a surface; it is particularly important in the use of these biocides that surfaces are clean prior to use.

Aldehydes are generally toxic and require special handling precautions, including adequate ventilation during their use. Formaldehyde is explosive at concentrations > 7% in air. Removal of residues following treatment is important to consider.

Halogens

Chlorine

Chlorine (usually as household bleach – a dilution of sodium hypochlorite) demonstrates rapid virucidal, bactericidal, fungicidal and sporicidal activity. In dilution, a neutral pH is important to control; for example, activity is reduced by a factor of 10 every pH unit above 7. Typical in-use dilutions for surface disinfection are 0.1 to 1% sodium hypochlorite (equal to a 1 in 50 and 1 in 5 dilution of household bleach, at 5% sodium hypochlorite, respectively). Chlorine is a reactive and short-lived biocide. For this reason, only freshly prepared dilutions should be used and reuse should not be considered. The activity of chlorine solutions depends on the amount of active (free) chlorine measured, which can be monitored easily using a variety of commercially available methods. Water (and water system) disinfection concentrations also vary, with a typical recommendation at 0.5–5 ppm of free (active) chlorine. Chlorine, and chlorine-releasing agents, are widely used for surface and water disinfection. Due to its reactive nature, repeated use on surfaces can be damaging. Chlorine is considered safe for use and demonstrates low toxicity, but can be irritating at higher concentrations.

Iodine and iodophors
Iodine, or the more widely used iodophors (iodine-releasing agents), also demonstrate broad spectrum, including sporicidal, activity. Similar to chlorine, activity is dependant on the amount of 'free' iodine available. Iodophors should be diluted and prepared according to manufacturer's instructions, and will vary considerably depending on their formulation. Although less reactive than chlorine, their activity can be reduced due to the presence of inorganic soil. Iodine solutions are generally only used as antiseptics, as pre-operative preparations. Iodophors are used as surface disinfectants, antiseptics and footbaths. At typical used concentrations, iodine has low toxicity, but can be undesirable due to staining of surfaces and difficulty in rinsing.

Oxidising agents
The most widely used oxidising agents are hydrogen peroxide, peracetic acid, chlorine dioxide and ozone. Oxidising agents are potent, broad-spectrum antimicrobials, but vary in sporicidal activity and material compatibility.

Chlorine dioxide
ClO_2 is widely used as a water and surface disinfectant, with a better environmental profile than chlorine.

It can also be used at low concentrations as an antiseptic. Due to its reactive nature and rapid decomposition, it is generally generated at the site of use, through a variety of reactions. The most widely used method is by reacting sodium chlorite with chlorine. As a strong oxidising agent, ClO_2 is bactericidal, virucidal, fungicidal and sporicidal, depending on the concentration. Sporicidal activity has been shown at concentrations > 11 mg/litre. Limited activity against protozoal cysts and algae has also been reported. ClO_2 has had restricted use in gaseous form for fumigation (see p. 221).

Hydrogen peroxide
Liquid hydrogen peroxide (H_2O_2) is a stable, clear, colourless liquid with broad-spectrum, including sporicidal and cysticidal, activity. It has been used as a disinfectant, sterilant and antiseptic at concentrations up to 8% for sporicidal activity. Higher concentrations can be damaging to surfaces. Synergistic formulations in combination with peracetic acid are available. Much lower concentrations are required in a gaseous form; vaporised hydrogen peroxide is widely used for fumigation (see p. 220). Hydrogen peroxide has an excellent safety profile, as it breaks down in the environment to water and oxygen. Similar to other oxidising agents, it is also sensitive to the presence or soil of other interfering substances.

Ozone
Ozone (O_3) has been used for water disinfection (at pH 6–7) and for area deodorisation. O_3 is a short-lived, powerful gaseous biocide with a slight blue colour and distinctive (fresh) smell. Ozone can be simply produced by reacting dry air or oxygen (O_2) with an energy source, generally UV light or, more commonly, a corona discharge. Ozone is an effective bactericide, virucide, fungicide, but has limited sporicidal activity at typical use concentrations. Activity has also been shown against protozoal cysts. Environmentally, ozone rapidly breaks down into oxygen and water vapour, with no concerns of toxic residues. As one of the most reactive oxidising agents, ozone can be damaging to surfaces at higher concentrations and is very sensitive to interfering substances.

Peracetic acid
Peracetic acid (PAA; CH_3COOOH) is bactericidal,

fungicidal, virucidal and sporicidal at relatively low concentrations (~0.3%). Formulation of the biocide is important to its activity and material compatibility, where increased temperatures can dramatically increase its biocidal activity but also its decomposition. PAA also decomposes into safe, non-toxic products (water and a low concentration of acetic acid, or vinegar). Unlike other oxidising agents, PAA retains activity in the presence of organic and inorganic soils. PAA formulations are widely used for device disinfection/sterilisation and high-risk surface disinfection.

Phenolics

Phenol derivatives are widely used due to their biocidal activity, including bactericidal, fungicidal and virucidal activity. Many formulations have limited activity against small, non-enveloped viruses (like parvoviruses) and mycobacteria, highlighting the importance of formulation and the choice of phenolic derivatives used to optimise activity. Phenolics are not sporicidal. Formulations will vary in toxicity, can be corrosive and have an 'institutional' odour. Certain animals are particularly sensitive to phenolics. They are widely used as general surface disinfectants, including walls, floors and cages.

A small group, referred to as *bis*phenols are used as antiseptics. The most widely used is triclosan, which has limited activity (bactericidal and to a lesser extent virucidal), but demonstrates very low irritation to the skin.

Quaternary ammonium compounds

Quaternary ammonium compounds (Quats or QACs) are cationic surfactants (surface active agents) which combine bactericidal/virucidal (generally only against lipid-enveloped viruses) activity with good detergency, and therefore cleaning ability. As for other biocides, the activity of QAC-based formulations will vary significantly. Limited formulations can have some activity against mycobacteria and are sporistatic. Activity can be affected by hard water (used for dilution), fat-containing substances and anionic surfactants. QACs have a pleasant odour, are not aggressive on surfaces and have low toxicity. They are widely used as cleaners/disinfectants on general, non-critical surfaces, including the removal of gross soil. Some QACs are also used at low concentrations as antiseptics.

Fumigation

Formaldehyde

Formaldehyde gas has been used for area fumigation for over one hundred years, due to its broad-spectrum biocidal activity. The gas may be conveniently generated either by heating paraformaldehyde (a white crystalline powder), or a 37% formalin solution. It is imperative that high humidity levels are maintained (for example by boiling an equal volume of water) during formaldehyde fumigation, to the point that surfaces should actually be physically wet, in order to ensure effectiveness. A concentration of at least 0.05 g of formaldehyde per m^3 is recommended, with soaking times long (18–24 hours) to ensure adequate decontamination, depending on the area size, desired level of decontamination, and area contents. At higher concentrations formaldehyde is explosive (>7% by volume in air). Formaldehyde is toxic and carcinogenic, characteristics which have limited its use. It is also important to note that toxic residues (in the form of a white powder) can remain on surfaces following fumigation and need to be safely removed prior to allowing re-entry into a given area.

Formaldehyde, like other aldehydes, has a cross-linking mode of action and can fix organic soils onto surfaces; this can inhibit the fumigation efficacy and is difficult to remove. A typical cycle consists of humidification (surface wetting), gassing and purging/clean-up. Aeration of an area is a challenge and can be achieved by controlled venting to atmosphere (discouraged), neutralising by ammonia, or adsorption onto activated charcoal.

Hydrogen peroxide

Vaporised hydrogen peroxide (VHP) is an odorless, colourless gas produced by vaporisation of liquid hydrogen peroxide to give a mixture of hydrogen peroxide and water vapour. When the concentration is maintained below its dew point VHP is a 'dry' process, and demonstrates rapid, broad-spectrum activity and material compatibility. VHP is virucidal, bactericidal, fungicidal, cysticidal and sporicidal. VHP, as a dry process is compatible and safe for use on a wide range of materials, including metals, plastics, and other materials (including artwork and

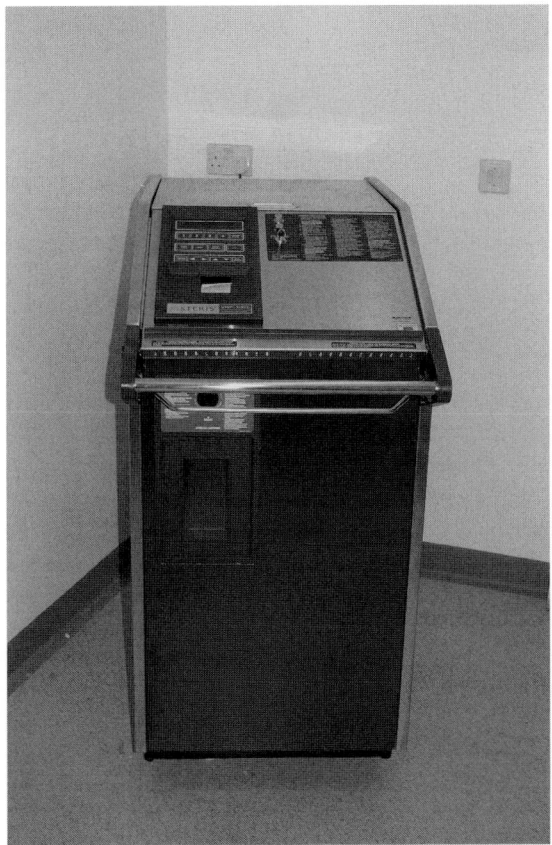

Figure 29.2 Vaporised hydrogen peroxide (VHP) decontamination system attached to a room.

electronics). Systems are available which control the decontamination (conditioning, fumigation and aeration) for enclosed areas, including isolators and rooms (Figure 29.2). In contrast to other fumigation methods, the area is generally dehumidified below 40% relative humidity and then VHP introduced to achieve sporicidal conditions (generally 0.1–3 mg/litre). Alternative 'wet' or condensed systems are also available, but should be considered as liquid peroxide fogging processes.

Chlorine dioxide

When in the gaseous form, chlorine dioxide is very reactive at low concentrations and demonstrates broad-spectrum efficacy. A typical fumigation cycle consists of conditioning, gassing and aeration phases (to non-toxic residues). A minimum concentration of 500–550 ppm (at 65% humidity) for twelve hours contact time has been recommended for broad-spectrum activity. High humidity (60–75%) levels are required for antimicrobial activity. Due to light sensitivity, fumigation should be conducted in the dark. Breakdown products include chlorine, which can be destructive on surfaces.

Ozone

Ozone generators have been used for area deodorisation, with activity against bacteria and fungi. There is limited activity against viruses and spores, with higher concentrations and humidity being required (0.5–3 mg/litre at 70–80% humidity). At these concentrations, ozone can be very damaging to surfaces.

Sterilisation

It is important to note that many methods can be considered sporicidal, referring to the ability to ability to kill spores, but may not necessarily provide sterilisation. Sterilisation is an absolute term which describes the complete destruction or removal of all viable micro-organisms in a validated process. Sterilisation processes can be classified as heat, chemical, radiation and filtration methods.

Wet heat (steam) sterilisation

Steam sterilisation is performed in a pressure vessel (autoclave) which exposes a load to saturated steam at a specified temperature, pressure and time. Saturated steam refers to holding as much water as possible, without allowing condensation to occur. Typical sterilisation cycles used are:

121 °C for 15 minutes
134 °C for 3 minutes

These cycles are given as minimum times, when the chamber and its load are up to the specified temperature. Steam, produced from boiling water, is an effective antimicrobial – as the temperature increases, so does the antimicrobial efficacy. Under pressure, the temperature can be raised above that at atmospheric pressure, thereby allowing shorter sterilisation times. An important consideration is the removal of air both from the chamber and its load, as air will inhibit the effectiveness and penetration of steam. Autoclave designs can therefore be classified based on the mechanisms of air removal.

Upward displacement autoclaves

These are traditional, small, laboratory autoclaves. Water is placed at the base of the vessel and boiled to produce steam. Air is then expelled from the vessel under pressure, through a safety valve on the lid, for a given time and closed. Heating continues during the sterilisation time, and then the vessel is allowed to cool.

Downward displacement autoclaves

These can vary in size from small, bench-top to larger-scale autoclaves. In a typical model, steam is introduced at the top of a pressure vessel and, because it is heavier than air, forces the air out through a valve at the base of the chamber. When the required temperature and pressure are achieved, the valve is closed and the load held for a given sterilisation time. Air is then introduced into the chamber and the contents allowed to cool (generally to below 80 °C). These autoclaves are widely used for liquid and surface (devices, cages, vessels, etc.) sterilisation. They should not be used to sterilise porous materials (like foodstuffs, towels, etc.) due to the difficulty of air removal.

Pre-vacuum autoclaves

A variety of designs and sizes are available for porous and non-porous loads. These sterilisers use a vacuum pump which removes the air from the chamber. Steam is generally pulsed into the chamber, to aid in the removal of air and allow for even penetration of steam through the load. Following sterilisation, the steam is evacuated and the contents allowed to cool (see Figures 30.5 and 30.6).

In all cases, it is recommended that defined loads and cycles are used, to ensure reproducible sterilisation. Cycles can be developed and verified periodically by performing routine tests which include (for steam sterilisation) air removal tests (e.g. Bowie–Dick test), temperature mapping, pressure/temperature probe calibration, leak testing and biological indicators.

Dry heat sterilisation

Dry heat can be an effective antimicrobial, but in contrast to steam requires exposure to extended periods at elevated temperature to ensure sterilisation. These methods are limited in their application due to their destructive nature.

Incineration

Incineration (combustion or burning to ashes) is essentially a destructive method, which is used for the disposal of contaminated wastes. Incinerators are fuelled by gas or oil and typically operate from 800 to 1000 °C. Control of emissions (biological and chemical) is important in their use. At a laboratory level, flaming (or passing a small device through a flame, usually a Bunsen burner) is used but can be unreliable.

Hot air sterilisers

Temperature-resistant surfaces (like some metals and glass) and materials (powders, some oils) can be sterilised by dry heat, but longer times are required as air is not effective at heat transfer. Typical dry sterilisation cycles used (minimum) are:

160 °C for 120 minutes
170 °C for 60 minutes
180 °C for 30 minutes

Gaseous chemical sterilisation

There are three major gaseous chemical sterilisation methods widely used for low temperature sterilisation.

Ethylene oxide (EO)

EO is a stable, colourless gas used for device sterilisation. Its activity is based on the air removal, EO concentration, temperature (30–60 °C), humidity (30–70%) and exposure time. EO demonstrates broad spectrum activity, but is significantly inhibited by the presence of soils. Due to the carcinogenic and mutagenic nature of EO, particular attention should be paid to occupational safety (e.g. adequate ventilation) during the sterilisation cycle and any subsequent material aeration, due to absorption of the gas into device materials/packaging. The toxic nature of the gas has restricted its widespread use in facilities; however, correct ventilation and gas monitors allow for exposure control.

Formaldehyde

Formaldehyde is used primarily as an area fumigant

Figure 29.3 Diagram showing a VHP generator connected to a room.

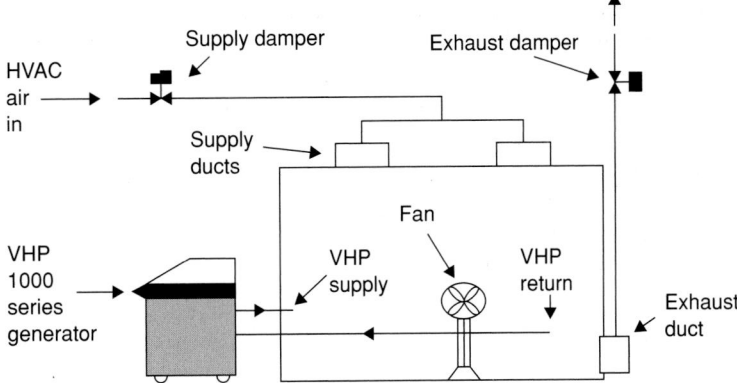

(see p. 220), but has also been used in combination with low-temperature steam (typical process temperatures of 70–80 °C) for sterilisation. The biocide is bactericidal, virucidal, fungicidal and sporicidal. Similar to EO, activity is dependent on correct control of humidity (generally 70–100%), and temperature (usually 50–80 °C). Formaldehyde is toxic, carcinogenic, and a strong irritant.

Hydrogen peroxide
Hydrogen peroxide is a powerful oxidising agent and is antimicrobial, including rapidly sporicidal, in its gaseous form at low concentrations in contrast to liquid peroxide. It has been widely used for area fumigation, as previously discussed (see p. 220). Device sterilisation with hydrogen peroxide is performed in the presence or absence of plasma (which is formed using electromagnetic fields). Typical sterilisation cycles involve drawing a vacuum (to remove air, which can inhibit the penetration of the biocide), exposure to gaseous peroxide (usually a series of pulses) and aeration by evacuation. Due to the breakdown of peroxide into water and oxygen, the safety profile is more desirable than for other gases.

Figure 29.3 shows a VHP generator connected to a room. A fan is placed in the centre of the room to circulate the vapour. Care must be taken to isolate the room's ventilation system from the VHP to prevent it spreading to other rooms. The room needs to be preconditioned by a method that varies with the type of system. Normally a sensor, which is connected to the generator, is placed in the room. External doors to the room may also need sealing.

Liquid chemical sterilisation
Liquids can provide the same sterilisation level as gases, but have the significant disadvantages of requiring rinsing following treatment and not allowing for packaging/sterile storage. As for any sterilisation process, a knowledge of and control of the process limitations is important to consider. These include ensuring all surfaces are contacted for the minimum contact time, broad-spectrum efficacy, predictable efficacy, defined loads, etc. These liquids are considered under disinfection and include aldehydes, halogens and oxidising agents.

Irradiation

Irradiation is the process of exposing a product or material to ionising radiation, emitted in the form of γ-rays (e.g. from a ^{60}Co source) or electron beams (E-beam). These methods are rapidly antimicrobial by directly attacking nucleic acids and indirectly through the generation of damaging free radicals and other reactive molecules that attack other cellular constituents. Due to safety risks, specific and expensive installations are required. Radiation is restricted in its use to wrapped and/or packaged materials and, to a lesser extent food preservation.

Filtration

Micro-organisms can be physically removed from liquids, powders and air using a variety of filtration methods. These include depth or surface filters (e.g. ceramic, sintered glass), and membrane filters (e.g.

High Efficiency Particulate Air Filters (HEPA) (see Chapter 32) or cellulose). Depth filters are generally used for pre-filtration and membrane filters for terminal filtration. Membrane filters are rated on their pore (exclusion) size, typically 0.8 to 0.1 μm; critical, sterilising-grade filters are usually ≤ 0.22 μm. Filters should be routinely checked for integrity and can be prone to contamination downstream if not controlled and maintained sterile.

Prion decontamination – a special consideration

Prions are proteinaceous infectious agents, which are widely accepted as the causative agents in transmissible spongiform encephalopathies (TSEs), including scrapie and bovine spongiform encephalopathy (BSE). These infectious agents are notoriously resistant to routine disinfection and sterilisation methods, including steam sterilisation. No single method has been shown to be 100% effective against prions. Cleaning of surfaces is probably the most important factor in reducing the risks of cross-contamination, followed by recommended decontamination methods:

- Chemical treatment with sodium hydroxide (generally > 1N for 1 hour) or sodium hypochlorite (2% available chlorine for 1 hour). Treatment with some phenolic disinfectants has also been shown to be effective. For devices, combining these chemistries with steam sterilisation is not recommended due to the production of noxious fumes, and device/steriliser damage.

- Extended steam sterilisation at ≥ 121 °C for ≥ 30 minutes (gravity displacement) or 134 °C for ≥ 18 minutes (prevacuum). Devices should be immersed in water during these cycles.

Further reading

Russell, A.D. (2003) *Principles and Practice of Disinfection, Preservation and Sterilisation*. Blackwell Science, Oxford.

30

Animals with Defined Microbiological Status

Robert W. Kemp

Introduction

Until the early 1950s, animals were housed in units with crude environmental controls, disease was rife and in addition to the effect of this on animal welfare, it gave rise to animal wastage, unreliable experimental data, wasted time and effort. Specific (or Specified) Pathogen Free (SPF) units were conceived to improve the situation by excluding the organisms responsible for laboratory animal disease.

The term SPF is gradually disappearing from use and instead animal units tend to be described according to the stringency of the barriers operated in order to define very closely the microbiological status of the animals produced or used within it.

The following terms are used in connection with barrier units:

- *Conventional*: Animals bred or maintained in the unit where routines are employed to reduce the rate of infection from other sources. This would probably include the wearing of some protective clothing and, for example, regular washing of staff hands. The animals housed may harbour undefined microflora which may include pathogens.

- *Minimal disease unit*: A unit where animals are housed which have been produced disease free and subsequently good standards of hygiene are used to minimise the risk of infectious disease. This term is quite often used for units where farm animals are housed.

- *Part barrier unit*: A unit in which only the high risk entry points are protected or the degree of protection may be less than a full barrier unit (e.g. partial rather than absolute air filtration). However, steps are taken to reduce contamination by full change of clothing for the staff, restricting traffic, sterilising materials or purchasing them with low levels of microbial contamination.

- *Full barrier unit*: An animal unit with procedures designed to reduce the risk of contamination of its occupants, e.g. by pathogens or harmful chemicals. All points where pathogenic organisms could gain entry to the unit are protected either physically (e.g. filters or autoclaves) or chemically (e.g. dunk tank).

- *Specific (specified) pathogen free*: As stated above, this term is now falling out of favour however its literal meaning is animals that are free from named pathogenic organisms but not necessarily free from those not named.

- *Hysterectomy derived*: The surgical removal of the intact gravid uterus. The young are released from the uterus under strict aseptic conditions and either reared by hand or fostered on to a gnotobiotic foster mother. Since the placenta acts as a barrier to most micro-organisms the young will be free of many, if not all, pathogenic organisms carried by the donor mother.

- *Gnotobiotic (known life) animal*: An animal in which all the life forms are known. These are animals which were originally germ free and housed in isolators, and then, to improve their ability to utilise food, or for experimental reasons, a known microflora is added.

- *Germ free or axenic*: An animal which is free from all demonstrable forms of life.

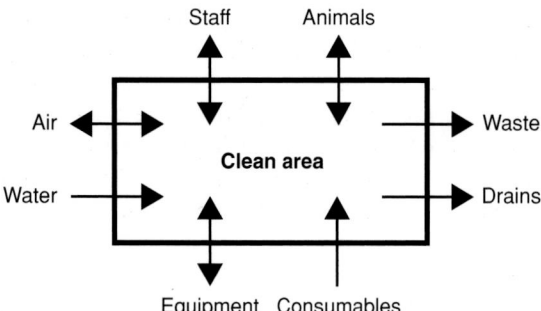

Figure 30.1   Movement across the barrier providing the opportunity for possible ingress of pathogenic organisms.

Barrier units

Routes of entry for pathogens

Pathogenic organisms can gain entry to an animal unit by various routes as indicated in Figure 30.1. All potential portals of entry for pathogens must be considered at the building design stage and careful consideration should be given at that stage to the methods of excluding these pathogens.

Design options for a full-barrier animal unit

Position of unit

The unit should be sited as far as possible from potential sources of contamination such as other laboratory animal units. Distance reduces the challenge to the barrier. A dusty external environment should be avoided as barrier units incorporate sophisticated, expensive filtration systems. Overloading them with an air supply carrying large quantities of particulate material will reduce the life of the filters, and place an unnecessary burden on the filtration system. Airborne chemical pollution on for example, busy roads, should also be avoided.

Fabric of the unit

The integrity of the outer shell of the unit is essential to prevent the introduction of pathogens. Walls act as physical barriers and should be constructed of materials which will not easily be breached by accidental or deliberate damage caused through impact, settlement or by the activities of gnawing vermin. Ideally, the unit should be windowless; however, if windows are installed, they should be well protected, e.g. by a vandal proof plastic shield. Particular care should be taken to seal all gaps at the junctions between walls, doors, windows and at the points where service pipes breach the barrier.

The drainage system should be carefully designed and maintained. The possibility of vermin gaining access to waste pipes as they enter man-holes must be eliminated. One way of achieving this is to incorporate a 'cascade system' where the waste pipe enters at a high level and protrudes from the wall of the man-hole.

Water traps (U-bends) should not be allowed to dry out. This may sometimes occur as a result of damaged or faulty materials or when the air pressure within the animal rooms becomes too great. All drains opening into the animal room must be provided with secure, well-fitted covers to finally thwart any adventurous and determined rodent managing to reach this far into the unit.

Single or double corridors

Clean and dirty materials must be kept separate. This can be achieved in two ways; they can be separated physically or be separated by time. If they are separated by time, clean materials (e.g. bedding, food) are delivered to rooms first and waste materials are removed from rooms later. After waste material has been transported down corridors they are disinfected before more clean materials are transported through them.

The unit can be designed with a 'clean' and 'dirty' corridor system. Each room has two doors, one opening onto a 'clean' corridor and one to a 'dirty' corridor.

Ventilation system

The use of forced ventilation in animal rooms offers a convenient entry route for pathogens. All air taken into the unit via the ventilation system should be filtered using High Efficiency Particulate Air Filters (HEPA) which are capable of removing virtually all sizes of airborne particles (see Chapter 32).

HEPA filters are expensive. It is usual to prolong their life by first passing the air through coarser filters to remove the larger particles. This will keep costs down by obviating the need for too frequent filter changes and the attendant contamination risk while this procedure is being carried out. It is possible to prolong the life of the HEPA filters for 2.5 to 5 years by using good primary filtration.

The ventilation input and extract can be balanced so that air inside the unit is at a slightly higher pressure to that of the outside air. This positive air pressure within the animal area results in a continual flow of air out of the unit through open doors and any gaps in the building fabric thus making it more difficult for airborne organisms to enter via these routes.

A mechanical breakdown will result in a loss of air pressure but for a short period this is unlikely to cause any problems. The worst situation would be a failure of the intake fan with the extract fan continuing to function. This would result in the reversal of pressures to a negative system with the risk of unfiltered air being drawn into the unit. The fitting of a fail-safe device which automatically turns off the extract fan should the intake fail will prevent this from occurring.

In large units operating a 'clean'/'dirty' corridor it is usual to have a gradient of positive pressures – 'clean' corridor to animal rooms to 'dirty' corridor to outside (Figure 30.2).

When operating a positive-pressure system consideration must be given to the leakage of unfiltered air and the possibility of exposing staff working in non-animal areas to the risk of laboratory animal allergens.

Water supply

Although most animal units are provided with water fit for human consumption, it must not be assumed that the supply is free from all pathogenic organisms. Most units use header tanks in animal drinking-water systems and these should be regarded as a potential source of contamination. Treatment of the water should be seen as an important part of the barrier and may be achieved in a number of ways. All systems require alarms in case of failure.

Filtration
Micro-organisms may be removed physically by a series of filters. A typical filtration system will incorporate initial 'rough' filters (usually 10 micron) secondary filters (1 micron) and finally a sterilising filter (0.2 micron).

If the water supply to the animals is gravity fed the pressure drop occurring across the filter(s) must be taken into account when deciding on the head of water needed to ensure an adequate supply at the drinking nipple. Some automatic systems incorporate pumps and valves to counter this problem.

Exposure to ultra-violet (UV) light
Water is passed slowly along special glass or plastic pipes which allow penetration of the UV light. The water flow must be reduced to allow adequate exposure time for any organisms to be killed. This method of water treatment is not usually suitable in barrier units housing large animal populations because of its inability to cope with heavy demands. It can, however, be combined with another treatment method, such as filtration, to speed up the treatment process and provide a plentiful supply of high quality drinking water.

Acidification
Measured quantities of hydrochloric acid (HCl) are manually added to containers of water from which the water bottles are filled. At a pH of about 2.5,

Figure 30.2 Diagram of a 'clean'/'dirty' corridor system. By employing a positive pressure gradient the flow of air inside the unit is always from 'cleaner' to 'dirtier' areas, so reducing the risk of cross infection between rooms.

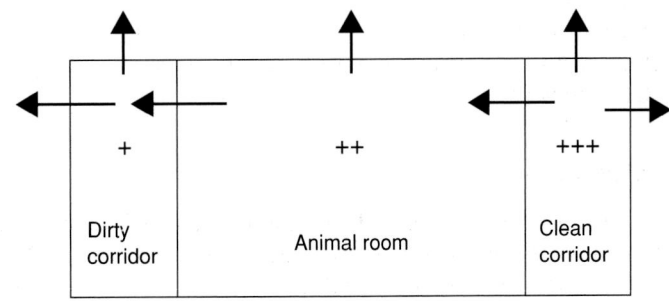

organisms are killed and the palatability is (perhaps surprisingly) increased. Automatic systems in which the acid is metered into the header tank have been used.

Additional chlorination

It is possible to use an automatic system to increase the level of chlorine in the incoming tap water to 20 ppm (super-chlorination) to kill any remaining organisms.

Choice of water treatment

The choice of water treatment will depend on several factors. These include:

(1) the potential effect of the treatment on the experiment;
(2) the cost of dosing and monitoring equipment;
(3) the availability of space for equipment;
(4) maintenance costs and down time.

Some units treat all water supplied behind the barrier rather than confining treatment to animal drinking water only. Supplies to hose points which are not to be used as sources of animal drinking water, may be treated chemically without fear of affecting the animals (see Chapter 27).

Air locks and pass locks

These may be incorporated in the unit on entry or exit routes for the passage of staff or materials. The lock is doubled doored, separates 'clean'/'dirty' areas and will normally incorporate an interlock system

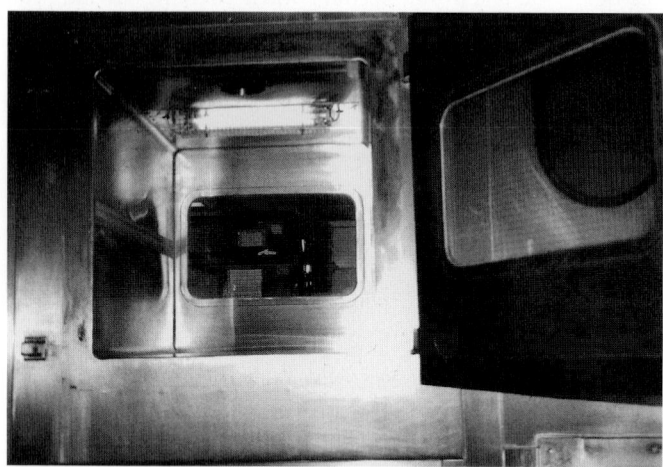

Figure 30.3   An open, double-doored ultra-violet hatch. (The UV light would normally be switched off automatically with the door open but the safety switch has been over-ridden for the purposes of this photograph only.)

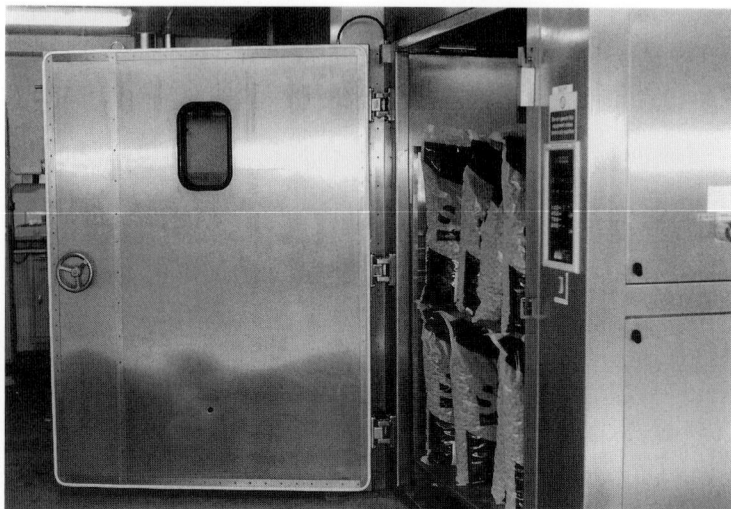

Figure 30.4   A large, double-doored fumigation chamber containing bags of diet. The diet has been irradiated and is sealed within polythene bags. Formaldehyde is used to sterilise the outside of the bags.

for ensuring that both doors cannot be open simultaneously. The lock will assist in reducing the pressure drop in positive-pressure areas when doors are opened, and will reduce the risk of flying insects gaining entry.

Entry locks may be used for the passage of goods into or out of a barrier unit. Some method of disinfection must be incorporated in the transfer system. Ultra-violet light or liquid disinfectant from a spray or 'fogger' are commonly used though neither of these methods are as effective as autoclaving (Figures 30.3 and 30.4). UV light has limitations as a disinfection agent as it will only treat exposed areas. Any surface in shadow will remain untreated and for this reason its use is often restricted to the sterilisation of the inner surfaces of the transfer hatch following a transfer rather than the goods being transferred. Any items which are to pass through the barrier via a transfer hatch should be heat sealed in a double layer of polythene and be pre-sterilised by, for example, gamma irradiation prior to entry. Immediately before placing the article in the transfer hatch, the outer protective cover is removed by an operator wearing clean or, preferably, sterile gloves. This ensures that any contamination is left on the 'dirty side' of the barrier. The package, now in its inner wrapper, can be disinfected within the lock to remove any organisms which may have contaminated the inner surface during the process of removing the outer wrapper.

Autoclaves

The bulk of the material passing through the barrier will do so via the autoclave. This is the most efficient method of decontaminating heat-stable materials. Autoclaves are available in various sizes the largest of which can accommodate cage racks. Although some of the older units are still equipped with downward displacement autoclaves modern buildings incorporate the more efficient high-vacuum type (see Chapter 29). The autoclave is situated so that one door opens on the 'clean' side and the other door and the machinery are located on the 'dirty' (Figure 30.5).

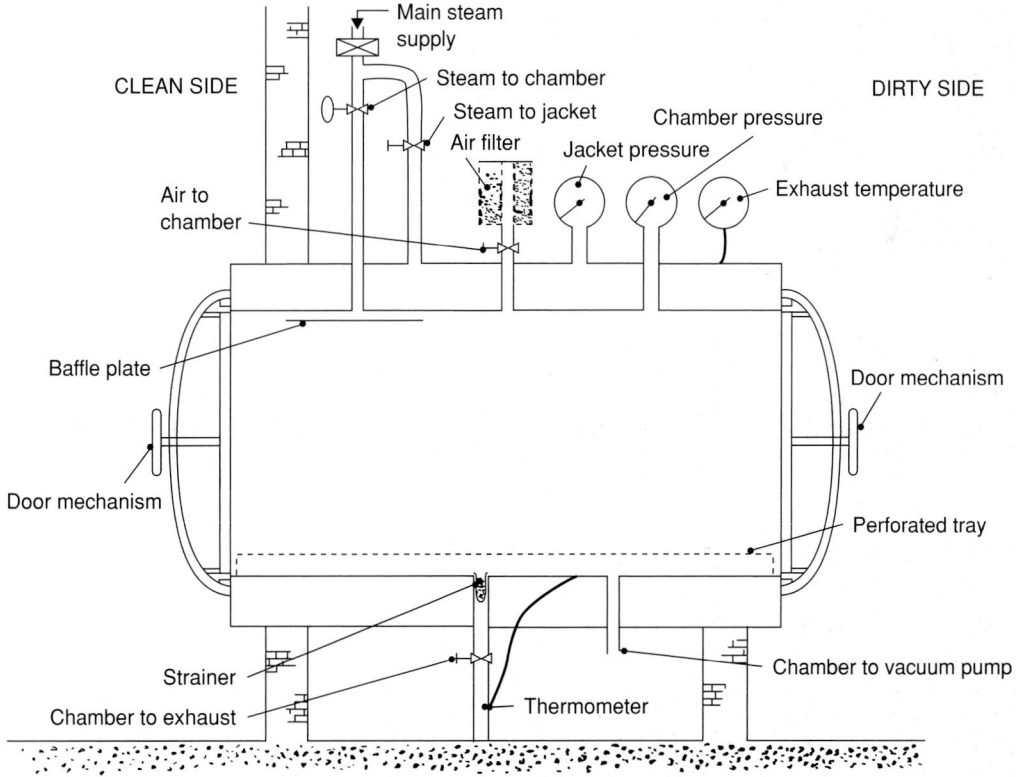

Figure 30.5   Cross-section of a through-the-wall autoclave. (Permission to reproduce this figure, previously published in *A Guide to Laboratory Animal Technology* by Martin D. Buckland, Lynda Hall, Alan Mowlem and Beryl F. Whatley, from Heinemann Medical Books Ltd.)

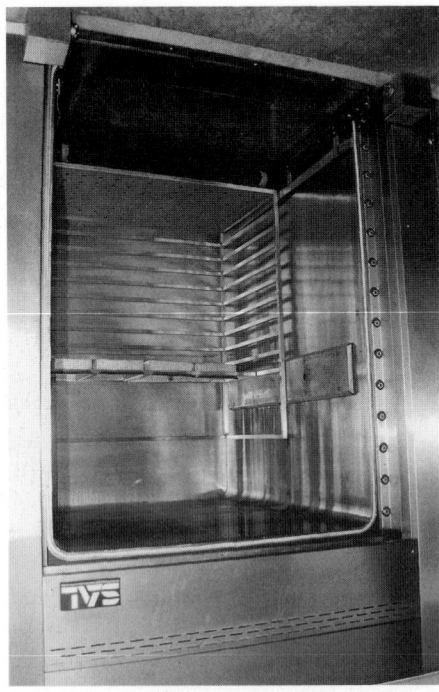

Figure 30.6 A double-doored, stainless steel, high vacuum auto-clave sufficiently large to take two cage racks. The double shell structure can be seen, separated by a rubber strip which seals against the inside of the door on closure.

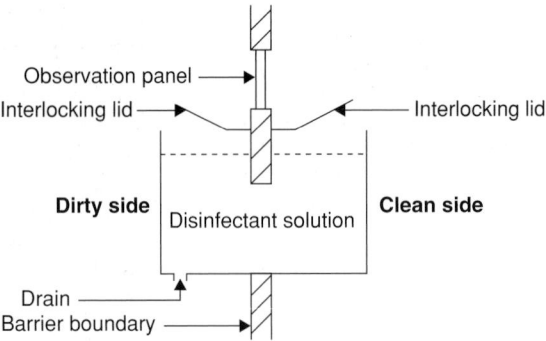

Figure 30.7 Disinfectant dunk tank straddling the barrier between 'clean' and 'dirty' areas.

Equipment required behind the barrier is loaded via the 'dirty' door (Figure 30.6). This door is closed and the appropriate sterilising or pasteurising cycle is selected. On completion of the cycle, the 'clean' door is opened and the treated material is removed from the chamber. The autoclave may then be used as a pass box for the removal of items from the unit.

Great care should be taken to avoid overloading the autoclave as sterilising efficiency will be impaired. Ideally, the maximum loading of the chamber should be ascertained for different types of porous materials during a series of commissioning trials using several thermocouples placed into the least accessible areas of the load. A standard operating procedure can be written detailing loading instructions. Each run should be monitored and recorded.

Dunk tank

This is used to pass previously sterilised, heat-labile materials into the unit. As disinfection is the method of decontamination, it must be regarded as a less efficient method than autoclaving.

The dunk tank is a large plastic or metal container which is set into the barrier wall. Half of the tank is on the 'dirty' side and half on the 'clean' side (Figure 30.7). The wall continues down into the tank so that when filled with a disinfectant solution, the integrity of the barrier is preserved. It is desirable to have both visual and verbal two-way communication at this point in the barrier. A reinforced glass observation panel can be used for written messages as well as manual indications in addition to a telephone or intercom (Figures 30.8 and 30.9).

The length of time that articles are held submerged in the disinfectant solution will depend on the disinfectant used and the nature and cleanliness of the articles. Two hours is usually sufficient for most articles. Pre-soaking in a separate container is sometimes implemented particularly for plastic objects.

It will be necessary to change the disinfectant solution before it becomes inactivated. The frequency of change will depend on:

- the type of disinfectant used;
- the cleanliness of the articles being passed through;
- the amount of use.

It is important that the barrier is not breached during the draining and refilling process. Normally an air-tight lid is lowered into place on the dirty side of the tank and the drain cock opened. Once the tank is empty an air-tight lid is used to seal the tank from behind the barrier. The dirty-side lid can now be opened to allow for the cleaning and re-filling of the

Figure 30.8 Stainless steel disinfectant dunk tank with lid open. The telephone intercom and view panels to the clean side can be seen above the tank. The circular port above the tank is for transfer of animals from the inside of the unit. Specially designed transport containers are hermetically locked onto the port. On the left of the dunk tank is an ultraviolet lock.

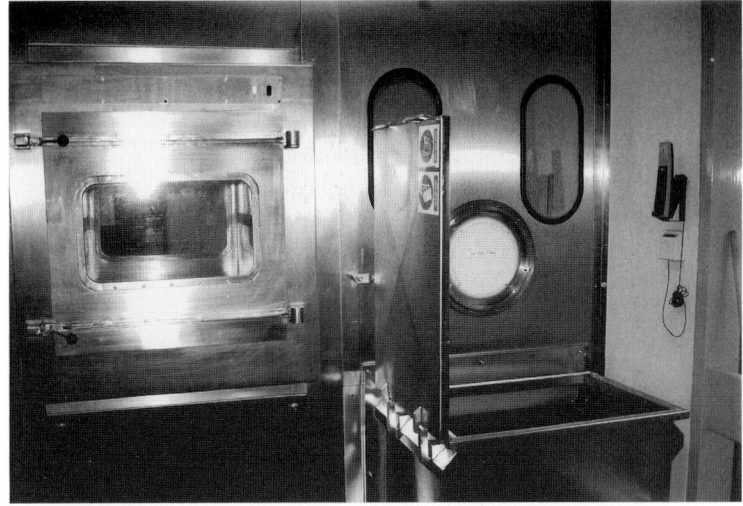

Figure 30.9 An open dunk tank showing the basket device aimed at keeping floating objects totally immersed in the disinfectant solution.

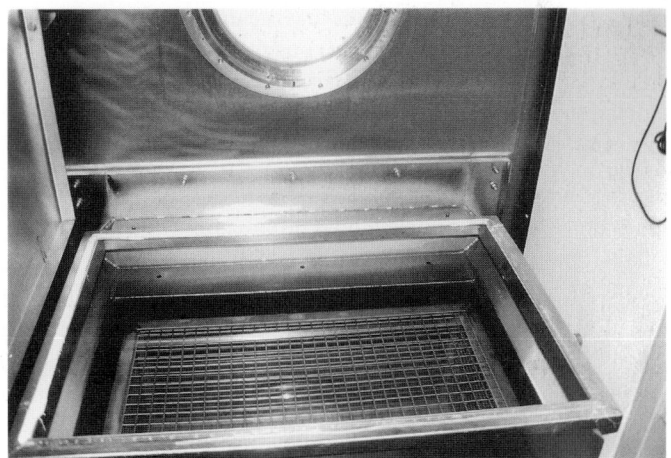

tank without pathogenic organisms gaining access through the barrier.

It is advisable to select a disinfectant with a wide spectrum of activity and which is rapid in action and long lasting. Kits are available for checking the strength of some disinfectants in use. Exposure of staff to the disinfectant solution should be avoided. When using the tank, eye protection should be worn, hands and arms may be covered by elbow-length waterproof gloves and a full-length apron worn to protect clothes from accidental spillage. Staff must be made aware of the hazards of the chemicals they are dealing with and a COSHH risk assessment must be made.

Staff decontamination

Perhaps the greatest risk to the integrity of a barriered unit is people, including:

- staff working in the unit;
- maintenance staff who may visit occasionally to service, replace or repair equipment;
- visitors, either from within or outside the organisation.

A rigorous changing and decontamination policy must be enforced to reduce to an absolute minimum the risk of any of these people introducing pathogenic organisms behind the barrier.

People present a risk in the following ways:

(1) They can act as mechanical vectors of infectious agents. These may be carried on the clothes or skin having been collected from pets at home or from casual contact with other laboratory, domestic or wild animals. The likelihood of pathogens entering by this route may be reduced by implementing a strict changing and/or showering regime. While it is difficult (though not impossible) to prohibit staff from keeping pets they should be made aware of the potential threat that their animals represent especially if their animals become ill.

(2) Humans can pass on their own diseases to the animals within the barrier. This risk may be reduced by ensuring that all staff report any infections, particularly sore throats, respiratory problems or diarrhoea, before entering the unit. A senior member of the unit staff in consultation with medical and veterinary staff can then make the decision whether or not they pose an infection hazard.

(3) Visitors to a unit may have visited other animal units and not allowed sufficient quarantine time to elapse before passing through the barrier. Quarantine times vary from unit to unit with a range from twenty-four hours to fourteen days.

(4) Perhaps one of the greatest risks involving people is that of complacency. The longer a barrier unit operates the greater the risk of contravention or bending of the rules or shortcuts being taken. Staff should be kept fully reminded of the consequences of such action. Any rule contravention must be dealt with quickly and the offender disciplined.

All staff and visitors must change their clothing and undergo a thorough wash or shower procedure prior to entering the unit. There are differences of opinion as to whether full showering is necessary. In some units stripping to underclothes followed by a thorough washing of hands, arms and face is deemed to be sufficient while other units insist on a thorough shower including hair wash before passing through the barrier. This is followed by dressing in sterilised clothes which may include T-shirt, trousers, socks, shoes, hat (covering all hair), mask and gloves. In units insisting on a full shower sterilised undergarments are provided and some units forbid the wearing of jewellery and also provide inside spectacles where necessary. The wearing of beards is not tolerated in some units as they can harbour micro-organisms. Full protective cover for beards is difficult but is essential if beards be permitted.

Rodent barriers

There are numerous ways in which vermin such as mice and rats can gain access to any animal unit. The consequences of such a breakdown of the barriers are dire. These animals are living, mobile cultures of many of the pathogenic organisms that we are trying to keep out of units. In theory it should be relatively easy to prevent their access but the determination of these animals to find food and warmth, particularly in the winter months, should not be underestimated. Outer unit walls should be of a smooth finish to a height of at least 600 mm and should be barriered to prevent access to roof areas. Walls will normally be rodent proof but it must be remembered that these are not continuous and will be breached at several points for the access of materials, staff and services. It is at these points that special care must be taken. All doors, windows and pipe accesses must be properly sealed into the wall. The bottom portion of doors should be metal clad to minimise the risk of accidental damage or gnawing and doorways should have step-over rodent barriers (Figures 30.10 and 30.11).

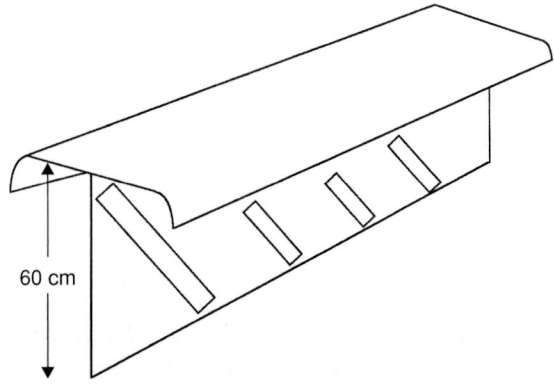

60 cm

Figure 30.10 Typical rodent barrier – note the 'T'-shape design to prevent animals jumping over. It is important that the barrier fits tightly to the walls and floor. Warning flashes on the sides help to avoid accidents to staff.

piliforme (formally known as *Bacillus piliformis*), the cause of Tyzzer's disease, and larval forms of higher parasites.

Preparation and operation of a full barrier unit

Fumigation

Prior to the introduction of animals into the unit, it will be necessary to clean and decontaminate the interior of the building to eliminate all pathogenic organisms. One of the most effective methods of decontamination is the generation of an atmosphere of formaldehyde. This gas is effective against a wide spectrum of micro-organisms. Its efficiency is however impaired by the presence of organic material, therefore the interior surfaces of the unit must be thoroughly cleaned prior to fumigation. Detergents or disinfectants used for cleaning must be thoroughly rinsed to avoid incompatibility with the formaldehyde.

Great care must be taken to keep the exposure of staff to formaldehyde to an absolute minimum, as it is highly toxic and irritant even at very low concentrations. Specialist contractors are available if staff are not sufficiently expert.

If fumigation is to be performed using the unit's own staff a safe and effective protocol must be followed. There are legal limits of human exposure to these chemicals.

Formaldehyde is most effective when temperature and relative humidity (RH) are raised – ideally above 24 °C and 80% RH. The gas can be generated by boiling commercial formalin, which is about a 40% w/v solution of formaldehyde gas in water. The usual amount for fumigation is about 35 cm^3/m^3.

The formalin may be boiled in a vessel, often a metal drum set off the floor to avoid surface damage. The vessel is fitted with an electric kettle element with a boil-dry cut out (Figure 30.12). The power supply to the kettle should be controlled from outside the area to be fumigated. Extra water may be added to the formalin to provide more steam which will raise the humidity and help to maintain the temperature.

Alternately, formalin may be generated by adding potassium permanganate crystals to formalin. Extra formalin is required to produce the heat-generating reaction. The quantity of formalin and potassium

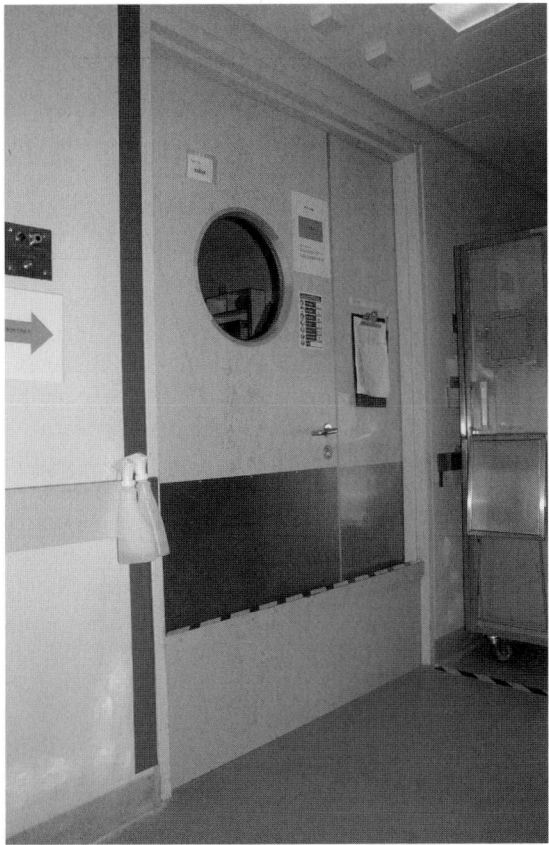

Figure 30.11   Rodent barrier in place.

It is advisable to paint warning markings on such barriers to prevent injuries to staff.

Insect barriers

Flying or crawling insects are potential carriers of pathogens. Closely fitting, self-closing doors should prevent ingress of both types. Defences in the entrance lobby could include 'insectocutors', insecticidal sprays or stick mats for crawling insects.

Placental barrier

The derivation of germ-free and full barrier animals by hysterectomy is reliant on the maternal placenta which acts as a barrier by preventing most micro-organisms present in the mother from infecting the unborn young. Unfortunately a small number of organisms can cross the placental barrier, notably *Clostridium*

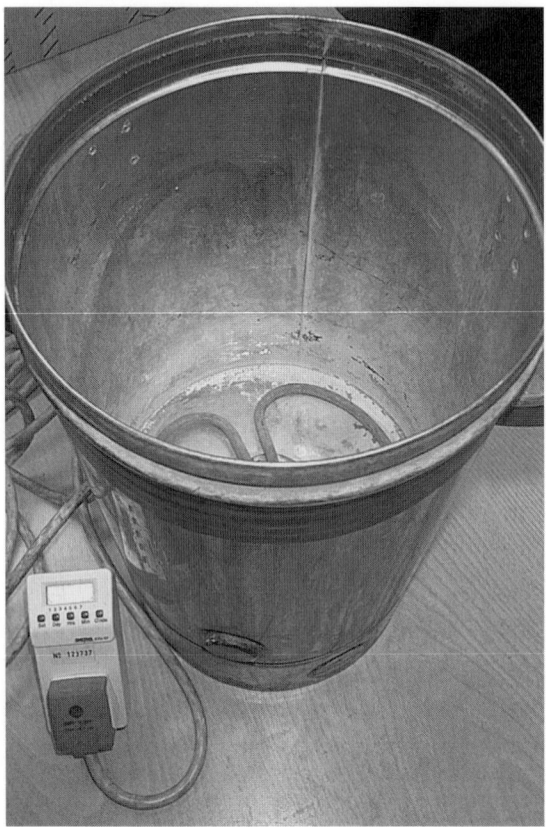

Figure 30.12   Formalin fumigation kettle.

permanganate required to fumigate a room is calculated as follows:

- Calculate the amount of formalin needed to fumigate the room by the kettle method and multiply that figure by two. The amount of potassium permanganate needed is equivalent to half the amount of formalin required.

Great care must be taken with this method as some of the gas is generated quickly. Extra water cannot be used with this method because it would interfere with the boiling reaction and impair gas generation. An alternative method for raising relative humidity to an optimum level may have to be sought. All methods of fumigation are dangerous and should only be carried out by trained personnel according to the establishment's standard operating procedure.

Formaldehyde may also be generated using a polymer such as formagen prills, which look like beads of plastic. These are heated on an electric hot plate.

Again the electricity supply needs to be controlled from outside the area. The room should be damped down prior to fumigation as it is a 'dry' method.

In order to control the formaldehyde for both efficacy and safety it is necessary to seal the unit as completely as possible. Any windows and doors to the area can be effectively sealed with polythene sheets and masking tape. Spore strips or scatter plates should be used to check the efficiency of the sterilisation process.

Ventilation ducts are best sealed by metal blanking plates inserted into the filter housings. If this is left until just before gas generation then the temperature within the unit can be maintained. It is essential to advise staff of the dangers involved and to inform them that the procedure is under way. Access to the vicinity should be restricted and warning notices displayed.

Once the gas has been generated, the unit should be left sealed for twenty-four hours. In many cases it is convenient and possibly safer to generate the gas after the working day on a Friday and ventilate the unit over the weekend.

Before the ventilation is turned on a check must be made to ensure that the gas dispersed will not affect animals or staff in the vicinity. It will be necessary to ventilate for at least twenty-four hours before the gas levels are reduced to an acceptable level for re-entry

Full barrier conditions are now instituted for the unit. Paraformaldehyde (a white powder) is often found on the surfaces which were wetted or which became wet due to condensation during fumigation. This may be washed off, but staff must wear respiratory protection from any regenerated gas.

A recently introduced method of fumigation uses vaporised hydrogen peroxide (see Chapter 29).

Once fumigation is complete items treated by other means may now be introduced e.g. cages via the autoclave.

Summary of formaldehyde fumigation
Actual procedures will vary between units. The following list is a guide only:

(1) unit equipped with bulky items which cannot be sterilised by other means;
(2) surfaces physically cleaned, disinfected and well rinsed;
(3) siting of the formaldehyde generators planned;

(4) total volume for fumigation and amounts of formaldehyde calculated;

(5) temperature and humidity kept high;

(6) microbiological monitors (e.g. spore strips) put in agreed sites;

(7) staff informed of procedures. Personnel working in the vicinity should be informed;

(8) unit sealed;

(9) gas generated;

(10) room left sealed for twenty-four hours;

(11) the room is ventilated;

(12) barrier status instituted;

(13) room unsealed;

(14) microbiological monitors covered and removed;

(15) paraformaldehyde is washed off;

(16) room stocked with other equipment and animals.

Introduction of new stock by hysterectomy derivation

The techniques described here relate to mice, rats, guinea pigs and rabbits.

Hysterectomy involves the removal of the whole uterus from the dam, using aseptic techniques, to avoid the contamination of the enclosed young which would occur during normal birth. The intact uterus may then be either transferred via a bath containing a warm disinfectant solution into the barrier unit or it may be delivered directly through the floor of a flexible film isolator. The young animals are then reared either by hand or by the more usual and less labour-intensive method of fostering.

In recent years, there have been great advances in the field of isolator technology. It has become more commonplace, therefore, to use isolators in the derivation procedure. A particular advantage is that newly derived stock may be held in the isolator while microbiological screening is performed, to ensure there has been no pathogenic contamination.

Preparation and sterilisation of the isolators

A small isolator in which the animals are to be delivered is linked to a larger, holding isolator by means of a flexible sleeve. All materials required for the hysterectomy and subsequent fostering of the young are assembled in the isolators prior to steril-

isation (Figure 30.13). Both isolators are sterilised with either ethaneperoxoic acid (peracetic acid), formaldehyde gas, vaporised hydrogen peroxide, or other chemical sterilant. After ventilating the isolators thoroughly, swabs of internal surfaces are taken and submitted for microbiological examination.

Introduction of gnotobiotic foster animals

Gnotobiotic animals are introduced into the holding isolator. Care must be taken to avoid microbiological contamination of these animals during the transfer process. It would be prudent to take faecal samples from these animals or submit a whole animal for microbiological examination.

Timed mating of foster and donor animals

Foster mothers should litter down three days before the hysterectomies are to be performed on the donor animal. Account must be taken of inter strain differences in gestation.

The hysterectomy operation

(1) The donor animal is killed by cervical dislocation (this causes minimal disturbance to the young).

(2) Hair is removed from the abdominal region, either by shaving or the use of depilatory cream.

(3) The shaved area is soaked in iodine/alcohol and dried with sterile swabs.

(4) The ventral surface of the donor female is pressed firmly against the cling film which forms part of the surgical isolator floor and is held firmly in place.

(5) An incision is made through the cling film, the skin and the abdominal wall, just large enough to remove the gravid uterus.

(6) The uterus is ligated at the cervix and at the ovarian end of each uterine horn.

(7) The entire uterus is lifted gently and separated from its connections.

(8) The uterus is placed into a disinfectant dunk tank located in the port separating surgical and

resuscitation isolators. An electrical heating element ensures that the disinfectant is maintained at body temperature and a heating pad is placed under the resuscitation isolator to keep the pups warm.

(9) The intact uterus is transferred to the resuscitation isolator.

(10) Both horns of the uterus are opened with a pair of scissors and each foetus with its attached placenta is removed and placed on the heated pad. Mucus is removed from the mouth and nose using cotton swabs and the fetus massaged gently to stimulate breathing.

(11) The umbilical cords are severed by crushing and stitching to prevent bleeding.

(12) Once the young are breathing well and are showing no signs of cyanosis they are ready to be transferred to the isolator containing the foster mother. The foster mother is taken from her cage and her offspring removed prior to the transfer. If the foster mother's own young are a different colour one can be kept as a 'sentinel' for microbiological examination.

(13) The new foster litter is placed in the vacated nest and mixed with the bedding to acquire its smell. The foster mother is returned to the nest after ten to fifteen minutes. Rejection of the young is unusual. It is possible to leave one to two of the original pups with the new litter if they are of a different colour. It helps if some urine from the original litter is smeared around the perineal region of the fostered litter.

Introduction of fostered animals into the barrier unit

Before transferring animals from the isolator into the barrier unit, samples should be submitted for microbiological examination. If no specified pathogens are detected the young, once weaned, may be moved into the barrier unit. Transfer may take place using one of two methods:

(1) The young are transferred to plastic filtered boxes which are then sealed hermetically, passed out of the isolator and transferred to the barriered unit via the disinfectant dunk tank.

(2) The holding isolator is locked on to a compatible transfer port in the barrier wall and the animals transferred directly.

It is important to keep accurate records of animals during the hysterectomy procedure so that the identity of both foster mothers and their fosterlings is known. This is particularly important if both are to be transferred to the unit and/or both are phenotypically identical.

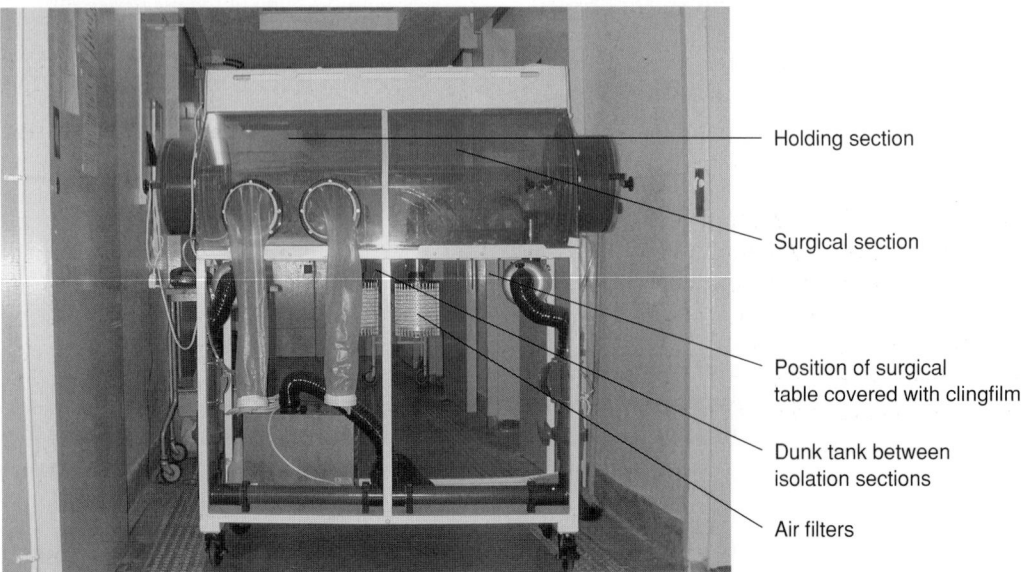

Holding section

Surgical section

Position of surgical table covered with clingfilm

Dunk tank between isolation sections

Air filters

Figure 30.13 Hysterectomy isolator.

The fostering of the young of one strain to females of a different strain could result in young which may respond differently to their parents. An example of this phenomenon is the C3H inbred mouse strain.

Females of this strain have a high incidence of mammary tumours caused by the *Bittner virus* which is transferred from mother to offspring in milk. Young fostered onto a Caesarean-derived mother of a different strain, however, will not receive the virus and although remaining genetically identical to the parent strain will have a much lower incidence of mammary tumours. This could affect experimental results or render the fostered C3H animal unsuitable for some types of work.

Monitoring of animals within the unit

Routine monitoring in a barriered unit is essential in order to ensure that the barrier has not been breached in any way. Routines will vary from unit to unit as will the samples which are taken. Examples of samples which may be taken are listed below.

Animals

Representative animals may be removed at intervals, autopsied and subjected to microbiological examination. All unexpected mortalities are treated in a similar manner. Faecal samples may be collected routinely and examined for parasites or bacterial pathogens. Experimental groups may use sentinel animals to detect infection (i.e. gnotobiotes placed in an experimental room to pick up any pathogens).

Air

Agar plates are placed near ventilation inlets for set time periods (settle plates) and/or placed randomly (scatter plates) in animal or other rooms. These are then incubated and the number of organisms counted (total viable count). This gives a rough guide as to the efficiency of the air filtration system together with the general hygiene standard within the unit.

Staff

Staff may have nose and throat swabs routinely taken and cultured.

Water

Microbiological examination of water will assess the efficacy of the water-treatment system. The presence of *Pseudomonas* and coliforms will indicate water contamination.

Dunk-tank fluid

Samples of disinfectant from the dunk tank may be taken for microbiological examination or, as mentioned previously, kits are available for checking the strength of some disinfectants. Many units rely on a routine replacement of the dunk-tank fluid, with a frequency of seven to fourteen days.

Conclusion

Even with the most stringent and sophisticated barrier system there is always the risk that some pathogens will gain entry to the unit. The greater the number of organisms penetrating the barrier defences, the greater the risk that contamination of the animals will occur. However, before these organisms can present a health problem, contact with the animal must be made. Maintenance of high standards of hygiene within the unit, using standard cleaning techniques and a good disinfection regime, will ensure these unwanted visitors are killed or removed before they have the opportunity to multiply, infect the animals and cause an outbreak of disease.

It cannot be overemphasised that the majority of breakdowns of the barrier will in some way be attributed to people, either working in or servicing the building. An enquiry will often highlight staff malpractices or complacency as the likely causes. Due to human nature, the longer the unit is in operation the greater these risks will become.

31

The Isolation of Laboratory Animals which are a Potential Infection Risk

Peter Gerson

Introduction

The term isolation unit is commonly used in the field of laboratory animal technology, however misinterpretation of the functions of these units is possible if the term is not clearly defined.

There are two categories of animal isolation unit, those which protect animals from potential hazards entering the unit from outside (positive air-pressure isolation units), and those which prevent potential hazards escaping from the unit (negative air-pressure isolation units).

Positive air-pressure isolation units

Laboratory animals requiring protection of their health status may be housed in isolation units which, through a variety of barriers, prevent the entry of potential hazards. The number and type of barriers used to protect the animals will vary, depending on the level of protection which is required. Fully barriered units (or Specified Pathogen Free Units) have well defined and commonly understood functions, as do flexible film and rigid isolators, which are able to protect gnotobiotic and germ-free animals. Fully barriered units are described in other chapters (see Chapter 30) and therefore, it is not necessary to describe them here although, there are similarities between positive air-pressure isolation units and negative air-pressure isolation units.

Negative air-pressure isolation units

Quarantine units

There are two types of quarantine facility associated with laboratory animals:

(1) those for animals obtained from within the UK;
(2) those for animals imported into the UK (Rabies Quarantine).

The first type is discussed in Chapter 33; the second type is referred to in this chapter.

Quarantine units which house animals recently arrived from a source outside the UK are subject to the quarantine conditions of the Department of Environment, Food and Rural Affairs (DEFRA), the Department of Agriculture and Fisheries for Scotland and the Welsh Office Agriculture Department, and also to the requirements of the Animal Health Act 1981 (HMSO 1981), as described in the Rabies (Importation of Dogs, Cats and other Mammals) Order 1974 (as amended) (see Chapter 28 for the legal requirements of importation of animals). Animals housed in quarantine units may carry naturally occurring infections which may be hazardous to other laboratory animals and/or humans, but usually they will not be experimentally compromised and will remain 'normal' throughout the quarantine period.

Due to the potential risk of zoonotic disease, primates are often associated with this type of isolation unit, however many other species are imported and housed in quarantine units.

The source of the animals is obviously important when assessing the potential risk they may present. Animals may be obtained from a commercial breeder, from another animal unit which has a closed breeding colony, or be supplied from a holding station where the history of the animals is known and documented. The potential risk from these animals is less than those which may be supplied from a commercial supplier which has caught the animals recently from the wild (rarely allowed), or where standards and/or records are poor.

Irrespective of their history, all animals in quarantine premises must be regarded as a risk to other animals in the animal department and in some cases also a risk to the personnel looking after them.

EEC Directive 92/65 (Balai Directive) (EEC 1992) allows certain categories of rabies-susceptible animals originating from within the countries of the EU to enter the UK without undergoing quarantine, but under tightly controlled conditions (see Chapter 28).

The main purpose for holding animals in a laboratory quarantine unit is to contain micro-biological hazards while assessing the health and general condition of the animals and treating them whenever necessary. The quarantine unit must be designed, staffed and operated to standards which minimise potential hazards.

DEFRA's *Definition of Premises* (HMSO 1985) outlines the standards required for quarantine units; they are uncomplicated and should present no difficulties for compliance by a modern animal facility. They are as follows:

- the premises must be maintained in a good state of repair;
- no changes must be made to the structure of the premises or in the arrangements for the isolation and detention of animals unless such a change is authorised by DEFRA;
- no person shall have access to premises or to animals therein unless that person is there in the course of his authorised business;
- notices warning of the quarantine status of the animals must be placed where they can be seen by

anyone who intends to gain access to the animals. The wording on the notices should be 'Danger! Rabies Quarantine only trained staff should handle the animals';
- where primates are quarantined, suitable protective clothing must be available at all times for the use of authorised officers of the DEFRA carrying out inspection of the premises; this clothing should consist of complete bodily covering such as an overall suit, mask, eye goggles or face visor, rubber boots and gloves.

Special consideration must be given to both the premises and the working protocols if animals housed under quarantine are to be used for scientific procedures of a hazardous nature. The minimum design requirements of a quarantine unit are unlikely to meet the more stringent requirements of an isolation unit used to house animals experimentally infected with hazardous material. Therefore, the quarantine unit will have to comply with these requirements as well as complying with DEFRA's regulations before the work can commence.

Scientific isolation units

Conditions regarding the site of the unit, the equipment and materials used and the work routines adopted are influenced by local circumstances and may differ between units, however, the broad concepts will be similar because they have to meet legislative guidelines.

If a scientific project requires animals to be infected with a substance which may be hazardous to health it will be subject to a variety of legislation, regulation and guidance including:

(1) The Animals (Scientific Procedures) Act 1986 (ASPA);
(2) The Health and Safety at Work etc. Act 1974 (HSW);
(3) The Control of Substances Hazardous to Health 1994 (COSHH);
(4) The Advisory Committee on Dangerous Pathogens (ACDP);
(5) European Union Directive 93/88/ EEC (EUD).

Categorisation of biological agents

Biological agents are listed and categorised within hazard groups and then subdivided between bacteria, viruses, parasites and fungi. Holding facilities appropriate to containing the hazard group are then chosen based on the ACDP guidelines. Therefore, when work is being considered which may be of a hazardous nature, it is essential that the hazard group into which it falls is known to ensure appropriate facilities are available for the work to be performed.

The Advisory Committee on Dangerous Pathogens (ACDP) has published *Categorisation of biological agents according to hazard and categories of containment* (HMSO 1995). This publication defines the hazard groups as follows:

(1) Hazard Group 1: A biological agent unlikely to cause human disease.

(2) Hazard Group 2: A biological agent which can cause human disease and may be a hazard to employees; it is unlikely to spread to the community and there is usually effective prophylaxis or effective treatment available.

(3) Hazard Group 3: A biological agent which can cause severe human disease and presents a serious hazard to employees; it may present a risk of spreading to the community, but there is usually effective prophylaxis or treatment available.

(4) Hazard Group 4: A biological agent which causes severe human disease and is a serious hazard to employees; it is likely to spread to the community and there is usually no effective prophylaxis or treatment available.

Biological agents are listed in their respective hazard groups except for Hazard Group 1. Hazard Group 1 consists of all the organisms which do not appear in Hazard Groups 2, 3 and 4. Therefore, the organisms in Hazard Group 1 would be far ranging, but would not require containment within isolation units.

Animal containment levels

The accommodation in which animals are housed is appropriate to their Hazard Group and is categorised as Animal Containment Level 1, 2, 3 or 4. This accommodation is usually referred to as Category 1, 2, 3 or 4 accommodation.

Animal containment level 1

The ACDP gives detailed descriptions of Category 1 accommodation which in the main, relates to a very basic type of accommodation, such as school or training/teaching facilities, where the animals are housed without any intention to challenge them with a pathogenic biological agent. However, some agents in this group may be pathogens of animals and additional precautions may have to be taken to prevent their release into the environment.

Animal containment level 2

There is little difference between the conditions for Category 1 and Category 2 accommodation. Category 2 conditions, which are listed below, are taken from the ACDP's *Categorisation of Biological Agents According to Hazard and Categories of Containment* (HMSO 1995). Modern laboratory animal facilities are expected to accommodate all animals to a minimum of Category 2 conditions.

Note the significance of the words 'must' and 'should' in the lists below.

(1) Access to the room must be limited to authorised people.
(2) The animal room must be easy to clean. Bench surfaces must be impervious to water and resistant to acids, alkalis, solvents and disinfectants.
(3) There must be specified disinfection procedures.
(4) If the animal room is mechanically ventilated, it must be maintained at an air pressure negative to the atmosphere.
(5) Efficient vector control measures (for example for rodents and insects) must be taken.
(6) Where necessary, there must be facilities for safe storage of biological agents.
(7) For the procedures which involve the handling of infected material (including any infected animal) or where an aerosol may be created, a safety cabinet, isolator or other suitable containment must be used.
(8) An incinerator for the disposal of animal carcasses must be accessible.

(9) Personal protective equipment, including protective clothing must be:
   (a) stored in a well-defined place;
   (b) checked and cleaned at suitable intervals;
   (c) when discovered to be defective, repaired or replaced before further use.

(10) Personal protective equipment which may be contaminated by biological agents must be:
   (a) removed on leaving the work area;
   (b) kept apart from uncontaminated clothing;
   (c) decontaminated and cleaned or, if necessary, destroyed.

(11) Suitable protective clothing and footwear should be worn in the animal room and cleansed, or removed, when leaving. A face shield or visor should be worn when inoculating animals.

(12) All manipulations should be performed so as to minimise the production of aerosols.

(13) The animal room should be adequately ventilated and, where mechanical ventilation is used, the air from the room should be extracted to the atmosphere. The word atmosphere in this context may be taken to mean the external and/or other parts of the building. In effect, this means maintaining an inward flow of air to the room.

(14) The door to the animal room should be closed when infected animals are present and should be labelled with a sign indicating the level of the work.

(15) Eating, chewing, drinking, smoking, taking medication, storing food for human consumption and applying cosmetics should be forbidden in the animal room.

(16) Mouth pipetting should be forbidden.

(17) Facilities should be provided for hand washing, preferably in the animal room.

(18) Hands should be decontaminated immediately when contamination is suspected and before leaving the animal room.

(20) All waste material, including animal bedding, should be rendered non-infective before disposal.

(20) An autoclave for the sterilisation of contaminated waste materials should be accessible on site.

(21) Materials for autoclaving or incineration and used animal cages should be transported without spillage.

(22) 'Access to an incinerator for the disposal of animal carcasses' may be taken to mean an incinerator at another site but, whether local or distant, carcasses and any other material for incineration must be transported in secure containers.

(23) Used animal cages should be rendered non-infective by disinfection, fumigation or heat treatment (steaming or autoclaving).

(24) Work surfaces should be disinfected after use.

(25) If floor drains are installed, the traps should always contain water. Drain traps should be inspected and cleaned regularly.

(26) All accidents and incidents, including animal bites and scratches, should be reported to and recorded by the person responsible for the work or other delegated person.

Animal containment level 3

The animal containment level 2 accommodation and work routines described are those expected and normally seen in 'conventional' animal departments not requiring special housing conditions. The following, as described in the ACDP's *Working safely with Research Animals: Management of Infection Risks* (HMSO 1997), are itemised changes from the requirements for Level 2 accommodation to that required for Level 3.

In addition to the requirements/recommendations itemised for Animal Containment Level 2, the following apply to Animal Containment Level 3.

Security and access

(1) The animal room must be separated from other activities in the same building. It should be separated from any main thoroughfare by an ante-room with two doors or be sited within an animal suite or animal unit. The ante-room should have facilities for the storage of protective clothing. Showering facilities should be provided in the ante-room or within the animal suite or unit.

(2) There must be an observation window, or an alternative, so that occupants can be seen. It is recommended that this be installed so that all occupants can be seen wherever they are working in the room, this may require one or more windows. Such windows should be positioned on exterior walls in such a way that those outside the facility may see into the animal suite, for example use one-way glass.

(3) The room is to contain its own equipment, so far as is reasonably practical.

(4) A specific biohazard sign indicating the level of work within the unit should be posted at the entry to the room and the room or suite should be locked when members of staff are absent.

(5) A suitable system should be instituted which signals occupancy of the room or suite by an employee. This is particularly important for weekend or out-of-hours work. Arrangements for lone working in animal facilities should be considered in the local rules. For some out-of-work hours, for example feeding of small animals, there may be a minimum risk. However, for work with larger animals, for example primates, or for more complex tasks, it is recommended that accompanied working should be undertaken.

Disinfection and disposal procedures

(6) In addition to bench surfaces, the walls and the floor must be impervious to water and resistant to acids, alkalis, solvents and disinfectants.

(7) The animal room must be sealable to permit disinfection. While the definition of disinfection may be widely interpreted, in practice it may be necessary to decontaminate by fumigating the accommodation when, for example, a spillage has occurred at the end of an experiment or when maintenance work is to be carried out.

(8) There should be means for the safe collection, storage and disposal of contaminated waste.

(9) The autoclave should be sited in the same building as the animal room or animal suite.

(10) Safety cabinets and isolators should be fumigated after use.

(11) The room should be disinfected or fumigated at the end of each experiment.

(12) Where floor drains are installed, the drain traps should be kept filled. The drain traps should be disinfected and cleaned regularly and at the end of each experiment.

(13) Infective materials taken into the animal room, or removed from it, should be transported in sealed containers.

Air handling

(14) The room must be maintained at an air pressure negative to the atmosphere. Extracted air must be filtered using a HEPA (high efficiency particulate air) filter (or equivalent) (see Chapter 33). The word atmosphere in this context may be taken to mean the external air and/or other parts of the animal suite or unit. In effect, this means arranging engineering controls so that a continuous inward airflow into the room is maintained. Provision should be made for comfort factors for both animals and staff, i.e. supply of fresh air and temperature control. Air should be extracted through a HEPA filter via ducting or by extracting air with a fan and HEPA filter sited in a wall or window. The ventilation system should incorporate a means of preventing reverse airflows. The supply and extract systems should be interlocked to prevent positive pressurisation of the room in the event of failure of the extract fans. Further guidance on alternative means by which the inward flow of air may be achieved is given under the ACDP's Laboratory Containment Level 3 in the *Categorisation of Biological Agents According to Hazard and Categories of Containment* (HMSO 1995).

Protective equipment and procedures

(15) Animals infected with Hazard Group 3 agents should be housed in some form of primary containment, for example isolators or safety cabinets which are provided with HEPA-filtered exhaust ventilation or equivalent. However, where it is not reasonably practical to use primary containment for animals, personnel should wear a complete change of clothing and use high performance respiratory protective equipment (RPE) at all times.

(16) When undertaking procedures with infected materials which are likely to give rise to aerosols (inoculation procedures, post-mortem examinations and harvesting infected tissues and fluids), a Class I or Class III microbiological safety cabinet (BS 5726: 1992, or a unit offering an equivalent level of protection), an isolator or other suitable means of containment is to be used. The containment unit used must exhaust to the outside air or to the room air-extract

system via a HEPA filter (or equivalent). If exhausting to the open air causes major problems, recirculation of exhaust air through two HEPA filters in series may, in exceptional circumstances, be considered as an alternative. In this case, the maintenance of a continuous airflow into the animal room during work with infectious material will be of particular importance and such an option should not be considered without prior consultation with the Health and Safety Executive (HSE).

(17) Protective clothing, including footwear and gloves, supplemented where necessary by heavy duty or waterproof clothing, should be worn in the animal room. The clothing should be disinfected or autoclaved after use. Gloves should be worn for all work with infective materials and hands should be washed before leaving the animal room. Gloves should be washed or preferably removed before touching items which will be touched by others not similarly protected, e.g. telephone handsets, paperwork etc. Where practical, equipment controls should be protected by a removable flexible cover which can be disinfected.

(18) There should be a wash hand basin fitted with taps which can be operated without being touched by hand.

Animal containment level 4

Written instructions must be prepared for work at this level, and a safety officer should be appointed and be accountable to the person identified as being responsible for the work. Personnel should be over the age of eighteen years, and must have had specific training in the handling of the animals infected with Hazard Group 4 biological agents and in the use of the safety equipment and controls of the animal room. The work should be closely supervised. The person responsible for the animal experiment must ensure that all those having contact with the animals and waste materials are made aware of the nature of the agent in question and of any specific precautions and procedures which may be required.

In addition to the requirements set out for Containment Levels 2 and 3, the following apply to Containment Level 4.

Security and access

(1) A key procedure must be established so that entry is restricted at all times. Entry must be through an airlock. The 'clean' side of the airlock should be separated from the restricted side by changing and showering facilities and preferably by interlocking doors. The outer door should be labelled with 'work in progress' sign.

(2) At all times during work in the animal unit there should be a second competent person available to assist in case of emergency.

(3) High performance RPE (two or more units) should be available in the 'clean' side of the animal unit for use in an emergency.

(4) There should be a telephone or other means of outside communication inside the animal unit.

Disinfection and disposal procedures

(5) In addition to the surfaces mentioned at Containment Levels 2 and 3, the ceiling must also be impervious to water and resistant to acids, alkalis, solvents and disinfectants.

(6) An incinerator for the disposal of carcasses must be available on site.

(7) A double-ended autoclave with interlocking doors with entry in the animal room and exit in a clean area should be provided. An additional ventilated airlock which can be fumigated may be required for passage of equipment which cannot enter the animal room through the personnel airlock or double-ended autoclave.

(8) All waste materials should be rendered non-infective before being removed from the animal room and should be autoclaved. Animal bedding and carcasses should be incinerated immediately on removal. A double ended dunk-tank filled with an effective disinfectant may be required for the removal of materials which cannot be autoclaved. Removal of materials in this manner should only be undertaken with the authorisation of the safety officer and under conditions defined in the local code of practice. The dunk tank should be sealed during fumigation if the disinfectant is incompatible with the fumigant. All effluent, including that from the shower, should be rendered safe before discharge.

(9) Where floor drains are installed, the drain traps should be kept filled and sealed until required. The effluent from traps must be rendered non-infective before discharge to a sewerage system. The drain traps should be disinfected and cleaned regularly and at the end of each experiment.

Air handling

(10) Input air must be HEPA-filtered and extract air is to be double HEPA-filtered (or equivalent) before it is ducted to the outside air or to the room-air extract system.

(11) The supply and extract airflow should be interlocked to prevent positive pressurisation of the room in the event of a failure of the extract fan and an emergency electricity supply should be provided to cut in automatically in the event of a power failure. The ventilation system should incorporate a means of preventing reverse airflows. Emergency power should provide for adequate lighting (not simply standard dim emergency lights) because, if a power failure occurs whilst a procedure is being carried out, the animal may become more difficult to handle, increasing the risk of injury or escape.

(12) A negative pressure of at least 70 pascals (7 mm of water) should be maintained in the animal room and a negative pressure of about 30 pascals (3 mm of water) in the airlock. An alarm system should be fitted to detect any unacceptable change in air pressure and manometers should be displayed which can be read from both inside and outside the unit.

Protective equipment and procedures

(13) Infected material, including any animal, is to be handled in a Class III safety cabinet or cabinet line in an isolator, or in other suitable containment in which exhaust air is double HEPA-filtered or equivalent. In principle, the primary containment of hazards implicit in Control of Substances Hazardous to Health (COSHH) (1998) should always be applied to controlling the risks from infected animals. However, in some circumstances the nature of the species (size and disposition) and the operations to be performed are such that this form of close

containment may not be practical. It may be appropriate, for example, for small mammals such as mice but not for larger animals. Where this is the case and the risks involved have been adequately assessed, 'other suitable containment' may be taken to include use of alternative engineering controls or, as a last resort, the use of RPE of proven efficacy.

(14) A complete change of clothing should be worn, i.e. staff should change into protective clothing before entering the animal suite. After work, the clothing should be removed in the 'dirty' side of the changing area and placed in a container for autoclaving. A shower should be taken before leaving the unit.

(15) There should be a programme of regular validation of the continuing safe operation of control systems (for example checks on airflows, filter integrity, sensors and indicators) coupled with routine servicing and maintenance of all safety equipment and plant. COSHH Regulation 9, in referring to maintenance, examination and testing of control measures and specifically to 'local exhaust ventilation' must be observed. This means that, for example, HEPA filters and their fittings and seals must be thoroughly examined and tested at intervals not exceeding fourteen months. In practice, depending on the frequency of use, these tests are commonly carried out at shorter intervals, for example six monthly.

(16) Infective material should be stored in the animal room, but where this is impractical such material taken into the room (or removed from it to another Containment Level 4 room on site) should be transported under the supervision of the safety officer, in sealed containers which have been disinfected externally.

The intention to perform work with microbiological agents in Hazard Groups 3 and 4 requires compliance with a great number of recommendations and regulations as described above. The following are some of the factors which must be considered.

The site of the isolation unit

The unit may be sited either inside an existing facility,

or situated outside as a discrete, independent building. There are advantages and disadvantages to both situations. It may well not be possible to site isolation units outside an existing facility because the requirement for such a facility, or the funds, or the land was not available at the planning stage.

Category 4 work is required by the Health and Safety Executive (HSE) to be separate from all other activities in a facility. Therefore, it has to be conducted in an isolation unit, which will present particular problems if attempting to add such a unit to an existing building. This often necessitates that Category 4 accommodation is sited separately.

An isolation unit situated outside the main facility

In the unlikely event of a breach in the barrier of a Category 3 or 4 unit, a facility separate from the main building would present less of a potential hazard than one situated within or near to the main animal department. However, there are problems associated with running a separate unit with regards to staffing, supplies and regular monitoring, particularly if the size of the unit does not warrant staff working full time in the unit.

An isolation unit situated within an existing facility

The unit should be situated in a discreet position away from unauthorised personnel or passing 'traffic', although it may be situated within or adjacent to the main animal facility. Therefore, the potential hazard to other animals is greater than that from a separate unit because the safety factor of distance is lessened.

Staffing

Staff must be fully conversant with the safety regulations before they enter the unit. There will be a rigorous code of practice in place which they must read and understand. New members of staff should not be allowed to work until they have been fully trained. A formal training programme should be in place requiring trainees to be 'signed off' for each aspect of work satisfactorily completed.

The hazardous nature of the work gives any accident a higher risk factor than if it happened in a 'conventional' area of the animal department. Therefore, it is recommended that staff never work unaccompanied in a unit. If this is unavoidable 'lone worker alarms' are useful devices to alert staff outside the unit of potential problems.

The unit is isolated and therefore, if assistance is required as a result of an accident the response time may be slower than if it occurred in the main facility. There must be sufficient personnel trained to respond to an accident and who are available at times staff are working in the unit. Part of this team should include members of the occupational health department.

Staff should not work in an isolation unit if they feel unwell or are suffering from an illness which may affect their immune system (such as a cold). Staff must be fully vaccinated against the micro-biological hazard associated with the work; if the work changes then additional vaccinations may be necessary. If the work is at Level 4 it is possible that a vaccine will not be available.

The type of unit, the rigorous codes of practice, the safety precautions and the requirement to have specific vaccinations, tends to focus the staff on the hazards involved and the necessary safety precautions to be taken. However, staff may continue to be concerned about working in such a unit, therefore, to allay these concerns it is important that the nature of the work, the potential hazards and the safety precautions are fully explained. A periodic update on the progress of the work, together with re-emphasising its importance is recommended; often this can have most impact if performed by a senior scientist directly involved in the work.

Once new work is underway, staff become accustomed to the routines and reassured by the safety precautions. However, reassurance must not be allowed to become complacency, consequently it is necessary to re-affirm safety precautions and the potential hazards of the work regularly.

Barrier systems in an isolation unit

The staff changing and showering system which will operate in an isolation unit will depend on the type of protection required for the staff. In Category 3 accommodation, where the unit houses animals in isolators (primary containment) only selected protective clothing items need be worn, such as gowns and gloves. Showering out of the unit need not be obligatory. In Category 4 isolation units, even though the animals are in isolators or safety cabinets, a complete change of clothing and a shower out is obligatory.

If it is not possible to house a particular species in isolators or safety cabinets satisfactorily, the emphasis for staff protection moves to protective clothing and respiratory protective equipment (secondary containment). The HSE much prefers primary containment as it is regarded as the safest form of personnel protection. This area is currently being looked at with a view to housing more species in primary containment systems however, at the time of writing, these systems are still being developed and are not yet available. Therefore, secondary containment remains the most extreme type of working environment likely to be encountered by animal technicians within Category 3 or 4 accommodation, and as such it is worth spending a little time to review it.

Changing routines where respiratory protective equipment (RPE) is required

Entering the unit

Initially, there may be a lobby which houses the 'clean' side of the autoclave, dunk tank, fogging (very fine spray) and formaldehyde chambers. In Category 4 accommodation it is obligatory that there are 'pass through' methods for sterilising materials out of the unit. This area may be chosen to be security locked, or alternatively, left available for access to other staff who can assist with processing materials in and out of the unit from the 'clean' side. The lobby will then lead to a changing area which must be security locked; an electronic key coupled with a pass number is one of the most secure methods. In case of emergency all security locked doors are easily operated from the inside for quick exit.

The main entry door into the changing rooms should be interlocked with the next door within the unit so that both cannot be opened at the same time (Figure 31.1). Whichever system is employed for entry into the animal accommodation, pairs of doors should always be interlocked.

In the first changing room (outer changing room),

all clothing, including jewellery, will be removed. Clean working clothes are then put on, which consist of underwear (disposable), socks, tops and trousers. At this point surgical gloves or similar hand protection will be put on.

Staff then pass through to the next changing room which will necessitate either passing through, or passing by a shower area, via two doors which are interlocked to prevent both opening at the same time. The second changing room (inner changing room) acts as a barrier between the shower area and the animal accommodation, while the shower area separates the inner changing room from the outer changing room. In the inner changing room other protective clothing is put on such as shoes, gowns and extra gloves. At this point respiratory protection will also be put on. The outer changing room is regarded as 'clean' while the inner changing area is regarded as perfectly safe but is still within the unit.

Respiratory protection

Respiratory protection can be achieved by either mechanically aided respirators (Figure 31.2 (a) & (b)) or non-mechanical half and full masks.

Mechanically aided respirators

Filtered air is delivered via a fan unit which can be either an integral part of a protective helmet, or can be worn separately, fitted to a belt. The fan unit supplies either a helmet or hood, or a hood with an attached half suit which protects the upper body. The helmet, or hood, encompasses the head and face to which is delivered filtered air. The air is exhausted slower than it is delivered thus giving a positive pressure to atmosphere.

The airflow of this type of respiratory protection must be checked each time it is used to ensure the fan unit is operating within set safety parameters. The main filters, which are protected by pre-filters, must be changed at pre-determined times. During use it is obvious to the operator that the fan unit is working, if it should fail then the operator must leave the animal accommodation immediately. The fan unit is operated by a re-chargeable battery which is usually coupled to the fan unit. A battery is usually able to run the fan unit for about eight hours before re-charging is necessary, however, it is common practice to keep the batteries on charge permanently when not in use.

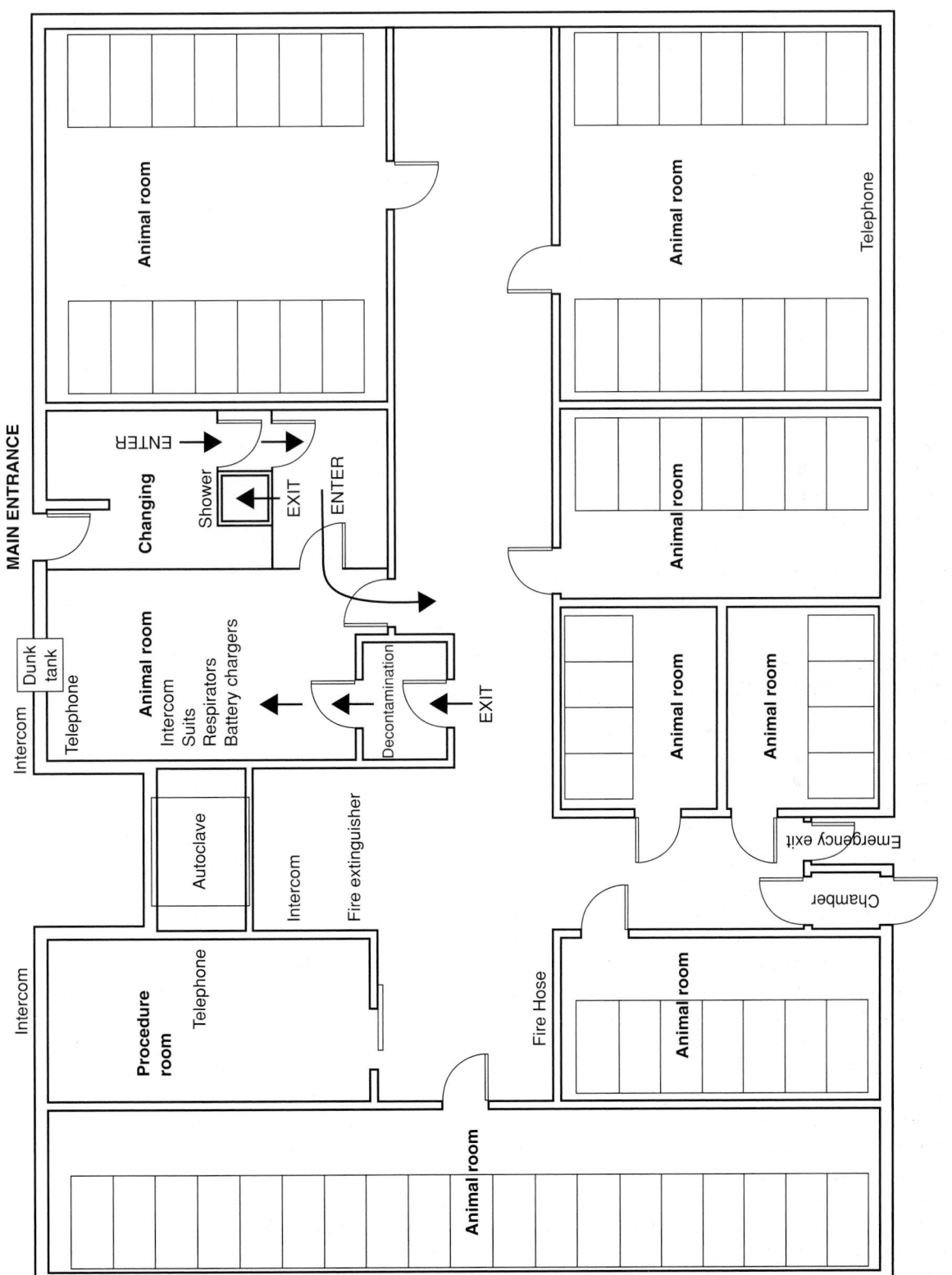

Figure 31.1   Plan of a Category 4 isolation unit.

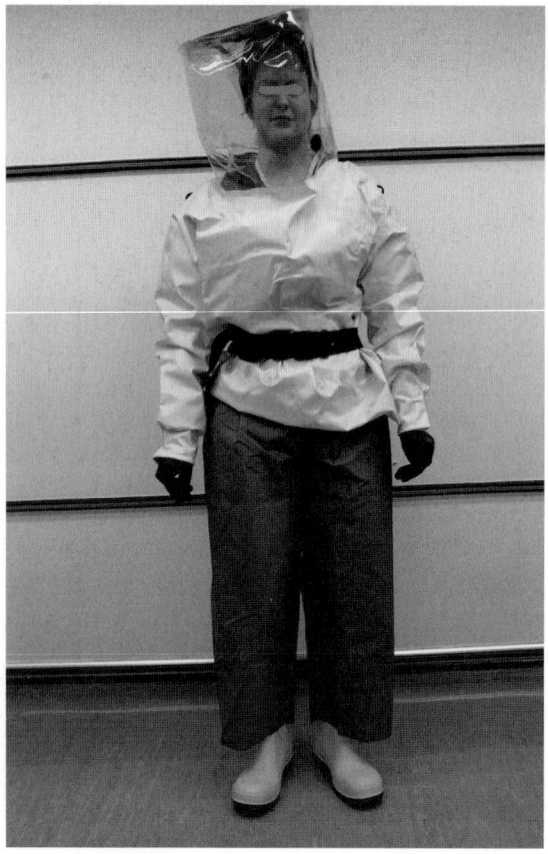

(a)

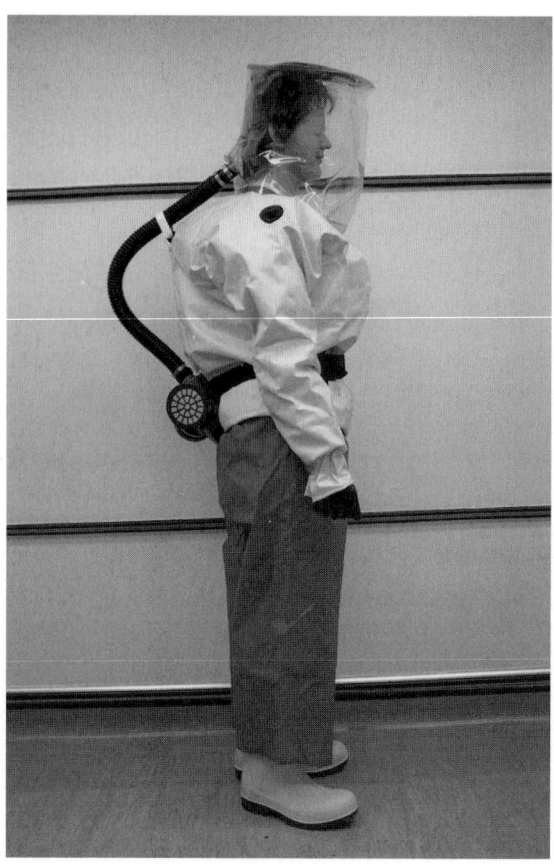

(b)

Figure 31.2 (a) & (b)   Protective clothing showing mechanically ventilated blouse with power unit and integral battery together with gloves, boots and trousers.

Face mask respiration

Masks are made of non-disposable material, often either silicone or natural rubber. They are designed either as half masks, which protect the nose and mouth, or full face masks which also protect the eyes. Air is breathed in without mechanical aid through filters situated either on the front, or on the sides of the mask; added protection to the head area can be provided by a plastic or cloth hood.

The safe use of these masks depends on their correct fit to the face of the operator by means of adjustable head straps. This can be determined by a colleague who can check for correct fitting each time it is worn. (Courses are available to learn the correct way for the safe fitting of face masks.)

Periodically, it will be necessary to leak-test the mask. This is best done during routine servicing and checking of the masks by accredited engineers (every six months is recommended). Breathing is made easier with the incorporation of inhalation and exhalation valves, which also prevent 'steaming up'. Filters, as with the mechanically aided respirators, are easily changed and should be done regularly within set parameters of use or time.

The mechanically aided respiratory protection system allows longer, more comfortable use than does the unaided system, however, the unaided system is less cumbersome to use and does not rely on mechanical support.

After putting on the respiratory protection equipment in the inner changing room the member of staff may enter the animal accommodation.

Exit from the animal accommodation

Before leaving the animal accommodation re-useable

equipment (respiratory masks, suits, gloves, etc.) will have to be decontaminated with an appropriate chemical disinfectant. Respirator masks can be wiped over with a disinfectant-soaked cloth, however, other items of protective wear will also have to be decontaminated and this task is made much easier if a mechanical sprayer is used. A hand-operated pressure spray similar to those used in the garden, or larger versions which incorporate a lance are suitable.

It may be regarded necessary to give operators an all-over spray of chemical disinfectant before leaving the animal accommodation. For this procedure the operator must be wearing protective wear which is at least shower resistant; this would be put on in the inner changing room and would consist of a pair of over trousers and Wellington boots. The worker would have to wear something to protect his upper body against the disinfectant. This is most comfortably achieved by wearing the mechanically aided respiratory half-suit.

Whichever method is chosen to decontaminate it must be situated immediately before the exit from the animal accommodation. This may take the form of a spraying device, a hand and foot bath, together with a cloth for the visor. Alternatively, a spray booth which gives a disinfectant drench for a prescribed time can be sited at the exit. All items to be disinfected must be able to withstand regular wetting of disinfectant; this includes clothing protection, respiratory protection equipment, the walls and floors affected, and/or the spray booth. Account must also be taken of the potential hazard of slippery floors at the site of spraying and the areas immediately adjacent which will be subjected to dripping suits and footwear. Tray liners are good temporary non-slip absorbent surfaces.

After decontamination, staff enter the inner changing room where the respiratory equipment together with outer gloves are removed and hung up to dry in readiness for re-use. (This room is safe in so far as all protective clothing has been decontaminated, but it is still within the Category 4 barrier). Staff then move towards the shower where all items of wear are then discarded and divided between 'disposables' and those for re-use such as tunics and trousers. Clothing will not be reused until it has been sterilised and laundered.

The area prior to the shower (between the shower and inner changing room), should be separated by a door to allow a little privacy, to separate it from the

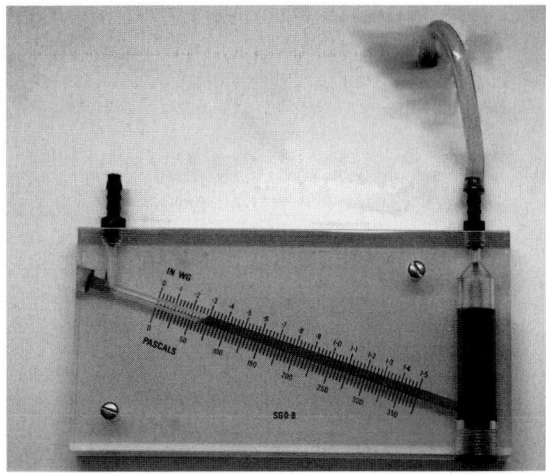

Figure 31.3 Manometer.

area which will have wet items dripping on the floor and to speed showering if there are mixed sexes. Staff then pass into the shower area and have a drench shower, which may be on a timed cycle, after which they pass into the clean changing room where they put on their outer clothing and leave the unit.

Ideally, separate changing facilities for the sexes are recommended, this speeds changing in and out of the unit and can prevent potentially embarrassing situations. However, with a little organisation both sexes can share the same changing and showering facilities.

The conditions within an isolation unit can be oppressive due, in the main, to the respiratory protective items which have to be worn. Consequently, the animal department staff find a shower a pleasant experience, albeit an obligatory one.

Working in the unit (Category 3 and 4)

Initially, the Health and Safety Executive (HSE) will have to ratify the suitability of the accommodation and the work routines for the work proposed. Following this they will have to be contacted regarding any significant proposed changes either to the accommodation or the work carried out.

Working protocols will have to be established which are general to the working of the unit while others will have to be written especially for specific work. Normally it is the leading scientist who will write up the safety protocols directly associated with the use of the hazardous material, while senior staff of the animal department will contribute the working protocols for the husbandry of the animals and associated procedures.

Material being worked with may necessitate extra, specific protection for the staff which may require variations to existing guidelines from the ACDP. For example, those working with infectious microbiological agents where the particular hazard is transfer of infection in blood, would have to pay particular attention to the use of needles and the potential risk of needle-stick injury during injections and bleedings. Alternatively, infections which may be transmitted through animal excreta would necessitate extra precautions being taken when handling animal waste products.

Ventilation and air pressure differentials

The isolation unit must run its ventilation system at a negative air pressure to the outside. That is, the ventilation system mechanically expels more air than it supplies to the unit therefore, air is naturally drawn into the unit through doors and any small breaks in the unit's perimeters, such as seals which may have lost their integrity. If, due to malfunction, the unit becomes positive, then there is a risk that air-borne micro-organisms, some of which may be hazardous, could escape from the unit.

The principle of air pressure differential is to have areas or rooms which are increasingly 'negative' the further into the unit they are situated. A minimum negative differential of 70 pascals (HSE 1997) is recommended for the animal rooms. Airlocks which separate two areas by an interlocked two-door system are useful for maintaining pressure differentials. They can be ventilated separately and are recommended to be negative by 30 pascals (HSE 1997).

Pressure differentials must be monitored continually. Manometers (see Figure 31.3) placed on the outside of the unit to monitor areas or rooms within the unit can give an early warning of any potential problem and should be checked and recorded regularly, as should internally placed manometers. Alternatively, or in addition to, automated monitoring can be achieved by computerised environmental monitoring systems which will give a read-out of any area or room and alarm if there is a problem. Certainly, there

must be alarms coupled to the ventilation systems which will alert of any failure, particularly to the extract system. In the event of ventilation failure an emergency extract fan and motor must be operational which can maintain the unit at a negative pressure until the problem is resolved.

Communication

The unit is isolated and therefore, ease of communication to the outside is essential. The telephone system will serve the unit well provided numbers and persons to be contacted are continually being updated and are clearly displayed within the unit. An intercom system within the unit may be of use if staff are restricted to certain areas, or if the unit is very large. If ventilated head-gear is being worn then noise may make it necessary to have the intercom system fitted with a call light indicator. Intercoms are more user friendly than telephones when talking to staff immediately on the outside of the unit. Alternatively it may be possible to incorporate sound enhancers into the respiratory head apparatus.

A telephone specifically for emergencies should be installed; this will give staff, on lifting the handset, immediate connection to an appropriate source of assistance, such as security. This can be of particular use for out of hours working. A panic button can also be installed which when struck emits a very loud siren outside the unit. This may be used to summon immediate assistance if, for instance, a serious accident has occurred where a member of staff had to be evacuated from the unit.

Staff of the occupational health department must be aware of the nature of the work performed in the unit and be prepared to enter if their services are required. Similarly, maintenance staff must also be prepared to enter the unit when required. From a different perspective it is essential that external emergency services, such as the fire brigade, are advised that these units are 'no go' unless informed otherwise.

It is inevitable that paperwork will be produced in the unit. This can cause problems of safe transfer if it is required for archiving, which is often the case when working to regulated standards such as Good Laboratory Practice. In such circumstances it is likely that any form of sterilising out of the unit will cause damage. The exception is the use of ultraviolet, which may be used in a Category 3 accommodation, providing the animals are kept in 'primary' containment. For the transfer of all other information where a written record is required, then the use of internal fax, scanning and email are invaluable. Local rules may dictate that original documentation is archived, in which case it can be stored in the unit.

Supplies

Supplies to an isolation unit have to be organised and processed, in part, independently of the main animal department. The isolation unit's requirements for items will probably be slightly different to those of the main department. For instance, the unit will probably use more disposable items and clothing than the main animal department; different disinfectants may be used and the sterilising process of moving items out of the unit may necessitate modifications to design, or choice of materials used for items of equipment and clothing.

The unit would be best served if it had its own store situated outside but nearby the unit, which could supply items as required. The isolationist nature of the unit requires that supplies have to be organised with care, as items forgotten by staff once inside the unit are not so readily obtained at short notice. A means of identifying items belonging to the isolation unit, such as colour coding, is advantageous.

Barriers (Category 3 and 4 containment)

Autoclave

The new generation of autoclaves can allow movement of items from the 'clean' to the 'dirty' side of the unit relatively easily if a short 'pass through' or decontamination sterilising cycle is incorporated in the programmes. After a cycle has been run to take goods inside the unit the autoclave is 'dirty'. If no items need to be sterilised out but further items require to be brought in and the chamber is empty, a short 'pass through' cycle lasting approximately fifteen minutes can be run. After this the 'clean' door can be opened safely and further items placed into the autoclave, the 'clean' door closed, then the inner door on the 'dirty' side can be opened and goods

immediately taken inside the isolation unit. Most items can be brought into the unit using this method.

The autoclave is of course also used for sterilising items out of the unit. The cycle times and temperatures are approximately as follows:

cage cycle = 134 °C for 3 minutes

bedding and waste cycle = 134 °C for 10 minutes

carcass cycle = 134 °C for 15 minutes

Duration and temperature of each cycle depends on the type of autoclave and the user's requirements. It may be necessary to have other cycles such as a fluid cycle. It is common practice to place a probe in the autoclave immersed in fluid, which through trial, represents the longest time the centre of any given load takes to reach sterilising temperature. The probe is an integral part of the autoclave sterilising cycle and therefore, ensures that a cycle cannot complete without all items having been sterilised.

Fogging chamber (Category 3 containment)

This is a convenient alternative method of transferring items into a unit if the autoclave is not available or if its size is restrictive. The chamber is double ended and is made of stainless steel or other suitable robust material able to withstand regular chemical fogging of chemical disinfectants.

A port on the inside door allows the nozzle of a fogger to inject a chemical disinfectant agent into the chamber. A pressure release escape port opens on the inside to compensate for the quick build up of pressure. Alternatively, a more automated system can be used which has both the disinfection injection apparatus and a filtered pressure-release fan unit incorporated.

The doors are interlocking to prevent both being opened at the same time. A fail-safe system is required whereby the outer or 'clean' door cannot be opened if the inner or 'dirty' door has been opened and a fogging cycle has not been completed.

The use of the fogging chamber allows immediate transfer of items and animals into the unit after a fogging cycle is complete; a cycle will take approximately thirty-five minutes – five minutes to fog and thirty minutes to allow action time for the disinfectant. Thus, once the cycle is complete the chamber is available at any time providing the inner door has not been opened. The size of the chamber can be custom made to the user's requirements.

Fumigation chamber (Category 3 and 4 accommodation)

A fumigation chamber is a double-ended vessel similar to a fogging chamber. Formaldehyde (40% formaldehyde vapour solution in water), is the usual sterilising agent used and is the method by which heat-sensitive materials are transferred out of the unit. Once a cycle had been completed and the sterilised items removed, the fumigation chamber could be used to transfer items into the unit in a similar way to the fogging chamber. However, unlike the fogging chamber the procedure for fumigation is a long process and would not be conducted merely for transferring items into the unit, except in an emergency.

Dunk tank

This is a convenient way to get small items quickly out of the unit. Mainly used for tissue or blood samples which are to be analysed in the laboratory. A tank of chemical disinfectant is situated on the wall between the 'dirty' and 'clean' side of the unit at a site which is most useful and practical. If specimens are to be transferred from the procedure or post-mortem room then direct access from this area would be particularly convenient, however, for general items a more common area would be preferable. Often, the site of the dunk tank is dictated by the design of the unit and the most readily available wall which 'straddles' the 'dirty' and 'clean' sides.

A central partition divides the 'dirty' and 'clean' sides of the dunk tank. Care has to be taken to ensure that the level of chemical disinfectant remains above the partition. Items are slid underneath this partition so that they are totally immersed for a pre-determined time. Materials which cannot be exposed to the disinfectant are enclosed in a heat-sealed bag then placed in a disinfected container which is sealed, and only opened in a safe and secure area such as a safety cabinet.

The disinfectant chosen will be that which is active against the hazardous agent being worked with in the unit. Periodic changing of the disinfectant is necessary to ensure that the disinfectant stays active. The intervals between changes will depend on usage, but approximately once a month is normal. All contents

are drained to the inside of the unit, the dunk tank cleaned and then refilled. During this process a means by which the dunk tank can be sealed from the outside is necessary. A fan which draws air into the unit situated adjacent to the dunk tank is of benefit in ensuring that the airflow moves into, and not out of the unit.

Port systems (similar to those used on isolators), which allow the spraying out of items with a chemical disinfectant are suitable alternatives to dunk tanks. They are cleaner to use and negate the need to use large quantities of chemical disinfectant at one time in one place.

A laboratory facility within the isolation unit which could process all samples would minimise the numbers of transfers of potentially hazardous material out of the isolation unit. However, it is unlikely that a laboratory would be equipped to fulfill all requirements and therefore, efficient and safe procedures for the transfer of hazardous material to destinations outside the units are essential.

Maintenance of unit (Category 3 and 4 accommodation)

The maintenance department will require access to the unit to carry out running repairs, for servicing and for emergencies. Therefore it will be necessary to ensure that there are maintenance personnel who are willing to enter the isolation unit, who have had the necessary training, have been vaccinated, have been advised of the work in the unit and are aware of the unit's safety regulations. They should be shown around the unit to familiarise themselves with the procedures for entry and the locations of equipment and apparatus which they may be expected to work with. Ideally, they could arrange for suitable tools and equipment to be housed permanently in the unit. This lessens the time that maintenance takes and prevents possible damage to pieces of equipment during the sterilising out process.

Releasing part of the unit to outside (Category 3 accommodation)

A major aid to the maintenance of the unit is the capability to separate off specific areas and open them up to the outside. This can be achieved by incorporating a second door to an animal room(s) which can be opened up to the outside. This door is sealed against any leakage of air and is security locked. To open it up, the room is first cleared and prepared for fumigation, the inside door sealed and the room then fumigated. After fumigation the inside door is kept sealed and security locked; the outside door can then be opened from the outside, after which the necessary work can be conducted by the maintenance staff without the restrictions imposed on Category 3 isolation units. Usually the room would only be opened up for major works such as decoration, installation of electrics, plumbing etc. On completion, the outside door is sealed and security locked, the inner door can then be opened and the room used again as Category 3 accommodation.

Similarly, it is possible to open up larger areas than just one room by housing temporary sealing doors in the main corridor. Planning is necessary to ensure that the sealing doors which separate the unit are sited in the most appropriate position and that the servicing of the functioning part of the isolation unit can continue satisfactorily while the maintenance work is being carried out; changing areas, showers and autoclave being the most important.

Account must be taken of the fact that any exclusion and subsequent return of a room, rooms or areas within the isolation unit will affect the ventilation and therefore, the air pressure differentials will have to be balanced accordingly.

Category 4 accommodation has to be completely fumigated before it can be opened up. Parts of the unit can not be separated off to outside while the unit is in use.

Changing of filters

In negative air-pressure isolation units it is the extract filters which present the main hazards, however, due to particular circumstances, such as breakdowns, it is possible that supply filters may also be contaminated. Therefore, the safest option is to assume that all filters to be changed are contaminated and present a hazard to the health of the operators changing them and, in some cases, to the environment, if changed incorrectly.

Filters are fumigated before changing is allowed. Areas for fumigation must be slightly negative or neutral to other areas to prevent fumigant drift; this will necessitate the use of the extract system both during and at the end of the fumigation cycle and therefore, the extract filters will be fumigated as a matter of course. However, this does not apply to the supply filters which will also have to be changed periodically. Irrespective of fumigation, the filters must be regarded as hazardous. Local rules will dictate PPE (personal protective equipment) and RPE and the methods to be used, but generally the systems employed will be similar to those described below.

Changing filters in the main ventilation ducting

Filters are usually housed in 'safe change boxes'. The filter is accessed via a heavy panel secured by turn keys. The panel is removed to expose a box attached to the ducting. Fixed to the outside of the box is a large, folded, heavy-duty polythene bag which is attached to the box by a heavy-duty rubber ring. Within the ducting is the filter which has a handle, the filter is pulled out of the ducting by the handle, which is grasped using the polythene bag, the filter is pulled into the polythene bag. The bag is then heat sealed while still attached to the box, or alternatively, removed from the box whereupon the rubber ring automatically seals the bag which can then be heat sealed. A new filter is fitted into the ducting and a new bag and rubber ring is fitted to the box and the ducting closed up with the panel.

Where there is a potential risk to the environment of contaminated air escaping from the isolation unit during the time taken to remove one filter and replace it with another, a double bank of filters is installed, one bank remains empty until it is time for changing, the new filters are installed before the old ones are removed. Thereby the air is always filtered during the changing process. For Category 4 accommodation, extract air has to be double-HEPA filtered so no escape will occur.

Changing filters in a room

This operation is similar to the procedures for the main ducting, but it is unlikely that there will be a double-bank situation available due to lack of space, and possibly no 'safe change box' for the same reason. In this case, after the protective grill has been removed, a bag can be sealed into the ducting by tape and the filter pulled into it. The bag can then be heat sealed before the bag is removed from the ducting.

Filters must be incinerated as soon as possible. In the case of those coming from 'live' Category 4 accommodation they will first have to go through an autoclave or a fumigation chamber to exit the unit.

Disposal of waste (Category 3 accommodation)

In a Category 3 unit, waste may be transferred to an autoclave providing it is within easy access and the materials are transferred safely. Safe transfer can be achieved in a sealed container, which can be disinfected out of the unit and put directly into the autoclave. Filter protectors, which allow disinfection of the container without damaging the filters, are removed just prior to sterilisation which will allow steam penetration into the container while preventing escape of hazardous material during transfer. Waste emanating from isolators will be disinfected out via the ports, double bagged, and taken for incineration.

Category 4 accommodation requires that all waste is autoclaved out of the unit via a double-ended chamber and incinerated on site.

Disposal of liquid waste (Category 4 accommodation)

The isolation unit would normally be dry, that is it would not have floor drains. Methods of cleaning are adopted which leave little surplus water.

In Category 4 units all liquid waste, including that from the showers, must be rendered safe before discharge into a drain. Common practice when working with viruses is to hold all liquid waste in tanks and heat it to between 95–100 °C for a minimum of two hours before discharge. When working with bacteria then either pressure vessels are used to enable the liquid to be heated above boiling point or, if this is not possible, sterilisation will be performed by chemical means.

It is advisable to have two tanks for liquid waste to allow continuous use of liquids in the unit and for back-up in case of break down. The size of the tanks depends on the amount of liquid waste to be discharged, but must be of sufficient size to prevent

interruptions in the working of the unit, but not so large as to make sterilisation of the contents impracticable. Two tanks, each holding 1200 litres, is a guideline for a small unit of one animal room, one laboratory and associated services.

Fumigation

Fumigation is the method of sterilisation used for safety cabinets, isolators, rooms or areas within the isolation unit, and for sterilising items out of the unit which would be damaged by other methods of sterilisation.

The most commonly used fumigant is formaldehyde vapour which is readily available as a 40% solution of fomaldehyde in water, or in the solid state as paraformaldehyde in either powder or prill form. All are heated to generate a gas which is the sterilising vehicle. For large areas, apparatus is available to heat the sterilising agent for prescribed periods and incorporates all the necessary safety features. Alternatively, there are commercially available formaldehyde generating kits which are also useful for fumigating isolators and safety cabinets. Formaldehyde gas generators (heating boxes) are incorporated into the design of safety cabinets and isolators which after preparation, only require that the formaldehyde vapour solution is added and the generator turned on.

Ideal environmental conditions for formaldehyde fumigation is a temperature of 30–33 °C and a humidity level of approximately 70%. An appropriate concentration level is 3000 ppm with a contact time of six hours, although the fumigant is usually left overnight before venting takes place, usually over a 24-hour period. The room can then be checked for residual vapour with a gas sensor via a small porthole in the door.

Staff should work in pairs when carrying out fumigation procedures to ensure assistance is available in case of mishap. Great care must be taken to ensure that no leakage of the fumigant occurs from the area being sterilised. Operators should monitor the fumigation process (when the gas is being given off). The area being fumigated should be under slight negative pressure to prevent leakage to outside. Room, cabinet or isolator filters should be exposed to the fumigant.

Staff respiratory protection equipment with suitable filters can be used if there is a slight leakage of fumigant. However, if high concentrations of gas are involved, such as those generated during the fumigation process, then only breathing apparatus with an independent source of oxygen would give adequate respiratory protection.

Fumigation of any area will require closing some dampers to the ventilation system to prevent escape of gas. The supply damper should be closed first and the extract damper second. After fumigation, when the room requires venting of vapour, the procedure is reversed and the extract damper is opened first. Alterations to the damper settings may affect the air-pressure differentials between areas within the unit which will require checking and balancing as appropriate.

Hydrogen peroxide (H_2O_2) is regarded as a suitable alternative to formalin for fumigation as it is more controllable, more easily monitored, gives a quicker sterilising cycle and breaks down to oxygen and water. Unfortunately, the equipment required to use this fumigant is, at present, very expensive.

Working protocols will have to be devised to suit local conditions and may vary a great deal between establishments. However, providing the work is conducted in appropriate accommodation, in a safe manner and within the HSE's general guidelines approval will normally be given.

Statutes, regulations and directives

Animal Health Act (1981) *The Rabies (Importation of Dogs, Cats and Other Mammals) Order 1974*. Dd 5065222 4/96 C3 1731 ON 341616. HMSO, London.

Animal Health Act (1981) *The Rabies (Importation of Dogs, Cats and Other Mammals) Order 1974 (Amendment No. 5 July 1985)*.

Schedule of Standard Conditions – Research Establishments. ADJAAC. HMSO, London.

ACDP (1995) *Categorisation of Biological Agents According to Hazard and Categories of Containment (1995)* (4th edn). HMSO, London.

EEC (1992) Council Directive 92/65EEC of 13th July 1992.

References

HSE (Health and Safety Executive) (2002) *The Control of Substances Hazardous to Health Regulations 2002. Approved Code of Practice and Guidance L5* (4th edn). HSE Books, Sudbury, UK.

HSE (1995) *Control of Substances Hazardous to Health Regulations (1994). General COSHH ACOP, Carcinogens ACOP and Biological Agents ACOP (L5)*. HSE Books, Sudbury, UK.

HSE (1997) *Working Safely with Research Animals: Management of Infection Risks*. HSE Books, Sudbury, UK.

Further reading

Advisory Committee on Dangerous Pathogens (ACDP) (1997) *Working Safely with Research Animals: Management of Infection Risks*. HSE Books, Sudbury, UK.

Health and Safety Commission (2005) *Control of Substances Hazardous to Health (5th edn): The control of substances hazardous to health regulations 2002 (as amended). Approved code of practice and guidance*. HSE Books, Sudbury, UK.

HMSO (1995) *Categorisation of Biological Agents According to Hazard and Categories of Containment* (4th edn). HMSO, London.

Smith, M.W. (1987) Chapter 11. In: T. Poole (Ed.) *The UFAW Handbook on the Care and Management of Laboratory Animals* (6th edn). Longman Scientific & Technical.

COSHH and ADCP guidance is constantly being updated, readers are advised to consult the following websites for the latest guidance: www.hse.gov.uk/aboutus/meetings/acdp and www.hse.gov.uk/coshh

32

The Environment

Gerald Clough

Introduction

The environment can be defined as the physical, chemical and biological conditions of the region in which an organism lives. Those conditions closest to the animal, for example within a nest or inside a cage or pen are referred to as the micro-environment. The area containing the micro-environment such as the cage (around a nest), an animal room (containing the cages in their racks) or animal building (in the case of farm animals in their pens) is then referred to as the macro-environment. From the fact that a cage can be regarded as either a micro- or a macro-environment it can be seen that these are relative terms.

Other aspects of the environment in laboratory animal buildings include procedures such as routine cleaning, feeding and watering which can affect the animals through disturbance. Thus, although such procedures are essential it is important to ensure that they are performed in a way which will minimise the degree of disturbance.

In nature, each species has become adapted to its environment. Many, particularly very successful species such as the rodents which are widely used as laboratory animals, can tolerate a wide range of conditions. The inherent physiological adaptability which permits them to do so can itself be a source of variation in such animals' response to experimental treatments.

The capacity of a species to thrive in captivity may depend on the similarity of the artificial environment to the natural environment from which the animals were obtained. Therefore, the more that is known about the natural environment of a species, the more likely it is that the artificial environment created for it will be conducive to its survival and its ability to live as normally as possible. Even with such knowledge, however, it is difficult to replicate the natural environment of a species since it will have been perceived through the senses of man and not those of the animal. Good examples of this 'problem' are the very different ways in which the eyes and ears of animals and man interpret their surroundings. For example while most animals can hear a far greater range of sound frequencies than man can, in contrast the eyes of man have greater acuity and can see many more wavelengths of light (colours) than most animals can. Thus, conditions which might seem to people quiet and with 'restful' colours could simultaneously appear very noisy and grey to an animal.

Over recent decades, as the use of laboratory animals has progressed, the demand for well-defined organisms with constant, reproducible responses has arisen. This is because it is important for investigators to be sure that any responses they see in their animals are due to the experimental procedures and not due to the inherent variability within the animals themselves.

It is well recognised, however, that the standardisation of living organisms is not a simple matter. This is particularly so since normal physiological processes such as growth, maturation and reproduction are themselves influenced by environmental factors such as temperature, lighting, noise, nutrition, infections and methods of husbandry.

It is for these reasons that in modern laboratory animal facilities considerable efforts are made to control at least those environmental factors which are known to influence experimental investigations adversely. The relationship between the macro- and micro-environments is clearly important in this respect as most regulatory requirements and methods of environmental control are aimed at controlling the macro- rather than the micro-environment.

As man's perception of the environment is different from that of animals it is not possible to list all the factors which make up their environment, but they certainly include:

- the cage, bedding, diet, water, other animals;
- temperature, relative humidity, day length, light intensity;
- air (oxygen, carbon dioxide, water vapour, ammonia, particles);
- routine care procedures, noise, personnel;
- breeding system;
- parasites, micro-organisms;
- prophylactic and therapeutic measures;
- experimental procedures.

Some of these factors are easy to control others are more difficult. Those factors listed above which are not discussed in detail in this chapter are covered in other chapters of this manual.

Interactions with man

The importance of man in the artificial environment varies with the species in question. Most species used in the laboratory live in close association with man though some (for example wild-caught primates, farm animals in 'open' situations) are more removed. Through selective breeding, domestic breeds have been created which exhibit the minimum of behavioural or physiological changes in man's presence.

From an animal's point of view, a person in the animal room may play a variety of roles depending on the person's activity – from predator to social partner or just part of the inanimate environment. If man is only an occasional visitor and becomes associated with 'unpleasant' experiences (e.g. by poor handling or restraint techniques) then he/she will become a negative aspect of the environment and will be avoided if possible. If, on the other hand, man becomes a familiar part of the environment and associated with 'pleasant' experiences (e.g. providing food, water or social interaction) then he/she will be approached rather than avoided; this is part of the process known as taming. This process is greatly facilitated if animals are reared with people from a very young age, hence the need for the 'gentling' of animals in the laboratory (Price 1976).

Interactions with other animals

The relationship of animals with others of the same or a different species is to a large extent dependent on their natural characteristics; in the wild they may be solitary or gregarious, territorial or non-territorial, predator and/or prey. Thus, individuals of a normally social species will react more negatively to being housed singly than will a solitary species; territorial species are unlikely to have enough space to establish a territory in a laboratory environment and prey animals will be affected adversely by the presence of a predator.

It should be remembered that when animals are housed in groups the groupings are 'unnatural' insofar as they are set up by man and not by the animals themselves. This can easily lead to the development of behaviour patterns such as bullying which a wild animal would more likely be able to avoid.

A common form of organisation is for animals to establish a social hierarchy wherein each individual becomes either subordinate or dominant to each other member of the group. In the wild state, this system is associated with a relatively low rate of aggression which is clearly an advantage in the laboratory situation. The fact that gregarious species will tolerate higher stocking densities than solitary ones means that this hierarchical system is the commonest form of social organisation among domesticated species, including those used in biomedical research. The artificial selection for docility, which has gone on for many years, has yet further facilitated the housing of laboratory animals at greater densities.

From a purely practical point of view it is clear that excessive stocking densities (overcrowding) will increase both the amount of waste produced within an enclosure as well as the temperature and relative humidity; such conditions increase the risks of infection.

This may to some extent be counteracted by the fact that the artificial environment pertaining in many laboratory animal buildings is likely to support a smaller variety or number of secondary hosts or vectors (indeed under barriered conditions they may be absent altogether) than would be present in the wild state. Because of this, the number of diseases infecting captive animals may be considerably reduced compared to those likely to infect their wild counterparts.

Is environmental control necessary for laboratory animals?

Very many experimental procedures rely on various responses of animals to provide a 'measure' of the effect of whichever treatment may be applied. In considering what is required of such animals, a useful (though perhaps rather simplistic) analogy is to consider what is required of a device such as a balance or a thermometer which might also be used as part of a procedure. It is well accepted that if a worker here in the UK, another in Rome and another in New York or Tokyo each weighed out 1.005 g of anything on a balance, each of them would have available the same amount of that substance; that is, the results are reliably reproducible. The reason for this is that equipment such as balances and thermometers are made to an agreed standard and are well maintained and calibrated. Ideally, therefore, experimental animals should also be in a sense made to an agreed standard, and should be well maintained and calibrated. The achievement of this ideal end point, however, is obviously complicated by the fact that animals are living entities which are not only sensitive to but can also respond to changes in their surroundings. The matter is further complicated by the fact that their sensitivity and response can vary with age, their physiological state and even their previous experience. It is for all these reasons it has often been said that environmental factors constitute the broadest and possibly most significant set of variables that confront biologists working with animal models.

Some effects of temperature (T) and relative humidity (RH)

As ambient relative humidity (RH) is of major importance to the heat balance of animals, the two topics of temperature (T) and RH are linked together. In relation to temperature and RH effects it is worth noting that the mammals and birds commonly used in research keep their deep body temperature (T_b) at a steady value, as does man which they are so often used to model. This ability is called homoiothermy. Every homoiothermic species has a range of ambient temperature over which it can maintain its T_b at a constant level by mechanisms involving heat loss and heat production. This temperature range, which varies from species to species, represents the limit of homoiostasis. Within this broad range there is a much smaller temperature range within which the body is at rest, the metabolic rate is constant and heat production and heat loss are at a minimum level; this is known as the zone of thermal thermoneutrality. The thermoneutral zone is delimited by the lower critical temperature (T_{cl}) and the upper critical temperature (T_{cu}). If ambient temperature falls below the T_{cl}, then the metabolic rate increases to maintain homoiothermia. If ambient temperature rises above the T_{cl}, there is also an increase in metabolic rate due to stimulation of the chemical processes within the cells.

The RH of air is the ratio (expressed as a percentage) of the actual amount of moisture in that air to the moisture it would contain if it were saturated (100% RH) at the same temperature and pressure. The higher the air temperature, the more water it can carry. Hence if warm, wet air is cooled, water is deposited on surrounding surfaces in the form of condensation (e.g. on the bathroom mirror and windows when you shower).

With laboratory animals to 'model' man, it should be remembered that whereas most of the animals used are relatively small, hair covered, non-sweating and crepuscular (active at dawn and dusk) or nocturnal in their habits, man is relatively large, basically hairless, profusely sweating and mainly diurnal in his habits.

The following are examples of known effects of temperature and RH on laboratory animals:

- *Changes in food and water intake*: these are relevant to the dose consumed by animals of any substances which may be supplied to them in their food or water.
- *Changes in drug activity*: in some cases increasing, in others decreasing their toxicity. As little as 4 °C change in ambient temperature can cause large (tenfold) variations in toxicity. Even larger variations (several thousand-fold) can be caused by an animal's previous thermal experience.
- *Increase/decrease in fertility, lactation and teratogenesis*: repeated short exposures to extremes can have cumulative effects, particularly on the development of the nervous system of some species.
- *Incidence of disease*: this may be direct (e.g. incidence of ringtail in rats related to low RH levels) or indirect and related to bacterial survival and

activity (e.g. ammonia production and its relevance to the induction of respiratory disease).

Some effects of air quality

The quality of the air is related to both its physical state (T, RH) and the 'pollutants' it can convey (gases, charged particles, pathogenic microbes etc.):

- temperature and RH effects already mentioned;
- aromatic substances, including pesticides and herbicides, some potentially carcinogenic, arising from sawdust bedding and affecting liver function;
- presence of (particularly pathogenic) microbes – of obvious relevance to disease;
- presence of positively or negatively charged ions – affecting survival of microbes and activity/behaviour of some animals.

Some effects of light

As most of the species used are crepuscular or nocturnal their eyes are adapted to dim light conditions and very few of them have colour vision; man's eyes are adapted to bright light conditions and have excellent colour vision. The following are examples of some effects light can have on animals:

- intensity (brightness) – relevant to retinal pathology especially in albinos – relevant to oestrous cycle length in some mouse strains;
- wavelength (colour) – age of sexual maturity in rats – relevant to wheel-running activity in mice;
- photoperiod – relevant to circadian and circannual rhythms, stimulating and synchronising breeding cycles, gastrointestinal function and motility of the rabbit (Jilge 1980), critical effects in 'photoperiodic species' including the hamster (Ellis & Follett 1983);
- the amount of light which 'leaks' into a room through the viewing panel from adjacent areas which may be lit at night for safety reasons (e.g. corridors) can have significant effects. Such contamination of ~30 lux is known to cause ovarian changes in albino rats (Beys et al. 1995) and as little as 0.2 lux during the dark phase has been shown to inhibit melatonin secretion in rats and adversely affect the outcome of tumour growth investigations (Dauchy et al. 1997).

Some effects of sound including ultrasound

There are two aspects of any sound which are important in relation to the functioning of the auditory system – its intensity (or loudness) and its frequency (or pitch). (For further background information on sound see Monitoring methods p. 278.)

The ears of most mammals respond to a much wider range of frequencies than do those of man. Rats and mice, for example, can hear (and also communicate using) sounds as high as 30 000–40 000 Hz (30–40 kHz). The upper cut-off frequency for most people is around 18–20 kHz. All 'sounds' above that frequency we refer to as ultrasound because they are too high pitched for us to hear. Whether or not a sound is 'damaging' depends not only on its intensity, frequency and duration, but also on the hearing ability of the species concerned, the age and physiological state of the animal at the time of exposure and possibly its previous auditory history. It should also be remembered that animals can 'hear' during sleep and under deep anaesthesia.

The relevance of sound in relation to experimental work is very extensive and the following effects are a few examples:

- physical damage to the cochlea resulting in temporary or permanent deafness to specific or multiple frequencies;
- hypertension;
- changes in bodyweight, immune response and tumour resistance;
- changes in blood chemistry and cellular distribution;
- cannibalism;
- increases or decreases in fertility;
- audiogenic seizures;
- audioconditioning, related to atypical drug responses.

The relevance of environmental factors

There are numerous well-documented examples of how environmental factors can interfere with experimental work and these have been reviewed from time to time (e.g. Clough 1982). Detailed observations made in a recent publication (Gärtner 1990) have demonstrated that reducing environmental variability through highly standardised husbandry does not greatly reduce the 'normal' random variability which can be observed in a number of quantitative biological traits including gravimetric, morphometric, haematological and biochemical characteristics of rats and mice.

As described earlier, however, there is also very considerable evidence showing that the environmental factors discussed can affect the outcome of experiments in most fields of biomedical research, certainly including studies of animal behaviour, cancer research, immunology, pathology, pharmacology, psychology, reproduction and associated areas. In conclusion it is suggested that it would be negligent to ignore the evidence and that for the majority of workers – and perhaps particularly for those involved with long-term work – at least those environmental factors known to be relevant to their work should be controlled. Although the degree of environmental control necessary may vary from one laboratory to another, it is only by considering all the information available relative to the work in hand that a reasoned assessment of individual needs can be made.

Finally it is of course necessary for anyone using animals as research tools to be aware of and comply with relevant national and international regulations. This will ensure not only compliance with the law, but also maximise the likelihood that the results obtained will be comparable with those of (and accepted by) workers in other laboratories.

The physical environment

Regulatory requirements – can they be justified?

Table 32.1 provides a summary of the current recommendations from twenty-eight countries for environmental control in rat and mouse rooms. Details of individual country's regulations are published.

In the UK, the most relevant and important regulatory authority is the Home Office Inspectorate operating under the Animals (Scientific Procedures) Act 1986. There are two Codes of Practice (CoP) attached to the Act, the first For the Housing and Care of Animals Used in Scientific Procedures (HMSO 1989) and the second For the Care and Housing of Animals in Designated Breeding and Supplying Establishments (HMSO 1995). Let us consider each factor in turn.

Temperature

Table 32.1 shows that although there are some minor differences between countries, a range of 23 ± 5 °C encompasses the recommendations of all the countries. Nevertheless, in the UK it is necessary to comply with the slightly more restrictive recommendations of the Home Office CoP (1989; 1995). This states that 'animal room temperatures should be carefully controlled and continuously monitored by instruments which are checked at least once daily.' The

Table 32.1 Range of environmental recommendations for the housing of rats and mice derived from the guidelines published by Canada, the Council of Europe, Germany, Japan, Sweden, Switzerland, the UK and the USA.

Environmental factor	Species	Recommended ranges		
Temperature (°C)	Mouse	23.5 ± 1.5 to 23.0 ± 5.0		
	Rat	21.0 ± 2.0 to 22.0 ± 4.0		
Relative humidity (%)	Mouse	50.0 ± 10.0 to 55.0 ± 15.0		
	Rat	52.5 ± 2.5 to 57.5 ± 17.5		
Light	Mouse and Rat	**Intensity (Lux)**		**Light:Dark (hours)**
		150–400		12:12
		Care needed		to 14:10
		with albinos 'intensity and L:D must be controlled'		
Sound level	Mouse and Rat	'Minimise' to 'not > 85dB' to 'About 50dB(A), < NRC45 and no distinct tonal content'		
Ventilation rate (air changes/hour)	Mouse	8–20, draught free		
	Rat	10–20, draught free		

Table 32.2   UK codes of practice guidelines for room air temperature for stock animals and during scientific procedures (Home Office 1989).

Adults	Optimal range (°C)	Possible settings (°C)
Non-human New World primates	20–28	* 22–26 ± 2
Mouse, rat, hamster, gerbil, small birds	19–23	** 21 ± 2
Guinea pig, quail	16–23	**, *** 18–21 ± 2
Rabbit	16–20	*** 18 ± 2
Non-human Old World primates, pigeon, cat, dog, ferret, pig	15–24	*, **, *** 17–22 ± 2
Domestic fowl and duck	12–24	*, **, *** 14–22 ± 2
Goat, sheep, cattle, horse	10–24	*, **, *** 12–22 ± 2
The target should be to maintain the room temperature in a band width of 4 °C, the whole of the band lying within the optimal range indicated		*, ** and *** indicate species which can be kept at the same T

recommended temperature variation limits for each species are shown in Table 32.2 and in addition it is stated that the '. . . design of the building should be such as to ensure that these temperatures can be maintained in both winter and summer.'

Commonly used ambient design temperatures for buildings in the UK are −2 °C and +27 °C; that is, the air conditioning system should be designed to maintain the temperature required inside the building as long as the ambient temperature does not go below −2 °C or above +27 °C.

The CoP (1989) also states, 'temperature regulation should ensure that there are no undue fluctuations within or between rooms. . . . In the majority of establishments it is desirable to provide a cooling system for . . . rodents and rabbits to comply with the upper limitations for room temperatures (see discussion below). If this is not available ad hoc methods, such as reduction of stocking densities, may be necessary to avoid heat stress.'

In practical terms reduction of stocking densities can present problems since animals moved out of a room to reduce its stocking density will then have to be placed in another area which is also designated under the Animals (Scientific Procedures) Act 1986 for that use. In reality, there are few ad hoc methods available to help in such a situation. If it is not possible to increase the ventilation rate, then probably the most practical solution is to increase air movement within the room by the use of a free standing fan.

As far as justification for the recommended temperature levels is concerned, the most relevant information is from Japan. Workers there have looked at the effect of room temperatures (at 2° intervals from 12–32 °C) on two generations of both rats and mice in relation to a variety of more than twenty parameters. On the basis of their results, the authors suggest that although the optimum temperature for both these species seems to be 23 ±3 °C, 23 ±5 °C is 'permissible' for their breeding and rearing.

It is worth noting that the recommendations from Europe state that 'under the climatic conditions prevailing in Europe it may be necessary to provide a ventilation system having the capacity both to heat and cool the air supplied' (Council of Europe 1986). When the relevant data are examined psychometrically, however (Clough 1999), they reveal that in any animal building with rooms containing different stocking densities of the same species, or indeed species with differing temperature requirements, then rather than '. . . may be necessary . . .', the wording should be '. . . it will be essential . . .' to have both heating and cooling if the stipulated temperature and RH conditions are to be maintained at all times.

Relative humidity

Recommendations for RH control (Table 32.1) also show quite close agreement between countries centring around 55%. The UK CoP (1989) recommends that:

'The relative humidity in animal rooms should normally be maintained at 55 ± 10%. Prolonged periods below 40% or above 70% should be avoided. In most cases some form of humidification will be required. Chickens are more tolerant than mammals and a range of 30–70% is acceptable.'

Consideration of the data presented in Table 32.3 shows that the RH levels currently recommended

Table 32.3   Relevance of ambient relative humidity (RH) to laboratory rodents and survival of some airborne pathogens.

Relative humidity (RH) (%)	Relevance and reference(s)
17–25	*Best survival of influenza, parainfluenza type 3, Vaccinia and Venezuelan equine encephalomyelitis viruses (Hemmes et al. 1960; Harper 1961; Miller et al. 1967)*
<30	*Initiation of ringtail in the pouched mouse (Ellison et al. 1990)*
<40	*Increased incidence of ringtail in rats (Njaa et al. 1957; Totton 1958; Flynn. 1967)*
~40	*Increased pre-weaning mortality and reduced growth rate in mice (Donnelly, 1989)*
40–45	*Increased transmission of Sendai virus in mice (van der Veen et al. 1972)*
	Reduced transmission of influenza virus in mice (Schulman et al. 1962)
>45	**Reduced incidence of ringtail in pouched mouse (Ellison et al. 1990)**
~50	**Overall viability of airborne micro-organisms lowest (Anderson et al. 1967)**
45–55	**Reduction in ammonia production in cages (Clough 1976; Gamble et al. 1976)**
	Reduction in rat respiratory mycoplasmosis (Broderson et al. 1976)
60–70	**Reduced transmission of Sendai virus in mice (van der Veen et al., 1972)**
	Increased transmission of influenza virus in mice (Schulman et al. 1962)
~70	**Decreased pre-weaning mortality and increased growth in mice (Donnelly 1989)**
65–75	*Increase in ammonia production in cages (Clough 1976; Gamble et al. 1976)*
	Increase in rat respiratory mycoplasmosis (Broderson et al. 1976)
74	*At 23 °C increases specific airway resistance in rats (Melville. 1972)*
80–81	*Best survival of poliomyelitis and adenoviruses types 4 and 7 (Hemmes et al. 1960; Harper 1961; Miller et al. 1967)*

RH in bold = current recommendations
Adverse effects of RH shown in *italics*
Beneficial effects of RH shown in **bold** text

correspond reasonably well with those levels of RH found in the literature to be 'beneficial' to animals. Hence, at the present state of knowledge the recommendations appear to be justifiable. In relation to the various recommendations summarised in Table 32.1 (see p. 260) it would seem that 55 ± 10% should create fewer problems than 55 ± 15%.

It will be noticed that much of the evidence available is indirect and there is a need for more specific investigations in this field.

Lighting

The CoP (1989) states:

'(1) Intensity – 350–400 lux at bench level is adequate for routine . . . activities. Care may be required to avoid undesirably high levels inside cages, especially for albino animals.

(2) Wavelength – there is no evidence to indicate that either fluorescent or incandescent lights have adverse effects.

(3) Photoperiod – For the majority of laboratory animals a daily cycle of 12:12 hours is suitable.

The circadian "clock" of some species [e.g. hamsters] may be affected as much by light pulses of less than one second during the dark phase as by a long photoperiod; in this case it may be important not to turn on lights during the dark period.

(4) Dawn and dusk – for some species of primates, birds and fish, a simulated dawn and dusk may be required.'

Table 32.4 shows some scientific data relevant to the recommendations for lighting levels in rodent rooms. In this case it can be seen that the currently recommended lighting levels (350–400 lux) do not coincide with those scientific findings listed as 'beneficial' to the animals. This suggests that the lighting levels currently recommended might be unjustifiably high, particularly at eye level for albino animals; clearly, additional specific information is required before more detailed recommendations can be made.

There is no evidence that photoperiod control of L:D (light:dark) 12:12 or 14:10 is likely to be stressful or have adverse effects on any of the common species.

It should be remembered, however, that in those species which are photoperiodically sensitive (e.g.

Table 32.4   Known effects of light intensity on rats and mice

Lux	Effect and reference(s)
<5	*Increases oestrous cycle length in LACA mice (Clough et al. 1984)*
10–20	**< 5% pre-weaning mortality in LACG mice (Porter et al. 1963)**
15–20	**Shorter oestrous cycle length in pigmented mice (Donnelly et al. 1993)**
20	**No depression of productivity in wild mice (Bronson 1979)**
>~25	*Albino rats experience distress (Schlingmann et al. 1993)*
>~60	*Pigmented rats experience distress (Schlingmann et al. 1993)*
30	**Maximum true weight gain of pregnant albino rats (Weihe et al. 1969)**
	Maximum growth of albino rat litters (Weihe et al. 1969)
32	*Retinal degeneration in albino rats exposed up to three years (Weisse et al. 1974)*
60	**Highest number of young/litter born in albino rats (Weihe et al. 1969)**
	Retinal degeneration in albino rats after thirteen weeks (Stotzer et al. 1970)
85	*Retinal atrophy in albino mice after 24 months (Greenman et al. 1982)*
145	*Retinal atrophy in albino mice after 18–24 months (Greenman et al. 1982)*
155	*Retinal atrophy in albino mice after 18–24 months (Greenman et al. 1982)*
200	*Increased vaginal cornification in LACA mice (Clough et al. 1984)*
240	*Retinal atrophy in albino mice after 18–24 months (Greenman et al. 1982)*
220–290	*Increased oestrous cycle length in pigmented mice (Donnelly et al. 1993)*
250	Maximum number of litters born in albino rats (Weihe et al. 1969)
335	*Retinal atrophy in albino mice after 18–24 months (Greenman et al. 1982)*
500	*> 50% pre-weaning mortality in LACG mice (Porter et al. 1963)*
1000	*Minimum growth rate in albino rat litters (Weihe et al. 1969)*
1000–2000	*Depressed productivity in wild mice (Bronson. 1979)*
2010	*Retinal atrophy in albino mice after 12 months (Greenman et al. 1982)*
5000	*Causes retinal degeneration within one hour, even during surgery (Schlingmann et al. 1993)*
20 000	*Damage to albino rat eyes in a few hours (Gorn et al. 1967)*

Emboldened **lux** = current recommendations
Adverse effects of light shown in *italics*
Beneficial effects of light shown in **bold**

hamster, see above) it can be very important not to turn on any lights during the dark phase of the 24-hour L:D cycle. As discussed earlier, care should be taken if light 'leakage' into animal rooms can occur during the dark phase of the 24-hour cycle.

Although very little work has been done on the relevance of the wavelength of light (colour) to laboratory animals, there is no indication that fluorescent or tungsten lights of the type commonly used in animal rooms have adverse effects.

There is little evidence to show that artificial dawn and dusk is essential to animal welfare. Nevertheless, it probably is justifiable for primates, birds and any other species likely to be in mid air when the lights go out at night time – purely from the practical point of view that such species rely heavily on sight for a safe landing! It may also be justifiable for any particularly light sensitive species such as some reptiles, amphibia and fish.

Animal rooms are not usually provided with windows because they:

- allow daily fluctuations in light intensity;
- allow fluctuations in photoperiod depending upon the time of year;
- interfere with air temperature control, particularly during sunny weather;
- reduce the security of the building.

Sound levels

It is in the area of sound control that the least information is available for guidance as to the levels needed in order to provide the most suitable conditions. It has already been noted that there is wide variation in the ability of different species to hear different frequencies and that all the common laboratory species can hear sounds which, because they are 'above' the hearing range of man, are referred to as ultrasounds. The CoP (1989) states:

'...The control of noise is important in the care of laboratory animals. Loud, unexpected and unfamiliar sounds are probably more disruptive than constant sounds. There is no indication that constant background noise, such as that generated by air-conditioning and similar equipment, is harmful to animals provided it is not too loud. The ability of such sounds to mask other noise is, however, unproven...it is not possible to give firm recommendations for noise levels...

'...However, it has been found empirically that if the general background sound level in an empty animal room can be kept below about 50 dB(A); below a noise rating curve (NRC) of 45; and free from distinct tonal content, then it is unlikely that there will be damage to animals or personnel when the room is in use...'

(For an explanation of the units dB(A) and NRC see Monitoring methods p. 278). From the author's experience of monitoring the environmental conditions in many laboratory animal buildings in the UK it is known that it is not uncommon for them to fail to meet this requirement, in particular that not to exceed NRC 45. The damaging effects of many audible sounds are well known (see p. 259 above). It is now known that some ultrasounds can have similar effects which can be disadvantageous to scientific investigations using animals (Clough 1982) and that there can be many sources of ultrasound present in animal facilities (Sales et al. 1992).

How much of a problem such sounds might cause depends upon the nature of the work for which the animals are being used. Certainly, in several laboratories with which the author is familiar, extraneous ultrasounds arising from electronic devices (including VDUs and video recording equipment) have caused significant interference with studies involving automated recording of rodent behaviour and activity.

Ventilation rates

The CoP (1989) states:

'...The ventilation rate of the room should be related to its stocking density....In fully stocked rooms for rodents and lagomorphs, 15–20 changes of...air per hour distributed throughout the room are normally

adequate. For cats, dogs and primates, 10–12 changes per hour may be adequate. Fewer air changes may be acceptable where stocking densities are low....The air distribution system should deliver as even a proportion of air to each cage or animal as possible whilst avoiding draughts...etc.'

As indicated in Table 32.1 (see p. 260), the recommendations for ventilation show considerable variation probably arising from the different stocking densities used in various parts of the world. There is also something of a conflict in this field between the needs for animal welfare (in terms of protecting the animals from airborne diseases) and staff safety (in terms of protection of personnel from animal allergens). This problem has been addressed specifically by some Japanese workers who developed what they have called the 'one-way airflow system' for animal rooms in order to try and solve the staff allergy problem (Yamauchi et al. 1989).

An earlier system (the so-called PIV or Positive Individual Ventilation system) of supplying and exhausting air directly into and out of each cage can also serve the same purpose. The original PIV rack was developed many years ago at the Jackson Laboratories in America (Cunliffe-Beamer & Les 1983) and was later taken up and produced commercially by the American cage manufacturer Thoren Caging Systems Inc., Hazleton, USA (Clough et al. 1995). Both the Japanese and American versions are very refined air-distribution systems which ensure that the conditioned air is delivered directly to each cage.

The principle of the Japanese system has now been superseded by specifically modified racks which do not require the modification of the whole room. In the PIV system, the rack shelves are divided internally to form separate plenum chambers. One of these carries HEPA-filtered supply air directly into each cage, the other carries the spent air away from each cage to be exhausted either back into the room or directly into the room exhaust system, again through HEPA filters. Because of the highly efficient way the air is distributed in these systems, they can allow considerable savings in capital and running costs of the building air-conditioning system as a whole. In both, even with the room ventilation rate set at only 8 ac/h (air changes per hour), cage air is changed 50 to 100+ times per hour. Using such systems, large savings in cost should therefore be expected.

Control of the physical environment

Temperature, relative humidity and air quality

The most common method of controlling these factors is by the use of an air conditioning system. For discussion see section on Air conditioning, ventilation, distribution and filtration (p. 266).

Light

For the reasons already stated above animal rooms are not usually provided with windows. The most common form of illumination is provided by tubular, fluorescent lights suspended from or attached to the ceiling. This results in a grading of light intensity from ceiling to floor so that animals in the top row of cages may be subjected to light intensity several hundred times higher than those in the bottom row (Clough 1984). When considering lighting installations there are again the same three aspects that need to be taken into account.

Intensity
The published recommendations have already been noted (Table 32.1, p. 260). More recent studies (Schlingmann et al. 1993) concur with those and suggest that a room light intensity of 210 lux at working height is quite adequate for personnel and reduces the likelihood that albino animals in the room will be exposed to undesirably high levels. In view of the extreme sensitivity of albino animals, however, the same authors also consider that they should have access to areas within the cage with a light intensity less than 25 lux.

In order to achieve these levels it is necessary to install sufficient light sources to give, as far as is practical, an even spread of the light being created. To ensure albinos in upper cages are protected from undesirably high levels, it will be necessary to provide some sort of shade – the most common system being to install an 'extra' shelf of opaque material above the top row of cages on each rack.

Wavelength
It has been noted that both fluorescent and incandescent lights appear to be equally acceptable. Though few species of laboratory animal have the ability to see

colour, there is some evidence that they can be affected by light of different wavelengths. From this point of view, consideration should also be given to cage materials that are translucent or transparent and this may assume some importance in this respect. Plastics such as polypropylene and polycarbonate, for example, tend to yellow with age and repeated sterilisation, especially if this is carried out by gamma irradiation. It is up to individual investigators to assess the significance of such factors to the work being undertaken.

It is generally recommended, therefore, to avoid using light sources with a strong colour and bias ensure that lights of the same colour and temperature are used throughout an animal facility. This will ensure that the occupants are not exposed to different colours of light as they move (or are moved) around the building or from one building to another. For the same reason, efforts should be made to ensure that when a bulb 'goes', it is replaced with another of a similar spectral output. From a purely human point of view it is worth selecting a light source which provides a colour rendering similar to that of daylight and which creates a diffuse 'soft' effect rather than one which is 'hard' and gives sharp contrasts.

Photoperiod
A daily cycle of 12 hours light:12 hours dark is suitable for the majority of laboratory animals. This is most easily obtained by providing windowless animal rooms in which the lights are controlled by automatic time switches.

Because the 'leakage' of very low levels of light into animal rooms during the normally dark part of the cycle can interfere with physiological responses it can be important:

- to prevent the leakage of light from adjacent areas into animal rooms through any viewing panels or door security windows (use either a blind or dark red glass);
- not to turn on the room lights during the 'night';
- not to open the door of any animal room during the 'night' if the adjacent area is lit.

Sound

It has already been noted that different species have different hearing abilities. Because of this, and the almost infinitely variable combinations of sounds which can occur in animal houses, it is impossible to give specific recommendations for permissible sound levels.

The design of the building (in particular the air-conditioning system) should be such as to ensure compliance with the UK CoP (1989) (see p. 264). From this point of view it is clearly sensible to include features in the design of the building which will minimise the transmission of sound from obvious sources such as plant rooms, cage wash and other noise-generating areas – including barking dogs and noisy primates.

Remembering that ultrasounds can have the same disadvantageous effects on animals as sounds audible to man, it is also sensible to avoid or shield any known sources of such sounds. These can include items such as computer monitors, various types of electronic equipment, squeaky doors, chairs and wheels, bells (including alarms and telephone bells), water running into stainless steel sinks and the friction of one metallic object on another (metal cage sliding into a metal rack; grid floors being inserted into cages; metal cage doors being manipulated).

Air conditioning, ventilation, distribution and filtration

The terms 'air conditioning' and 'ventilation' are often used incorrectly as though they were synonymous; this is probably because a ventilation system is often used to carry conditioned air from the plant room to the areas which need to be 'air conditioned'. Ventilation involves merely the introduction of (generally fresh) air into a space (either by natural or mechanical means such as a fan), air conditioning as the term implies involves the conditioning or treatment of the air before it is introduced. The form of treatment involved will depend on the requirements but, as far as laboratory animal buildings are concerned, it is likely to include heating, cooling, humidification, de-humidification and filtration. After 'conditioning', the air must be delivered to the occupants without at the same time creating problems of draughts, smells or other undesirable characteristics. In such buildings, ventilation is most often maintained by mechanical means using fans to distribute the air through ductwork. With such a system

it is possible to maintain a constant air change rate irrespective of external conditions

Air conditioning

The history of the application of air conditioning to laboratory animal housing can be followed from various publications (Firman 1969; Blood 1976; Brader & Sutter 1988; White 1991; Hughes & Reynolds 1995; Hughes et al. 1996; Clough 1999).

Figure 32.1 (from Clough 1999) shows a layout typical of an air-conditioning system (often also referred to as an air handling unit or AHU) for a modern animal house illustrating many of the desirable features. Let us consider and comment upon the function of each part by following the route of 'outside air' to the animal rooms beneath.

Outside air

The quality of the outside air is important in terms of its physical state (T, RH, speed of movement) and the fact that it can act as a vector for other materials (freezing fog, gaseous and other pollutants, particles – some of which may be infectious – insects etc.).

Fresh air inlets are usually sited at high level in order to minimise some of the above. Air taken in at low level, for example, is nearer sources of obvious pollution such as:

- vehicle exhaust gases;
- particles of dust, dirt and soil, all of which can carry infectious organisms and may themselves be allergenic;
- contaminants arising from wild animals, particularly those of the same species as the occupants of the building (because they are the most likely to be carrying pathogens of that species);
- ants, other ground living insects and arthropods which may act as vectors of disease.

Outside air damper

This usually takes the form of louvres, some sort of grille or adjustable vanes. These help to direct the flow of air and, if adjustable, can be used to control the volume of air entering the air conditioning system. They also prevent birds, large insects and other airborne objects from being dragged into the air conditioning system.

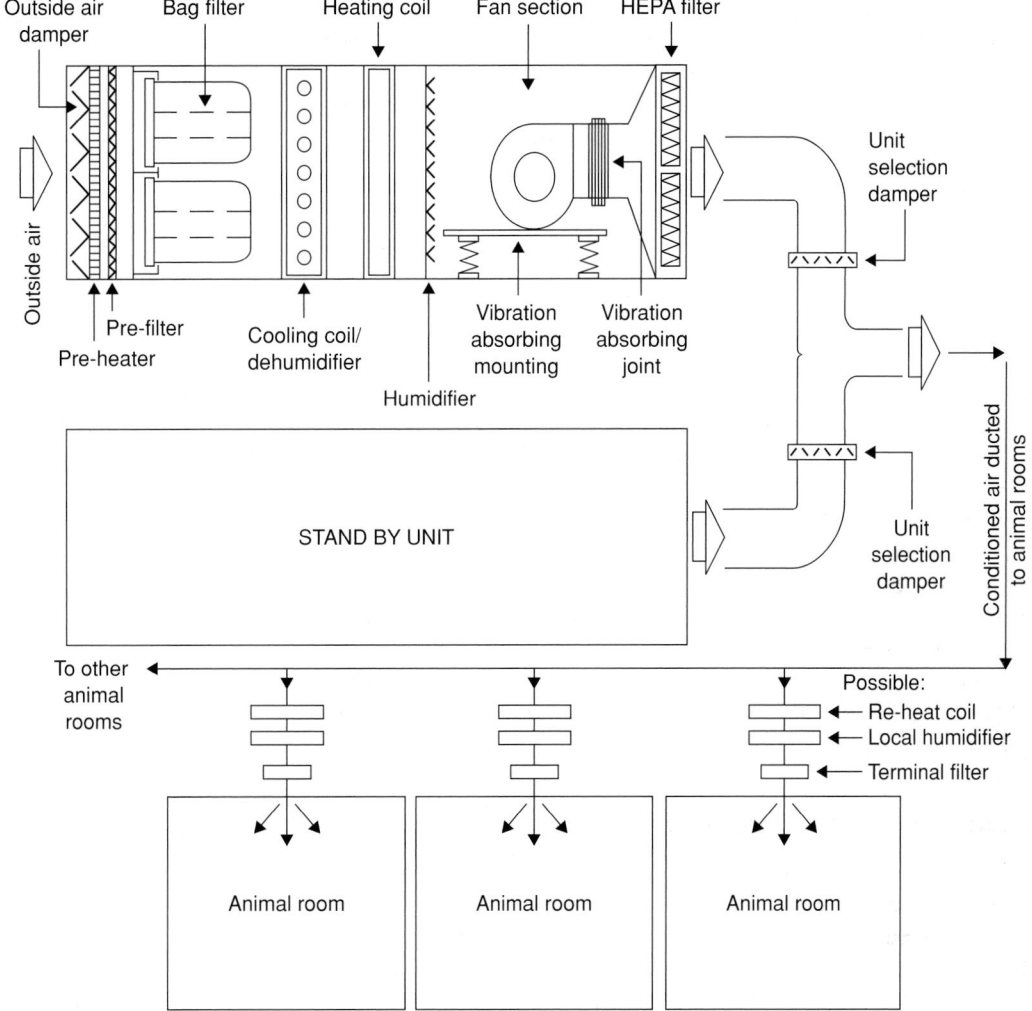

Figure 32.1 Typical animal house air-handling unit. Reproduced with permission from Poole (ed.) (1999) *UFAW Handbook on the Care and Management of Laboratory Animals: Terrestrial Vertebrates Vol. 1* (7th edn), Chapter 8 'Animal units'. Blackwell Publishing, Oxford.

Pre-heater/s

Depending on the type of heating (electric, hot water, steam) the pre-heater/s is/are likely to be either tubular electric elements or a system of finned, hollow pipes (rather like a car radiator) carrying warm or hot water. The primary function of the pre-heater/s is to prevent the ingress of freezing fog which would otherwise quickly block up the pre-filter.

Pre-filter

This is usually a relatively coarse filter in the form of:

- throw-away, removable panels which can be replaced as they become clogged;
- stainless steel 'wool' (rather like a domestic pan scourer) mounted in panels which can be hosed or washed down and sterilised if necessary;
- an automatic roll filter; this is rather like a giant film cartridge (Figure 32.2) on which a roll of filter medium is automatically 'advanced' (either manually or by electric motors) as it becomes clogged; once the roll is used up a new one is put in its place.

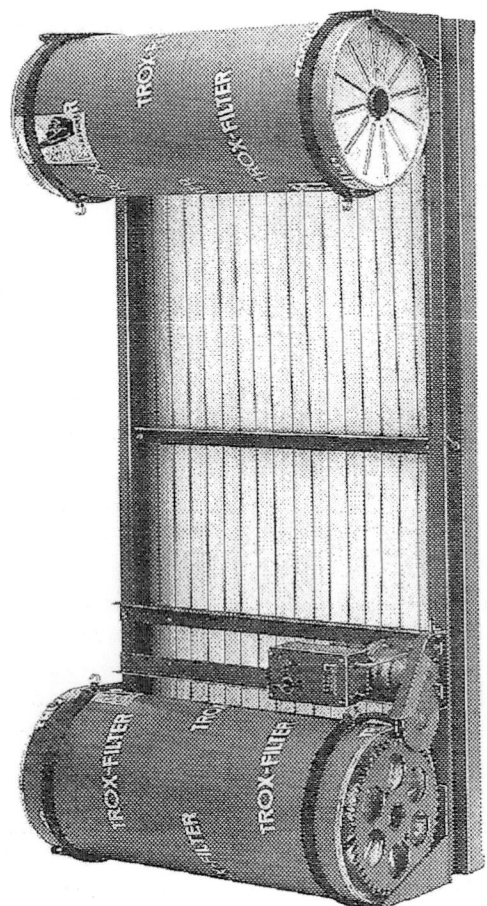

Figure 32.2   Automatic roll filter.

In order for any filter to work efficiently, it must be used within the range of conditions specified with the documentation which accompanies it. For example, a filter will only carry out its function correctly within limited linear air velocities (e.g. 1.75–2.5 m/s); its efficiency will be reduced at either lower or higher air speeds. Similarly they are designed to work within a certain range of air pressures; for example, a coarse filter may need the air to be at a pressure of 25–75 Pa before it will pass through. As the filter becomes loaded with dirt the resistance rises to 125 Pa, and it will need to be changed, otherwise the airflow rate will be reduced to an unsatisfactory level. The specifications usually also indicate the dust-holding capacity of the filter – coarse filters generally holding 2–4 kg dust/m^2 of filter surface.

The function of the pre-filter is to remove the larger particles of dust, dirt and other air-borne

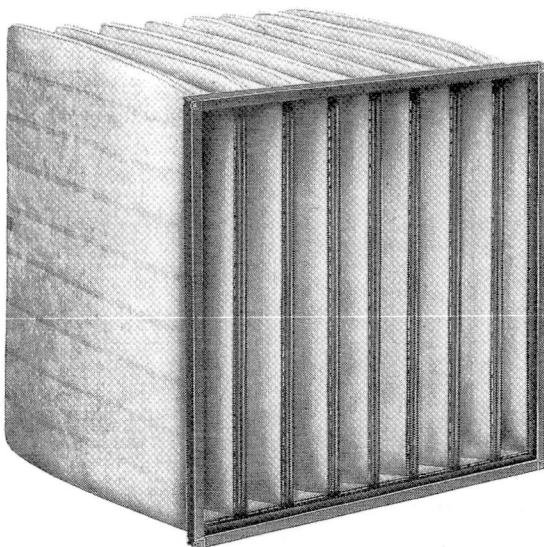

Figure 32.3   Typical bag filter.

objects such as insects, leaves etc. and so protect the finer and more expensive filters downstream from becoming clogged too quickly.

Bag filter

The filter media used at subsequent stages of filtration are usually more efficient than those used in pre-filters. This means that their resistance to airflow is also greater. Hence, in order to allow the same volumes of air to flow through, it is usually necessary to have filters with a larger surface area. This can be achieved in several ways:

- expanding the ductwork to a larger size;
- using bag filters (rather like a series of pillow cases supported at their open end upstream so that the air has to flow through them to pass along the ductwork) (see Figure 32.3);
- using duct filters in which 'normal' square filter panels are mounted in the ductwork (as shown in Figure 32.4) which effectively doubles or quadruples the area of filter face available within the same sized ductwork.

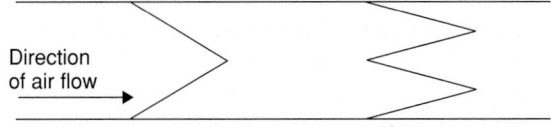

Direction of air flow

Figure 32.4   Increase in filter area gained by oblique mounting of panels.

Cooling coil/dehumidifier

Like some pre-heating coils, the cooling coil/s usually consist of a system of finned hollow pipes built into a frame which fits inside the air handling unit – again similar to a car radiator. Chilled water (or an antifreeze-like fluid) is circulated through the tubes and in this way the air is cooled as it passes over the fins. The 'depth' or thickness of the cooling unit is related to the cooling capacity required and the temperature of the chilled fluid passing through it. If the coolant is too cold, then there is a danger of moisture in the supply air condensing onto the coils and freezing; hence the size (surface area available for heat exchange) needs to be such that the maximum volumes of air required can be adequately cooled whilst the temperature of the coolant is high enough to prevent the freezing of any condensate.

As indicated by the discussion above, the cooling of the air as it passes over the coil necessarily results in its de-humidification. This is because, as already mentioned, the water-carrying capacity of air is related to its temperature; the higher the temperature the more water can be carried, hence cooling of a body of air results in condensation. It is for this reason that underneath the cooling coil will be a tray or similar collecting device in which the condensate will collect and from which it can be drained away into the drainage system.

Heating coil

This is usually of a similar construction to the cooling coil already described. In this case, however, the fluid circulated through it is usually low pressure hot water – like the radiators in many domestic central heating systems. Again, its capacity must be related to the rate of airflow and the temperature difference required between the air supplied to it and leaving it. In winter, for example, the incoming air having already passed through the pre-heater, may be at a temperature of, for example, 3–7 °C; as it passes through the heating coil it may be necessary to heat that air up to around 20 °C. If limited space in the building restricts the size of the air conditioning unit, then an alternative solution is to supply the heating coil with steam or high pressure hot water so that more energy is available to heat up the air as it passes through the coil. Remember that air leaving the heating coil (having been de-humidified as it passed through the cooling coil) will have a very low RH by the time it is heated up to the required level.

Humidifier

This provides water in order to raise the RH of the passing air to the required level. There are several ways of introducing water into the air:

- by spraying it directly from jets;
- by atomising the water to create an aerosol; for example by directing a jet of water at a spinning disc;
- by introducing steam from a bath or lance.

It should be noted that following the risks associated with Legionnaire's disease, so-called 'humidifier fever' and other problems associated with high humidity and wetness inside ductwork maintained at around room temperature the spraying and atomizing methods have fallen from favour. Direct injection of steam from a lance at least ensures that the water supplied is sterile. Nevertheless, care needs to be taken to ensure that the likelihood of condensation occurring downstream of the steam lance/s is minimised.

Fan section

This is the part of the AHU which houses the fan. The latter is often mounted on a sprung platform which minimises the transmission of vibration and noise from the motor to the casing of the AHU and surrounding atmosphere. For similar reasons there is usually a flexible, vibration-absorbing joint between the fan and the downstream ductwork.

HEPA filter

In many animal facilities, particularly those in which the aim is to minimise the risk of undesirable organisms gaining access to the animals, e.g. barrier-maintained or SPF buildings, the supply air is passed through what are commonly referred to as 'absolute' HEPA (High Efficiency Particulate Air) or HESPA (High Efficiency Sub-micron Particulate Air) filters. In practice, because of their high resistance to airflow, such filters increase both capital and running costs of the air conditioning system. This is because a more powerful fan is required to push air through them and service life is reduced because they block up more quickly than those of a lesser efficiency; hence the need to 'protect' such expensive filters by the use of coarser filters upstream which remove the larger particles.

Because of their high resistance to airflow, it is again important to maximise the surface area available to the passing air so as not to reduce the ventilation rates. HEPA filters are usually very deep as the medium is packed into the frame in deep pleats (see Figure 32.5 (a) and (b)). Care must be taken when handling this type of filter as dropping one can break the air-tight seal between the filter medium and the frame in which it is supported.

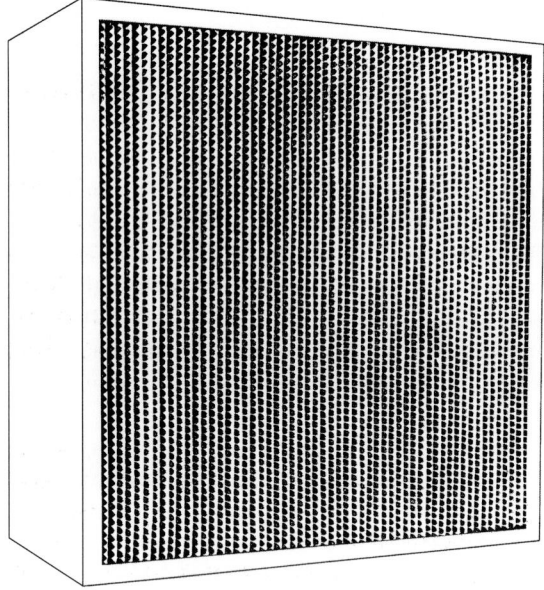

(a)

Figure 32.5 (a)   Typical HEPA filter panel.

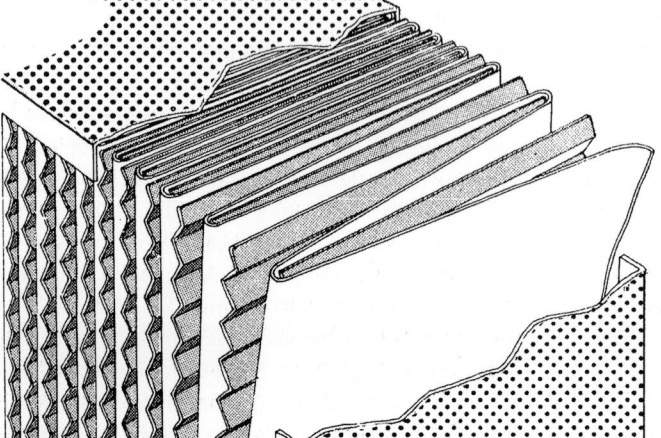

(b)

Unit selection damper

When a stand-by AHU is included in a facility, dampers are required to control which unit supplies air into the ventilation system. In a situation as illustrated in Figure 32.1 (see p. 267), only one of the two sets of unit selection dampers is open at any time. It is possible to have an automatic switching system included so that if the AHU in use fails, then the stand-by unit cuts in automatically and the relevant unit selection dampers open and close accordingly. In practice this situation is likely to arise only infrequently. Hence, in order to prevent the 'main' AHU wearing out well before the stand-by it is common practice for the maintenance schedule to include planned switching from one AHU to the other at regular intervals (e.g. monthly, three- or six-monthly) so that both units get an equal amount of wear.

Conditioned air ducts

The conditioned air is carried to the animal rooms through ducts. These may be made from metal, plastic, 'fibreglass' (GRP or glass reinforced plastic) or any other suitable material. Corrugated flexible trunking is commonly used to accommodate corners and joints between lengths of rigid ductwork. This is usually circular in section and consists of what looks like a very long coiled spring covered in flexible fabric.

While the ductwork at the plant-room end of the system is relatively large in cross section, it reduces in

Figure 32.5 (b)   Detail of pleated construction.

size as branches leave it to supply the various areas being conditioned. The ductwork may contain:

- dampers at various points along its length to direct and control air flow;
- gas-tight dampers (to bring into use when various areas of the building are being gas 'sterilised'), these may be manually or electrically operated;
- vanes to direct airflow and minimise turbulence (particularly at sharp bends in the ductwork);
- sound attenuating devices ('silencers') to reduce noise.

In working to achieve the desired level of environmental control it is important to bear in mind the following:

- All the factors mentioned above (including bends and the corrugated walls of flexible ducts) will increase turbulence, reduce airflow along the ducts and will have an effect on noise generation. Excessive noise in air conditioned buildings is very often caused by the ductwork being under-sized for the volume of air being pushed through it.
- As air moves through the ductwork, it is likely to lose its 'condition' – particularly when long distances are involved. Heat will be lost or gained depending on the temperature of the air surrounding the ductwork. This will, in turn, affect the RH. Hence long runs of ductwork usually have to be insulated to minimise this effect.
- Long runs similarly increase the risk of condensation occurring on the walls of the ductwork. This can result in increased maintenance problems. It is of particular concern where ductwork runs vertically so that any condensation is likely to fall back and pool at the bottom of the vertical run.

Terminal (booster) treatment; re-heat coil/s; local humidifier/s; terminal filter/s

As noted above (particularly in systems including long duct runs) the condition of the air is likely to deteriorate by the time it reaches its destination. Under such circumstances terminal treatment ('extra' treatment just before the air enters the animal room/s) will be required to 'top up' the T, RH and cleanliness to the required levels. If this is the case, then extra heating coils, humidifiers and filters will have to be installed within the ductwork just before it discharges into the animal room.

Such a system of terminal air treatment is often installed by choice rather than by necessity. This is because it makes it easier to control the conditions within individual animal rooms; especially important where species in adjacent rooms have different environmental requirements or where stocking densities are likely to vary considerably. The use of terminal filters can also help to reduce the risk of cross-contamination between rooms in case of a failure in the air supply caused by power, plant or any other breakdown.

Animal room/s – air distribution

As has already been noted the CoP (1989) recommends that, 'The air distribution system should deliver as even a proportion of air to each cage or animal as possible whilst avoiding draughts.' Bearing this in mind, as well as the cost and effort which goes into delivering conditioned air to an animal room, it is clearly important that having arrived there it should be distributed as effectively as possible. This matter is discussed in considerable detail by Clough (1999) with the conclusion that:

'Unfortunately it is not possible to recommend a specific air distribution layout which would be satisfactory for every animal room. This is because, to achieve maximum efficiency, the arrangement of the supply and exhaust points must be related not only to both the density and arrangement of the animals within the room but also to the size and shape of the room itself; all these factors are likely to vary.'

It is also concluded, however, that a system involving several air-distribution points within each room is likely to perform better than a system with a single air-supply point. This is confirmed by other workers using new computer-based technology to model airflow and heat transfer in rooms. This technique was used on a typical animal room to obtain predictions of the likely airflow patterns and temperature distribution. Hughes et al. (1996) then confirmed the computer predictions by carrying out tests on a full-scale model of the room. From this, they recommended the arrangement shown in Figure 32.6 as being the most satisfactory for general use in typical animal rooms; they defined a 'typical' animal room as being rectangular with the animal cage racks arranged along the long walls.

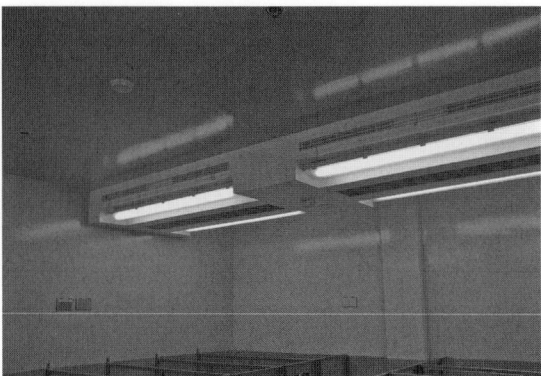

Figure 32.6   'Bulkhead' air distribution system recommended as the most satisfactory for use in typical rooms.

Animal rooms – local barrier systems

In connection with:

- the increasing use of 'clean' animals;
- the increasing use of immunologically comprom-ised and transgenic animals;
- the use of 'containment' facilities to protect per-sonnel from hazardous procedures (infectious, radioactive, toxic, carcinogenic, etc.);
- the need to protect staff from airborne allergens (aeroallergens) arising from the animals

there has been an increase in the development of technical devices aimed at increasing and main-taining greater separation between animals and staff. The correct operation of many of these has significant implications on the distribution of air in the rooms in which they are used. Such devices include the following.

Filter caps and bonnets

These are simple protective microbiological filters fitted to individual cages. The major problem likely to be encountered when using filter caps is the effect they can have on the micro-environment. This is because they reduce the ventilation of the cage result-ing in higher levels of temperature and RH as well as a build-up of carbon dioxide and ammonia. Indeed Serrano (1971) concluded that the increase in envir-onmental variability caused by their use could have a greater effect on experimental results than would the microbes they are designed to keep out! Conditions within filter top cages can be improved by blowing air over the filters, although the benefits derived from this will depend on a number of factors including:

- the stocking density of animals in the cage;
- the length of time since the cage was cleaned out;
- the surface area of the filter material;
- the density of the filter material and its resistance to airflow;
- the speed of the air blowing over it.

Environmental chambers

These are enclosed chambers designed to provide control of factors such as T, RH, air speed, air pres-sure, light and noise. These are most commonly used for experimental purposes.

Filter racks

A self-explanatory term used to describe any animal cage racking system fitted with a means of surround-ing the cages with clean air. They operate in a similar way to a clean bench or safety cabinet. That is, they take air from the room, filter it and then direct it around the cages. The air inside them is usually positive to that in the room, as they were first developed in order to protect clean animals from contamination.

Ventilated cabinets

These are enclosed, ventilated cabinets in which the cages are kept (see Figure 32.7). Such cabinets are most commonly used as containment systems with the air pressure inside negative to that of the air around them.

Individually ventilated caging systems (IVCs)

These can be very sophisticated, the rack itself acts as the air delivery and exhaust system (see Figure 32.8). They typically deliver high air change rates (often 50–100 ac/h) directly into each cage. Some can be operated under positive, negative or ambient pres-sure depending on the purpose for which they are being used. Some are reported to protect the animals from contamination whilst simultaneously protect-ing the personnel operating them from aeroallergens and other airborne contaminants arising from the animals.

Perhaps their most important facility is that their air supply and/or exhaust points can be connected directly to those of the room/s in which they are housed. Under these conditions (whereby cages

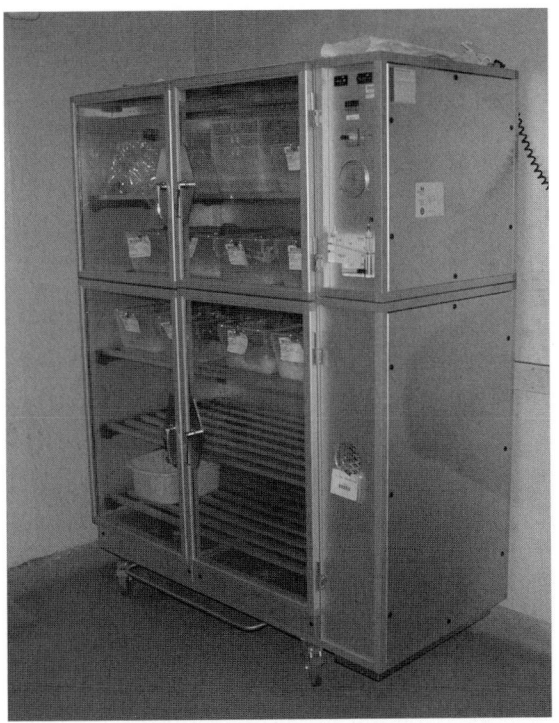

Figure 32.7 Example of a typical ventilated cabinet.

receive 50–100 ac/h but the room air change rate can be reduced to 4–8 ac/h) they can reduce the volumes of air required by up to 50% thus having a significant effect on both installation and running costs of the air conditioning system.

Cubicle systems

A cubicle, as the name suggests, is a small room or compartment often partitioned off from a larger room. All or some of the air may be supplied to the cubicle by a separate inlet but often it is merely drawn from the room itself by locating an exhaust duct in the ceiling of the cubicle so that it operates very much like a 'fume cupboard' (see Figure 32.9). Their use has been studied (Hessler 1991; Hughes 1994; Curry et al. 1998), the main conclusion being that they can be very useful in increasing by four to five times the number of animal housing spaces within a given area. It is worth noting that they are accepted by authorities such as the American Food and Drug Administration (FDA) and the UK and Japanese Good Laboratory Practice (GLP) regulators as a means of running several studies within a limited area. As with IVCs, their use requires careful planning because of their relevance to the distribution of air within the building.

Isolator systems

Probably the most reliable and effective form of local barrier is the flexible-film, germ-free isolator originally described by Trexler and Reynolds (1957; see also Trexler 1976) and primarily developed for the housing of gnotobiotes (Figure 32.10).

It should be noted that the same techniques can be used for the housing of SPF and other microbiologically defined animals. With appropriate modifications such isolators can also be operated under negative

Figure 32.8 Examples of racks with individually ventilated caging systems (IVCs).

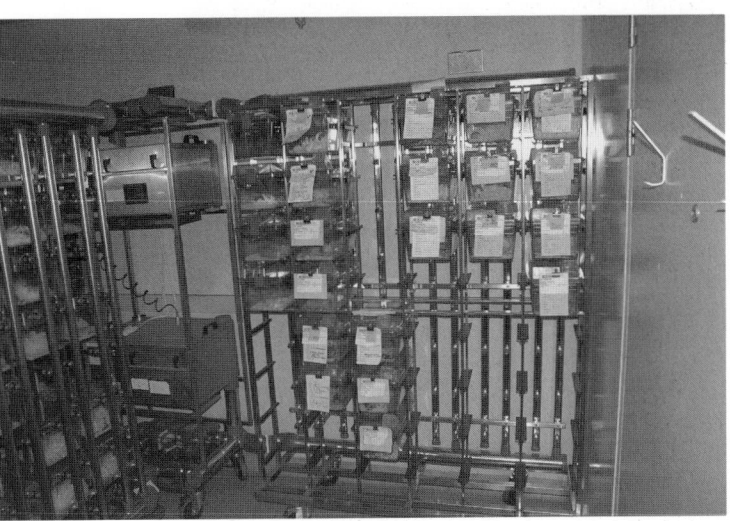

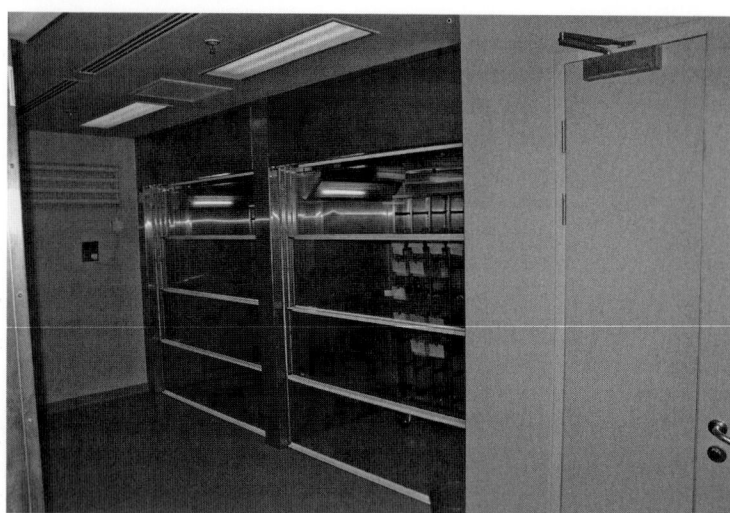

Figure 32.9 Typical cubicle system with vertically sliding sash 'doors'.

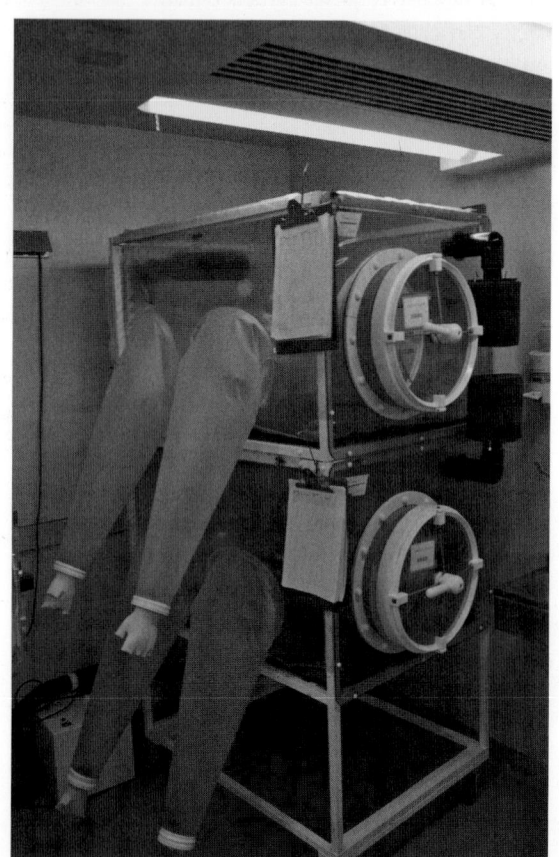

Figure 32.10   Flexible film isolator.

pressure. In these circumstances, the isolators can form a secure system for the containment of animals carrying various forms of hazard. Whilst such a system may initially appear expensive in both space and labour, for small-scale procedures it can provide a relatively cheap and practical solution, ensuring safety and unimpeded experimentation of a hazardous nature in what would otherwise be conventional animal accommodation.

If an isolator suite is to be created, as with all the other devices mentioned above, detailed consideration must be given to it in the early design stage so that appropriate provision can be made for the specialised air supply/exhaust system/s which will have to be provided. In the case of a 'hazard suite', it is advisable to contain the entire procedure, including cage washing and waste disposal or possibly pre-disposal treatments, within the containment area.

Environmental monitoring

Anyone involved in biomedical research should control at least those environmental factors which are most likely to influence the work being carried out. In most situations such work will, in any case, be controlled by regulatory authorities such as the UK Home Office, the FDA and GLP all of which make it incumbent upon users to ensure certain specified levels of control. This being so, it is strongly recommended that a quality control programme should be established to provide either continuous or periodic checks to ensure that the required standards are being met.

There are many instruments available commercially which are suitable for environmental monitoring and some of these are described below in Monitoring methods. There are also companies whose business it is to check those aspects of the environment which require more sophisticated instrumentation than is usually available in the average animal house. This applies particularly to such aspects as sound levels, air distribution efficiency and balancing of the ventilation system. With all monitoring techniques, it is important to establish standard methods of taking the measurements so that they are routinely comparable.

UK Guidelines require that air temperature and RH are monitored continuously in each animal room. Less frequent checks are required for areas such as photoperiod control, light intensity (including that in cages – particularly of albino animals) sound levels, ventilation rates and the efficiency of air distribution systems. Routine, preventative maintenance checks (with occasional specialist advice when necessary) should ensure that the air-conditioning system works according to specification. Particular attention should be paid to the condition of the filters. It is important to be aware that obstructing air supply or exhaust grilles with room furnishings and alterations in rack layout within a room can significantly alter air movement patterns.

Monitoring methods

Air temperature and relative humidity

The most popular way to monitor room temperature has been to use a maximum–minimum thermometer which is re-set every 24 hours. Monitoring RH has always been much more of a problem, for although checks can be made fairly simply with devices such as a whirling hygrometer, these only allow a spot check and give no indication of the rapid fluctuations in RH which can occur with changes in the weather and husbandry procedures such as floor washing and hosing down.

With recent advances in electronics, however, there are now a number of solutions to this problem. The simplest is a hand-held, digital thermohygrometer which can memorise the maximum and minimum of both factors over any period until the device is re-set. This can be used in exactly the same way as a max./min. thermometer but has the additional benefit that it also records the max./min. relative humidity as well.

This makes it ideal for use in individual rooms to ensure that the temperature and RH are staying within the guideline requirements. Such devices usually have an optional, plug-in external probe, which can be sited remotely from the meter. Some can also be linked into a central scanning device which will monitor the readings being input to each probe and give a warning when conditions go outside pre-set tolerances. Remember, however, that the sensors on these devices (particularly that for RH) are affected by dirt and moisture and can give misleading results.

For more detailed checking of the temperature and RH distribution within rooms to ensure, for example, that there are no undue fluctuations a data logging device will be required. These are available as mains or battery operated and are capable of logging the output from one or several T/RH probes at varying time periods. The memory can hold large numbers of records and so can usually be left running for several weeks before it becomes full. The printout can be formidable, however, with many thousands of numbers. For this reason the data from such devices is usually downloaded into a computer with suitable software and reproduced in graphic form which is much easier to understand.

Although there is an infinite number of points within an animal room from which recordings can be made, it is generally most useful and informative to put one probe in the supply air, one in the exhaust air and one each at the top and bottom of an animal rack. This can yield information about the adequacy (or inadequacy!) of the mixing of the air within the room as well as about the temperature and RH of the air around the cages in which the animals are living.

The sensitivity and accuracy of these devices depends largely on the quality of the sensors. Temperature is usually accurate to within $\pm0.5\ °C$. RH is less accurate, usually $\pm3\%$ RH between 40 and 60% RH but only $\pm5\%$ at higher and lower levels of RH.

Ventilation

Probably the most common method used to assess ventilation rates is to measure the volume of air being delivered to or removed from a room over a period. By comparing this with the volume of the room the

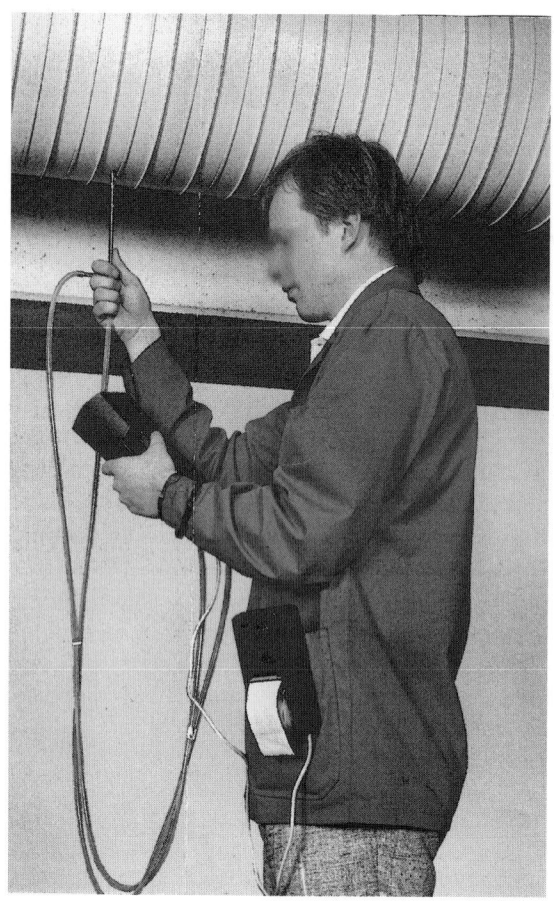

number of air changes per hour can be calculated. One method frequently used to determine such volumes is to use a manometer with a Pitot tube inserted into the air stream in the ductwork through sampling points specifically provided for this purpose (see Figure 32.11).

Using this technique, it is necessary to take the average of several readings inside the ductwork in order to allow for the variation in speed across the duct due to the drag effects of the duct walls. The proximity of bends, dampers, sound attenuators or other devices within the ductwork will all affect the readings and these must be taken into account when interpreting the results.

Another common method is to use a wind vane or hot-wire anemometer. The former is basically a propeller linked to a meter calibrated to convert its rotational speed to linear air speed. The latter relies on the cooling effect of air moving over a heated wire to act as the sensor, again linked to a meter to convert the temperature change to the corresponding air speed. Either of these can be used to determine the average speed of air entering/leaving the supply/exhaust grille(s) in a room and this is converted mathematically to a volumetric measurement.

Both methods are very prone to operator error as well as to errors which can easily be introduced by the geometry of the ductwork and grille face(s). Such methods rarely give better than ±10–15% accuracy,

Figure 32.11   Taking a reading of air speed in ductwork using a Pitot tube.

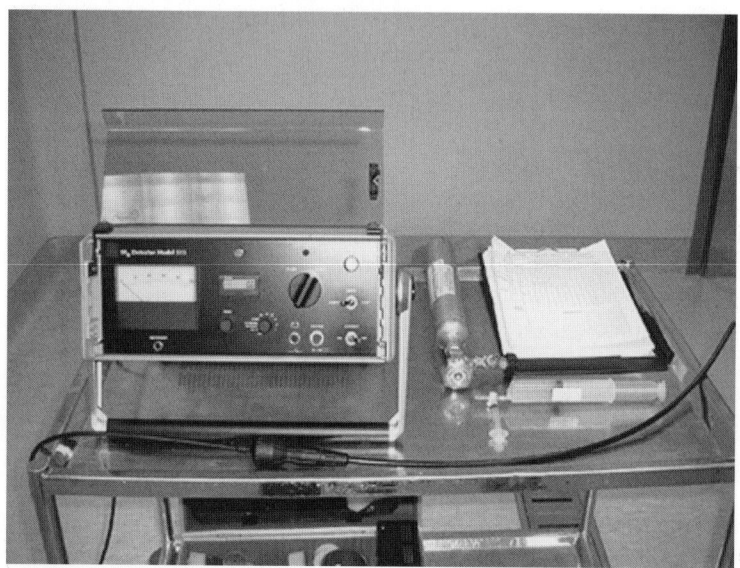

Figure 32.12   An SF$_6$ detector chromatograph ventilation rate meter.

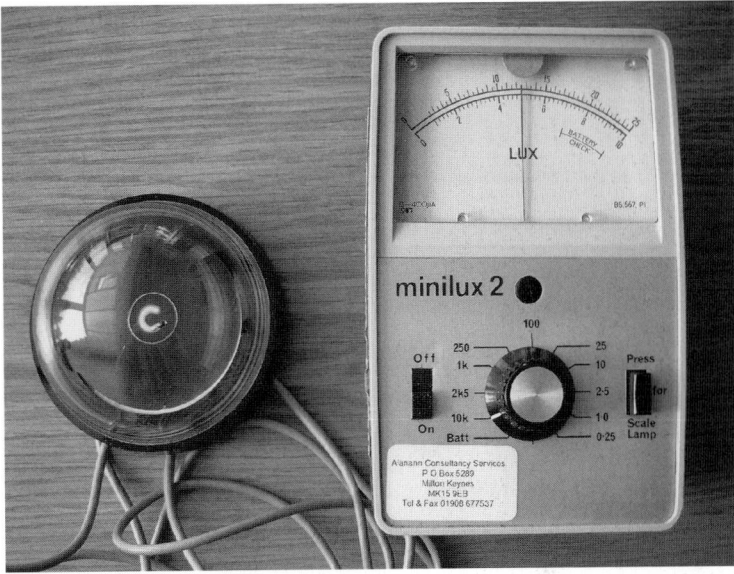

Figure 32.13 A typical light meter with colour-corrected cell.

though a carefully standardised technique helps in comparative measurements and can be useful for routine monitoring purposes.

A quicker method, which is considerably less prone to operator error, is to use an anemometer in conjunction with a 'hood' which fits over the supply/exhaust grille being measured. The anemometer and hood are pre-calibrated to provide a direct volumetric measurement of the air flowing through them. Again this must be compared with the room volume to give a calculated air change rate.

Even more accurate (can be as good as ±3–5%) is the Ventilation Rate Meter (VRM). This can be used to compare the ventilation rates within different parts of the same room and even within individual cages, provided it is used correctly. Because of this, it is currently the most practical device for assessing the efficiency of air distribution systems. It is a gas chromatograph specifically modified to detect a chosen tracer gas such as sulphur hexafluoride (SF_6) (see Figure 32.12).

The principle of operation is that a quantity of the tracer gas is released into the space to be measured. The rate of decay of the tracer, due to its removal with the ventilating air, is monitored over a timed period by the VRM. The rate of removal is, of course, correlated with the ventilation rate and this can be calculated from the results.

Although some years ago it was common to use a radioactive tracer, it is now much more common to use a non-radioactive gas such as SF_6. This has all the characteristics of the 'ideal' tracer gas. It is:

- not present in the atmosphere;
- colourless;
- odourless;
- tasteless;
- non-metabolisable;
- non-toxic;
- non-inflammable; and
- detectable in such small quantities (less than 1 part per billion) that in the average animal room it is only necessary to release about 0.5 cc; this means it can be used quite safely with animals and people in the room.

Light

The unit of illumination is the lux. It is possible to read a newspaper by moonlight at a level of < 5 lux, while a sunny day may provide illumination of 25 000 lux or more.

For absolute measurements, a properly calibrated meter, preferably with a colour-corrected sensitive cell suitable for all common types of artificial light is most useful (Figure 32.13). To allow for all circumstances likely to be found in animal rooms it should have a range from 0 to about 10 000 lux. It is usual to measure the light intensity 1 metre from the floor at the centre of the room. Further measurements can be made at a various points to give some indication of

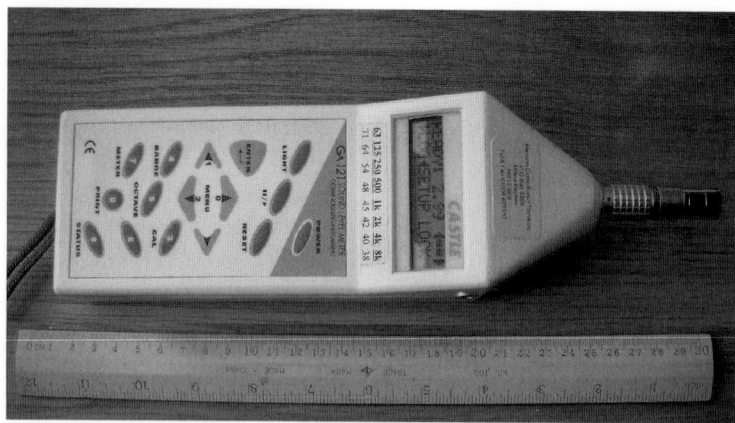

Figure 32.14 A typical integrating octave band sound level meter.

the variation in light intensity throughout the room. This can be very great, especially in rooms with windows, hence the need for the apparently high upper limit recommended.

Sound

The unit of sound is the Bel (it has a capital letter because it is named after Alexander Graham Bell, the inventor of the telephone). As an increase of 1 Bel represents a tenfold increase in sound intensity, however, the most commonly used unit is the decibel (dB), which is 1/10th of a Bel. The two aspects of any sound which are important in relation to hearing are its intensity (or loudness) which is measured in dB and its frequency (or pitch) which is measured in hertz (Hz) or cycles per second. The lowest note on a standard piano is 27.5 Hz and the highest 3520 Hz (3.52 kHz). The Greenwich mean-time 'pips' on the radio have a frequency of 1 kHz. Frequencies too low for humans to hear are referred to as infrasound, those too high as ultrasound.

Although the human ear responds to frequencies in the range 15–20 000 Hz the response is non-linear. Hence for a 100 Hz note to be heard at the same loudness as a 1 kHz note at 60 dB, the 100 Hz note needs to be at 66 dB. When sound levels are measured, this variation in the sensitivity of the human ear can be taken into account by incorporating weighting networks in the meter; these are termed A, B and C. Of these the A network is by far the most widely used and this is the meaning of the letter A in the unit dB(A) very often associated with sound level measurements.

Sound can be measured by its intensity in Watts per m^2 (W/m^2) but is more commonly measured by the pressure changes it causes in the air in Newtons per m^2 (N/m^2); hence the letters SPL which mean sound pressure level. Confusingly, a doubling of sound intensity at any point on the dB scale gives an increase of 3 dB; however, because sound pressure only doubles at half the rate that sound intensity does, a doubling in sound pressure at any point on the dB scale gives an increase of 6 dB. To add to the confusion, due to the peculiarities of the human ear, a subjective doubling of the loudness of any sound is represented by an increase of about 10 dB(A)!

Now, whereas so-called 'pure tones' consist of sound of only a single frequency (e.g. the Greenwich mean-time 'pips' at 1 kHz) most sounds consist of a variety of frequencies distributed throughout the frequency range; this is termed broadband sound.

Noise rating curves (NRC) and their American equivalent, noise criterion curves (NCC), were developed as a means of assessing the annoyance value of intrusive noises such as might interfere with normal speech. Such rating procedures are merely attempts to predict the likely response of a typical (human) population to such an intrusive sound. In order to establish an NRC, the meter used must be capable of measuring the frequency content of the sound over eight different octave bands. As a matter of interest, the highest frequency in an octave is twice that of the lowest. In NRC (or octave analysis) mode, what the meter does is to measure separately those parts of the broadband sound which occur in each of the eight frequency bands. The centre frequencies of these bands are 63, 125, 250, 500, 1000, 2000, 4000 and 8000 Hz. In other words, when the meter is measuring the sound content in the 1000 Hz octave band

Table 32.5   Examples of noise rating curves (NRC).

NRC Number	Octave band mid-frequency (Hz)							
	63	125	250	500	1 k	2 k	4 k	8 k
35	63	52	45	39	35	32	30	28
40	67	57	49	44	40	37	35	33
45	**71**	**61**	**54**	**48**	**45**	**42**	**40**	**38**
50	75	65	59	53	50	47	45	43
55	79	70	63	58	55	52	50	49

it automatically filters out all the other frequencies which are occurring simultaneously.

In order to achieve the UK CoP (1989) requirement of NRC 45, the dB level at each of the eight octave bands must not exceed those shown in Table 32.5 for NRC 45.

It is for this reason that the guideline requirements for sound demand fairly sophisticated sound measuring equipment. Figure 32.14 shows a typical sound level meter of the type required.

The measurement of sound levels is very prone to operator interference and it must always be remembered that different room dimensions and construction and the presence of other equipment (whether silent or not) can markedly affect the acoustics of the area being studied. It is important, therefore, when making sound measurements, to standardise the method of use, always holding the meter at the same distance from the body, in the same orientation and at a standard height from the floor. It is convenient in routine monitoring to have it 1 metre from the floor in the centre of the room as is used for standard light measurements.

Integrated systems

There is a variety of proprietary systems available which can be built into an animal house which will completely automate environmental monitoring. Some are modular in nature and can be extended as and when necessary by adding on new 'units' according to requirements. Most of these are custom-built at the time the building is constructed and usually link into a central, computerised, programmable, analysis, storage and control system, often forming part of the so-called BMS (building management system). Most of them can be arranged to monitor all the common factors at whatever frequency is selected by the user. Some of these systems have the drawback that they use the same sensors as a source of environmental data for monitoring purposes as are used to control the air-conditioning equipment. If such a twin-function sensor malfunctions this can lead to errors which may go undetected and it is clearly more satisfactory to have separate sensors related to control and monitoring functions.

Monitoring problems

With the right equipment, due care to the technical procedures involved and equal care in interpretation of the results obtained, environmental monitoring is not a difficult matter.

Conversely, some of the commonest problems relate to poor maintenance, poor technique (including poor or incorrect siting of sensors) and incorrect interpretation of data. An example will perhaps illustrate this point. At one establishment, it was the practice to monitor the ventilation rates of a group of six rooms by measuring the volumes of air being taken into the air-conditioning plant supplying them. A simple mathematical calculation (volume of air supplied divided by the volume of the rooms) provided the reassuring figure of 15 ac/h/room. A subsequent check on the air volumes actually entering/leaving each room, however, showed that the average air change rate was only 7–8 ac/h/room. This was due to a combination of severely clogged filters, inadequate seals around the filter mounts and badly leaking ductwork.

Those readers who use word processors will no doubt be familiar with the term WYSIWYG used to describe those devices where the output from the printer is exactly the same as the display on the screen; in other words, 'What You See Is What You Get'. In relation to environmental monitoring it is tempting to suggest another acronym WYMIOWYTYG meaning What You Measure Is Only What You Think You're Getting!

It should always be remembered that the reason for checking the environment is to ensure that the animals are being kept in appropriate conditions. Hence monitoring should, as far as possible and within the realms of practicality, always be carried out in the animals' rooms and as close to the animals as is reasonable – it is their welfare with which we are concerned.

Table 32.6 Relationship between currently published environmental requirements for the comfort and wellbeing of laboratory rats and mice.

Factor	Published range	Relevance to comfort and wellbeing
Temperature	$23 \pm 5\,°C$	Not likely to be stressful or have major adverse effects.
Relative humidity	$55\% \pm 15\%$	As above if achieved in cages. $55\% \pm 10\%$ (already adopted by some authorities) allows greater margin for removal of water from cages.
Ventilation rate (air changes/hour)	8–20	Not < 15 air changes/hour in fully stocked rooms probably satisfactory provided it is associated with efficient air distribution systems. New systems may allow fewer changes in rooms.
Light intensity	60–400 lux	350–400 lux satisfactory for staff working. Care needed to avoid retinal damage to albinos in upper cages.
Photoperiod	12 hours light:12 hours dark	Not likely to be stressful or have major adverse effects.
Wavelength		Lack of information on wavelength effects but no evidence that fluorescent or tungsten lights are disadvantageous.
Sound	~50 db(A), not > NRC 45 to < 85 dB	Current recommendations are all related to human ear function. This factor is the one most likely to give rise to discomfort and lack of wellbeing in these species

Conclusions

Table 32.6 summarises the relationship between the various physical factors we have discussed and the comfort and wellbeing of rats and mice and provides comments indicating that, although most of the available guidelines seem to be broadly acceptable, further data on most of the areas would be helpful in confirming or refuting this.

References

Anderson, J.D. and Cox, C.S. (1967) Microbial survival, pp. 203–206. In: P.H. Gregory and J.L. Monteith (Eds) *Airborne Microbes:* 17th Symposium of the Society of General Microbiology, Cambridge University Press.

Beys, E., Hodge, T. and Nohynek, G.J. (1995) Ovarian changes in Sprague-Dawley rats produced by nocturnal exposure to low intensity light. *Laboratory Animals*, **29:** 335–338.

Blood, D.C. (1976) Heating methods (pp. 247–276). In: T. McSheehy (Ed.) *Control of the Animal House Environment* (Handbook 7). Laboratory Animals, Huntingdon, UK.

Brader, W.R. and Sutter, J.W. (1988) Clean animal room HVAC systems. *Pharmaceutical Engineering*, **8:** 13–18.

Broderson, J.R., Lindsey, J.R. and Crawford, J.E. (1976) The role of environmental ammonia in respiratory mycoplasmosis of rats. *Am. J. Path.*, **85:** 115–130.

Bronson, F.H. (1979) Light intensity and reproduction in wild and domestic house mice. *Biol. Reprod.*, **21:** 235–239.

Clough, G. (1976) The immediate environment of the laboratory animal (pp. 77–94). In: T. McSheehy (Ed.) *Control of the Animal House Environment* (Handbook 7). Lab Animals, Huntingdon, UK.

Clough, G. (1982) Environmental effects on animals used in biomedical research. *Biol. Revs.*, **57:** 487–523.

Clough, G. (1984) Environmental factors in relation to the comfort and well-being of laboratory rats and mice (pp. 7–24). In: *Proc. Symp. Laboratory Animal Science Association and Universities Federation for Animal Welfare: 'Standards in Laboratory Animal Management'.* UFAW, Hertfordshire, UK.

Clough, G. (1999) The animal house: design, equipment and environmental control (pp. 97–134). In: T. Poole and P. English (Eds) *The UFAW Handbook on the Care and Management of Laboratory Animals* (7th edn), Vol. 1 Terrestrial Vertebrates, Blackwell Science, Oxford.

Clough, G. and Donnelly, H.T. (1984) Light intensity influences the oestrous cycle of LACA mice (pp. 60–64). *Proc. Symp. Laboratory Animal Science Association and Universities Federation for Animal Welfare: 'Standards in Laboratory Animal Management'.* UFAW, Hertfordshire, UK.

Clough, G., Wallace, J., Gamble, M.R. et al. (1995) A positive, individually ventilated caging system: a local barrier system to protect both animals and personnel. *Laboratory Animals*, **29;** 139–151.

Council of Europe (1986) European Convention for the Protection of Vertebrate Animals Used for Experimental and Other Scientific Purposes; Appendix A, Guideline for Accommodation and Care of Animals. Council of Europe, Strasbourg.

Cunliffe-Beamer, T.L. and Les, E.P. (1983) Effectiveness of pressurised individually ventilated (PIV) cages in reducing transmission of pneumonia virus of mice (PVM). *Laboratory Animal Science*, **33:** 495.

Curry, G., Hughes, H.C., Loseby, D. and Reynolds, S. (1998) Advances in cubicle design using computational fluid dynamics as a design tool. *Laboratory Animals*, **32:** 117–127.

Dauchy, R.T., Sauer, L.A., Blask, D.E. and Vaughan, G.M. (1997) Light contamination during the dark phase in 'Photoperiodically controlled' animal rooms: Effect on tumour growth and metabolism in rats. *Laboratory Animal Science*, **47 (5):** 511–518.

Donnelly, H.T. (1989) Effects of humidity on breeding success in laboratory mice (pp. 17–24). *Proc. Symp. Laboratory Animal Welfare Research – Rodents.* UFAW, Hertfordshire, UK.

Donnelly, H.T. and Saibaba, P. (1993) Light intensity and the oestrous cycle in albino and normally pigmented mice. *Laboratory Animals*, **27:** 385–390.

Ellis, D.H. and Follett, B.K. (1983) Gonadotrophin secretion and testicular function in golden hamsters exposed to skeleton photoperiod with ultrashort light pulses. *Biology of Reproduction*, 29: 805–818.

Ellison, G.T.H. and Westlin-van Aarde, L.M. (1990) Ringtail in the pouched mouse (*Saccostomus campestris*). *Laboratory Animals*, 24: 205–206.

Firman, J.E. (1969) Animal houses, part 2: Heating and ventilation of animal accommodation (Ch. 2). In: D.J. Short and D.P. Woodnot (Eds) *The IAT Manual of Laboratory Animal Practice and Techniques* (2nd edn). Crosby Lockwood Staples (Granada Publishing), UK.

Flynn, R.J. (1967) Notes on Ringtail in rats (pp. 285–288). In: M.L. Conalty (Ed.) *Husbandry of Laboratory Animals*. 3rd Intl. Symp. of ICLA. Academic Press, London.

Gamble, M.R. and Clough, G. (1976) Ammonia build-up in animal boxes and its effect on rat tracheal epithelium. *Laboratory Animals*, 10: 93–104.

Gärtner, K. (1990) A third component causing random variability beside environment and genotype. A reason for the limited success of a thirty-year-long effort to standardise laboratory animals? *Laboratory Animals*, 24: 71–77.

Gorn, R.A. and Kuwabara, T. (1967) Retinal damage by visible light. *Archs Opthal.*, 77: 115–118.

Greenman, D.L., Bryand, K., Kodell, R.L. and Sheldon, W. (1982) Influence of cage shelf level on retinal atrophy in mice. *Lab. Animal Sci.*, 32: 353–356.

Harper, G.J. (1961) Airborne micro-organisms: survival tests with four viruses. *J. Hyg., Camb.* (England), 59: 479–486.

Hemmes, J.H., Winkler, J.C. and Kool, S.M. (1960) Virus survival as a seasonal factor in influenza and poliomyelitis. *Nature*, 188: 430–431.

Hessler, J.R. (1991) Section 2.4: Animal cubicles (pp. 135–154). In: T. Ruys (Ed.) *Handbook of Facilities Planning* (Vol. 2). Laboratory Animal Facilities, Van Nostrand Rheinhold, New York.

Home Office (1989) *Code of Practice for the Housing and Care of Animals used in Scientific Procedures*. HMSO, London.

Home Office (1995) *Code of Practice for the Housing and Care of Animals in Designated Breeding and Supplying Establishments*. HMSO, London.

Hughes, H.C. (1994) The use of containment cubicle systems in preventing airborne cross-contamination (pp. 145–147). In: J. Bunyan (Ed.) *Welfare and Science*. Proc. of the Fifth Symp. Federation of Laboratory Animals Science Associations, London. Royal Society of Medicine Press, London.

Hughes, H.C. and Reynolds, S. (1995) The use of computational fluid dynamics for modelling airflow design in a kennel facility. *AALAS Contemporary Topics*, 34: 49–53.

Hughes, H.C., Reynolds, S. and Rodriguez, M. (1996) Designing animal rooms to optimise airflow using computational fluid dynamics. *Pharmaceutical Engineering*, **March/April**: 46–65.

Jilge, B. (1980) The response of the caecotrophy rhythm of the rabbit to single light signals. *Lab. Animals*, 14 (1) 3–5.

Melville, G.N. (1972) Water content level in inspired air: effects on specific airway resistance in rats. *Respiration*, 29: 127–134.

Miller, W.S. and Artenstein, M.S. (1967) Aerosol stability of three acute respiratory disease viruses. *Proc. Soc. Exp. Biol. Med.*, 125: 222–227.

Njaa, L.R., Utne, F. and Braeckkan, O.R. (1957) Effect of relative humidity on rat breeding and Ringtail. *Nature*, 180: 290–291.

Porter, G., Lane-Petter, W. and Horne, M. (1963) Effects of strong light on breeding mice. *J. Anim. Tech. Ass.*, 14: 117–119.

Price, E.O. (1976) The laboratory animal and its environment (pp. 7–23). In: T. McSheehy (Ed.) *Control of the Animal House Environment*, (Handbook 7). Lab Animals, Huntingdon, UK.

Sales, G.D., Milligan, S.R. and Khirnykh, K. (1992) *The Acoustic Environment of Laboratory Animals: A Survey of Ambient Sound Levels with Particular Reference to High Frequency Sound* (p. 79). UFAW, Hertfordshire, UK.

Schlingmann, F., Pereboom, W.J. and Remie, R. (1993) The sensitivity of albino and pigmented rats to light. A mini review. *Animal Technology*, 44: 71–85.

Schulman, J.L. and Kilbourne, E.D. (1962) Airborne transmission of influenza infection in mice. *Nature*, 195: 1129–1130.

Serrano, L.J. (1971) Carbon dioxide and ammonia in mouse cages: the effect of cages, covers, population and activity. *Lab. Animal Sci.*, 21: 75–85.

Stötzer, H., Weisse, I., Knappen, F. and Seitz, R. (1970) Die Retina Degeneration der Ratte. *Arzneimittel-Forsch.*, 20: 811–817.

Totton, M. (1958) Ringtail in newborn Norway rats – A study of the effect of environmental temperature and humidity on incidence. *J. Hyg., Camb.* (England), 56: 190–196.

Trexler, P.C. (1976) The development of isolators. *Postgrad. Med. J.*, 52: 545.

Trexler, P.C. and Reynolds, L.I. (1957) Flexible film apparatus for the rearing and use of germfree animals. *Appl. Microbiol.*, 5: 406.

Van der Veen, J., Poort, Y. and Birchfield, D.J. (1972) Effect of relative humidity on experimental transmission of Sendai virus in mice. *Proc. Soc. Exp. Biol. Med.*, 140: 1437–1440.

Weihe, W.H., Schidlow, J. and Strittmatter, J. (1969) The effect of light intensity on the breeding and development of rats and golden hamsters. *Int. J. Biometeorol.*, 13: 69–79.

Weisse, I., Stötzer, H. and Seitz, R. (1974) Age and light-dependent changes in the rat eye. *Virchows Arch. Path. Anat. Physiol.*, 362: 145–156.

White, B. (1991) Section 7.3: Mechanical systems (HVAC) (pp. 308–320). In: T. Ruys (Ed.) *Handbook of Facilities Planning* (Vol. 2). Laboratory Animal Facilities, Van Nostrand Rheinhold, New York.

Yamauchi, C., Obara, T., Fukuyama, N. and Vedi, Y. (1989) Evaluation of a one-way air flow system in an animal room based on counts of airborne dust particles and bacteria and measurements of ammonia levels. *Lab. Animals*, 23: 7–15.

33

Disease

Stephen W. Barnett and R. Ian Porter

Introduction

Care routines carried out in experimental units include measures designed to keep animals free from disease. The reason for this effort is obvious, animal disease causes suffering, invalidates experimental results, leads to economic loss and can result in human disease. Control of disease is therefore essential. A knowledge of the principles of the disease process enables early identification of specific conditions and can assist in devising protocols to eliminate them from the unit.

Disease may be defined as, 'any condition which interferes with the normal well-being of an animal'. Diseases are divided into two major groups depending on their causes, which are either infectious or non-infectious.

Infectious disease

An infectious disease is one that is caused by a specific, pathogenic agent capable of being trans-mitted from one individual to another by direct or indirect means. Where transmission is by direct contact the disease is said to be contagious. The agents responsible for infectious disease are viruses, bacteria, fungi, protoctista, invertebrate parasites and prions.

Non-infectious diseases

Non-infectious diseases are those which cannot be attributed to an infectious agent, examples of these are given in Table 33.1.

Stress

An important component of disease is stress. It can occur for a variety of reasons, for instance:

- environmental change – high stocking densities, noise, transport;
- experimental procedures;
- as a result of infectious disease.

Table 33.1 Examples of non-infectious disease.

Cause	Description	Example
Nutritional	Insufficient or excessive supply of one or more nutrients, imbalance of nutrients	Obesity, avitaminosis (see Chapter 26 on Nutrition)
Metabolic	Failure of normal metabolic processes	Hypocalcaemia, pregnancy toxaemia
Genetic	Genetic mutations which may be inherited from parents	Hydrocephalus, immune deficiency
Chemical	Variety of conditions caused by contact with harmful chemicals	Poisoning, chemical burns, mutation
Trauma	Physical damage	Fight wounds, broken limbs, surgical wounds
Environmental change	Adverse alteration of the physical environment	Extremes of temperature, low humidity, noise
Radiation	Exposure to ionising or non-ionising radiation sources	Burns, damage to DNA causing tumours, death if dose is high enough.

Stress is a perfectly normal reaction to unusual or potentially threatening situations. The initial response is one referred to as the 'fright, fight and flight' response, initiated by stimulation of the sympathetic nervous system and the release of adrenalin and noradrenalin from the adrenal medulla. In time, a further group of hormones is released from the adrenal cortex (mineralocorticoids and glucocorticoids) which help to return the body to normal.

Stress becomes a problem when the stressors persist and the body is exposed to the hormones long term. Blood pressure, metabolic rate and heart rate remain elevated. In addition, one of the functions of glucocorticoids is to switch off the inflammatory response when there is no need for it, thus preventing damage to healthy tissue. However if stress is caused by an environmental stressor, such as overcrowding or transport, and an animal is then exposed to an infectious organism, the elevated glucocorticoid levels can impair the response of the immune system and so lower resistance to the disease.

Animals cope with stress in various ways and some are common when an animal is sick or in pain. They include:

- overeating or refusing food;
- lack of grooming or excessive grooming;
- isolation;
- aggression;
- stereotypies (stereotypy is a repetitive behaviour pattern with no obvious purpose); examples of this are:
  — pacing: where animals walk up and down along exactly the same path for long periods
  — tumbling: where animals tumble repeatedly, placing their feet and hands in the same place with each tumble;
  — bar chewing.

Single or multiple disease factors

Sometimes disease is caused by a single infectious or non-infectious factor, but more often it is caused by a number of factors acting at the same time e.g.:

- a mouse may inherit a susceptibility to audiogenic seizure but it is not until it is exposed to a particular environmental stimulus that it will exhibit the condition;

- an adverse environmental condition which puts an animal under stress will impair its immune system and will therefore increase the likelihood of infection leading to disease;
- ammonia in the air, produced by the breakdown of nitrogenous compounds in urine, will damage cells lining the respiratory tract which reduces the ability of the body to resist invasion by infectious organisms;
- stress is evident in all disease conditions.

Diseases of unknown aetiology

Occasionally, the exact cause of a disease is not clear; for example it may be caused by an infectious agent but the precise one has not been identified. These are classified as diseases of unknown aetiology.

The effect of age on the development of disease

Animals are at more risk from certain conditions at specific ages, e.g. very young or very old animals, are more likely to be affected by infectious disease. Arthritis and cardiovascular disease are more commonly seen in old animals than those of younger age.

Infectious agents which cause disease

Bacteria

Bacteria belong to the kingdom Prokaryotae, they are small, primitive, single-celled organisms which consist of a protoplast surrounded, in all cases except the *Mycoplasmas*, by a cell wall. The cell wall contains a mucopeptide which gives it rigidity. Some bacteria contain large amounts of mucopeptide (above 50%) others have low amounts (less than 10%). The two types of cell wall can be identified by the Gram staining reaction. Those with small amounts of mucopeptide are classified as Gram negative and those with large amounts are classified as Gram positive. This distinction is an important aid to identifying bacteria.

In bacteria, the nuclear material is a single, circular chromosome which is not separated from the rest of the protoplast by a nuclear membrane; this feature distinguishes them (Prokaryotes) from other organisms (Eukaryotes) in which there is a nuclear membrane. Bacteria have a wide variety of modes of life: only a very few of them seriously compromise animal health. Some are capable of utilising simple inorganic molecules (autotrophic bacteria) using either the energy of external chemical reactions, or solar energy; all of the pathogenic types need a source of organic carbon and nitrogen and may have specific requirements for other nutrients. Many bacteria, like mammals, require a supply of oxygen (aerobic bacteria). Others, however, stop multiplying when oxygen is present (anaerobic bacteria). A few bacteria, called facultative anaerobes, are capable of surviving and multiplying in both aerobic and anaerobic conditions.

The shapes of bacterial cells are few: there are spheres, straight rods, curved and spiral rods, a few are filamentous (Figures 33.1, 33.2). Dimensions vary between 1 μm and 10 μm, so a large bacillus (rod) might be 10 μm long and 2 μm in diameter, while a small coccus (sphere) may be as small as 1 μm in diameter. The *Mycoplasmas*, are even smaller than this, being approximately 0.3 μm.

The cell wall of most pathogenic bacteria (those capable of causing disease) is supplied with a means of attachment to other cells. Usually the attachment is via thin protoplasmic extensions called fimbriae. Some bacteria have one or more long, hair-like structures called flagella which allow them to swim. A number of species of bacteria produce a mucilaginous capsule outside the cell wall which hinders the destructive action of phagocytes and antibodies. Two bacterial groups (the *Clostridia* and *Bacillus*) withdraw their protoplast inside a protective spore when conditions become less than ideal. The spore is capable of withstanding highly adverse conditions for long periods.

Most bacteria are capable of multiplying very rapidly by simple fission and can increase their numbers logarithmically (double their numbers per unit time) under ideal conditions. Some can also reproduce sexually by a process called conjugation. Some fimbriae develop into sex fimbriae which connect to other bacteria and provide a route for DNA to be transferred. The DNA exchanged in this way does not come from the main chromosome but is an extra store found in structures called plasmids. Antibiotic and disinfectant resistance can be passed from one bacterium to another by conjugation.

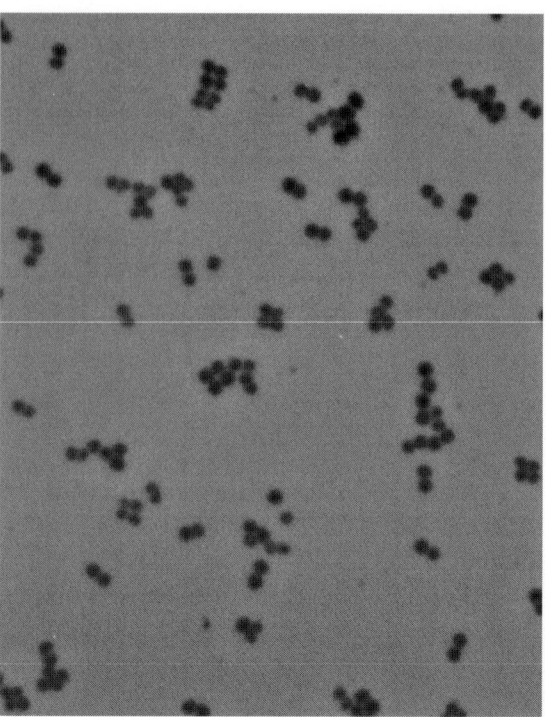

Figure 33.1 Slide showing cocci in different arrangements: (a) diplococci (pairs); (b) staphylococci (bunches); (c) streptococci (strings).

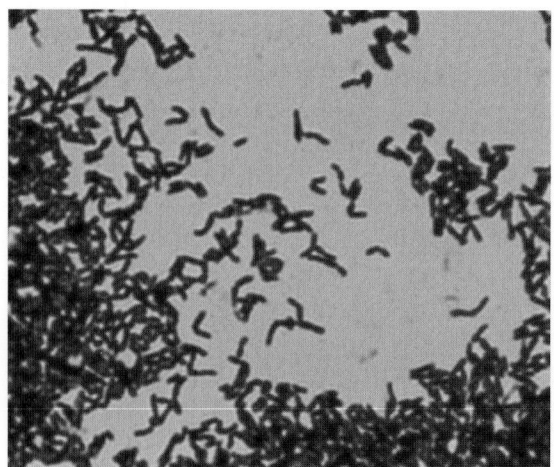

Figure 33.2 Bacilli.

Pathogenic bacteria have quite a narrow optimum range of environmental conditions. They multiply most rapidly at 35–40 °C. Temperatures below this slow down reproduction and at freezing point it usually stops altogether. Higher temperatures also slow down reproduction, but at 65 °C most of the cells die. Spores are much more resistant to heat although exposure to steam at temperatures of a minimum of 121 °C for fifteen minutes will destroy most of them (see Chapter 29).

Examples of bacterial diseases

Salmonellosis

Agent: *Salmonella enteriditis* (*typhimurium*); Gram negative, non spore-forming rod.
Hosts: rats, mice, guinea pigs, other rodents, primates. This organism is a zoonosis.
Route of infection: oral.
Clinical signs:

- *Acute*: anorexia, weight loss, dull coat, gastro-enteritis (but not always diarrhoea); in some cases conjunctivitis, enlarged liver and spleen causing abdominal distension.
- *Chronic*: anorexia, weight loss. Bacteria may remain in liver, spleen and lymph nodes and re-infect the intestines, e.g. by passing down the bile duct.

Pasteurellosis

Agent: *Pasteurella multocida*; non spore-forming, Gram-negative rod.
Host: rabbit.
Route of infection: aerosol or contact. Naso–pharynx is site of infection. Organism may lay dormant for long periods. Relatively common in conventionally housed rabbits. Outbreaks are more prevalent in summer and when ventilation is inadequate.
Clinical signs: different regions of the body are affected. The primary infection usually occurs in the upper respiratory tract and either stays there or spreads.

- Upper respiratory tract (snuffles or rhinitis) – noisy breathing, discharge of grey mucus around nose. Wiped off discharge may also be seen on medial aspect of fore leg.
- Lower respiratory tract – laboured breathing, breathlessness, lethargy. Fever in late stages (pneumonia).
- Conjunctivitis – eye inflamed, watery to creamy discharge (infection occurs via the nasolacrimal duct).
- *Otitis media* and *interna* (middle and inner ear inflammation) – head held to one side, unable to move in a straight line, loss of balance (infection occurs via Eustachian tube).

Mycoplasmosis

Agent: *Mycoplasma pulmonis*.
Hosts: rats and mice.
Route of infection: respiratory route, by contact. (There are other forms, including mycoplasmosis of genital organs where transmission is by venereal route.)
Clinical signs: chattering, respiratory distress, discharge from eyes and nose. Can develop into *otitis media*.

Anthrax

Agent: *Bacillus anthracis*; Gram-positive, spore-forming rod.
Hosts: all mammals including man.
Route of infection: contact with soil (usually through breaks in the skin or mucus membranes) or from eating contaminated animals.
Clinical signs:

- Peracute – very sudden onset. Staggering, respiratory distress, trembling, collapse, convulsion and death. Often the first sign that is seen is death (the dead animal will appear bloated with black discharges (blood) oozing from nostrils and anus).
- Acute – as peracute but is preceded by a rise in body temperature and a period of excitement followed by depression and cardiac distress. Pregnant animals may abort and lactation cease. A bloody discharge from anus may be present.
- Chronic – local lesions any occur in the throat and on the tongue. In some cases animals may survive a mild, chronic attack.
- Cutaneous – swellings in various parts of the body. This manifestation is seen when the organism lodges in skin abrasions.

Anthrax is classified as a notifiable disease under the Animal Health Act 1982. If the presence of a notifiable disease is suspected, the Department of Environment, Farming and Rural Affairs (DEFRA) must be notified by the quickest possible route. This usually means either informing a police officer or the divisional veterinary officer. A list of notifiable diseases can be found on the DEFRA website (www.defra.gov.uk).

Action that should be taken: the dead animal and all contacts must be isolated. Entry on to the land must be prevented. Quarantine, disposal of the carcass and cleaning procedures must be carried out as directed by DEFRA veterinary officers.

Viruses

Viruses are non-living entities. They consist of a strand of nucleic acid which is protected by an array of protein molecules, normally arranged in a symmetrical way. Sometimes the protein coat, called the capsid, is surrounded by a membrane or envelope. Viruses are much smaller than bacteria, ranging from 10 nm to 300 nm in size. They are incapable of multiplying outside living cells. When a virus attacks a cell it usually attaches itself to the cell membrane so that its nucleic acid can pass into the cell. The viral nucleic acid then takes over the synthetic mechanisms of the host cell and programmes it to produce viral nucleic acid and viral protein. New virus particles are released by sudden rupture of the host cell or by gradual release through the host cell membrane.

Examples of diseases caused by viruses

Sendai virus
Agent: Sendai is a paramyxovirus.
Hosts: mice, rats, hamsters and guinea pigs.
Route of infection: aerosols (finely disseminated droplets) or contact.
Clinical signs: these vary with species and strains. Rats, hamsters and guinea pigs are usually asymptomatic. Some strains of mice are also very resistant to the disease. Susceptible mice strains show staring coat, laboured breathing, rapid weight loss. Death follows in severe cases. There is a high mortality in pre-weaner mice.

Parvovirus
Agents: Canine parvovirus.
Hosts: dogs.
Route of infection: oral route.
Clinical signs (in dogs): can affect all dogs, but puppies are more susceptible. Dehydration, lethargy, diarrhoea (haemorrhagic), vomiting. Pain in anterior abdomen. Body temperature is normal to subnormal in adults, very high in pups. Pups under eight weeks may die rapidly with heart failure and pulmonary oedema.

Fungi

Fungi are eukaryotic organisms which have a cell wall. Most fungi are saprophytes and live by digesting dead organic matter and absorbing the simple products of digestion. Some can be pathogenic. Parasitic fungi behave in a similar way except that they penetrate and digest living or dead tissue on the body (skin and claws).

The yeasts are single-celled fungi which reproduce asexually, and often respire anaerobically. Other fungi consist of a network of branching threads or hyphae which can spread through the substratum on which they live and feed. The network is known as the mycelium. Sometimes the hyphae are divided into individual cells by cross-walls, but frequently there are no cross-walls and the mycelial strands are filled with multi-nucleate cytoplasm called a syncytium. From time to time, a form of sexual reproduction takes place. Sporangia are formed, in which the spores which will enable the dispersion of the fungus will develop.

Example of fungal diseases

Ringworm
Agent: *Microsporum* sp. and *Trycophyton sp.* (among others).
Host: all mammals.
Route of infection: skin, on contact with an infected animal or fungal spores.
Clinical signs: these may vary slightly with each species but generally include facial dermatitis, circular areas of alopecia, may involve feet. Infection may be self limiting or persist for years. To control this organism it is necessary to isolate infected animals, and clean the environment (spores can exist up to thirteen months off host).

Prions

Prions are abnormal proteins which can be passed from animal to animal. They appear to have the ability to affect normal proteins altering their structure, resulting in a breakdown of normal tissues. They affect the brain and cause the normal brain architecture to be destroyed resulting in gaps, giving a sponge-like appearance when observed under the microscope. Prions are associated with a group of diseases called transmissible spongiform encephalopathies (TSEs) which include scrapie in sheep, bovine spongiform encephalopathy (BSE) or 'mad cow disease' in cattle and Creutzfeldt–Jakob disease in humans. The disease does not occur normally in small laboratory animals but a great deal of research is being carried out on these agents and many mice and others rodents are experimentally infected.

Unlike normal proteins, prions are very resistant to chemical and heat treatments. When used experimentally animals must be housed in Category 4 isolation units.

Invertebrate parasites

Invertebrate parasites are major causes of disease in animals and are dealt with in Chapter 34.

Transmission of infectious disease

Infectious organisms can be transferred from an infected animal to the environment of a healthy one by the following routes.

Transmission by animals

A pathogenic organism grows and reproduces in an infected animal and is shed by that animal. If it is brought into contact with an uninfected animal, particularly one which has been reared in the microbiologically clean surroundings of an experimental animal unit, the infection will be passed on readily.

The signs of infection may be obvious or *overt*, in which case it should be possible to be identify its presence before the animal is brought into the animal unit. Alternatively the clinical signs of infection may not be apparent, in which case it is said to be a *latent* infection; the organism may be incubating in the animal and will develop into overt disease in a short time. Isolating animals in quarantine units for a period before allowing them to come into contact with other animals in the unit ensures animals incubating infections will not bring them into the unit. In some cases latent infection never develops into overt disease, but the organisms continue to reproduce and use the infected animal as a means of dispersal. Such animals are called *carriers*.

Wild and feral animals may be carriers, as they harbour a number of organisms to which they have developed immunity but which would cause serious illness in animals reared in a microbiologically clean experimental animal unit.

Transmission by vectors

Vectors are animals which transmit infectious organisms but are not affected by them. Humans can act as vectors of animal disease organisms, bringing them into the unit on their clothes and bodies. Changing into dedicated work clothes and good personal hygiene counteract this mode of introduction and spread.

Other examples of vectors are fleas, mosquitoes and ticks, all of which puncture the skin of animals to feed off blood and can transmit organisms directly into the circulatory system. Arthropods can also act as vectors of eggs of invertebrate parasites such as tapeworms. Filtered air conditioning and the use of insectocutors limit the entry of these vectors. Wild birds and vermin can also act as vectors and should be excluded from animal facilities.

Transmission by fomites

Fomites are inanimate objects capable of absorbing and transmitting disease organisms. Common fomites are food, water and bedding.

Transmission by intermediate hosts

Intermediate hosts are animals in which parasites must spend time in order to complete their life cycle. They are distinguished from the definitive host which is the host in which the parasite reaches sexual maturity. Transmission of disease by means of an intermediate host is an important factor if animals are kept outdoors (e.g. see Liver fluke, p. 298).

Transmission of infectious disease between human and animals

We have already considered humans acting as vectors of animal disease organisms but humans can also transmit their own diseases to animals. An example of this is human influenza which can be transmitted to and cause disease in ferrets.

Routes of infection

Infectious organisms can be introduced into the environment of an animal by the means mentioned above but in order to cause disease they must enter the animal's body. There are a limited number of routes by which this can happen.

Oral route (also known as the alimentary route)

Pathogenic organisms are ingested when contaminated food and water are consumed, bedding chewed or when animals lick each other when grooming. Once ingested, the organism can penetrate the epithelial cells of the gut causing local damage, or gain access to the circulatory system, so causing more widespread disease. Some organisms stay in the gut and produce toxins which may pass into the blood and are circulated around the body (e.g. *Clostridium perfringens*).

Respiratory route

Organisms can be inhaled into the respiratory tract and cause respiratory disease or, in some cases can spread to cause more general clinical signs. Sneezing and coughing by infected animals discharges droplets containing pathogens into the air. Even if the droplets evaporate quickly the infectious organisms remain in the air to be carried on air currents. Finely disseminated droplets, called aerosols, can remain in the air for long periods and are spread over a wide area. Some are small enough to escape the defence mechanisms in the respiratory tract and get deep into the lower respiratory tract where even small numbers can cause damage.

Pathogenic organisms can be dispersed into the air in other ways, e.g. movement of animals in cages raises dust which may contain pathogens.

Integumentary or transdermal route

This involves the transmission of pathogens through the skin. The whole of the exterior of the body (including the eye which is protected by the cornea, a transparent, skin-like membrane) is covered by skin and is very resistant to infectious organisms. In order to pass into the body by this route the skin must be breached, this can happen in three main ways:

(1) infection of a wound, e.g. caused by fighting or other accidental trauma, by a hypodermic or tattoo needle, ear punch or surgeon's knife;
(2) infection by an arthropod bite (e.g. tick, mite, flea, louse) – many pathogens are transferred in the saliva of arthropods (although this is likely to be a rare occurrence in laboratory animal facilities);
(3) infection by an active parasite – a few pathogenic organisms are able to penetrate unbroken skin to gain entry into the circulatory system.

Venereal route

Infections contracted as a result of sexual contact.

Transplacental route

Although the placenta is often considered to act as a barrier to infection this is not always the case, several viruses are known to have the ability to cross from the maternal blood to foetal blood in the placenta giving rise to congenital infections. In addition some parasitic worms have a larval stage which is designed to break through the walls of blood vessels and many of these may cross the placenta into the unborn foetus (see *Toxocara canis*, Chapter 34).

Body defence mechanisms

Animals have a number of defence mechanisms which inhibit invasion by pathogens. These include:

- *Physical barriers*: skin is hard and dry which makes it difficult for most organisms to penetrate. Hair prevents some organisms gaining easy access to the skin and guards some orifices such as the nose. Wax in the ears prevents entry to the auditory canal.

- *Mechanical barriers*: the whole of the respiratory tract is lined with ciliated epithelial cells interspersed with mucus-secreting goblet cells. The mucus makes the surface sticky, trapping the invading organisms and contains natural antimicrobial chemicals such as antibodies. The cilia waft trapped particles up and out of the tract. In addition, the nasal cavity contains a twisted network of thin bones (the conchae or turbinate bones) covered with a mucous membrane which increases the surface area covered by the mucus. Epithelial cells which are infected may be shed (a process called desquamation) removing the pathogens together with the damaged cell which can be rapidly replaced.

- *Anti-bacterial secretions*: many body fluids contain chemicals which destroy or inhibit the activities of pathogens. Sweat, tears and tissue fluid contain lysozymes which damage bacterial cell walls. Sweat, gastric juice and vaginal secretions are acidic and sebum and sweat contain unsaturated fatty acids all of which damage micro-organisms.

- *Commensal competition*: populations of micro-organisms reside in the mouth, upper respiratory tract, digestive system, vagina and on the skin. These keep pathogenic organisms under control by competition for food.

Immune response

If pathogens overcome the physical and chemical barriers and gain entry to animal tissues then a series of reactions are initiated by macrophages and follow a cascade designed to eliminate the pathogens and repair the damage that they have done. Chemical messengers (cytokines) are triggered by pathogens affecting the cells they or their toxins damage. In turn these original 'target' cells also influence other cells through these messages.

Present in the blood are the components of three immune response systems:

(1) the kinin system which affects blood vessels;
(2) coagulation/fibrin system also affecting blood vessels;
(3) the complement system.

The complement system is the most important as it is essential to bind antibodies to antigens and to facilitate phagocytosis of the invading organisms. It is the means by which most bacteria trigger the immune response. This cascade of chemicals has a direct effect on the capillaries in the area and also releases components of the immune system such as histamine, which is released from mast cells, and triggers a group of substances called vasoactive amines which may cause a range of processes such as capillary dilatation, but also, at the more extreme level, anaphylaxis. The combined effect of these chemicals is to dilate and increase the permeability of local capillaries so that

more blood flows to the area and more tissue fluid and white blood cells can pass through the capillary walls to the infected area. The mediators direct phagocytic neutrophils and monocytes (which are called macrophages when they leave the blood vessels and enter the tissues) and enable them to attach to, engulf and digest the pathogen. The extra tissue fluid which reaches the area helps to dilute toxins produced by the pathogen and brings proteins, such as fibrin, which initiates repair of damaged tissue.

The increased flow of blood to the infected area causes it to become warm and red. Increased fluid accumulating in the tissues causes swelling and pain. These four conditions, redness, pain, swelling and heat, are referred to as the 'cardinal' signs of inflammation.

If all goes well these events and their sequelae, all produced by chemical messengers, will destroy the infectious organism, repair the damage and return the animal to normal. This series of reactions is part of the innate or non-specific immune reaction, they work no matter which organism/s are causing the infection.

Some organisms are able to escape the non-specific immune system and go on to cause serious disease. They do this in various ways. For instance they can block the release of complement and so reduce the ability of phagocytes to attach and digest them. Specific immune responses have evolved to cope with many of these organisms. In outline this involves lymphocytes producing specific molecules, one end of which attaches to the pathogen and the other end to phagocytes or other elements of the immune system. The two are thus anchored together, making it more difficult for the pathogen to escape destruction.

These molecules are called antibodies or immunoglobulins. They are generated when a pathogen is detected in the body. The first time the pathogen is encountered it takes a few days to manufacture antibodies but after that the immune system carries a memory of the pathogen and produces antibodies very rapidly.

Pathogenesis of infectious disease

The way in which an infectious disease develops in an animal depends on the nature of the infective organism, the route of infection, the scale of the infection and the characteristics of the animal infected.

Virulence and amount of infective agent

In order to cause disease an infectious agent has to overcome the defence mechanisms mentioned above; its ability to do this is known as its virulence. Different strains of the same pathogen may have different degrees of virulence. Virulence also varies with the state of the host; an agent that has little effect on a healthy adult animal could be extremely virulent in very young, very old or immuno-compromised ones.

Genetic differences in host strains can also influence the susceptibility of the strain to the disease. An example of this is seen with the pneumonia caused by Sendai virus in mice. In some mouse strains the mortality is extremely high (e.g. 129/ReJ) whereas other strains are hardly affected at all (C57BL/6J).

In addition to virulence, the numbers of pathogens present influences the ability of infective organisms to cause disease. Generally, the more virulent an organism the fewer of them are needed to cause disease, but even low virulence organisms may be dangerous if enough of them are present.

The words morbidity and mortality are used to describe the effect of a disease on an animal colony. Morbidity refers to the number of animals which become sick and mortality refers to the number which die from the disease. So a disease which has a high morbidity and high mortality means many of the animals contract the disease and a high proportion of these will die from it. High morbidity and low mortality means the disease is very infectious but is not usually fatal.

Spread of the pathogen within the host

Organisms differ in the way they spread and cause damage within an animal body. Some do not spread far, but remain and reproduce at the site they initially invaded; they may produce toxins which are distributed through the circulatory system. The spore-forming bacteria *Clostridium tetani* is an example of this type of agent. It enters the body through a wound in the skin and reproduces in the warm, anaerobic conditions under the scab which forms over the wound. The toxin it produces enters the blood and circulates around the body, interfering with the junction between nerves and muscles causing a permanent muscle contraction, an often fatal condition commonly known as 'lockjaw'.

Some organisms spread directly from cell to cell. They enter a cell then feed, grow, reproduce and burst out of the cell. Each new organism produced then enters a new cell and repeats the process. *Eimeria*, the protoctistan parasite, is an example of an organism which spreads in this way (see Chapter 34).

Other organisms spread through the lymph and circulation system. They gain entry to the body and begin to reproduce, and are carried by the lymph to the local lymph nodes. In small-scale infections the phagocytic cells which colonise the lymph nodes usually destroy the organisms, but in heavy infections they escape destruction, pass through the lymph system and drain into the blood circulatory system. They are carried to internal organs such as the liver and spleen, where they undergo further reproduction, killing cells of the organs in the process and causing areas of necrosis (cell death). These additional pathogens also enter the circulatory system and some reach their target organ, that is the organ from which they can leave the host they are inhabiting so they can easily infect another animal. Organisms such as the bacteria *Salmonella* often target the intestines and pass out with faeces, whereas the virus Ectromelia (mouse pox) targets the skin and leaves the host through skin eruptions.

During the period of reproduction and spread, the host's immune system is operating and the progress of the disease depends on the effectiveness of the pathogen in escaping destruction. Other, less common, paths of spread include the nerves and nervous system (e.g. rabies) and the cerebrospinal fluid.

Terms used to describe disease

A number of terms are used to describe disease; some examples of these are explained in Table 33.2.

Control of disease

Prophylactic measures

The most satisfactory means of controlling disease is to prevent it entering an animal unit. Prophylaxis is the word used to refer to any measure which prevents an animal contracting a disease. It includes the

Table 33.2 Terms used to describe disease.

Acute disease	Disease with rapid onset and rapid resolution (either recovery, death or development to chronic disease).
Chronic disease	Disease of long duration.
Peracute disease	Very rapid onset.
Sub-clinical	Disease organism is present but at a level too low to cause identifiable clinical signs.
Sub-acute	Moderately rapid and severe.
Sequelae	This word derives from Latin and means 'to follow'. It relates to the pathological consequences of disease. In some cases tissue repair is complete following disease leaving no lasting effects. In other cases the disease leaves lesions which affect the organ permanently, e.g. mycoplasmosis causes damage to the lung which may not repair. The most drastic sequela is death.

barriers mentioned in Chapter 30, routine cleaning, sterilisation, disinfection.

Programmes of vaccination and worming are important prophylactic measures. Dogs, cats, ferrets and farm animals can be vaccinated against diseases considered a danger; they may also be given anthelmintics to protect them from endoparasites. Although vaccinations are available for some rodent and lagomorph diseases the practicalities and cost of vaccinating large numbers of small animals precludes their use in most cases.

Vaccinations may have an influence on experimental results in some types of studies therefore they should only be used in consultation with the scientist and the named veterinary surgeon.

Therapeutic measures

If animals do contract infectious disease a decision has to be made whether to treat it or not. The disease itself, or administration of treatment, may influence experimental results, in which case the animal may need to be withdrawn from the study. Animals may be sensitive to some drugs, for instance guinea pigs and hamsters are intolerant of many antibiotics. Antibiotics may improve the condition of one animal but the animal may continue to shed infectious organisms and therefore may be a source of infection to other animals. Infectious disease can spread rapidly in situations where large numbers of animals are housed together, so in many laboratory animal units it may be impractical to treat large numbers of animals. However, some conditions are relatively easily treated, e.g. pin worm infections of mice are often treated with drugs.

Radical measures

Where infectious disease cannot be prevented or treated, an individual animal may have to be killed to prevent it suffering or infecting other animals. In some circumstances the whole colony may have to be killed and the affected area decontaminated using sterilisation and fumigation techniques. However these measures are of no use unless the route by which the infection entered the colony is identified and blocked.

Radical measures are expensive in terms of animal welfare, life and economic cost; they are only used where no other measures are possible. They are rarely warranted in minimal barrier units unless the disease organism is a zoonosis.

It is part of the role of the named veterinary surgeon to advise on the use and effects of prophylactic, therapeutic and radical measures to control disease.

Zoonoses

A zoonosis is a disease which may be transmitted from animals to man. Zoonoses, therefore, present a hazard to all who work with animals and care must be exercised in dealing with them. These hazards present themselves in two ways:

- animals which are known to be infected with dangerous pathogens, either because they have been diagnosed to have contracted a disease, or because they have been deliberately infected as part of an experimental regime;

- animals whose microbial status is unknown and which could be infected with dangerous pathogens (newly arrived, wild-caught animals present the greatest risk in this respect).

When a disease is transmitted from an animal to a human, there are three possible outcomes:

- The disease may present the same signs and symptoms, and follow the same course in the human as it does in the animal.
- The disease may present a serious and life-threatening syndrome in the animal, but cause only mild, if any, symptoms in the human, causing little or no problem.
- The disease may be a mild and unimportant infection in the animal, but cause a serious, debilitating and possibly fatal syndrome in humans.

Many pathogens are host-specific, or nearly so, so are unlikely to cause problems in humans, but pathogens which do not demonstrate any specificity are likely to be hazardous. Diseases of non-human primates present particular risks. Because of the close evolutionary relationships between humans and other primates, they have many diseases in common, and any organism which is pathogenic in the monkey is likely to be pathogenic in the human also. This is reciprocal – laboratory primates may come into contact with human diseases which are capable of affecting them adversely.

In general, people handling animals should always be aware of the risk attendant on handling and working closely with laboratory animals. Precautions which should be taken are:

(1) a high standard of personal hygiene, e.g. washing hands after handling animals and especially before handling food;
(2) use of appropriate protective clothing;
(3) avoiding bites and scratches, using gauntlets if necessary;
(4) covering all skin abrasions with waterproof dressings;
(5) avoiding inhalation of potentially contaminated dust by using face masks and maintaining a dust-free atmosphere;
(6) it may be considered appropriate for high-risk staff to carry a card giving details of the animals with which they work, so that if a sudden illness occurs, medical practitioners will be assisted in diagnosis.

References and further reading

Fox, J.G. (Ed.) (1988) *The Biology and Diseases of the Ferret.* Lea & Febinger, Philadelphia, PA.

Fox, J.G., Cohen, B.J. and Loew, F.M. (1984) *Laboratory Animal Medicine.* Academic Press, Orlando, FL.

Laber-Laird, K., Swindle, M. and Flecknell, P. (1996) *Rodent and Rabbit Medicine* (Pergamon Veterinary Handbook Series). Elsevier, Oxford.

Roitt, I. (1991) *Essential Immunology* (7th edn). Blackwell Science, Oxford.

34
Parasitology

R. Ian Porter

Introduction

A parasite is an organism which forms a relationship with another organism, the host, on which it depends for all or part of its metabolic requirements. The relationship causes harm to the host while supporting the life of the parasite. In some cases, the parasite may have a complex life cycle in which it is dependant on two, three or more entirely different hosts at different stages in its development.

Parasites are commonly distinguished as:

- endoparasites, found inside the body of the host, in a body cavity, within the digestive tract or the host tissues; or
- ectoparasites, found attached to the outer surface of the host.

Characteristics of parasitism

The major problems facing parasites are:

- The harmful effect on the host: if a parasitic infection becomes very heavy, the host may die, and a parasite which kills its host could be considered to have failed.
- The difficulty of infecting new hosts: parasites which are completely dependent on the host usually have only a brief period during which they are infective.
- Living in a difficult and sometimes hostile environment: host tissues always react against the presence of the parasite and the parasite has to overcome these adverse reactions. In some cases the physiological needs of the parasite are not easily procured (e.g. most intestinal parasites have to survive in near anaerobic conditions).

Adaptations to the parasitic mode of life, whether total or partial parasitism, are of three kinds:

- *Structural adaptation*: The shape of the parasite is determined by its habits. Examples include the dorso-ventral flattening of lice to enable them to flatten themselves against the skin of the host; the large surface area of tapeworms which enables them to absorb digested food efficiently through the surface.

- *Physiological adaptation*: Modifications in metabolism enable them to cope with adverse conditions. Examples include the ability of most intestinal parasites to survive in conditions of very low oxygen concentration.

- *Reproductive adaptation*: The ability of many parasites to produce an enormous number of eggs, most of which will fail to reach maturity, e.g. the sheep liver fluke may produce up to 10 000 eggs per day. Many parasites are hermaphrodite and self fertile, so that reproduction is possible even when there is only a single parasite present in the host.

Endoparasites

The majority of endoparasites found in domestic and laboratory mammals belong to the Kingdom Protoctista or one of the following groups from the Kingdom Animalia:

- Phylum Platyhelminthes – flat worms, which include:
  — Class Trematoda – flukes
  — Class Cestoda – tapeworms;
- Phylum Nematoda – roundworms.

Kingdom Protoctista

The name of protozoa is often associated with this group of parasites. It has now fallen into disuse except as a non-taxonomic collective name for four of the phyla of protoctista: Rhizopoda, Zoomastigina, Apicomplexa and Ciliophora. Where the name is used it should always start with a lower case letter (IoB 1989).

Protoctists are primitive eukaryotic organisms consisting of a single cell without a cell wall. Most are free living, and totally harmless, but all protozoan phyla have some parasitic members. One phylum, the Apicomplexa (formally called Sporozoa), consists only of parasitic species.

Parasitic protozoans fall into three groups.

(1) *Enteric protozoa* infest the alimentary canal and its associated glands. They attack the cells lining the intestine (either the large intestine or the small intestine or both), or the cells of the liver. The parasitic amoebas, ciliates and flagellates have a simple life cycle, reproducing by fission and producing spores which are excreted in the faeces.

The enteric Apicomplexans (e.g. Coccidia) have a more complex life cycle, which includes alternating asexual and sexual phases. These organisms develop inside the cells they attack.

(2) *Blood protozoa* live in the blood, although they spend part of their life cycle in other cells, such as those of the liver. Some of these are Apicomplexans, with alternating sexual and asexual phases, but the Trypanosomes have a much simpler life history. Most of these blood parasites rely on insect vectors for transmission to new hosts.

(3) *Urogenital protozoa* infect the bladder and the reproductive tract. Most of them are flagellates with a simple life cycle and are transmitted by venereal contact.

Example of protoctista life cycle

Eimeria

There are a large number of species of *Eimeria* most of which live in the intestines of specific hosts. One species, *Eimeria stiedai*, colonises the epithelial cells lining the bile duct, it affects rabbits and infections are often fatal.

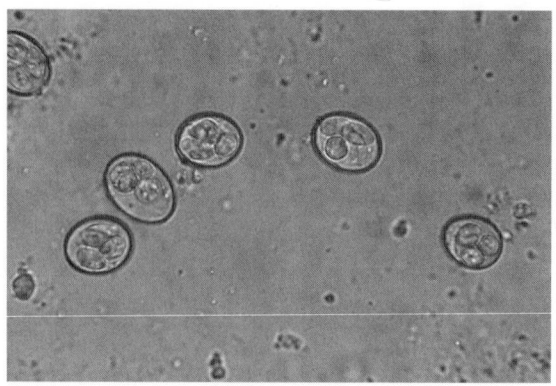

Figure 34.1   Eimeria sporulated oocyst.

Life cycle of *Eimeria spp.*

An oocyst containing a single cell is passed out in the faeces of an infected animal. Outside the animal it undergoes development to become a sporulated oocyst which consists of an outer shell containing four sporocysts each containing two sporozoites (Figure 34.1). When ingested by a suitable host the sporozoites are released from the oocyst and enter epithelial cells lining the intestine.

Asexual reproduction phase

The sporozoite grows within the epithelial cell to become a trophozoite, it then divides repeatedly to produce a number of merozoites. Merozoites burst out of the cell and each enters new epithelial cells to repeat the process. This cycle is repeated approximately three times.

Sexual reproduction phase

After a number of asexual reproduction generations some merozoites enter epithelial cells, grow and undergo repeated cell division to produce microgametes (male gametes). Other merozoites enter epithelial cells, grow and develop into single macrogametes (female gametes). When released the microgametes seek out macrogametes and fertilise them to produce a zygote. While still in the cell, a protective envelope develops around the zygote and development of the oocyst is completed.

Clinical signs

Many species of *Eimeria* are pathogenic only if present in large numbers. Heavy infestations cause severe enteritis and diarrhoea which may contain blood (haemorrhagic diarrhoea). Death is a possible outcome.

Kingdom Animalia – Phylum Platyhelminth

Class Trematoda (flukes)

Trematodes are usually small (2–5 mm), roughly oval, oblong or triangular in shape, very thin and flat. They are found in the intestines, bile ducts and liver and lungs of mammals. They attach themselves by means of suckers, one at the anterior end, and the other nearer the posterior end. The alimentary canal is very simple, usually consisting of a Y-shaped tube with only a single opening. Most trematodes are hermaphrodite, are self fertile and have enormous reproductive capacity. Many feed on blood which they extract from small blood vessels. The loss of blood, together with tissue irritation and the toxic effects of the parasite's excretory products are what cause the pathological effects of fluke infestation.

Life cycle of Trematodes

All flukes have a complex life cycle which involves an intermediate host – usually an aquatic snail. Eggs are shed into the fluke's environment and pass out of the host's body, usually in the faeces. They hatch into larvae which must, within a short time, find and enter the body of a snail. Within the snail, the larva develops and usually multiplies, so that one primary larva may give rise to many infective parasites. After a period within the snail, the next larval stage leaves the snail and forms a cyst which resists dehydration and may remain infective for a long time. When it is eaten by the primary host, the cyst opens in the gut and the young fluke makes its way to the location where it will spend the rest of its life. In some cases, the larva which leaves the snail infects a second intermediate host. Infection of the primary host takes place when this intermediate is ingested.

Class – Cestoda (tapeworms)

Cestodes are related to flukes, but are quite different in structure. They possess a tiny head (or scolex) which is equipped with a rostellum with one or more rings of hooks and an arrangement of suckers, for attachment to the intestinal wall of the host. Immediately behind the scolex is a zone of proliferation, where the production of segments (strobilisation)

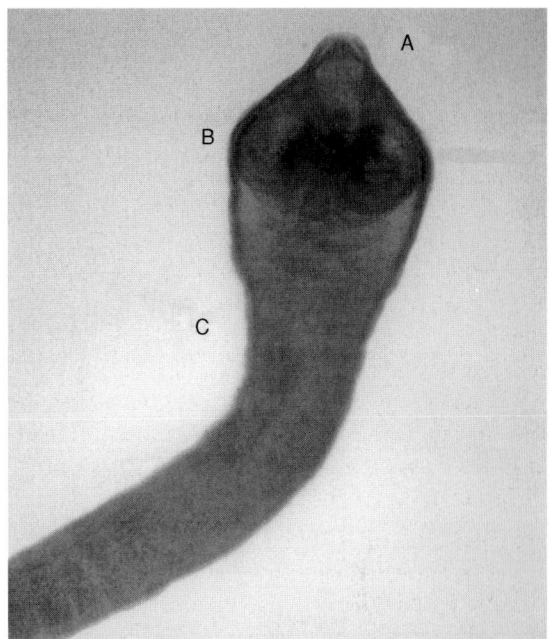

Figure 34.2 Tapeworm scolex (A = rostellum with hooks, B = suckers, C = zone of proliferation.

occurs (Figure 34.2). Rapid growth of these gives rise to a succession of identical segments (or proglottids) which means that, in many tapeworms, enormous length can be achieved. Tapeworms from larger host species may be several metres long.

As the proglottids are pushed further and further away from the scolex, each one develops a full set of reproductive organs, both male and female. Other internal organs are either very simple, or absent and the tapeworm feeds by absorbing digested food, with which it is surrounded, directly through its outer cuticle. When the organs are mature, self fertilisation occurs (with the worm folding up so one segment is able to mate with one in another region) and eggs start to be produced. These are not shed, but are stored in an egg container or uterus. Further development results in the atrophy and disappearance of the reproductive organs, and further growth of the uterus. The lower part of the tapeworm consists of a series of gravid proglottids (Figure 34.3), which comprise little more than the uterus which is swollen with eggs. The gravid proglottids break away from the end of the tapeworm and are shed in the host's faeces.

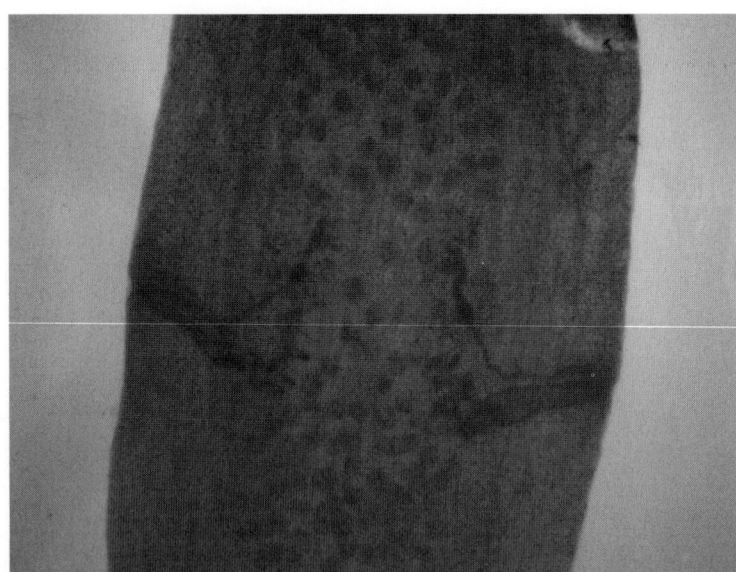

Figure 34.3   Gravid proglottid.

Life cycle of Cestoda

All tapeworms are intestinal parasites which are highly adapted to live in an environment virtually devoid of oxygen and which contains digested matter which they use as a source of food. The life cycle is complex. The eggs, either contained within the proglottid, or released after the proglottid has decayed, are passed in the faeces of the host and ingested by a mammal or, in some cases, by an insect. In a mammalian intermediate host, the egg hatches in the stomach or intestine and releases an embryo which has six spines (called a hexacanth). With the aid of the spines, the embryo penetrates the wall of the intestine and enters the mesenteric blood vessels from where it is carried via the circulation to the muscles, liver or central nervous system of the host. Here, the embryo matures into the infective stage called a cysticercus or bladder worm. This is a spherical, fluid-filled bladder with a scolex which is either suspended from the bladder or inverted inside it. At this stage, the tapeworm enters a long dormancy, which will last until the secondary host is eaten by the primary host.

In the intestine of the primary host, the bladder worm everts its scolex, which attaches itself to the intestinal wall and begins to develop into the adult form of the tapeworm. If the intermediate host is not eaten, no further development can occur. Those tapeworm species which use invertebrate intermediate hosts have a similar history, the cysticercus, or equivalent stage, developing in the body cavity of the insect.

One species of tapeworm of importance in laboratory animals, the dwarf tape worm (*Hymenolepis nana*), does not need an intermediate host.

Kingdom Animalia – Phylum Nematoda

Nematodes are more advanced than platyhelminths and have a well developed alimentary canal with a mouth at the anterior end opening into a muscular, sucking pharynx, and an anus near the posterior end. The body wall has four bands of longitudinal muscle tissue, contraction of which causes the characteristic side-to-side lashing movements of roundworms. The sexes are separate, and the ovaries and testes are both elongated, tubular structures filling the body cavity. In many species, females are considerably longer than males. The worms pair for copulation and the transfer of sperm; fertilised eggs which result from copulation are retained in the tubular uterus of the female while the yolk and shell are deposited on them. Nematode parasites of mammals are most frequently found in the intestine and in the lungs. Lung parasites and some of the gut parasites feed on blood, which they obtain by penetrating the capillaries running close to the surface. Other gut parasites use the digested food in the intestine.

Life cycle of nematodes

Life histories of nematodes differ considerably in detail, but in general, they all pass through several larval stages, one of which is the infective stage. With few exceptions, the larvae of nematodes undertake a remarkable migration within the primary host. The infective larva is usually ingested by the host but it does not remain in the gut where it will eventually reside. Instead, the larva penetrates the gut wall and enters the circulatory system. It is carried in the blood to the lung capillaries. Here, the larva breaks out into the lung alveolus and is coughed into the throat. From the throat the worm is transported to the intestine where it matures and begins its parasitic existence as an adult.

Pathogenicity of endoparasites

The damage which the endoparasite inflicts on its host depends on several factors including:

- *Physical effects of the presence of the parasite*: Heavy infestations of intestinal parasites, particularly roundworms, may physically occlude the gut so that the passage of digesta is markedly impaired and abdominal straining can lead to conditions such as rectal prolapse. These factors may occur in addition to any other effects.

- *Tissue damage*: All endoparasites cause some tissue damage, but this may not cause the animal to become clinically ill. Tapeworms attach themselves to the gut lining, and some species embed so deeply as to cause severe enteritis. Intestinal flukes always cause enteritis, since they burrow deeply into the mucosa. Liver flukes irritate the liver tissue and bile ducts causing scarring (cirrhosis), hardening and thickening. The signs of liver damage, such as jaundice and impaired liver function may be apparent. Lung flukes and lungworms have similar effects on the lung tissue, the affected animal may cough in the early stages and later exhibit signs of respiratory distress. Intestinal roundworms of the hookworm type burrow deeply into the intestinal mucosa and again cause enteritis. Damage is also caused by the migrating larvae of roundworms. Larval forms of tapeworms and roundworms which find themselves in the 'wrong' tissue can cause irritation and the host forms fibrous or calcified cysts around them. If these form in muscle, pain and stiffness can result.

- *Physiological effects*: Blood loss, either as a result of tissue damage and severe enteritis, or as a result of ingestion by the parasites, may result in severe, debilitating anaemia. This is a common sign of heavy endoparasite infestation. Parasite infestation often causes a rise in the proportion of eosinophils in white blood cells, for reasons which are not entirely clear. Parasites which feed on digested food in the intestine might be thought to increase the appetite of the host, to make up for the lost food. In fact, the opposite often occurs, and animals with heavy tapeworm infestations are frequently anorexic.

Identification of the presence of endoparasites

Worm and fluke infestations can be identified directly and by the behaviour of the host. Signs of worm infestation vary greatly, depending on the age and resistance of the host and the number of parasites present. In relatively heavy infestations, the animal will be in poor condition, showing loss of appetite, lethargy and often a swollen abdomen. Lungworms will cause coughing and choking. Blood smears may show a raised count of eosinophils. The animal may show irritation around the anus which it will attempt to alleviate by licking the area and by rubbing it against a hard surface. In tapeworm infestations, and in some roundworm infestations, the parasites may be visible in the faeces.

Flotation method

Positive identification can be made by observing the eggs of the parasite in faeces. A sample of faecal material is homogenised in a little saturated salt, the homogenate is placed into a centrifuge tube and topped up with saturated salt solution until there is a meniscus at the top. A cover slip is placed over the top and the tube is placed in a centrifuge set at the lowest revolutions for two minutes. This causes the eggs to float to the top and they can be floated off onto slides and examined under the microscope. It is easy enough to recognise parasite eggs in a faecal sample, but it is less easy to identify the species of parasite solely from the appearance of its eggs.

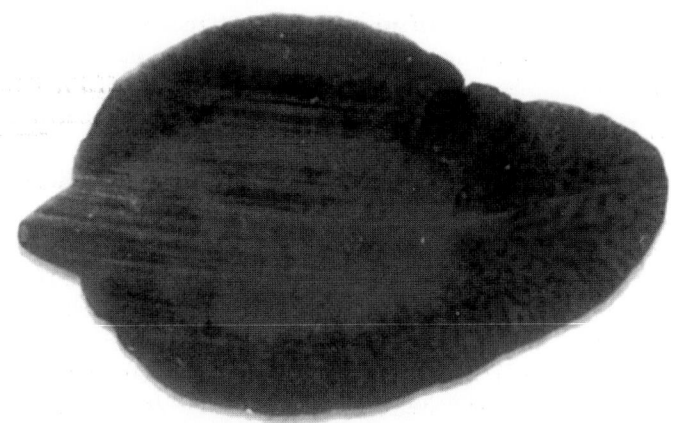

Figure 34.4   Adult *Fasciola hepatica* (liver fluke).

Examples of endoparasite life cycles

Fasciola hepatica: the sheep liver fluke

This is a large fluke, up to 30 mm in length, which is found in the bile ducts of the sheep and other ruminants, and less commonly in many other species (Figure 34.4). It is occasionally found in other locations. This fluke, like most other species, is hermaphrodite and fertilises itself. Eggs are shed into the bile and thence via the faeces to the exterior.

Life cycle

The eggs hatch releasing ciliated miracidia, which attempt to infect the intermediate host. The most common intermediate host is *Lymnaea truncatula*, the water snail, but other species of this genus are sometimes infected. The miracidium penetrates the body wall of the snail, shedding its ciliated epithelium as it does so, becoming a sporocyst larva. Germinal cells inside the sporocyst develop into secondary larvae called redia, and five to eight may form inside each sporocyst. Between four and seven weeks after infecting the snail, each redia gives rise to several cercariae (Figure 34.5), which leave the snail and normally within two hours attach themselves to leaves of grass or water plants where they lose their tails, secrete a cyst wall and become a metacercaria.

This is the infective stage of the fluke and the cysts are ingested by the definitive host along with the plant. The cyst wall dissolves in the stomach and liberates the immature fluke. The young flukes enter the abdominal cavity by penetrating the wall of the intestine. From the cavity they migrate through the liver tissue to the bile ducts where they remain.

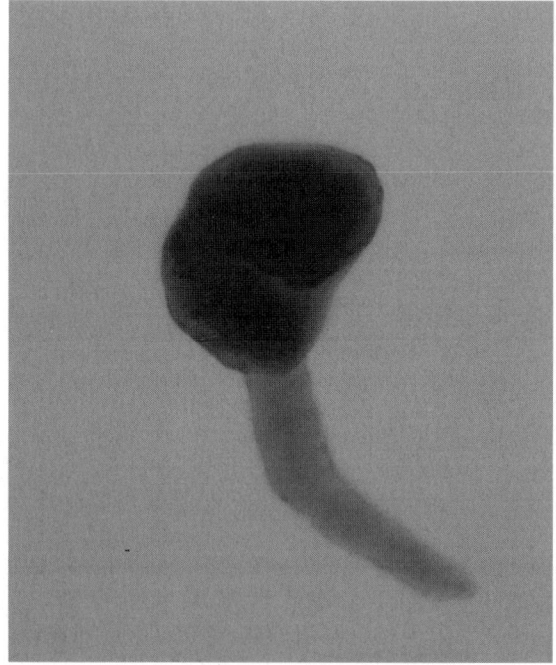

Figure 34.5   Fluke cercaria.

Eggs will start to appear in the host faeces about eight weeks after the initial infection.

Clinical signs

The effect of the fluke on the host may be profound. In the acute form, when the sheep has been infected with several thousand cysts, the liver is extensively damaged by the simultaneous migration of many immature flukes. The failure of liver function causes jaundice and ultimately the death of the host. A complication which may arise is secondary bacterial infection by *Clostridium* species which develop actively in the anaerobic conditions of the necrosed tissue.

Identification

Presence of the fluke can be confirmed by identification of eggs in faeces or the adult flukes in the liver at post mortem.

Control

Sheep could already have been infected before being brought into an animal unit or the parasite could be introduced into an experimental animal unit on vegetation (e.g. hay), so it is wise to autoclave hay before feeding. Infestations should not be a continual problem because of the absence of the intermediate host. Sheep kept outdoors should be kept off damp land. The named veterinary surgeon will prescribe treatment for infected sheep.

Taenia taeniaeformis: the cat tapeworm

This flat worm is found in domestic cats and other felids. The intermediate stage, the cysticercus, is found in rodents. Adults can be 15–60 cm long and 6 mm wide. The rostellum on the scolex has two rows of hooks. The eggs are spherical and once they have undergone some development the hexacanth embryo can be seen within the shell. In this species the cysticercus has its scolex outside the bladder. It is called a bladder worm or *Cysticercus fascicularis*.

Life cycle

The embryonated eggs are ingested by the rodent intermediate host where they hatch in the small intestine. They pass to the liver and develop into infective larvae in about thirty days. They appear as relatively large white cysts (Figure 34.6). The cat becomes infected when it eats the rodent or its liver. Once in the intestines of the cat the scolex attaches to the gut wall and the bladder is shed. Proglottids begin to be produced from a zone (the zone of proliferation) immediately behind the scolex. As the proglottids are pushed further from the scolex they develop and mature. Each proglottid has both male and female sex organs and once these are developed the worm folds on itself so that a proglottid from one region mates with a proglottid from another region. The resulting eggs are released, still within the proglottid, with faeces of the host.

Clinical signs

In the definitive host, light infestation may cause no apparent clinical signs. Heavy infestations cause chronic diarrhoea, weight loss and, occasionally, a

Figure 34.6 Cyst containing a cystercercus from the liver of a rodent intermediate host.

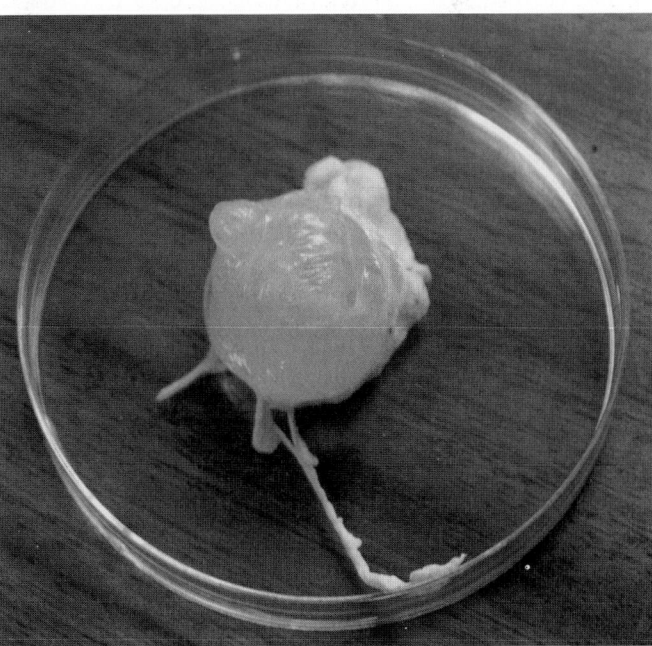

perforated gut. In the intermediate host, white cysts are seen in the liver at post mortem but often there is no other effect.

Identification

Adult worms can be seen in the intestines of the cat at post mortem. Eggs and proglottids can be recovered from faeces.

Hymenolepis nana: the dwarf tapeworm

These, as their common name suggests, are small tapeworms. They are from 25–40 mm long and less than 1 mm wide. The rostellum has a single crown of hooks. The eggs are oval (44–62 µm × 30–55 µm). They infest mice, rats, hamsters and gerbils and have been found in Old World primates and man.

Life cycle

Hymenolepis nana is unique among tapeworms in not requiring an intermediate host.

Production of eggs follows the same pattern as *Taenia*. Eggs passing out of the host are directly infective to another host. Embryos are released from the egg in the small intestine and penetrate the villi where they form a cysticercus. In four to five days they re-enter the lumen of the intestines, attach to the wall and develop into a mature worm. The life cycle takes fourteen to fifteen days to complete.

Eggs can hatch in the intestines of the host in which they were produced, this is called auto infection. Insects such as beetles and fleas can act as vectors, the host being infected when they ingest the insect.

Clinical signs

In light infections clinical signs are not seen. In heavy infestations there is weight loss, retarded growth and enteritis.

Identification

Eggs and proglottids can be recovered from faeces. The adult worm can be seen in the intestines at post mortem.

Toxocara canis: the dog roundworm

Toxocara canis is a roundworm which has a wandering larval stage. The adult worms inhabit the small intestine, sexes are separate, with the males reaching 10 cm in length and females 18 cm. They mate in the small intestine and the female produces eggs which

pass out of the host with faeces. A female may produce 1000 eggs a day.

The eggs are small (85 × 75 µm) with tough, sticky shells. They can survive in the environment for long periods and are very difficult to eradicate because they are resistant to most hygiene measures. The eggs are carried on dogs coats, human shoes and clothing and by wind. Flies, worms and rodents ingest second stage larvae which they are then able to spread (these are called parentenic hosts).

Life cycle

Outside the dog the eggs start to develop to become first stage larvae (L1), which are harmless, then second stage larvae (L2) which will cause infection if ingested. The time taken to develop into an L2 larva depends on the environmental temperature, two to three weeks in the summer but longer as the temperature drops.

Once ingested the shell is digested away and the L2 larva is released. It burrows through the gut wall and passes by way of the circulatory system to the liver, heart then to the lungs. In the lungs, the L2 larvae develop into L3 larvae. These pass up the trachea, cause irritation and are coughed up and swallowed. Back in the intestines the worms develop into L4 larvae then adult worms which mate and produce eggs.

The life cycle described above, called the hepatic-tracheal route, occurs in all dogs. In bitches over five weeks of age some of the L2 larvae from the lungs pass to the circulatory system to be distributed to muscles and other tissues around the body. They stay, inactive, until the bitch becomes pregnant. In the sixth week of pregnancy the larvae become mobilised and re-enter the circulatory system. Some are deposited around the placenta where they burrow through the wall to enter the foetus and lodge in the liver and lungs. Others are deposited in the mammary glands from where they can infect the pup when it takes colostrum.

When the pups are born, the L2 larvae recommence their development. Pups can be shedding eggs by the time they are three weeks old.

Clinical signs

Migration of the larvae through tissues and their presence in liver, heart, lung and intestines produce widespread damage in foetal, immature and adult dogs. Nasal discharge, diarrhoea, vomiting, reduced

Figure 34.7 Head and tail of a *Syphacia obvelata*.

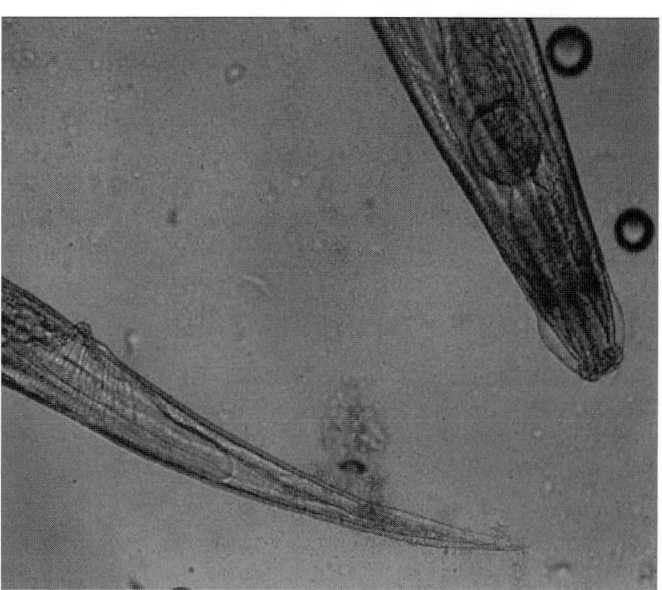

growth rate and neurological signs may occur. The severity of the signs increase with the severity of the infestation.

Presence of the worm can be confirmed by identifying eggs in faecal samples or finding adult worms in the intestines post mortem.

Control

Eggs are extremely persistent and will survive many disinfectants and cleaning agents, they are therefore very difficult to clear from the environment. Prenatal transmission adds to the difficulty of control. Scrupulous hygiene and regular worming to prevent adult *Toxocara* surviving long enough to breed is the usual way to effect control.

The named veterinary surgeon will devise a suitable worming programme.

Zoonosis

There is risk of humans being infected by L2 larvae; they cannot complete their life cycle in humans but they can cause damage. The larvae migrate through tissues (the condition is called visceral larva migrans) and target the liver or the eye, where they can cause blindness. Personal hygiene and control of the worm in dogs should prevent the infection of humans in animal units.

Syphacia obvelata: the mouse pinworm

These worms are thought to be very common in conventional animal units. In addition to mice, they are found in rats, hamsters and other rodents. The females are 3.4–5.8 mm long and 240–400 μm wide. Males are less than half that (Figure 34.7). Eggs which are oval with one flat side measure up to 153 μm long × 55 μm wide.

Life cycle

The life cycle follows the pattern already described for nematode worms. Adult females lay eggs in the colon and on the perianal skin, these develop into L2 larvae and therefore become infective within a few hours.

New hosts become infected by licking the perianal area of an infected cage mate or by consuming contaminated food or water. Larvae may hatch from the eggs laid in the perianal area and pass back into the colon – a form of infection called retro-infection.

Clinical signs

Low numbers of worms in the gut will cause no clinical signs. Heavy infestation can block the gut (called impaction) and cause conditions which are associated with intestinal straining e.g. prolapse of the rectum and intussusception (telescoping of the gut).

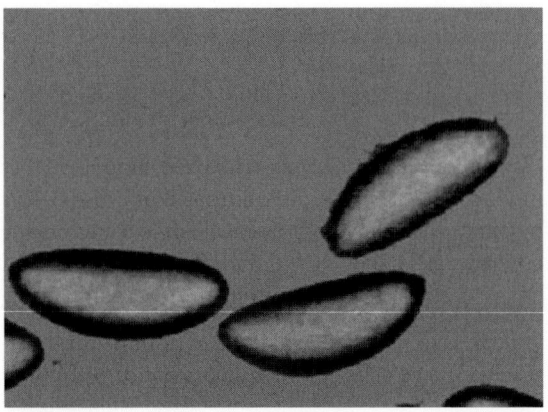

Figure 34.8   Eggs recovered from an infected rodent using the stick tape method.

Identification

Eggs can be identified in faeces (see Flotation techniques, p. 297) or by placing a piece of sticky tape over the perianal area. Any eggs present will be removed with the tape which can be transferred to a microscope slide for examination (Figure 34.8).

Control

Good routine hygiene measures should prevent entry of these organisms. There are drugs to treat the condition which can be recommended by the named veterinary surgeon when appropriate.

Ectoparasites

The majority of ectoparasites belong to the:

- Kingdom Animalia
  — Phylum Arthropoda
  — Class Insecta
  — Class Arachnida

The arthropods are characterised by the presence of an external skeleton composed of a complex polysaccharide called chitin. The body is divided into segments and each segment bears a pair of jointed appendages. In the more advanced arthropods these appendages are modified to fulfil a wide range of functions. Those on the head form the external jaws and the antennae, those on the thorax may be legs used for walking and pincers for grasping food,

while those on the abdomen may be modified to form swimming appendages or gills or both. In the more advanced arthropods there are many body segments without any appendages at all. The presence of a hard external skeleton restricts growth, so the animal develops in a series of moults. A new, soft skeleton develops under the old one, which splits, and is shed so that the animal can expand before its new skeleton hardens. Only the juvenile stages of insects and arachnids moult. The adults do not moult or grow at all. All the parasites dealt with in these notes are either insects or arachnids.

Insects

Insects have a body clearly divided into three regions, head, thorax and abdomen, and possess three pairs of legs on the thorax. The three pairs of jaws are often modified to accommodate different modes of feeding. Insects absorb oxygen from the atmosphere directly into their tissues through laterally placed spiracles which open into a network of fine tubes which ramify through the body. Most adult insects have one or two pairs of wings and most lay eggs. After the egg stage there are two distinct types of life history:

(1) *Exopterygota*: The egg hatches into a nymph, which is similar to the adult except that it is very much smaller and its reproductive organs are undeveloped. The nymph grows by a series of moults and at each stage, or instar, becomes more and more like the adult. Only after the final moult is the insect sexually mature.

(2) *Endopterygota*: The egg hatches into a larva, which is usually very different from the adult, often being wormlike, and sometimes devoid of legs. The larva usually undergoes several moults, then finally turns into a pupa. This instar appears to be a dormant stage, but in fact the insect undergoes a complete reorganisation during the pupal stage and eventually emerges as an adult.

Arachnids

Arachnids, or spider-like arthropods, are unlike insects in several respects. The body is either divided into two regions, the cephalothorax and abdomen, or is undivided. They have four pairs of legs, plus a pair of chelicerae used for seizing prey, although these may be modified into a piercing and sucking appendage, or into jaws which can chew food. They do not possess multiple spiracles just a single pair which opens into a cavity containing folds of thin vascular tissue called lung-books, across which gaseous exchange can take place. The smallest arachnids, the mites, absorb oxygen over their whole body surface. Arachnids never have wings. They lay eggs which, in the parasitic species, hatch into larvae. The larvae are similar to adults, but smaller, and only have three pairs of legs, so could be confused with an insect. After a single larval instar, the larva moults and becomes a nymph with four pairs of legs, although still immature. The adult appears after the nymph moults.

Examples of ectoparasites

Insecta

Lice (order *Anoplura* and order *Amblycera* formally called *Mallophaga*)

These are wingless insects which inhabit the skin and fur of mammals and the feathers of birds. Their entire life cycle is spent on the body of the host. The anopluran lice (sucking lice) have mouthparts adapted for piercing and sucking and they penetrate the skin and feed on blood and tissue fluid, causing intense irritation. The amblyceran lice (biting lice) feed on dead skin and hair in mammals and on feathers in birds and cause considerably less irritation. The sucking lice are very flat dorso-ventrally so that they can flatten themselves against the skin of the host to avoid dislodgement by scratching. The legs are equipped with strong hooks so that they can grasp the hair firmly. The amblyceran lice of mammals are also dorso-ventrally flattened, while those of birds, which often inhabit the feather shafts, are thin and elongated. Louse eggs (nits) are attached by a glue to the hairs of the host and they hatch into nymphs (exopterygote life history). Lice undergo three nymphal instars.

Fleas (*Siphonaptera*)

These are wingless insects which, in most cases, only inhabit the host in order to feed. All fleas have piercing and sucking mouthparts which are used to penetrate the skin and extract blood from the host. Adult fleas can survive for many weeks without food, but they are very sensitive to heat and can quickly detect the presence of a potential food source. Many fleas show some host specificity, but they will bite animals other than their normal food source, and may withdraw blood. Fleas need a blood meal before they are able to reproduce. They are flattened laterally, which enables them to move quickly and easily between the hairs or feathers of the host and they are equipped with strong legs and have the ability to jump long distances (Figure 34.9).

Fleas exhibit the endopterygote life history. They lay eggs in crevices in the floor and walls (Figure 34.10), and the eggs hatch into grub-like larvae which feed mainly on the droppings of the adult (Figure 34.11). Those species which remain attached to the host lay their eggs on the host in the lesions caused by the adults. When the larvae hatch they drop off the host. There is only a single larval instar, and it moults to form a pupa (Figure 34.12). After a period as a pupa, the length of which stage depends on ambient temperature, the adult emerges and is ready to feed.

Arachnids

Mites (order *Acarina*)

These are minute arachnids, mostly less than 1 mm long. There are both parasitic and non-parasitic mites. The parasitic types inhabit mammalian skin where they feed on dead skin and tissue fluid. The most important varieties of parasitic mite are:

(1) those which burrow into or puncture the epidermis causing intense irritation, hair loss, thickening and flaking of the skin and ulceration, a condition usually known as mange (the form of mange known as sheep scab, caused by the mite *Psoroptes ovis*, is commercially significant); and

(2) those which inhabit the external ear canal causing flaking and exudation of the lining, leading to occlusion of the canal, a condition usually known as ear canker.

The life cycle of mites is straightforward. The larval and nymph instars of the parasites feed on the same material as the adults, so all four stages are found together. The entire cycle lasts only a few days. Infection is by direct contact between infected and non-infected animals or by fomites.

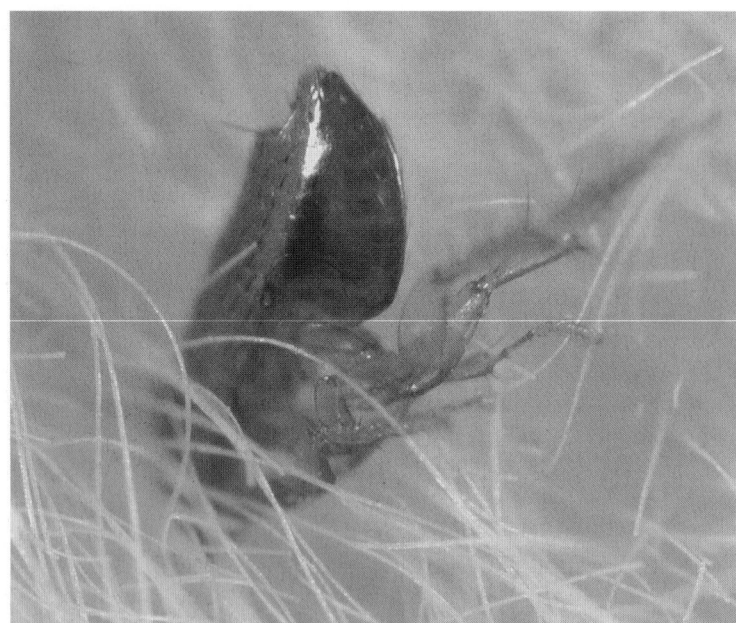

Figure 34.9   Flea feeding.

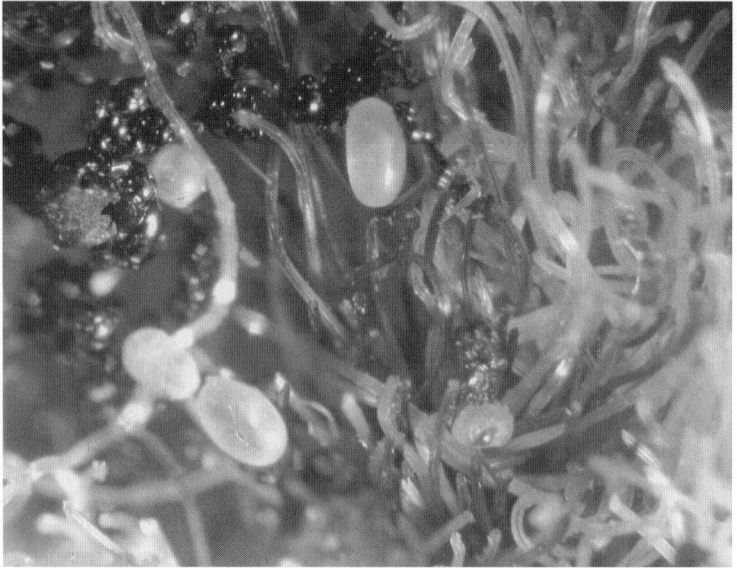

Figure 34.10   Flea eggs.

Ticks (order *Acarina*)

These are closely related to mites but are much larger and do not spend their entire life cycle on the host. Larvae, nymphs and adults have piercing mouthparts (called the hypostome) with which they penetrate the skin of the host animal and withdraw blood. A tick may increase its size several-fold as it feeds and becomes engorged with blood. When it has fed, the adult may stay on the host for a few days, but will eventually drop off after it has mated. Eggs are laid in a sheltered location (e.g. under a stone) and hatch into larvae, which climb to the top of grass blades or other vegetation, awaiting a passing host. When a suitable host brushes past the vegetation, the larval ticks attach themselves. Ticks are either one-host, two-host or three-host ticks. One-host ticks remain

Figure 34.11   Flea larvae.

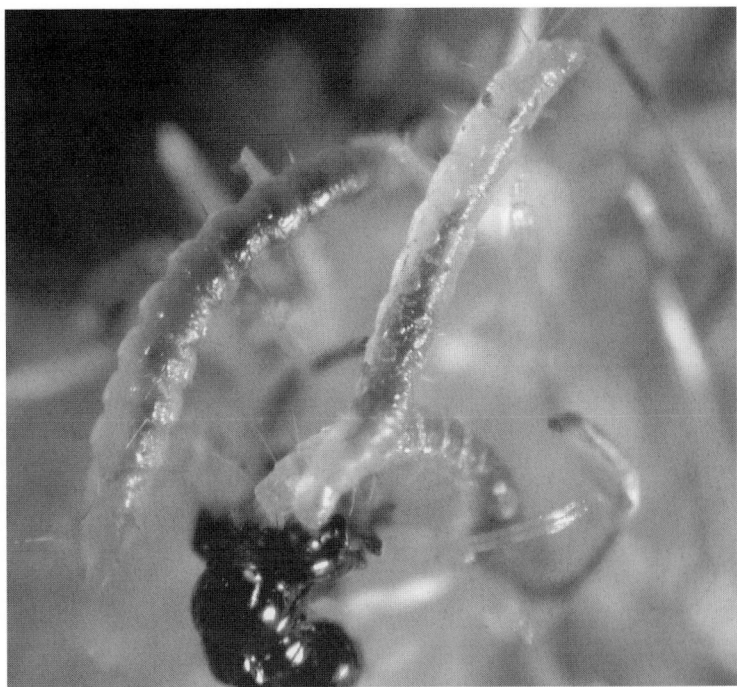

Figure 34.12   Flea pupa.

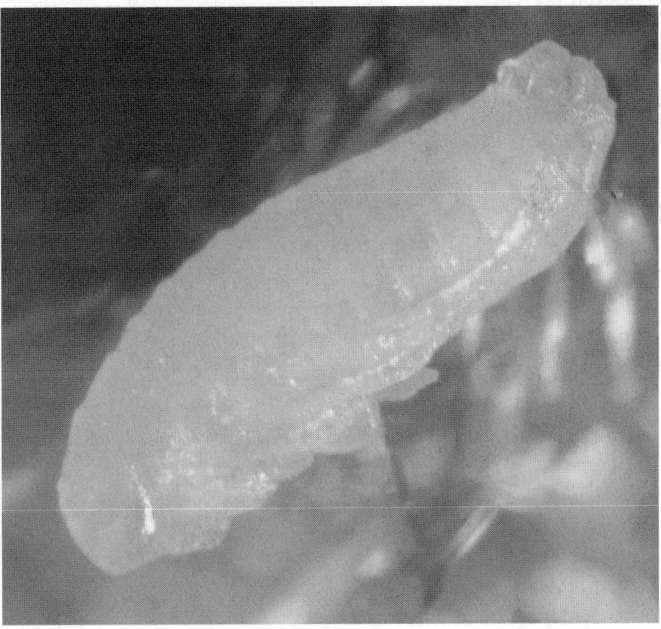

on the same the host through the larval, nymphal and adult instars. Two-host ticks moult once on the host, then drop off as engorged nymphs. Three-host ticks drop off after each engorgement, and after moulting, each instar finds a new host.

Pathogenicity of ectoparasites

The effects of ectoparasite infestation are:

(1) *Irritation*: The presence of any ectoparasite causes irritation which will lead to excessive

scratching and rubbing, to the extent that the affected animal may injure itself. The blood-sucking parasites introduce saliva into the bites to prevent the blood from clotting and this can cause local swelling as well as itching.

(2) *Hair and skin loss*: Mange mites in particular can cause large areas of alopecia and skin lesions which can become painful.

(3) *Blood loss and anaemia*: This is a complication which can arise if infestation with blood-sucking parasites is very heavy. The loss of blood can prove to be debilitating or even fatal in young animals.

(4) *Tick paralysis*: This is a form of paralysis which is probably an effect of the toxins present in tick saliva. Infestation does not need to be very heavy, as animals appear to become sensitised. The paralysis is progressive and can be fatal if it affects the respiratory muscles.

(5) *Secondary infection*: Often the most serious complication of ectoparasite infestation is the introduction of other infectious organisms. Some infections (e.g. rickettsial infections like typhus) are almost exclusively transmitted by tick bites. Any skin lesion caused by ectoparasites or by the animal itself seeking to alleviate the irritation has the potential to become infected. A common complication of ear canker is infection of the inner ear (*otitis interna*).

Identification of ectoparasites

The presence of ectoparasites is usually evident from the behaviour of the affected animal. Excessive scratching and restlessness are indicative of the presence of some irritating visitor. Close inspection may reveal specimens of the adult forms of the larger species. Nits are very small, but the use of a hand lens can make their detection easier. Areas of hair loss are always suspect. The presence of mites in such locations can be demonstrated by taking skin scrapings. If the material removed is mounted in 10% potassium hydroxide, skin and hair become transparent so that the mites can be observed under the low power of the microscope. Ear canker mites cause a typical sign: the animal holds its head on one side and will frequently shake its head. Inspection will reveal

partial or total occlusion of the passage by dead cells and dried exudate which, when treated like skin scrapings, should prove the presence of the mites.

Examples of ectoparasites

Phylum Arthropoda

Class Insecta

- Order Siphonaptera
  - *Ctenocephalides canis* Dog flea
  - *Ctenocephalides felis* Cat flea

Although the names of these fleas associate them with specific species they can be found in a variety of hosts. Adult females can reach 2.5 mm long, often more than twice the size of adult males (Figure 34.13). The life cycle is as described above in biology of ectoparasites.

Clinical signs
A number of signs indicate fleas are present. The animal scratches, is restless and the coat is ruffled. Wounds may be present as a result of the scratching. There may be an allergic response to the chemicals in flea saliva showing as red raised areas.

Fleas can act as vectors of the dog tapeworm *Dipylidium caninum* and the dwarf tapeworm *Hymenolepis nana*.

Identification
The host becomes restless and scratches. The flea or its excrement can be seen in the coat. Hair loss and signs of irritation on the skin.

Control
Drugs are available from the named veterinary surgeon. Adults and immature forms spend time off the host so it is necessary to treat the environment as well as the animal.

- Order Anoplura
  - *Polyplax serrata* Mouse louse

These sucking lice are associated with mice but may be present on other species. They are up to 1.5 mm long. Each egg is cemented to an individual hair near to the skin. They are transmitted by direct contact.

Figure 34.13 *Ctenocephalides canis* (dog flea).

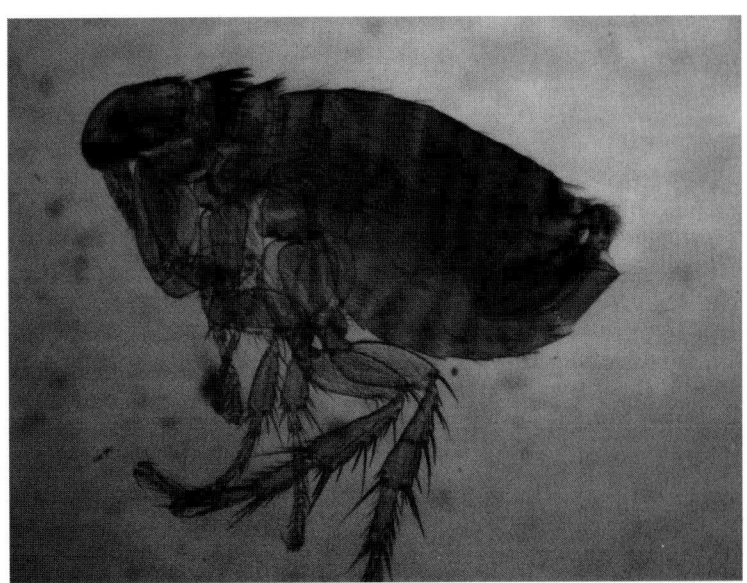

Life cycle

The life cycle is largely as described in the section on biology of ectoparasites (see p. 302). Nymphs hatch from the eggs in five to six days and undergo three moults to reach maturity and the complete life cycle takes approximately thirteen days.

Clinical signs

Presence of these lice causes intense irritation, so the host will be seen scratching and there may be traumatic damage resulting from this. In heavy infestations there will be anaemia and death.

Identification

Louse or nit on the host.

Class Arachnida

- Order Acarina
  — Family Psoroptidae
  — *Psoroptes ovis* the sheep scab mite

This mite, which is a serious parasite of the sheep, feeds on tissue fluid which it sucks through tiny punctures made in intact skin. Swelling of the skin around the bite occurs and serum exudes on to the surface where it dries and forms a crust. The mites cannot survive on the crust, so they move to the edges of the lesion, which increases in size as a result. The wool on the crusted areas becomes loose and is easily pulled out. The lesions are intensely itchy and the animal will scratch and nibble at the affected area, thus removing the wool. The discarded wool contains mites which will infect other sheep coming into contact with it.

Life cycle

After copulation, the mites lay their eggs at the edge of the lesion. They hatch in one to three days and the emergent larvae will feed for two to three days before moulting. Nymphs feed for two to three days, then rest for thirty-six hours before the final moult. The adults will copulate almost immediately after the moult. Two days later, the females moult again and start laying the following day. Females live for about thirty to forty days and lay a total of ninety or more eggs. The lesions caused by the parasite grow quite rapidly and are easy to see once the disease is established. The mite may be found on any part of the body, but the most usual locations are around the shoulders and along the flanks. Although the parasite normally attacks the sheep, it may be transmitted to other species.

Clinical signs

Infected sheep isolate themselves from the flock, they can be seen scratching on fences, posts or any other suitable object. Loss of wool is evident. Traumatic damage due to excessive scratching may become infected with secondary organisms. Untreated sheep scab can lead to death.

Identification
Inspecting samples from the lesions or discarded wool for mites.

Control
Various chemicals for external or parenteral application are available and can be used under the supervision of the named veterinary surgeon.

— *Psoroptes cuniculi* Ear canker mites of rabbits

This mite closely resembles the sheep scab mite and its life cycle is very similar (Figure 34.14). The difference is that *Psoroptes cuniculi* colonises the inner pinna of the ear starting deep in the ear canal. If left untreated the infection will spread upwards to cover the whole ear and head (Figure 34.15).

Clinical signs
A yellow/brown crust forms on the surface of the ear. The irritation causes the rabbit to scratch and shake its head which can cause secondary traumatic damage.

Control
The mite can live away from a host for several months. It can be brought into the unit on infected rabbits, by flies and in contaminated food and bedding. Normal quarantine practice and hygiene measures should prevent entry. Infected rabbits must be isolated and treated according to the advice of the named veterinary surgeon.

Order Acarina

• Family Ixodidae
  — *Ixodes ricinus* the Castor-bean tick

This is the most common tick in the UK. It can cause considerable discomfort and irritation, as well as more serious problems. Tick infestation in this country is not the problem it can be in warmer areas of the world, where the number of tick species is much greater. The Castor-bean tick is a large species; the adults are easily visible and when engorged with blood, may be 9–10 mm long. It is a three-host species (Figure 34.16).

Life cycle
The eggs are laid on the ground in suitable crevices in batches of several thousand. After laying, the female

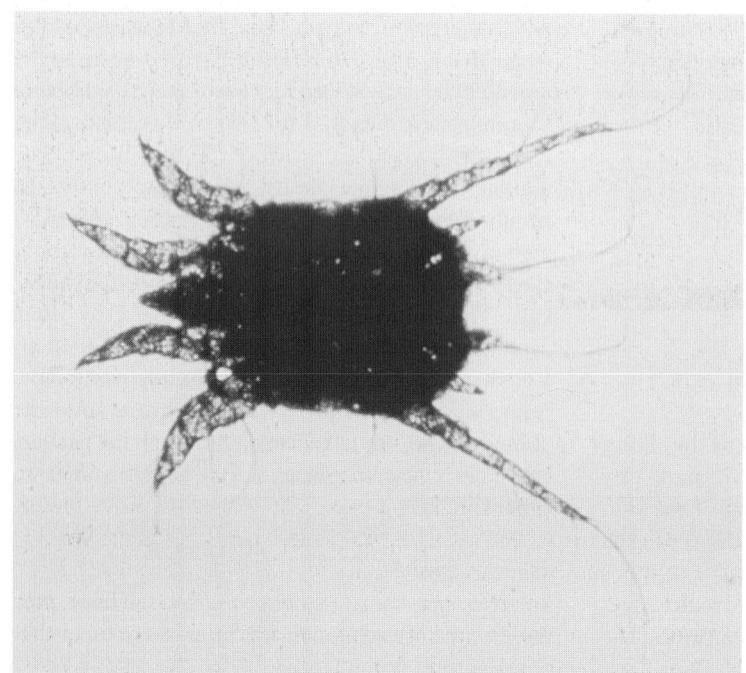

Figure 34.14 *Psoroptes cuniculi* (rabbit ear canker mite).

Figure 34.15 Rabbit's ear infected with the canker mite.

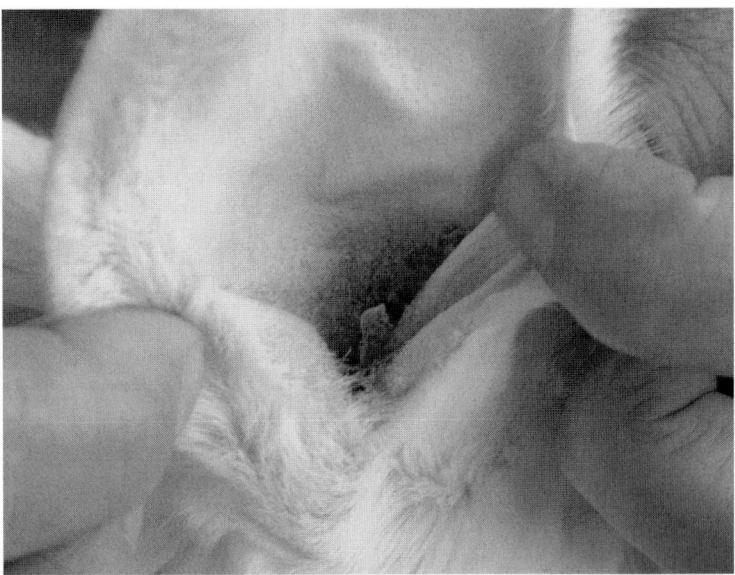

Figure 34.16 *Ixodes ricinus* (tick).

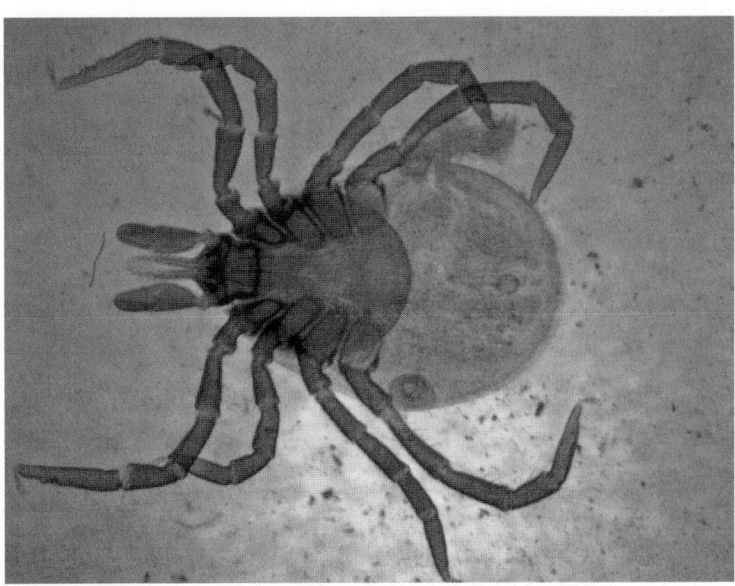

dies. Depending on the temperature, the eggs hatch in two to thirty-six weeks, and the emergent larvae climb to the tips of grass stalks or low shrubs where they are visible as clusters of small (1–2 mm), brown 'seeds'. This stage is often known as the 'seed-tick' stage. When a potential host brushes past the herbage, the larvae transfer to the animal, clinging with their claws. They start to feed immediately and in two to six days, they are fully engorged. They drop off the first host and hide away until they have moulted. This is another temperature-dependent process, and may take between four and fifty-one weeks. The nymphs repeat the process of finding a host and take between three and seven days to become fully engorged. The second moult also takes place on the ground in eight to twenty-eight weeks, and the adults wait for the third and final host. Copulation usually takes place on the host, and after the female has mated and engorged (five to fourteen days) she will drop off the host, find a suitable place, lay eggs and die. Males may stay on the host for any-thing up to four months, and it is during this period that large accumulations of ticks may occur. In the UK, there are two populations of ticks. Spring feeders emerge and feed in the period March–June, while autumn feeders are active during August–November. Both populations are present on the western side of the British Isles, but only spring feeders are found in eastern areas. Ticks will survive for remarkably long periods without food. Laboratory investigation has shown that unfed larvae can survive for nineteen months, nymphs for twenty-four months and adults for twenty-seven months. Normally, the complete life cycle lasts for three years.

Clinical signs

Tick paralysis is not common in the UK, but, apart from the irritation which can be caused, and the blood-loss which may occur in heavy infestations, the most serious effect of tick bites is disease transmission. Ticks are known to transmit pathogenic protozoa, rickettsiae and viruses and can be the vectors of red-water fever in cattle, 'louping-ill' in sheep and various forms of encephalitis and haemorrhagic fever.

Identification

Ticks can easily be seen on an animal.

Control

Individual ticks can be removed, taking care not to leave mouthparts in the animal. Chemical treatment is available on the advice of the named veterinary surgeon.

Zoonosis

Ticks can transmit disease to man. An example is Lyme disease caused *by Borrelia burgdorferi* (a spirochaete bacteria). The disease causes lethargy, headaches and arthritis.

References and further reading

IoB (1989) *Biological Nomenclature*. Institute of Biology, London.

Owen, D.G. (1992) *Parasites of Laboratory Animals* (Laboratory Animal Handbook No. 12). Royal Society of Medicine Press, London.

Flynn, R.J. (1973) *Parasites of Laboratory Animals*. Iowa State University Press.

35

Animals (Scientific Procedures) Act 1986

Kevin P. Dolan

Introduction

The use of animals for scientific procedures is controlled by the Animals (Scientific Procedures) Act 1986 (subsequently referred to in this chapter as ASPA or the Act). The Act is administered by the Secretary of State for Home Affairs who is responsible to Parliament for its operation. The Act is an enabling act; this means that the Home Secretary has the power to alter its provisions without having to pass a new law through Parliament. So the law is able to develop and change as new knowledge becomes available. The Home Secretary has exercised this power several times since the original law was enacted, an example being adding *Octopus vulgaris* to the list of animals protected by the Act.

The Act forms part of the criminal law and, like other parts of the criminal law, failing to comply with some of its provisions can lead to prosecution and imprisonment. Non-criminal breaches can be dealt with by a range of sanctions from a letter of admonition for minor lapses to revocation of licences or certificates of designation.

Guidance on the Act is given in the *Guidance on the Operation of the Animals (Scientific Procedures) Act 1986* (Home Office 2000) subsequently referred to as HOG.

The scope of the Act is clearly set out in the 1991 Report of the Animal Procedure Committee which states that it provides for the licensing of experimental and other scientific procedures carried out on protected animals. Thus the Act controls the whole range of scientific procedures, from major surgery to the many thousands of scientific procedures which are so minor that they do not require anaesthesia, e.g. the taking of a blood sample.

Regulated procedures

The Act defines a regulated procedure as any experimental or other scientific procedure applied to a protected animal which may have the effect of causing that animal pain, suffering, distress or lasting harm. Under the act, these terms include death, disease, injury, physiological and psychological stress, significant discomfort, or any disturbance to normal health, whether immediately or in the long term. The cumulative effect of procedures must be taken into account when deciding if they are regulated or not, for instance, procedures which on their own do not qualify may do so if they are applied as a series.

A procedure is also regulated if following or during a procedure an animal reaches the stage at which it becomes a protected animal and the procedure may have the effect of causing pain, suffering, distress or lasting harm. Similarly a procedure which may result in pain, suffering, distress or lasting harm to a foetus or immature form at or beyond the stage at which it becomes protected is regarded as a regulated procedure, irrespective of any effect on the parent animal.

Anything which may result in the birth or hatching of a protected animal with abnormalities which may cause it pain, suffering, distress or lasting harm; for instance, the breeding of animals with harmful genetic defects is a regulated procedure. It follows that the term regulated procedure includes genetic manipulation involving animals which will reach the stage at which they will become protected animals. The crucial term *may* in the definition of regulated procedure is of importance in this context.

A procedure is still regulated even if any pain, suffering, distress or lasting harm which would have otherwise resulted is mitigated or prevented by anaesthetics or other substances to sedate, restrain, or dull perception, or by prior decerebration or other procedure for rendering the animal insentient. Giving an anaesthetic, analgesic or other substance to sedate or dull the perception of pain of a protected animal for scientific purposes is itself a regulated procedure. Likewise, decerebration, or any other procedure to render a protected animal insentient, if done for scientific purposes, is a regulated procedure.

Procedures which are not regulated

Although appearing to have the three essential elements of a regulated procedure, i.e. scientific, protected animal and pain, some procedures are not regulated procedures because the Act specifically excludes them. Exempt procedures include:

- methods used solely for the identification of an animal if it causes only momentary pain or distress or no lasting harm;
- procedures carried out as part of normal veterinary and agricultural practice;
- methods of euthanasia which appear in Schedule 1 attached to the ASPA;
- clinical testing on animals carried out under the Medicines Act 1968.

If there is any doubt as to whether a procedure is regulated, the Home Officer inspector for the establishment should be consulted.

Protected animals

A 'protected animal' for the purposes of ASPA means any living vertebrate (other than man) and the invertebrate *Octopus vulgaris*.

An animal becomes protected when it reaches the following stages of development:

- mammals birds and reptiles from halfway through gestation or incubation periods;
- fish, amphibia and *Octopus vulgaris* from the time at which they become capable of independent feeding.

Under the ASPA, the Secretary of State may extend the definition of a protected animal to include 'invertebrates of any description' and to alter the stage of development at which an animal may become protected.

Living

For the purposes of the Act, an animal is regarded as 'living' until the permanent cessation of circulation or the destruction of the brain. Brain destruction is not complete in decerebrated animals, therefore these are considered to be living and protected under the Act.

Project licence

Definition

The official definition of a project licence is to be found in Section 5 of the Act itself.

> 'A project licence is a licence granted by the Secretary of State specifying a programme of work and authorising the application, as part of that programme, of specified regulated procedures to animals of specified description, at a specified place or places.' (Home Office 1986)

There are legal restrictions on the granting of a project licence. The Animals (Scientific Procedures) Act (S.5 (3)) stipulates that a project licence can only be granted for one or more of the following reasons:

(1) the prevention, diagnosis or treatment of disease;
(2) the study of physiology;
(3) environmental protection benefiting health and welfare;
(4) advancement of biological or behavioural sciences;
(5) education and training (factors such as the level of education, an in-depth consideration of alternatives and the level of severity (usually unclassified, see section on The severity of procedures, p. 313), enter into the consideration of the granting of a licence under this heading);
(6) forensic enquiries;
(7) breeding animals for scientific purposes (an application for a licence under this heading will not be concerned with the ordinary breeding of animals for research but will be associated with the production of mutant strains of animals expressing a genetic defect or breeding involving genetic manipulation).

This list is of the utmost importance because it lays down the motives for using animals in research which could justify that use, even though it may involve suffering, distress or lasting harm.

Justification (cost/benefit)

The establishment of justification of the programme must be the main theme of any application for a project licence. The requisite justification is arrived at by a careful weighing up of the relationship between the possible suffering of the animal and the desirable consequences which are the hoped-for results of the research – the cost/benefit assessment.

An assessment of the proposed severity limits and the potential benefits of the work is crucial to the granting of a project licence. In effect the Act requires that the likely adverse effects of the procedures be weighed against the benefit likely to result from the proposed programme of work. Although in some situations it is difficult to assess in advance the immediate benefit of work, e.g. fundamental research, where no immediate benefit is sought other than the increase in knowledge, this would not prevent the project licence from being granted. There is no intention of the Home Office to control research by ascribing greater intrinsic merit to one area of research than to another. In all cases, applicants for project licences must set out the potential benefits of their specific project. To this end, project licence applicants must assess the likely severity resulting from the procedures so that this may be balanced against the potential benefit. It is, therefore, necessary to distinguish between assessment of the potential severity of individual procedures (or series of procedures) and the overall severity of the project. No work, however mild will be permitted unless it can be justified.

The severity of procedures

The evaluation of the 'cost' within the cost/benefit assessment is expressed in terms of severity limits – unclassified, mild, moderate, substantial.

The Home Office Guidance (HOG) (Home Office 2000) is comprehensive and clear on this topic 'in assessing the severity of a series of regulated procedures, account should be taken of the effect of all the procedures (whether regulated or not) applied to each animal or group of animals; the nature of any likely adverse effects; the action taken to mitigate these effects; and the endpoints applying to the procedures.'

The crucial factor in the assessment is the maximum severity to be experienced by any animal. It represents the worst potential outcome for any animal subjected to the protocol, even if it may only be expressed by a small number of the animals to be used.

In practice assessing severity limits can present difficulty, guidance is given as follows.

Unclassified

Protocols performed entirely under general anaesthesia, from which the animal does not recover consciousness. This includes the preparation and use of decerebrated animals.

Mild

Protocols which, at worst, give rise to slight or transitory minor adverse effects. Examples include: small infrequent blood samples; skin irritation tests with substances expected to be non-irritant or only mildly irritant; minor surgical procedures under anaesthesia, such as small superficial tissue biopsies or cannulation of peripheral blood vessels. However, if used in combination or repeated in the same animal, the cumulative severity may be increased beyond mild. Protocols may also be regarded as mild if they have potential to cause greater suffering but contain effective safeguards to initiate effective symptomatic or specific treatment or terminate the protocol before the animal shows more than minor adverse effects.

Moderate

Protocols regarded as moderate include toxicity tests (which do not involve lethal end points) and many surgical procedures (provided that suffering is controlled and minimised by effective post-operative analgesia and care). Protocols which have the potential to cause greater suffering but include controls which minimise severity, or terminate the protocol before the animal shows more than moderated adverse effects, may also be classified within the moderate severity limit.

Substantial

Protocols which may result in a major departure from the animal's usual state of health or well being. These include: acute toxicity procedures where significant morbidity or death is an endpoint; some efficacy tests of anti-microbial agents and vaccines; major surgery; some models of disease, where welfare may be seriously compromised. If it is expected that even one animal would suffer the substantial effects, the procedure would merit a 'substantial' severity limit.

Assessing procedure severity

In any procedure, standard condition 6 attached to the project licence requires that 'the degree of severity imposed shall be the minimum consistent with the attainment of the objects of the procedure.'

Besides the assessment of individual procedures, the project licence holder must give an assessment of the overall severity of the whole project.

The assessment of the overall severity of a project will reflect the cumulative effect of each procedure; the number of animals used in each procedure; the frequency of use of each procedure; the proportion of animals which are expected to be exposed to each procedure; and the length of time that the animals might be exposed to the upper limits of severity. The assessment of overall severity will be used as part of the cost/benefit assessment.

If, during the life of the project licence, experience shows that an earlier endpoint would be equally acceptable scientifically, but would involve a lower level of suffering by the animal, applications may be made for the project licence to be amended to allow for modifications, both to severity limits and techniques.

However the project licence will be regarded as breached if the project licence holder does not inform the Home Office if a procedure causes an animal to suffer beyond the authorised severity band.

Some limiting clinical signs (rodents and rabbits)

As already indicated there are few clear criteria for deciding levels of severity but there are some publications which may prove useful, see *Laboratory Animals* (1990), UFAW (1989). John Finch and Tony Buckwell produced a useful relevant appendix of examples of appropriate clinical signs in respect to rodents and rabbits. Table 35.1 summarises their work.

Humane end points

The severity of a procedure may be able to be reduced by withdrawing an animal from the procedure or killing it humanely at an earlier stage, for instance as soon as discomfort is identified. This is referred to as a humane end point.

The proper fixing of humane end points is an essential aspect of the refinement of any procedure in

Table 35.1   Clinical signs of severity bands for rodents and rabbits. Adapted from Finch, J. and Buckwell, A.C. (1992) Limiting clinical signs appendices, *Laboratory Animal Science Association Newsletter*, **Winter**: 16–17.

Mild	Reduced weight gain.
	Food/water intake 40–75% of normal for 72 hours.
	Partial piloerection.
	Subdued but responsive – normal provoked behaviour.
	Hunched – transient, especially after dosing.
	Vocalisation – transient.
	Oculo–nasal discharge (mild/transient).
	Tremors – transient.
Moderate	Weight loss up to 20% of bodyweight.
	Food/water intake less than 40% of normal for 72 hours.
	Marked piloerection – staring coat.
	Subdued behaviour even when provoked, little peer interaction.
	Hunched – intermittent with pallor.
	Vocalisation – intermittent.
	Oculo–nasal discharge – persistent.
	Altered respiration.
	Tremors – intermittent.
	Convulsions – intermittent.
	Prostration – transient say less than one hour.
Substantial	Weight loss greater than 25%.
	Reduced food/water intake less than 40% for 7 days or anorexia.
	Marked piloerection – dehydration.
	Unresponsive to provocation.
	Hunched – 'frozen' with pallor and cold.
	Vocalisation – distressed and unprovoked.
	Oculo–nasal discharge – copious.
	Laboured respiration.
	Tremors – persistent.
	Convulsions – persistent.
	Prostration for more than an hour.
	Self-mutilation.

a realistic application of the principles of the 3Rs (see Chapter 36). The Act requires that applicants for a project licence specify the action to be taken to mitigate the effects of procedures on an animal. In practice, humane end points may vary greatly, e.g. geriatric status in regard to some primates in defined cases to much more specific conditions.

Project licence

Application for a project licence

In order to obtain a project licence the applicant must detail the intended work and its benefits. Full details are given in the Home Office Guidance (HOG 2000) and on the licence application form but required information includes amongst other things:

- the purpose and scientific justification for the work;
- a full description of the procedures involved;
- an estimate of the number of animals of each species which may be required;
- an assessment of potential severity;
- considerations which have been given by the applicant to reducing the number of animals used, refining procedures to minimise suffering and replacing animals with alternatives (i.e. the principle of the 3Rs).

Project licence applicants must have attended the Home Office training module for project licensees.

The completed application form must be considered by the local ethical review process at the establishment where the work is to be carried out before being sent to the Home Office for approval.

The managerial role of the project licence holder

Project licence applicants undertake to assume overall responsibility for the proper conduct of the programme of work specified in the licence. They are also responsible for ensuring all conditions attached to the licence are complied with.

Supervision is among the most onerous duties of the project licence holder. Project licence holders may be deemed to be aware of all occurrences within their programme of research. They may, consequently, be liable to sanctions for misdemeanours committed by others within the project. Particularly important in this context is the fourteenth condition of a project licence requiring supervision of personal licensees. Further information on this topic is given in HOG 5.32–5.39.

It is apparent from the wide responsibilities associated with a project licence that it is usually advisable that project licence holders have a deputy or deputies, since joint project licences are unacceptable. A Deputy project licence holder will be required where:

(1) the nature or scope of the project is such that control is best exercised through one or more deputy project licence holders;

(2) work is to be done at more than one place so that a deputy is available locally to supervise the work on the project licence holder's behalf;

(3) the project licence holder is likely to be absent from time to time;

(4) the project licence holder does not hold a personal licence (HOG 5.37).

The deputy licence holder must be in position to exercise day-to-day control over the work and his or her identity must be made known to those working on the project. A deputy licence holder will normally hold a personal licence. For further details see HOG 5.38.

Conditions of a project licence

All project licences have conditions attached to them. Eighteen are standard conditions and apply to all licences. Further conditions can be added to project licences by the Home Secretary should he/she think it necessary. The eighteen standard conditions are issued with all project licences and can also be found in Appendix D of HOG. Breaches of conditions 1–5, summarised below, constitute a criminal offence:

(1) only regulated procedures which are specified on the project licence may be performed and they must be performed by a suitable authorised personal licence holder;

(2) procedures can only be performed at the place stated on the licence;

(3) neuromuscular blocking agents must not be used in place of an anaesthetic;

(4) neuromuscular blocking agents can only be used with the permission of the Home Secretary;

(5) re-use of animals needs permission.

Duration of a project licence

A project licence is valid for five years. Application for renewal should be made well in advance of the expiry date. The licence is not transferable and terminates on the death of the holder. It may continue in force temporarily if the Home Office is notified within seven days, by an appropriate representative who has learned of the death of the licence holder.

If it is necessary to transfer the licence to another holder, a fresh application must be made and will be considered accordingly.

Re-use of animals

Animals which have been used for one series of procedures for a particular purpose authorised by a project licence may not be used for another series of procedures, for another purpose unless specific authority has been granted by the Home Secretary in advance.

The circumstances where authority may be given are as follows:

- Where an animal has been subjected to a series of procedures for a particular purpose but has not been given a general anaesthetic and that series is complete and the animal fully recovered.

- If the animal has been given a general anaesthetic it cannot be used in a second series of experiments unless:
  — the anaesthetic was given only for surgical preparation for the subsequent series of procedures;
  — general anaesthesia was for immobilisation only;
  — if during re-use the animal is terminally anaesthetised.

- If an animal undergoes a series of procedures for the same purpose this is not classed as re-use, e.g.:

  — if it is necessary to know how an animal responds to substances A, B and C before it is dosed with substance D;
  — if an animal has to be surgically prepared for a series of procedures, e.g. creation of a carotid loop which is subsequently used to measure blood pressure during a series of procedures.

Personal licence

A personal licence is the Home Secretary's endorsement that the holder is a suitable and competent person to carry out, under supervision if necessary, specified procedures on specified species of animals. Procedures can only be carried out if they form part of a programme of work authorised by a project licence (HOG 6.1–6.2).

Although new licensees are often restricted initially to particular projects (HOG 6.9), generally speaking experienced licensees are not restricted in this manner.

Most new licences carry a supervision condition and licensees will be expected to work under supervision until such time as the project licence holder considers them competent to work unsupervised (HOG 6.21).

Generally, personal licences remain in force indefinitely but are reviewed every five years. There are however exceptions to this, e.g. when issued to students for the purposes of study.

Application for personal licences

Applicants for personal licences must satisfy certain criteria including:

- They must be at least eighteen years of age.
- They must have appropriate education and training, which includes knowledge of the relevant scientific discipline and a knowledge of the handling and husbandry of the animals they are seeking to work on. They must be aware of the care an animal needs after the procedure.

  Minimum appropriate education will normally be five GCSEs or equivalent and successful completion of Home Office training modules 1, 2 and 3 (and in some cases 4). Exceptions can be made in these minimum education requirements on presentation of suitable evidence.

If the above criteria can be satisfied, the potential personal licensee will complete an application form which details the required regulated procedures and animals which are to be used. This application form has to be signed by a sponsor, who holds a position of authority at the establishment and who is an existing personal licence holder. The sponsor must certify that the licence applicant satisfies the character, education and training requirements and is suitable to carry out the work applied for.

If the applicant is a person who does not have English as a first language the sponsor has to certify that they understand their responsibilities under the Act.

Conditions on the personal licence

Twenty-two standard conditions are attached to all personal licences but the Home Secretary can add extra ones if it is considered necessary. Full details can be found in HOG Appendix E. A summary of conditions 1–10 are given below, breaches of conditions 1–9 and failure to comply with a requirement under condition 10 are criminal offences. Breach of any condition can result in the licence being revoked.

(1) Only procedures for which authority is given may be carried out.

(2) Only animals authorised on the licence may be used.

(3) Work may only be done if authorised by a project licence.

(4) Regulated procedures may not be performed as an exhibition to the public or on live television.

(5) Neuromuscular blocking agents must not be used instead of anaesthetics.

(6) Neuromuscular blocking agents may only be used if specifically authorised by the Home Secretary.

(7) Procedures may be performed only at the place/s specified.

(8) Any animal suffering or likely to suffer at the conclusion of a series of procedures must be humanely killed.

(9) The re-use of an animal is prohibited unless express authority has been granted by the Home Secretary.

(10) If an inspector requires that an animal be killed because it is undergoing excessive suffering it must be promptly and humanely killed.

In addition personal licensees must keep records of all animals they have carried out procedures on. These records must be maintained for five years.

Responsibilities of the personal licence holder

The guidance notes on the operation of the Animals (Scientific Procedures) Act 1986 makes the following points on the responsibilities of personal licence holders:

- 'It is particularly important for personal licensees to appreciate that they bear primary responsibility for the care of animals on which they have carried out scientific procedures.' (HOG 6.17)
- 'Personal licensees must be familiar with, and abide by, the authorities granted in the project licence under which they will be working: the objectives, plan of work, protocols, endpoints and the conditions of issue.' (HOG 6.14)
- 'Personal licensees should ensure that the cages, pens or places in which the animals are held carry labels indicating the project licence number, the protocol (19 b) number or short title, the personal licensee, the start date and any additional information which may be required by the inspector.' (HOG 6.20). Larger animals are identified individually.

Assistance to personal licensees

The law permits a personal licensee to request a non-licensed assistant to carry out certain procedures on their behalf (HOG 6.22–6.27). The procedures which be may carried out are those which do not require any technical knowledge or skill (they are also known as non-technical procedures) and would not be expected to result in any immediate welfare problems for the animals. Personal licence holders can only ask for this assistance if they have authority from the Home Secretary to do so. This authority is given as an additional condition on the personal licence. The personal licensee remains accountable to the Home Office for the animals.

There is no attempt to define these so-called 'non-technical procedures', rather it is a matter of giving 'for instances':

- filling food hoppers and water bottles with previously mixed diets or liquids of altered constitution or to which test substances have been previously added;
- placing of animals in some previously set-up altered environments, e.g. inhalation chambers, pressure chambers, aquatic environments;
- pressing the exposure button to deliver previously determined doses of irradiation to an animal;
- pairing/grouping associated with the breeding of animals with harmful genetic defects;
- withdrawing contents from an established ruminal fistula;
- operating automated machinery which carries out inoculation of eggs;
- placing animals in restraining devices (e.g. metabolism cages) as defined by the project licence;

- withdrawing food and/or water, as defined by the project licence;
- placing avian eggs into previously set chillers at the termination of a procedure.

The Home Secretary may consider giving permission to the delegation of other tasks but only in the presence of the licensee and on animals rendered insentient by decerebration or general anaesthesia from which the animal will not recover:

- administration of substance(s) or removal of body fluids through established cannulae or catheters as authorised by the project licence;
- administration or recording of electrical stimuli through electrodes implanted by a personal licence holder.

Designated establishments

The Act requires three types of designated establishment:

- designated scientific procedure establishments;
- designated breeding establishments;
- designated supplying establishments.

Scientific procedure establishments will include premises where animals are held, before, during and after procedures, but which are not bred. If animals, listed on Schedule 2 to the Act (Table 35.2), are bred for use in the same establishment or somewhere else, the premises will need certificates of designation as breeding establishments.

Establishments which do not breed animals but which house them before supplying them to scientific procedure establishments need certificates of designation as supplying establishments.

Establishments which qualify for more than one of the certificates must apply for each designation which is appropriate. An establishment which breeds animals with harmful genetic mutations or genetically manipulated animals or supplies surgically prepared animals must also be designated as a scientific procedure establishment.

The designation of establishments

The certificate of designation is issued to a person who represents the governing authority of the establishment and who is ultimately responsible to the Home Office for ensuring that the conditions of the certificate are observed. This person is commonly know as the certificate holder.

'Under Section 6(5) of the Act, all applicants for certificates must nominate:

(1) one or more persons responsible for the day-to-day care of the animals (since March 1997 the Named Animal Care and Welfare Officer – NACWO);
(2) one or more veterinary surgeons to provide advice on animal health and welfare.'

If the facilities provided are appropriate and those persons nominated for the care of the animals are suitably qualified, a certificate will be issued with certain standard conditions and, where necessary, additional conditions.

Limitations on, exemptions from and amendments of certificates

An overseas breeding or supplying establishment cannot be certified under the Act. Consequently, consent is required for the use of all imported cats and dogs and also for the use of imported Schedule 2 species unless they have been acquired from a supplying establishment (see Chapter 28). The Secretary of State can grant an exemption from the demands of Schedule 2 (cf. *Code of Practice for the Housing and Care of Animals used in Scientific Procedures* 3.5 (Home Office 1989) (referred to hereafter as CODHCASP)).

Table 35.2   Animals listed on Schedule 2 of the Act.

Animals which may be obtained from designated breeders or suppliers	Mice, rats, hamster, gerbil, guinea pig, rabbit, European quail (*Coturnix coturnix*), non-human primate, ferret, genetically altered pigs and sheep.
Animals which must be obtained from designated breeders	Cats and dogs

While there is no restriction in the Act on importation as such, it would be prudent to seek Home Office approval to ensure that animals may be used once they have been imported.

The importation of animals from overseas is controlled by the Animals and Animal Products (Import and Export) Regulations 1995 which is in keeping with the Balai Directive 92/65/EEC and the Animals (Post-Import Control) Order 1995. In some cases there may be involvement with the Endangered Species (Import and Export) Act 1976. Details about licences, health certificates, rabies and other quarantine requirements should be obtained from the Animal Health Division, DEFRA.

In some forms of research, particularly ecological studies, regulated procedures may need to be performed outside designated premises. ASPA S.6 allows for permission to be given for regulated procedures to be performed in a place other than a designated establishment (PODE).

This readiness of official variation of stipulations under the ASPA gives a welcome flexibility in its practical application. The availability of the staff of the inspectorate ensures the efficient achievement of this flexibility in practice.

Persons named on the certificate of designation

Three persons must be named on the certificate of designation:

- the certificate holder (CH);
- the named animal care and welfare officer (NACWO);
- the named veterinary surgeon (NVS).

The role of the certificate holder

ASPA S.8 imposes the obligation of paying the relevant fees on the certificate holder (CH). HOG 4.44 stresses that both the amount of and basis on which these fees are charged may be varied from time to time in line with any changes in the cost of regulatory arrangements. At present they are charged annually and consist of a flat rate annual fee on the designation/s of the establishment and a fee for each personal licensee.

Other responsibilities of the CH are given in detail in HOG 4.12–4.54. Amongst others they include ensuring that:

- the inspector is provided with reasonable access to all parts of the establishment;
- the NACWOs discharge their duties;
- the NVSs discharge their duties;
- the fabric of the establishment is maintained in accordance with the COPHCASP and other relevant codes, e.g. on euthanasia;
- the establishment is appropriately staffed and licensees trained;
- competent persons are available to kill animals humanely;
- animals are obtained from appropriate sources.

An additional responsibility for the CH is to establish an ethical review process (ERP).

The CH is responsible for the operation of the local ERP and for appointing the members of a committee or group to implement the procedure.

The CH must ensure as wide an involvement of establishment staff as possible in a local framework acting to ensure that all animal use in an establishment is carefully considered and justified; that proper account is taken of all possibilities for the reduction, refinement and replacement (the 3Rs) (see Alternatives and the 3Rs, Chapter 36, pp. 337–344); and that standards of accommodation and care are maximised.

The involvement of outside people in the ERP of an establishment must be considered by the CH.

Conditions on the certificate of designation

There are twenty-six standard conditions on the certificate of designation of a scientific procedure establishment. They appear in full in HOG Appendix B (Home Office 2000).

HOG Appendix C lists the twenty-three conditions on the certificates for designated breeding and supplying establishments. The variations in the text are merely changes demanded by differing circumstances.

The role of the named animal care and welfare officer (NACWO)

This named person will often be a senior animal

technician. All new NACWOs must undergo and pass an accredited training course. Usually, several such persons will be named for each establishment. Each individual will be responsible for a discreet area of the establishment. These areas should be clearly defined and communication routes put in place to ensure a standard approach across the establishment. The daily responsibilities assigned by HOG to the NACWO implies a need to appoint deputies.

Responsibilities of the NACWO listed in HOG (4.58)

- Be familiar with the main provisions of the Act;
- have an up-to date knowledge of laboratory animal technology and be aware of the standards of husbandry and welfare set out in the code of practice and taking steps to ensure that these are met;
- be knowledgeable about relevant methods of humane killing listed in Schedule 1, together with any other appropriate methods listed in the certificate of designation, and either be competent in their use or be able to contact other competent people who are named on a register maintained at the establishment;
- know which of the areas of the establishment are listed in the Schedule to the certificate of designation and the purposes for which they are approved;
- ensure that every protected animal in all designated areas is seen and checked at least once daily by a competent person;
- know how to contact at any time the NVS or deputy, the CH or nominee, and, at scientific procedure establishments, all project and personal licence holders;
- be familiar with the main provisions of the project licences, particularly adverse effects expected for each protocol, the control measures and the humane end points specified;
- assist the CH in ensuring that suitable records are maintained, under the supervision of the NVS, of the health of the animals; the environmental conditions in the rooms in which protected animals are held; and of the source and disposal of protected animals;
- take an active part in the ethical review process (ERP) at the establishment, and advise applicants for licences and licensees on practical opportunities to implement the 3Rs.

IAT NACWO guidelines

The Institute of Animal technology has issued guidelines for NACWOs. These Guidelines supplement, with more practical details, the demands made upon the NACWO in respect to the requisite functions, re-sponsibilities and qualities associated with the office.

They identify the role as being the key by which CH properly discharge their obligations and responsibilities and that most of the statutory duties, performed by the NACWO are directed towards minimising suffering and optimising the welfare of animals being bred or used for scientific procedures at the establishment.

The guidelines also state that the contribution of the NACWO towards the 3Rs – refinement, reduction and replacement – can and should be made during the planning stage of project licences and as part of an ethical review process and that further opportunities to contribute will occur during the five-year life of the project. These may include improvements to care regimes, enhancement of housing standards, notifying the personal licence holder if the condition of an animal gives cause for concern, caring for sick animals and if necessary, humanely killing the animal.

The guidelines continue:

'the provision of the highest standards of animal welfare and husbandry is explicit in this often challenging and demanding role. The NACWO will be called upon to advise and assist others working under the legislation, including the certificate holder, personal and project licensees and the NVS. Expertise in all areas of animal care and husbandry is a pre-requisite and will include areas such as health, nutrition, caging and housing, biology, breeding and legislation. A certain maturity, coupled with tact and diplomacy, may be needed in some dealings.

'Selection of the right person with the right qualifications and the right attitude to animals and others within the establishment, coupled with management support and an opportunity to maintain and further develop the necessary skills and attitudes, is seen as key to the successful functioning of an individual in the NACWO role. Whilst it is vital to establish good lines of communication with all people working within the legislation, the provision of a means of direct access between the NACWO and certificate holder is particularly important.' (IAT NACWO guidelines November 2000)

The qualities listed in the guidelines acknowledge that 'the skills and knowledge required to fulfil this vital important animal welfare position are both numerous and varied'.

'An extensive knowledge of the welfare and husbandry requirements of the species housed at the establishment is essential. Such knowledge will include the accommodation needs for different group sizes, optimum environmental conditions including enrichment opportunities, nutritional requirements and expert knowledge of the physiological and ethological needs of the species maintained. The ability to recognise any variance from normal health and behaviour in the animals under his/her care is essential. NACWOs must be able to determine the action that must be taken along with its degree of urgency and be conversant with all methods of euthanasia listed under Schedule 1 of the Act, together with any other methods approved by the Home Secretary for use at that establishment.'

This person will normally be a qualified and senior animal technician but in some establishments may be an experienced stockman or a veterinary or biological graduate with the appropriate experience and training.

The post also requires a detailed understanding of the various legislation under which the use of animals at the establishment is regulated, together with the knowledge and ability to act as advisor to other individuals working within it, such as the CH, the NVS, personal and project licence holders etc. The NACWO may also be called upon to advise on local issues within the establishment including areas such as health and safety and the acquisition, transportation and disposal of animals.

NACWOs must be familiar with the content of project licences operating in their area of responsibility and, in particular, the types of procedures, severity limits, conditions and humane endpoints contained therein.

Also required are good communication skills, both verbal and written, and sufficient standing and authority at the establishment to enable them to access the appropriate persons, offer advice and obtain timely action whenever necessary.

It is a pivotal position and it is incumbent upon the person appointed to establish, and nurture, a culture of care within the establishment. The NACWO, irrespective of his/her position in the establishment, must promote the right caring attitude, amongst all those coming into contact with animals, regarding welfare and use of animals.

It is vital that the NACWO be not only appropriately trained and qualified but that he/she constantly updates this knowledge and skills base to remain at the forefront of new and emerging technologies. The organisation of training for all animal care personnel may also be delegated to the NACWO, thus guaranteeing best standards of animal welfare. He/she should also be prepared to make, and progress, improvements to the care and welfare of animals whenever the opportunity arises. The NACWO must, therefore, keep abreast of developments and advances in the field of laboratory animal science and welfare. This continued professional development is crucial to the role and can be achieved by regular attendance at scientific meetings or discussion groups, reading scientific literature and communicating with his/her peers. Membership of professional laboratory science organisations, such as the Institute of Animal Technology (IAT) and/or the Laboratory Animal Science Association (LASA) is strongly recommended. It is desirable for NACWOs to be registered animal technicians.

It is imperative the NACWO has access to all designated rooms within his/her responsibility at all times as the NACWO must be able to advise a licensee which rooms in his/her area of responsibility are authorised for animal use and the types of procedures and species which may be used within them.

In summary the NACWO will make an important contribution to the control of severity of procedures by:

- advising the certificate holder and project licensee on matters of animal welfare and husbandry during the construction of the project licence;
- alerting the appropriate individual to an animal which is experiencing, or is likely to experience, pain and suffering.

The NACWO must have the necessary status, authority and management support within the establishment to ensure high standards of welfare are maintained and that the terms and conditions of all licences are strictly adhered to. In short the NACWO must be acknowledged and accepted as a valued expert on animal husbandry, care, welfare and legislation.

The role of the named veterinary surgeon

The responsibilities which indicate the particular functions required on the part of the NVS are clearly listed in HOG 4.61–4.64. (Home Office 2000)

The NVS should:

- be familiar with the main provisions of the Act;
- ensure that adequate veterinary cover and services are available at all times, and that the necessary contact details are known to those with relevant responsibilities for the care and welfare of protected animals;
- visit all parts of the establishment designated in the certificate at a frequency which will allow the effective monitoring of the health and welfare of the animals under their care;
- notify the personal licensee whom is charge of a protected animal if they become aware that the health or welfare of an animal is giving rise to concern (if there is no licensee, or if one is not available, the NVS must take steps to ensure that the animal is cared for and, if necessary, that it is humanely killed using an appropriate method; if there is any doubt about what action should be taken a Home Office inspector should be notified);
- be familiar with the relevant methods of humane killing listed in Schedule 1 to the Act, together with any additional approved methods set out in the conditions of the certificate of designation;
- have a thorough knowledge of the husbandry and welfare requirements of the species kept at the establishment (including the prevention, diagnosis and treatment of disease); and be able to advise on quarantine requirements and health screening, and the impact of housing and husbandry systems on the welfare and needs of a protected animal;
- control, supply and direct the use of controlled drugs, prescription only medicines and other therapeutic substances for use on protected animals in the establishment;
- maintain health records to the required professional standard relating to all the protected animals at the establishment, including advice or treatment given; and ensure that such records are readily available to the NACWO, the certificate holder and (if requested) the Home Office;
- certify that an animal is fit to travel to a specified place;

- have regular contact with the certificate holder and the NACWO;
- take an active part in the ethical review process at the establishment.

The NVS should nominate deputies and make sure they are known to other relevant members of the establishment.

Overlapping responsibilities of the NACWO and NVS

The NACWO and NVS are closely associated in both Sections 6 and 7 of the Act. On both of them is laid the responsibility of dealing with an animal the health or welfare of which gives rise to concern. Both the NACWO and the NVS are obliged to notify the relevant personal licence holder, if appropriate, or care for the animal or see that it is killed. Subsection (7)s of Section 6 and 7 of the Act suggests the NACWO might notify the NVS when there is concern about an animals health and welfare. It also suggests either the NACWO or the NVS might notify the inspector in such circumstances.

The very nature of the roles ascribed in law to the NACWO and NVS imply involvement one with the other as well as an amount of overlapping of the duties assigned to either of them. The most onerous duty of the NACWO, the daily checking of every animal, is a prerequisite for the NVS to adequately fulfil his/her main responsibility of monitoring the health and welfare of the animals. The awareness of the NACWO alerts the NVS to attend immediately to the care of specific animals.

- The NACWO must ensure health records are maintained in a form determined by the NVS.
- The NACWO must know how to contact the NVS or her/his deputy.
- The duties of the NACWO and NVS regarding euthanasia overlap.
- The NVS must have regular contact with the NACWO.
- The NVS should make the health records available to the NACWO.
- The NVS should make known the identity of nominated deputies to the NACWO.

Background literature on both the NACWO and NVS reinforce the need for these two named persons to be closely associated. It is particularly in the area of training that the duties overlap.

> 'The NACWO may also be given delegated authority for the organisation of training for all animal care personnel.' (NACWO guidelines, p. 5, IAT 2000)

> 'The NVS is in the best position to advise on improvements in anaesthesia, surgical techniques and the control of pain and will be expected to do so. An NVS will also be expected to advise on methods of humane killing and train technicians and scientists in these and other skills.' (Guide to Professional Conduct 3.7.6)

> 'The NACWO will be called upon to advise and assist others working under the legislation including . . . the NVS.' (NACWO guidelines, IAT 2000)

> 'The NVS should be familiar with the range of scientific procedures carried out under project licences and may take part in training of technicians and personal licence holders on animal welfare and health.' (NVS Guidance 20, RCVS 2004)

> 'Commonly a senior animal technician holds the position of NACWO and is the main point of contact on matters relating to the general care and husbandry of animals in the establishment. He or she is likely to be the person who contacts the NVS in cases where the health or welfare of an animal gives rise to concern. The NVS should foster a good working relationship with the NACWO(s) and other animal care staff' (NVS Guidance 37, RCVS 2004).

Ethical review process (ERP)

The Act requires the certificate holder (CH) to establish and maintain a local ethical review process (LERP). The CH is responsible for appointing members to the process and should ensure as wide an involvement of establishment staff as possible. HOG Appendix J (Home Office 2000) advises that at all establishments membership must include the NVS and representatives from among the NACWOs. Project licensees and personal licensees should also be represented at user establishments. Generally speaking, as many people as possible should be involved in the ethical review process and some of the other suggestions for suitable classes of members include:

- Where possible, the views of those who do not have responsibilities under the Act should be taken into account.

- One or more lay persons, independent of the establishment, should also be considered.

Home Office inspectors should have the right to attend any meetings and have access to the records of the ethical review process.

Aims

The aims of LERP are:

- to provide independent ethical advice to the certificate holder, particularly with respect to project licence applications and standards of animal care and welfare;
- to provide support to named people and advice to licensees regarding animal welfare and ethical issues arising from their work;
- to promote the use of ethical analysis to increase awareness of animal welfare issues and develop initiatives leading to the widest possible application of the 3Rs.

It achieves these aims by:

- promoting the development and uptake of the 3Rs (reduction, refinement and replacement) in animal use, where they exist, and ensuring the availability of relevant sources of information;
- examining proposed applications for new project licences and amendments to existing licences, with reference to the likely costs to the animals, the expected benefits of the work and how these considerations balance;
- providing a forum for discussion of issues relating to the use of animals and considering how staff can be kept up to date with relevant ethical advice, best practice, and relevant legislation;
- undertaking retrospective project reviews and continuing to apply the 3Rs to all projects, throughout their duration;
- considering the care and accommodation standards applied to all animals in the establishment, including breeding stock, and the humane killing of protected animals;
- regularly reviewing the establishment's managerial systems, procedures and protocols where these bear on the proper use of animals;
- advising on how all staff involved with the animals can be appropriately trained and how competence can be ensured.

Commonly, there should be a promotional role, seeking to educate users (in applying the 3Rs) and non-users (by explaining why and how animals are used), as appropriate. Ideally, there should be some formal output from the ethical review process for staff and colleagues in the establishment, made as widely available as security and commercial/intellectual confidentiality allow.

Members of the process must meet regularly and keep records of their discussions and advice. They should be open to attendance from all staff. It should be clear how submissions to the process could be made. The people involved should be regarded as approachable, dealing in confidence with complaints and processing all suggestions for improvement.

All project licence applications must go through the ethical review procedures because an application will not be considered for formal authorisation by the Home Office until the prospective project has been considered appropriately within the local ethical review process.

Receipt of a project licence application signed by the certificate holder will be taken by the Home Office to mean that the application has been through the ethical review process for that establishment.

The role of the Home Office inspector

Home Office inspectors are people with either medical or veterinary qualifications. The following extract from the APC 1992 Report (no.19) describes the role of the Inspector.

> 'Inspectors consider in detail applications for licences and advise the Home Secretary on how to ensure that only properly justified work is licensed. They carry out visits, mainly without notice, to establishments designated under the Act to ensure that its controls and the terms and the conditions of licences issued under it are being observed.'

It is obvious from the above that the role of the inspector is multifarious. Besides other commitments, e.g. dealing with correspondence from members of the public concerned about the use of animals in research, she/he advises, reviews, inspects and reports.

Section 18 of the ASPA stipulates in detail the legal status and duties of the inspector. It empowers the Home Secretary to appoint inspectors; sets out their duties to visit establishments and advise and report to the Secretary of State; and empowers inspectors to order the killing of an animal.

The various roles of the inspector

The inspector advises
The inspector advises on the welfare of protected animals and offers advice to project and personal licensees on their applications, for example, on amendments of their licences. Consultation with the inspector can prove to be a most fruitful source of direction in respect to animal experimentation. Such counselling may be the most beneficial result of an inspector's visit. The inspector's advice can also be sought by telephone.

The inspector reviews
The inspector reviews applications for licences and certificates and may also review applicants for a personal licence.

The inspector inspects
Most visits by an inspector to a designated establishment are usually for the purposes of an inspection, though as indicated above, visits may be for purposes of advising licensees, named persons, certificate holders or other personnel.

The purposes for the visits of inspectors are clearly laid down in law. Section 18(2) of the ASPA states that it shall be the duty of an inspector:

- to visit places where regulated procedures are carried out, for the purpose of determining whether those procedures are authorised by the requisite licences and whether the conditions of those licences are being complied with;
- to visit designated establishments for the purpose of determining whether the conditions of the certificate in respect of those establishments are being complied with.

Both of these paragraphs would indicate that the visiting inspector would be concerned, during the inspection, with the welfare of the animals.

The inspector reports
Section 18(2) states that it shall be the duty of an inspector to report to the Home Secretary any case in which any provision of this Act or any condition of a

licence or certificate under this Act has not been or is not being complied with and to advise him on the action to be taken in any case.

The animal procedures committee

Under the Act, the Secretary of State must establish a committee called the Animals Procedures Committee (APC) which is an independent advisory body. The duties of the APC are as follows.

- They must advise the Home Secretary on matters concerned with the Act referred to it by him / her or on their own initiative.
- In their discussions, they must balance the legitimate requirements of science and industry with protection of animals from suffering and unnecessary use in procedures.
- They may promote research relevant to its functions and obtain advice from experts.
- They may carry out their functions by establishing sub-committees and may co-opt extra members.
- They must make a report to the Home Secretary every year, who presents the report before Parliament.

Specific responsibilities

Most project licence applications are considered by Home Office inspectors and granted on their advice. Some project licence applications which are particularly sensitive are considered by the APC. The APC is involved in considering and advising the Home Secretary on granting project licences in the following areas:

- the use of primates in procedures of substantial severity;
- the use of wild-caught primates;
- microsurgical training;

- they may also be asked for advice on any other project application if the Home Secretary feels it would be useful.

Membership of the APC

Membership consists of a chairman and at least twelve other members.

- At least two thirds must be registered medical practitioners or veterinary practitioners or hold relevant biological qualifications and experience.
- There should be at least one barrister, solicitor or advocate.
- At least half should not have held a licence under the Act for at least six years.
- There should be adequate representation from animal welfare groups.
- Members are appointed for four years and cannot be re-appointed more than once.

References and further reading

Association of Veterinary Teachers and Research Workers (1989) *Guidelines for the Recognition and Assessment of Pain in Animals.* UFAW, Hertfordshire, UK.

Home Office (1989) *Code of Practice for the Housing and Care of Animals used in Scientific Procedures.* HMSO, London.

Home Office (2000) *Guidance on the Operation of the Animals (Scientific Procedures) Act 1986.* HMSO, London.

Institute of Animal Technology (IAT) (2000) *Guidance to Named Animal Care and Welfare Officers.* IAT, Oxford.

LASA Working Party (1990) The assessment and control of the severity of scientific procedures on laboratory animals, LASA Report, pp. 97–130. *Laboratory Animals,* **24.**

Webliography

Home Office publications on the Animals (Scientific Procedures) Act 1986 can be accessed at the Home Office website (www.homeoffice.gov.uk/ccpd/aps.htm).

36

The Ethical Implications of the Use of Animals in Scientific Procedures

Kevin P. Dolan

Introduction

This section is not intended to be a course in ethics but is concerned with the ethical discussions surrounding the use of animals in research, ethical theories dealing with the use of animals and the application of accepted ethical theories to the use of animals in research.

There is, however, some need to put this subject, 'ethical implications', within a more general framework of moral philosophy within which it belongs and to distinguish it from law with which it is closely related and which looms large in the use of animals in scientific procedures.

Terms such as 'moral philosophy' may startle but the phrase means the same as ethics and merely implies thinking about what is right and wrong in respect of our actions. Throughout the media there is indiscriminate use of such terms as ethics, morality and mores. It is sufficient in this text to concentrate on ethical implications, on the general assumption that ethics is a sort of science of conduct.

Ethics explores and for some delivers satisfactory answers about what constitutes right or wrong behaviour and produces persuasive arguments about the acceptability or unacceptability of human actions. It must be appreciated, however, that ethics is in no real sense of the word a science. Sciences are empirical, they depend for verification on experience, e.g. by experiment or observation. Ethics is speculative; its currency is the value judgement – a considered opinion, maybe – but not an established fact.

These characteristics may make ethical discussion appear somewhat inadequate at the interface with reality. In spite of its rarefied nature, however, it has some value. It can help to provide a common consensus for popular support for legislation on controversial issues, a relevant and practical factor in respect to the Animals (Scientific Procedures) Act 1986 (ASPA). Ethical arguments are important in evaluating the rightness or wrongness of laws themselves; whether they are good or bad laws. There have been bad laws; not even law can be judge in its own case. Law is not its own criterion of righteousness. It is not, *per se*, a norm of morality.

This distinction between what is legal and what is considered ethical is crucial. No doubt there are those who have scant respect for correct conduct who talk cynically in terms of 'it doesn't matter if it is not honest as long as it is legal'. Most law-abiding citizens see a real difference between the two concepts. Even among practitioners in the field of animal experimentation some immediate reactions to particular propositions clearly indicate this difference. There are research workers who would not perform some procedures even though they are legal under licence, e.g. some researchers, while happily operating under ASPA, positively condemn the LD50 test or use of any primates. They distinguish strongly between what is allowed by law and what, for them, is ethically unacceptable.

The salient distinction between ethics and law is that ethics is 'exhortation without enforcement' whereas law is 'an order, command or directive by authority backed by a sanction, penalty or punishment'. It would be wrong, however, to regard ethics as having no clout; accepted attitudes within the group, the mores within a community and the particular ethical slant given by society to education, can have strong persuasive powers. It could be argued that peer pressure within the scientific community by such institutions as the Institute of Animal Technology (IAT), the Laboratory Animal Science Association (LASA) and the Universities Federation for Animal Welfare (UFAW) has evolved a more benign ethical attitude to the use of animals in research during this century. A useful survey of this progressive ethical attitude has been carried out by Barley (1999).

The close association of the ethical and the legal in dealing with concern about the use of animals in research is evident from various official statements:

- The European Convention on Animal Experimentation of 1986, although a political document with legal implications introduces into its preamble an ethical dimension, '. . . . recognising that man has a moral obligation to respect all animals and exercise due consideration for their capacity and memory.'

- When introducing the second White Paper (1985) of the ASPA, the then Parliamentary Under-secretary of State at the Home Office said, 'One of the tests of a civilised society is its treatment of animals.'

- The marked entwining of ethical and legal considerations concerning animal experimentation has been highlighted by this Home Office Letter (Ref. 3–4.98):

'6.1 Establishments now have a year in which to devise or revise local processes and to demonstrate to the Home Office how they will be effective. The aim is for establishments to have met the requirements, as set out in the Annex, by April 1999. A condition should then be added to the Certificate of Designation.
'6.2. This condition will require that an appropriate Ethical Review Process is in place which demonstrably meets the needs of the establishment and the aims of the policy. The ultimate sanction for not complying with this condition will be revocation of the certificate, subject to the right to make representations.'

From the above the moot point regarding whether justification of a regulated procedure, allowing a person to use animals in research, is in the main legal or ethical becomes even more complex.

The ethical controversy

That there is a controversy in this area is beyond dispute, the necessarily strict security surrounding any animal unit bears witness to this undeniable fact. The contenders fall roughly into three groups:

(1) Some anti-vivisectionist societies are extreme in their opposition to the use of animals. Ingrid Newirk of People for the Ethical Treatment of Animals (PETA) regards the use of animals even in painless research as fascism. Some of these extremists even regard the keeping of pets as unacceptable, as a form of supremism – challenging an animal's individuality. Among the extreme opponents to animal experimentation are some who are not averse to the use of violence to press home their views.

(2) There are moderate movements unhappy with the use of animals in experiments, as indeed, aren't we all? They concentrate on eliminating as far as possible the use of animals in research while accepting that animal experimentation does produce benefits for both animals and humans.

(3) Finally there are societies which accept the justification of using animals in research and have contributed greatly to drawing attention to the need for high standards of care of the animals used.

Sentiment and speciesism

Two important factors in this ethical debate are sentiment and speciesism.

Sentiment

This human phenomenon is to the fore in any public debate or private discussion on animal use. It can be described as thought or reflection coloured by emotion.

Sentiment influences opinions, such as moral judgements, by basing decisions on feelings and emotions rather than on reason and logic. This does not mean that such decisions lack validity in every day life. Humans are not mere computers. We share the rich appetites of vibrant life with the rest of the animal kingdom. We are motivated by complex forces which reflect reality more closely than does cold intellectual speculation.

Sound consistent humane sentiment, as opposed to a weak irrational indulgent sentimentality, may form a valid basis for moral judgements. The humane feelings of animal technologists rather than spurious moral outrage, does and will continue to maintain the care and welfare of laboratory animals. Sentiment as an expression of the emotional influences on our behaviour is an essential element in the human condition. It serves a purpose throughout life to attune us to our surroundings. Even David Hume, the greatest sceptic among moral philosophers, in his *An Enquiry concerning the Principles of Morals* talks in terms of a 'sentiment of humanity' as being a potent force in the development of morality.

Undiscerning sentiment

Over-concern is frequently expressed for furry cuddly mammals accompanied by an indifference to less appealing rats or scaly reptiles. Such expression of sentiment is reprehensible, especially if misinformed, inconsistent and illogical. Examples of inadequate expressions of sentiment are not uncommon. Anti-vivisectionists have been known to release both rabbits and ferrets from the same establishment with unfortunate consequences to both species because the laboratory ferrets were ill-equipped to survive in the wild. There are those who express outrage at the use of 2.3 million rodents (1996) used in research but make no mention of the 8.5 million (approx) wild rodents professionally exterminated annually. Britain's cats kill approximately 100 million small birds and mammals every year according to a survey carried out by Professor Robert May of Princeton University (May 1988). It appears that many who are deeply concerned about the loss of animal life in laboratories, an insignificant figure in comparison with the havoc wrought by the well fed British tabby, tacitly accept this mass slaughter.

Sentiment is bound to play its part in attitudes to our treatment of animals. It is a powerful instrument of propaganda for either side in any polemics but particularly telling in the debate on medical benefits from the use of animals in research. It must however be used with caution and viewed with suspicion; rhetoric is a noble art but has frequently been used by the unscrupulous to deceive the unwary.

Speciesism

The essence of speciesism can be summed up in the phrase 'the boundary of my group is the boundary of my concern'. A consequence of this attitude in the past was that animals were regarded as expendable in whatever manner served the purposes of human beings. David G. Porter (1992) claimed that there existed among research workers an inarticulated acceptance that they were justified in giving priority to the needs of man above those of other animals particularly in respect to the health and survival of humankind. That supposition in its extreme unqualified form is an expression of speciesism.

Peter Singer, the philosopher loudest in the condemnation of speciesism (a term he adopted from Richard Ryder), does not deny the distinction between ourselves and animals. He admits as we all do the existence of species in the animal kingdom, marked differences between the different species and a certain gradation of sentience among species. Singer argues, that if possessing a higher degree of intelligence does not entitle one human to use another for his own ends, how can it entitle humans to exploit non-humans?

Other philosophers have also considered our attitude to those outside the accepted group of concern whether other races and, perhaps surprisingly to us in this day and age, all those of the female gender. They rightly argued the case for individuals of deprived groups excluded from equal treatment. Jeremy Bentham, an early advocate of Utilitarianism (1748–1832) was one of the few who was ready to apply the principle of equal consideration of interests also to animals.

'The day may come when the rest of the animal creation may acquire those rights which never could have been witholden from them but by the hand of tyranny. The French have already discovered that the blackness of the skin is no reason why a human being should be abandoned to the tormentor. It may one day come to be recognized that the number of the legs, the villosity of the skin or the termination of the *os sacrum*, are reasons equally insufficient for abandoning a sensitive being to the same fate. What else is it that should trace the insuperable line? Is it the faculty of reason? But a full-grown horse or dog is beyond comparison a more rational, as well as a more conversable animal than an infant of a day or a week, or even a month old. But suppose they were otherwise, what would it avail? The question is not, Can they reason? nor Can they talk? but, Can they suffer,' (*Introduction to the Principles of Morals and Legislation* ch. XVII, 1789)

In this passage Bentham points to the capacity for suffering as the vital characteristic that gives a being the right to equal consideration. The capacity for suffering – or more strictly, for suffering and/or enjoyment or happiness – is not just another characteristic like the capacity for language. The capacity for suffering and enjoying things is a pre-requisite for having interests at all.

Singer points out that it would be nonsense to say that it was not in the interest of a stone to be kicked along the road. A stone does not have interests because it cannot suffer. Nothing that we do to it could possibly make any difference to its welfare. A mouse, on the other hand, does have interest in not being tormented, because it will suffer if it is.

If a being suffers, there can be no moral justification for refusing to take suffering into consideration. No matter what the nature of the being, the principle of equality requires that its suffering be counted equally with like suffering, in so far as rough comparisons can be made, of any other being. If a being is not capable of suffering, or of experiencing enjoyment or happiness, there is nothing to be taken into account. This is why the limit of sentience (using the term as a convenient, if not strictly accurate, shorthand for the capacity to suffer or experience enjoyment or happiness) is the only defensible boundary of concern.

It should be pointed out that while Bentham and Singer would agree that concern should extend to all sentient beings, Bentham, unlike Singer perhaps, but like many members of the human race, did not consider that the rightful concern for animal suffering completely ruled out the use of animals which might involve pain. In spite of his obvious sympathy for animals, Bentham was blatantly carnivorous. He believed, as obviously other people do, that his relish for meat justified the killing of the animal. Arguing, of course, with due concern for animal suffering, that the pain to the animal must be kept to the minimum. Using the same ethical approach it would seem easier to justify the use of animals for the greater good of the health of humans and animals alike. As long as there is a constant striving to replace animals; that the balance of the benefit and the suffering of the animal is of an acceptable level and that any suffering or even discomfort is kept to a minimum.

Ethical theories

It is a truism to state that there is no universal ethical accord concerning the use of animals in research. Not only are there differing schools of thought on the matter but there is a variety of conflicting arguments. Those arguments depend on the ethical theories of their proponents.

Stretching far back into the past, even to the time of Aristotle (384–322 BC) and reaching even to the time of Descartes (1596–1650), who spoke in terms of; 'animals can't talk, therefore they can't think, therefore they can't feel'; there seemed to be little place for ethical disputations on the treatment of animals. They were beyond concern even considered as lacking consciousness and thus incapable of suffering, surely an attitude that ignored facts.

A general notion of the supremacy of man over brute nature engendered the attitude that lower animals were completely at man's disposal. Ancient and modern ethical theories that regarded 'might as right' had few scruples about either the use or abuse of animals, for whatever purpose, by human beings. How else could bear-baiting, etc. have been accepted within a society?

The Machiavellian ethical theory of consequentialism, implying that the end justified the means, could render acceptable any actions however abhorrent as long as the desirable goal was attained. This type of argument could easily be used to defend even the most outrageous abuse of either animals or humans.

Modern ethical theories which talk in terms of rights for animals produce a completely different ethical approach to the debate on the use of animals in research. Regan (1983), Rollin (1993), Ryder and Singer (1992) particularly in his devastating attack on speciesism, represent that side of the ethical divide.

Utilitarianism

Jeremy Bentham, a leading figure of Utilitarianism, propounded arguments on the need for concern for animals akin to those used by Singer in his condemnation of speciesism. Unlike Singer, however Bentham was prepared to justify the use of animals by humans even if it involved killing animals for food. While avoiding the extreme consequentialism of Machiavelli, Bentham, as a Utilitarian, assessed the ethical worth of any action in the light of 'the greatest happiness of the greatest number'. This maxim was, for Utilitarians, the criterion of the rightness or wrongness of human behaviour. This approach lends itself well to considering the acceptability of an action on the basis of a cost / benefit assessment. In other words, a weighing up of the desirability of a procedure by whether the resulting benefit contributes to the greatest happiness of the greatest number. Unlike Machiavellianism, however, always including in that weighing up process the cost, e.g. suffering and animal suffering at that, as a crucial consideration.

A basic tenet of Utilitarianism, 'the pursuit of pleasure is good in itself' implies that an act which may cause gratuitous suffering is morally undesirable. Bentham readily admitted this proposition. Consequently, Utilitarianism as an ethical theory commits those who hold this view to avoid causing suffering as far as is possible. This commitment can only be tempered by the desire to achieve the greatest happiness of the greatest number.

Utilitarianism as an ethical theory is committed to carefully calculating what benefits can justify procedures which may be unacceptable as such but may be seen as acceptable in the light of those benefits. With its hedonistic imperative – its compelling drive to increase pleasure (in a refined sense) and reduce pain and suffering wherever possible – Utilitarians are bound to be fully committed to the vigorous pursuit of the 3Rs (Replacement, Reduction, Refinement) in respect to animal experimentation. (For an explanation of the 3Rs, see pp. 336–337.)

Pain (and of course 'suffering, distress or lasting harm')

In the debate about the use of animals in research, pain (and what has been added above is to be understood as implied if appropriate in the situation) is, of course, the crucial issue. If pain, suffering, distress or lasting harm is not present then whatever animal use may be involved is outside the scope of the ASPA and so not directly relevant to this text. The ethical implication is very much the same whether we are considering pain, suffering, distress or lasting harm. The varying intensity of each of these states will however affect the ethical assessment of the cost / benefit. The concentration here is on pain, those who seek more details on the other undesirable states should consult *Guidelines on the recognition of pain, distress and discomfort in experimental animals and an hypothesis for assessment* (Morton & Griffiths 1985).

Universality of pain

Pain is one of the most vivid forms of awareness. Everyone knows by experience what pain is. There is no concept whose objective existence seems to have been so empirically and universally established yet all direct knowledge of it is necessarily subjective and a clear definition of it proves elusive. One working dictionary definition of pain is 'an adverse sensation experienced when the body is injured or afflicted in some way'. In a scientific setting pain is associated with such nociceptive systems as sensory, motor and memory systems. In this context, pain may be defined as 'an adverse sensory experience caused by actual or potential injury which is accompanied by protective somatic and visceral reactions and induces changes in behaviour including behaviour which can be specific for an individual animal' (AVTRW 1989).

Pain and suffering is rampant in nature. The slightest mistake in life or an inadvertent exposure to infection on the part of any creature can bring immediate, inevitable and dire consequences, even death.

Animal pain

The mechanisms responsible for pain are remarkably similar in all vertebrates. Anaesthetics and analgesics control what appears to be pain in all vertebrates and some invertebrates. The biological feedback mechanisms for controlling pain seem to be similar in all vertebrates, involving serotonin, endorphins, enkephalins and substance P. Endorphins have been found in earthworms. The existence of endogenous opiates indicates that animals are capable of feeling pain. They would hardly have neurochemicals and pain-inhibiting systems identical to ours and show the same diminution of pain signs as we do if their experiential pain was not being controlled by these mechanisms in the same way that ours is.

The many similarities between animals' and humans' anatomical and chemical pathways of pain perception are used to justify the validity of the use of animals in research for the benefit of humans. Therefore, conditions which are painful in humans should be assumed to be painful in animals until behavioural or clinical signs prove otherwise.

The cost of the cost/benefit

The cost of the cost/benefit (see Chapter 35) is the pain, suffering, distress or lasting harm to the animal. If any proportionality is to be arrived at between this cost and hoped-for benefit, some attempt must be made to measure that cost.

The measuring of pain, suffering and distress of experimental animals is not ethical but technical demanding specialised expertise. The scientific assessment of these phenomena has advanced and is still a matter for research in spite of doubts in the past even by experts on the subject.

The Littlewood Committee (1965) having researched the subject reported that 'It is not as a rule possible to assess degrees of real pain in animals.'

We have progressed from that position. 'Since a wide variety of biochemical, physiological and behavioural parameters must be considered and since adequate statistical analyses of the relative importance of each are not available for each species and type of pain, the overall assessment of welfare in individual cases can only be treated as a value judgement based upon the experience of those presented with the task.' (*The Veterinary Teachers and Research Workers' Guidelines* 1989).

No doubt a gradation in the degree of pain, suffering or distress can be recognised. At one end of the spectrum there is trivial and momentary pain, such as that evoked by a simple injection. However, technical incompetence or undue repetition could escalate the degree of suffering to one that could be considered more severe.

At the other end of the spectrum there is severe pain which has been described as that produced by procedures to which normal humans would not voluntarily submit without appropriate analgesia or anaesthesia. Such pain could result from extensive tissue injury or with certain malignant tumours. Severe distress, on the other hand, might be that associated with conditioned helplessness experiments, or with deprivation of food and water, or when deprived of social contact for long periods. In between trivial pain and severe pain there is a grey area, a moderate pain zone which may be relatively long lasting.

Acceptability of pain

Pain is the greatest disadvantage of using animals in experiments because of the distress caused to the animal. There is also a scientific reason to avoid pain in the use of animals in research. The reactions which it is intended to observe can be distorted by pain due to the high stress factor involved. In spite of these considerations many will concede that a certain amount of pain is acceptable to advance our knowledge particularly as regards medicine. This reflects human attitudes to pain throughout history. Painful procedures in the form of barbaric operations were performed to avert greater pain. The use of pain, sometimes grotesque, was employed as an instrument of law and order.

In fact pain is not all bad; it has its positive uses. It functions as a warning, indicating internal and external danger. Children whose pain mechanism is defective have a low survival rate. Pain also operates in the context of penalty/reward mechanisms involved in the process of learning in both animals and humans.

It must be stressed that in spite of the fact that pain has been regarded as an acceptable part of reality, most humans strive, and rightly so, from humanitarian motives to avoid inflicting pain on animals. This is particularly true of many involved in research. The corollary of such an attitude is that whatever pain is involved in the use of animals is not only controlled but restricted as much as possible. Pain can only be justified in these conditions when it is considered objectively to be a cost worth paying. Perhaps one can accept the proposition that we may hurt a little to help a lot.

Sapontzis in his book, *Morals, Reason and Animals*, introduces a special feature of concern for animals beyond the prevention of causing them pain, 'Life is necessary for enjoyment and fulfilment, this generates an interest for sentient beings in remaining alive as long as life holds the prospect or even just hope of sufficient enjoyment or fulfilment for them, and that our common moral goals include a concern with insuring that all those capable of enjoyment and fulfilment have a fair chance at achieving an enjoyable fulfilling life.' (Sapontzis 1987).

This would imply that animal life is of value in and of itself. We should even question the morality of killing animals even without pain. Perhaps pain should not be the major factor to be considered in our concern for animal well-being. Certain interests are of higher priority to animals than pain. Animals will chew off limbs to escape traps, implying that desire for freedom or life takes priority to the avoidance of pain. In some cases animals will choose sexual contact at the cost of pain.

Cost/benefit – the balancing act

Dr. Robert Watt, the former Chief Inspector, Home Office, pointed out that the big ethical decision – that animal experimentation should be allowed under specified conditions – had already been taken at a national level by the passing of the ASPA. Dr. Watt went on to indicate the role of the Secretary of State, acting through, and using the experience and expertise of, the Inspectorate, 'To weigh the likely adverse effects on the animals concerned against the benefit likely to accrue as a result of the programme to be specified in the licence. In difficult cases requiring specialized knowledge external assessors and the Animal Procedures Committee are consulted. Work is considered to be justified if the likely benefit exceeds the likely cost to animals in suffering'. (cf. LASA Newsletter pp. 14–16, Sept. 1994.) A model of the cost/benefit process is shown in Figure 36.1.

The Ethical Review Process

An obligatory and essential element has been introduced into the decision-making mechanism for justifying the granting of a project licence. This development, instigated by the APC, brings to the fore the ethical dimension in the approval of regulated procedures. This leaves in no doubt the ethical implications of the use of animals in scientific procedures (see Chapter 35).

Use of animals in research

While it is essential to use alternatives to animals wherever possible, it must be admitted that at our present stage of knowledge and technology the use of animals is a requisite for efficient progress in the conquest of illness. A consideration of the advantages and disadvantages of animal use in research is therefore appropriate to those working in this area. In most instances the advantage or disadvantage will be *vis-à-vis* non-sentient alternatives but it could be *vis-à-vis* human beings or have an element of both.

The advantages of live animals as tools for research

A true picture of biological reality

Although in mathematics the whole is equal to the sum total of the parts this is not true in all sciences and is incorrect in the living sciences. From experience we know that we have achieved much in research through the use of cell culture, tissue culture and organ culture. They are all parts of the whole

$$justification = \frac{benefit}{cost}$$

$$justification = \frac{importance\ of\ objectives \times probability\ of\ achievement}{cost\ to\ animals\ in\ suffering}$$

$$justification = \frac{background\ objectives/potential\ benefits \times scientific\ quality}{adverse\ effects\ and\ coping\ strategies}$$

$$justification = \frac{Section\ 17 \times Section\ 18}{Section\ 19}$$

Section 17 – background, objectives and potential benefits
Section 18 – description of plan of work (scientific quality)
Section 19 – protocol sheets (details of the procedure to be performed and possible adverse effects on the animals used)

Note: valid objectives must be original, realistic, current and potentially beneficial within the terms of the 1986 Act.

Figure 36.1 Project licence form. First published in the Animal Procedures Committee Report (1993), p. 27.

living entity – the organism, but putting those parts together cannot fully recreate the functioning, living organism. Not even collating all the knowledge we may have ascertained from a full investigation of each of those parts can provide a full picture of the biological reality of that organism. Each part or group of parts in isolation will react in ways that are different, sometimes fundamentally different, than when they are in a whole living organism. In such a setting, involving the interaction of all the various parts of the organism and the impact of metabolic cycles, the previously separately observed results can be completely different from what is discovered by observing the complete living organism.

In short, although using isolated cells or tissues can provide useful information, the living organism is more than all its parts put together. Consequently only by use of the living animals can we learn the complete truth about the variety of vital functions.

Statistically significant numbers of laboratory animals

To ensure changes seen as a result of experimental work are real and do not occur by chance, the change must be seen in sufficient numbers of animals. In experiments involving cancer research or toxicology, for example, the production of large numbers of inbred rodents means that a sufficiently significant number of individuals are available to support valid research, always presuming that the minimum number required is used and that the extrapolation is scientifically acceptable. Equally valid results are less likely if larger species are used because the cost of keeping them means fewer can be used. The same is true of using humans because humans vary in their backgrounds and there are insufficient numbers of suitable individuals.

Known health status

One of the essential features for successful research is the exclusion of any outside factors which may introduce variables. In the case of laboratory animals, health status can be more clearly defined than it can be if human subjects are used. By the use of barrier-maintained animals, disease, a major variable in biomedical studies, can be obviated. Human subjects of this type would not be available. In the case of gnotobiotic animals, the pathogenic effect of a particular species of micro-organism can be studied in depth.

It is impossible to make such studies, *in situ*, in any other way apart from the use of gnotobiotic animals.

Inbred animals

The importance of excluding as many variables as possible in any programme of research, has already been stressed. Until the coming of successful genetic manipulation techniques, inbred animals were the only available source of organisms which were almost genetically identical and as such were ideal for use in research. Such a need could not be met by selection from among the human population. Transgenic animals, 'knock-outs', for example, can now better fulfil this role so vital to areas such as cancer research (see Chapter 14).

Short generations

In studies involving reproduction and genetics there is a marked advantage in being able to draw data from a number of generations. This implies that the research should be able to be completed at least well within the working life of the experimenter, in fact, usually within a much shorter period. Consequently research of this type can only be successfully carried out using animals such as rodents, e.g. mice, which have postpartum oestrus. This means that one generation may be as short as approximately four months.

Ethical considerations

Some forms of research depend greatly on postmortem data. Given that appropriate humane endpoints are always adopted and that the ideal form of euthanasia is competently performed, it is preferable ethically to use animals rather than humans in such circumstances.

Ideal models

Some species have predispositions to particular diseases, e.g. the Chinese hamster with a susceptibility to diabetes. Likewise, some species have a specific characteristic which is of immense worth in some form of experiments, for example, the ample cheek pouches of the hamster have proved to be suitable sites for tumour transplants. The abundant epidermal tissue of the armadillo makes it valuable for research into and a development of a therapy for leprosy. In such instances the use of these animals could progress research far better than the use of human beings, other animals or alternative methods.

Results of these research programmes could be applied to all species including humans in need of the benefit of that type of research.

Veterinary medicine

Veterinary medicine has progressed tremendously both with regard to prevention and therapy as a result of the use of animals in research. Numerous vaccines have been developed, e.g. against rabies, through the use of laboratory animals. These advances have been made possible either by the use of ideal models, which have already been referred to, or by the use of conspecifics.

The advantages of using animals in this way for their benefit of other animals are probably more obvious than in other forms of animal experimentation.

Difficulty of validation

In spite of the efforts of ECVAM (European Centre for the Validation of Alternative Methods) progress has been slow in the development of adequate alternatives to animals in research. In addition it has been difficult to validate proposed alternatives to the satisfaction of all regulatory authorities. Usually, the assessment of the adequacy of an alternative to the use of live animals will need the further use of animals to validate the proposed new method.

In view of the advantages already described above, the preferable experimental model is at present most often the live animal.

Expertise in animal studies

On account of the vast experience of both technicians and scientists in the use of animals throughout the whole of this century, an immense reservoir of useful knowledge concerning animals, their husbandry needs, their biology and their behaviour has been amassed.

This particular advantage of animal use has increased the awareness of the need for animal welfare. It has contributed considerably to the refinements in the application of animal care. Experience of this extent is lacking in the use of alternatives.

The testimony of history

The advantages of using animals in research have been obvious to scientists for many centuries. As far back as the third century BC in Alexandria, philosopher–scientists like Erasistratus were advancing human knowledge and medical skills by using animals in their research. Erasistratus, an early anatomist, developed the catheter through his work with animals. Galen (c. 200 AD), the most renowned physician of the ancient world, used both pigs and apes to explore the functions of the blood in living organisms.

William Harvey (1578–1657) first described the circulation of the blood in his *De motu cordis et sanguinis in animalibus* (On the motion of the heart and blood in animals) (1628). The title itself indicates how he achieved this great advance in medical knowledge. He stated categorically the need to use animals in research. It is said that he used more than forty species of animals in his experiments.

Charles Darwin (1809–1882) who deplored some forms of animal experimentation testified to the Royal Commission (1875) that he thought that a ban on animal experimentation would be 'a great evil'. The implication of this remark was that he appreciated the many advantages which had accrued from the use of animals in research.

In this century knowledge of medical matters has not only progressed through the use of animals but has positively accelerated. This is not the place to reproduce long lists of achievements. It is enough to point out that had there been a mandatory moratorium on the use of animals in research at any time in the past there could have been dire consequences for the progress of medicine and the living sciences. Such a moratorium in 1910 could have deprived mankind in the years immediately following of extensive knowledge of vitamins. Such a moratorium in 1950 could have deprived that generation of the polio vaccine. The last few decades of animal use has produced new vaccines for animals and humans, new medicines, new forms of therapy, such as transplants, and most of all, advances in applied genetics, again for the good of animals and humans alike. These valuable contributions to the well-being of living creatures continues. A single injection which will protect against the dominant form of meningitis could soon be available thanks to genetically engineered vaccines (cf. IAT Bulletin Nov. 1997).

Disadvantages of live animals as tools of research

In the early 1970s, the then Minister of Education and Science stated:

'The government's view is that scientists always prefer alternatives where available for reasons of humanity, economy and convenience.' (Hansard vol. 814, No. 116, col. 1642–46).

Scientists agree with anti-vivisectionists that it is not desirable to use live animals in experiments. Scientists differ from anti-vivisectionists in accepting the need for animal experimentation, although the scientist is more aware of the practical disadvantages of using animals.

The following types of disadvantages are among the difficulties associated with the use of animals in research.

Ethical considerations

Pain, suffering, distress or lasting harm are not by any means desirable results of any venture. Whatever can be done to avoid inflicting such hardships on animals must be an ethical imperative. Only the expectancy of real proportionate benefits can possibly justify the use of animals in this way. Accepting that proposition may render such use acceptable but it is by no means desirable.

Cost

It may be a mercenary consideration but it is a most telling argument against the use of animals in research. Costs incurred, for example, in the use of gnotobiotic animals can be astronomical. An example from the 1980s illustrates how money can be saved through the use of alternatives. Sheep were used for specific export tests, the examination of each sample cost £50. A bench test was eventually adopted, which had previously not been acceptable internationally, with considerable saving in sheep, staff time and money. The cost of each test came down to £1.

Intrinsic dangers

Bites and scratches are a constant hazard in animal work and some large animals can cause serious injury. Also, the health hazards associated with zoonoses must not be ignored. Laboratory Animal Allergy (LAA) is now a recognised industrial disease. The danger of allergens in the animal laboratory is a serious matter. The long-term health and career prospects of young research workers can easily be jeopardised by reactions to fur, feathers, urine, etc.

Extrinsic dangers

The prospect of violence against staff and property in animal units is a real possibility. Irksome restraints are consequent upon the strict security needed to counter these threats.

Variations

Accurate calculations are crucial for the production of valid results from any experiment. Calculations vary in complexity in relation to the number of variables involved. Variables associated with experimental animals – age, heredity, health status, stress, etc. – are more numerous and more unpredictable than the comparatively simple parameters involved in other techniques such as cell culture. Some of the variables can be obviated and are, but only with great effort and at great cost.

Distortion

The ideal model for biological research would be an average, normal, unstressed animal. However, an average animal, almost by definition, does not exist in the real world. Such an animal is the creature of statistics – 'out of data by equation'. The normal is determined in relation to extremes – it is more an ideal projection than a real animal.

Analogous argument and extrapolation

The argument from analogy, probably the weakest form of logical argument, is based on the similarities found in two different subjects and progresses from these recognised similarities to posit other similarities. In analogy it is not a matter of simply comparing like with like. It is a matter of comparing 'part like' with 'part like'.

The many similarities to be found in the anatomy and physiology of various species can be used as a basis to presume that the way in which, for example, a drug acts in the body of one species of animal will be similar to the way it acts in another species. Obviously, the more similar the two species involved are to one another the more valid will be the conclusion that the drug will initiate the same reactions in each species. Deductions based on analogy are arrived at by the process of speculation known as extrapolation. It is upon the proper operation of this process of extrapolation that the validity of knowledge gleaned from animal experimentation depends. Many species of animal are similar but none of them are the same, otherwise they would not be separate species. The most assiduous extrapolation from numerous experiments using morphine on many other species could not predict the dramatic effect of this drug on cats. The development of, for example, penicillin could have been very adversely affected if it had depended on guinea-pig trials because of the toxic effect it has on this species. Likewise, the history of the use of thalidomide may have been different had there been more meticulous extrapolation involved in research and had it been tested on a greater variety of species. An indication of the importance of concentration on the method of extrapolation rather than depending on crude presumptions of analogy based on apparent similarities is illustrated by the usefulness of tissue culture. There are several instances where the extrapolation from human tissue culture to the human being is more reliable than from whole animals to humans since the species difference is eliminated. Tissue cultures react to most viruses affecting humans, whereas many species of laboratory animals are insensitive to a number of viruses. In short mice are not men.

The importance of direct relevancy of every detail of research using an animal model for proper extrapolation has been emphasised by the Animal Procedures Committee. Their Annual Report (1989) (3.12 and 3.13) noted that while strychnine-induced convulsions had been used as an experimental model for epilepsy it was known that the mechanism of convulsions produced by strychnine differed from the seizures which typically occur in epilepsy. The use of strychnine to simulate epilepsy could therefore not be justified.

Distaste

Experiments on animals usually demand that the animal is deprived of its freedom, is kept in a cage or even restrained. Operations may be part of the experimentation. No caring human being can be responsible for such a scenario without feeling reluctance to cause distress to a fellow creature. There is not only the distasteful task of disposing of carcasses but the ending of the life of any animal disturbs sensitive and caring technicians and scientists.

On a much lower level, sewer level in fact, animal units bring their own special problems of waste disposal. It is not without reason that the unofficial symbol of the animal technician is a scraper.

The sum total of these disadvantages of using animals in research is a powerful motive for a pursuit, as far as possible, to implement the 3Rs.

Understanding the need for and methods of reduction, refinement and replacement (3Rs)

This topic is a major feature in the debate, in the scientific community, on animal use. The striving for a fulfilment of the ideal of the 3Rs is a direct result of the hedonism (pleasure is desirable but suffering is undesirable) of a Utilitarian ethical approach to animal use employing a cost/benefit assessment.

It must not be assumed, however, that this is a purely ethical matter. The obligation to constantly seek for more acceptable expressions of the 3Rs in practice is solidly grounded in law.

> 'The Secretary of State shall not grant a project licence unless he is satisfied that the applicant has given adequate consideration to the feasibility of achieving the purpose of the programme to be specified in the licence by means not involving the use of protected animals,' (ASPA S.5(5))

> 'The Secretary of State requires that (project licence) applicants set out the measures they have taken to ensure that every reasonable effort has been made to incorporate replacement, reduction and refinement alternatives in the plan of work and protocols requested; and that named persons are consulted during the drafting of project licence applications.' (HOG 5.14)

> 'The Secretary of State will review, and may recall or revise, licence authorities should suitable replacement, reduction or refinement alternatives become available during the lifetime of the project licence.' (HOG 5.20)

A Home Office communication (HO/PCD-H Nov 1997) reiterates the significance of alternatives:

> 'This government will insist that applicants for licences demonstrate their efforts at finding alternatives before the use of animals is proposed' (Response to APC Report).

Finally,

> 'An experiment shall not be performed if another scientifically satisfactory method of obtaining the result sought, not entailing the use of an animal, is reasonably and practicably available.' (Directive 86/609/EEC Art.23)

The concept of the 3Rs presented by Russell and Burch in *The Principles of Humane Experimental Technique* (1959) has been presented in various ways over the last few decades. The most recent authoritative interpretation of and outline of the application of the 3Rs in practice is to be found in *Selection and Use of Replacement Methods in Animal Experimentation*. This publication was issued (1998) under the auspices of FRAME (Fund for the Replacement of Animals in Medical Experiments) and UFAW (Universities Federation for Animal Welfare). This booklet provides the basis of the presentation of this topic.

Marshall Hall's principles

The above praiseworthy approach to animal use is by no means new. Marshall Hall struck a similar humane note in 'A critical and experimental essay on the circulation of the blood' (1831).

- 'We should never have recourse to experiment in cases in which observation can afford us the information required.'
- 'No experiment should be performed without a distinct and definite object, and without the persuasion, after the maturest consideration, that that object will be attained by that experiment, in the form of a real and uncomplicated result.'
- 'We should not needlessly repeat experiments which have already been performed by physiologists of reputation.'
- 'An experiment should be instituted with the least possible suffering. In all cases the subject of the experiment should be of the lowest order of animals appropriate to our purpose as the least sentient; whilst every device should be employed, compatible with the success of the experiment, for avoiding the infliction of pain.'
- 'Every physiological experiment should be performed under such circumstances as will secure due observation and attestation of its results, and so obviate, as much as possible, the necessity for its repetition.'

Alternatives and the 3Rs

It is usual to accept the term 'alternatives' as not only referring to replacement methods, but as including all the 3Rs – reduction, refinement and replacement as defined by Russell and Burch (1959).

- *Reduction*: A means of lowering the number of animals used to obtain information of a given amount and precision.
- *Refinement*: Any development leading to a decrease in the incident or severity of inhumane procedures applied to those animals which have to be used.
- *Replacement*: Scientific methods employing non-sentient material which may replace methods which use conscious living vertebrates. (Russell and Burch wrote within the context of the Cruelty to Animals Act 1876.)

This 3Rs approach combined animal welfare with good science and best practice. Each of the 3Rs is not to be taken in isolation. To be most effective they should be considered as complimentary to each other – each employed in concert with the others. The use of non-animal alternatives does not only offer the possibility of reducing the number of animals which might have to be used subsequently, e.g. when screening candidate chemicals during the early stages of product development, but can also lead to refinement of such animal experiments, when their use is unavoidable.

There must always be the overruling caveat – the 3Rs should only be applied when attainment of the scientific objective of the proposed, and worthwhile, investigations will not be compromised.

Details of appropriate methods of replacement, reduction and refinement will be presented under their respective headings. It must be stressed that each of the 3Rs in some circumstances overlap. The exact interpretation of the precise scope of each of the 3Rs has varied somewhat in the literature over the last few decades. Similarly in some commentaries on the subject, the order in which the 3Rs are given differs. In his book *Alternatives to Animal Experiments* (1978), Smyth defines alternatives using the concept of the 3Rs but arranges these notions in the following order – replacement, reduction and refinement:

> 'Alternatives include any procedures which do away with animals altogether, lead to a reduction in the total number of animals used or lead to less distress to the animals employed.'

Replacement

Putting replacement as the initial 'R' seems preferable

both logically and ethically, especially as regards ethics because many opposed to the use of animals in research seem to be more concerned about the fact that animals are being used rather than about how they are used. Logically, it seems more appropriate to try to dispense with the use of animals if possible before going on to consider the reduction of the numbers required. Attention to the care and welfare of the animals comes within the scope of refinement. The requirement for refinement follows naturally from an ethical approach to animal experimentation but implementing the most appropriate form of refinement is a scientific and/or technical, not an ethical affair. These requirements need to be dealt with by the experts directly involved.

A realistic approach to the 3Rs in practice is not just an attempt to apply specific categories of alternatives but is rather an atmosphere in which all the following considerations are brought into play. There should be a careful selection of the species of animal and careful attention to the manner of their use. The species chosen must always be the most appropriate both biologically and ethologically.

Species which are regarded as having the least developed nervous system are to be preferred. The design of the experiment must ensure that the objective is achieved with as few animals as possible and with the least interference possible. The ultimate aim is always to replace the animal by an alternative wherever possible.

Some progress has been achieved in the use of alternative methods. A driving motive behind the ASPA has been the reduction of the number of animals used in research by whatever means possible. This theme was brought to the fore in the second White Paper to the ASPA as long ago as 1985:

'The total number of experiments on living animals in Great Britain fell from 5.6 million in 1971 to 3.6 million in 1983. There are many reasons why the number has fallen, but the development of alternative techniques has been an important one. There is more scope for further progress. The Government is keen to see the continued development of alternatives and, in order to encourage it, has already granted £50 000 towards the research of the Fund for the Replacement of Animals in Medical Research and plans to provide a further £100 000 over two years. No previous Home Secretary has provided funds for alternative research and the decision to do so now is an earnest of the

Government's determination to see progress made in this field as rapidly as possible.'

In 2003 the total number of experiments on living animals in the United Kingdom was 2.79 million. Unless the demands set by regulatory bodies for safety testing, etc. are reduced accordingly or amended in keeping with these ideals, it is difficult to see how even moderate reductions can be achieved in this figure.

It may be noted that even animals may not always be an adequate alternative to using humans. It was estimated for example that had practolol toxicity been detectable in the experimental animal, it would have needed 50–100 000 animal experiments to pick it up. Could such massive animal use be justified? Should the public accept that human beings are in some cases the most suitable test animal? Should the public become more accepting of the idea that drug treatment is not without risk in the same sense that surgery is risky? In this case a drug offers a lesser risk in place of a greater one – continuation of an undesirable condition.

Russell and Burch's (1959) definition that 'any scientific method employing non-sentient material which may, in the history of animal experimentation, replace methods which use conscious living vertebrates' is expanded in this text. Among the 3Rs 'replacement' is the term most closely associated with the concept of 'alternatives'. Consequently it appears more appropriate to include within this topic of replacement the requirement to select for experimentation the species regarded as being the least sentient which is adequate to the particular line of research. This is not strictly speaking a replacement of animal use but it is an attempt to reduce animal suffering. For this reason the choosing of a lower (the term is used with caution) species may be regarded by some as coming within the scope of reduction.

A salient feature of any comment on or discussion of replacement must be an acknowledgement of the complexity and fluidity of the subject matter. Since animal procedures are used in such a wide range of scientific areas, it is impossible to describe the possible replacement methods available to all scientists in all fields of work. New possibilities of replacement will continue to be developed and validated and it is the responsibility of those carrying out animal experiments to remain up to date in this area. It follows that any serious discussion of the value of any specific alternative method is a matter for experts in that line of research and will be conducted in the appropriate technical language.

Types of replacement

- *Relative replacement*: For example, the humane killing of a vertebrate animal to provide cells, tissues and/or organs for *in vitro* studies.

- *Absolute replacement*: Animals would not need to be used at all, for example, the permanent culture of human and invertebrate cells and tissues.

- *Direct replacement*: For example, when the skin of human volunteers or guinea-pig skin is used *in vitro* to provide information which would otherwise have been obtained from tests on the skin of live guinea-pigs.

- *Indirect replacement*: For example, when the pyrogen test in rabbits is replaced by the Limulus amoebocyte lysate (LAL) test or a test based on whole human blood.

- *Total replacement*: For example, taking a decision not to conduct an animal procedure because of lack of justification or reliability of the method, using a human volunteer instead of a guinea-pig, or testing a chemical on cells *in vitro* instead of on animals.

- *Partial replacement*: For example, the use of non-animal methods as pre-screens in toxicity testing strategies. A series of *in vitro* tests, called screening cascades, are used to identify potential problems with new compounds before animals are used.

Replacement methods

In vitro methods and tissue culture

In vitro (literally, 'in glass') appears to be a generic term not always clearly defined, but generally applied to systems of research using subcellular fractions, short-term maintenance of tissue slices, cell suspensions and perfused organs, and tissue culture (cell and organotypic culture), including human tissue culture. Similarly the phrase 'tissue culture' seems to be used in a generic manner covering the *in vitro* cultivation of organs, tissues, cells and embryos

(cf. the FRAME and UFAW publications mentioned above, see p. 337).

Cells, tissues and whole organs, as well as parts of organs, can now be kept alive outside the body. The cells are kept in buffered solution with nutrients under conditions which closely resemble their normal physiological situation. Consequently physiologists and pharmacologists make wide use of animal and human tissues. In toxicology, *in vitro* methods act as pre-screens, so that the most toxic compounds can be screened out before less toxic compounds are tested in animal experiments. This process not only complements animal studies but allows for the accomplishment of subsequent improved and more detailed *in vitro* work.

Advantages of *in vitro* systems

- Once validated, *in vitro* systems can provide information in a cost-effective and time-saving manner.
- *In vitro* systems can sometimes be used to produce data which are more reliable and more reproducible than data from animal studies. In other cases, they can be used to increase the efficiency of whole-animal studies and decrease the number of animals required.
- *In vitro* systems are ideal for mechanistic investigations at the molecular and cellular level, as well as for target organ and species toxicity studies.
- Human tissues can be used in *in vitro* systems. The use of human cells obviates the need for cross-species extrapolation, and thus is more relevant to the human situation.
- The use of *in vitro* methods can be done in the absence of complex body systems which might introduce confusing factors. This allows studies to be done which could not be conducted in animals.

Disadvantages of *in vitro* methods

- *In vitro* methods lack the complex interaction of the numerous factors within a living organism, e.g. immune responses, the endocrine system, the nervous system, the circulation of the blood, etc.
- Models are not yet available for all tissues and organs, or for all toxicity endpoints.
- It can be difficult to relate concentrations of drugs and test chemicals *in vitro* with those occurring in body fluids *in vivo*.

Cell culture

Primary cell culture

A primary cell culture involves the isolation of cells by the disruption of the tissue, often with proteolytic enzymes. The major advantages of primary cultures are the retention of the capacity for biotransformation and tissue-specific functions. One limitation of primary cultures is the necessity to isolate cells for each experiment. This may result in the loss of or damage to the integrity of the membrane and loss of cellular products. During the interval necessary to establish monolayer cultures, damage is often repaired.

Primary cultures have a limited life-span and changes in metabolism and tissue-specific functions will occur with time in culture.

Cell culture techniques are commonly used for monoclonal antibody production, virus vaccine production, vaccine potency testing, screening for cytotoxic effects and studying the function and make up of cells.

Cell lines

The use of cell lines provides a number of advantages for the study of many biological phenomena, including toxicity. A wide variety of cell types can be used, including human cells and those from specific tissues for investigations of target organ specificity.

Most cells lines can be stored at ultra low temperatures and they either have a finite life span, or they are capable of an unlimited number of population doublings (continuous cell line). However, the differentiated functions may be altered in cell lines depending on the culture conditions. The metabolic capacity of the cells may also decrease depending on the culture conditions. Although continuous cell lines offer the advantage of indefinite growth and ease of manipulation, finite cell lines are usually chromosomally abnormal and display *in vitro* ageing.

Isolated and cultured cells offer many advantages both in the study of mechanisms of cellular toxicity by chemical agents and for *in vitro* bioassays.

Established animal cell lines such as Chinese hamster ovary (CHO) and mouse lymphoma L5178Y, suffer from inter-laboratory variation, especially in basic properties like chromosome number. This is because they have been maintained for many years in culture collections. One attempt to minimise the problems of differentiation, senescence and instability has been to generate immortalised cell lines by introducing viral oncogenes into primary cells. Examples of cells which have been immortalised include rabbit kidney, mouse macrophages, rat liver and human lymphocytes.

Subcellular fractions

Fractionated organelles and membranes prepared from defined cell types can be used for specific cell-free investigations. These *in vitro* systems, which are usually prepared by differential centrifugation, include nuclei, mitochondria, lysosomes and membrane vesicles.

Organ culture

Organ culture refers to a three-dimensional culture of tissue retaining some or all of the histological features of the tissue and preservation of its architecture, usually by culturing the tissue at the liquid–gas interface on a grid or gel. Organ cultures cannot be propagated and experiments in organ cultures generally involve a large degree of experimental variation between replicates, making organ cultures less suitable than cell cultures for quantitative determinations. The production of organ cultures requires fresh tissue from the relevant organ, although one organ can provide material for several cultures.

Organ cultures can be used to study pharmacodynamics. The functions studied include oxygen consumption, glucose uptake and release, pyruvate release, lactate release, nitrogenous excretion and cell proliferation. Complex human skin models have been developed and some are available commercially. Test protocols have been developed for use with these human skin models, which enable topically applied aqueous and non-aqueous test materials to be screened for their skin irritancy potentials. (A summary of the advantages and limitations of tissue culture techniques is given in Table 36.1.)

Use of early developmental stages of vertebrates

There is a presumption in this context that there is less likelihood of the occurrence of animal suffering if we accept that the nervous systems of the organisms are not sufficiently well developed to arouse an awareness of pain. This method of research has special legal significance in the UK. The ASAP does not protect mammals, birds or reptiles before they reach a stage halfway through gestation nor other vertebrates

Table 36.1 Examples of advantages and limitations of tissue culture systems (from FRAME and UFAW 1998).

System	Advantages	Disadvantages
Organ culture	Retention of structural integrity. Maintenance of cell–cell inter-relationships.	Large degree of experimental variation. Short-term viability. Statistical sampling problems.
Primary cell culture	Retention of several differentiated functions.	Loss of tissue architecture. Requires recovery period owing to damage from isolation.
Continuous cell culture	Increased cell viability period. Easier to maintain than primary cultures. Can assume characteristics of transformed cells. Can differentiate *in vitro* to assume new phenotypes.	Loss of tissue architecture. Loss of differentiated organ functions. Significant loss of metabolising capacity.

and the *Octopus vulgaris* before the larvae become capable of independent feeding.

Tests based on mammalian whole-embryo culture systems are well developed for *in vitro* methods for the detection of reproductive toxicity and teratogenicity, and for elucidating mechanisms of teratogenesis. Chick embryos and frog tadpoles are also being used for these purposes. Chicken eggs have been used for identifying irritants, e.g. the CAM (Chorio-allantoic membrane) irritancy test.

Use of lower organisms
This method of research is acceptable on the basis that less suffering is being experienced by the organisms used because they are presumed to be less sentient than the more common experimental animal. Even more preferable is the use of organisms regarded as being completely non-sentient, e.g. bacteria, and algae. The following are instances of such forms of replacement.

- The AMES (Bruce) Test is well established for screening large numbers of chemicals for potential toxic effects. This assay utilises Salmonella bacteria to detect chemical mutagenesis. The AMES test has been validated for regulatory toxicology purposes as a screen for genotoxic chemicals.

- Certain species of light-emitting bacteria are being used in toxicity tests. The energy for their light production comes from respiration. As the biochemical processes of respiration are very similar in all organisms, then any chemical which disrupts respiration in bacteria may possibly do the same in humans and would therefore be toxic to humans.

- Since yeasts are eukaryotes their cells are more like mammalian cells than bacteria cells are. As their chromosome structure resembles that of mammals, yeasts are more suitable for revealing certain kinds of genetic damage. Yeasts are also used to detect substances which might cause skin damage in the presence of light.

- The coelenterate, *Hydra attenuata*, is used in pre-screening techniques for teratogenicity. This technique is commercially available. It is based on the ability of the hydra to rapidly regenerate from dissociated polyps, which are used as artificial embryos.

- The nematode, *Caenorhabditis elegans*, is widely used in genetic research and in fundamental studies in biology. Substantial progress has been made in complete sequencing of the genome of *C. elegans*. It is becoming clear that many of its genes are conserved in humans. Its use in research has made contributions to fundamental studies in neurophysiology and behaviour, developmental biology, including mechanisms of programmed cell death (apoptosis) and genetics.

- The fruit fly has proved invaluable in genetic research and in fundamental studies in cell biology. Studies with *Drosophila spp.* provided the first evidence that X-rays are mutagenic, and they are being used for pre-screening to test for chemical mutagens and carcinogens.

- One unusual piece of research had been designed to test the effects of narcotic drugs. Spiders were given controlled doses of a drug and the extent of their consequent deviant behaviour in web spinning was then carefully observed and recorded.

- A replacement of rabbits for testing pyrogenic endotoxins has been validated. In fact the LAL (Limulus amoebocyte lysate) Test is more sensitive, economical, convenient and reliable. Blood is taken from the horseshoe crab (*Limulus polyphemus*) and the Limulus amoebocyte lysate is extracted from the blood cells for the detection of endotoxins. Unfortunately, this particular alternative method has had an impact on the population of horseshoe crabs. Perhaps, in cases of this nature, attention needs to be paid to overall environmental considerations.

Assays using the organisms referred to can only give limited information. They cannot act currently as a complete replacement in toxicology. They are, however, useful as pre-screen systems for agrochemicals and environmental pollutants.

Physico-chemical methods

Assessment of the chemical properties of a substance will provide some information about its possible toxic effects, e.g. compounds with high or low pH values and low buffering capacities are likely to be irritant to the skin, so testing on animals is not necessary. Physical and chemical techniques can be used to study enzyme structures and the mechanisms of their action. In pharmacology and toxicology, physicochemical analysis can be used in predicting both the likely beneficial and harmful biological effects of chemical substances.

Progress has already been made in developing alternatives to the Draize eye (rabbit) test, e.g. EYTEX – a protein matrix is exposed to the suspected eye irritant. However, recent (1998) validation studies have shown that more *in vitro* test development is required if the Draize eye test is to be replaced by a non-animal testing strategy. Hen's egg test – chorioallantoic (HET – CAM) assay, isolated rabbit eye and bovine cornea have been proposed to replace this undesirable test.

Mice used to be used to check the purity of each new batch of insulin. HPLC (high performance liquid chromatography) is now used to analyse insulin for impurities.

Mathematical and computer models

Molecular modelling

In molecular modelling, the three-dimensional structural and electronic properties of a biological site are used to predict whether a novel molecule would interact with it, producing a biological effect. In some cases the detailed structures of such biological sites are known (for example from x-ray crystallography, or other studies). In other cases, the nature of the site of action is inferred from the structures of the molecules known to interact with it, compared with similar structures that do not (a technique known as pseudoreceptor modelling). Molecular modelling is restricted to making predictions about biological sites whose structures are reasonably well understood.

CADD (computer-assisted drug design)

This uses interactive graphics in the early stages of development of new compounds. Receptor sites of cells are explored. Once the shape of receptor sites are known attempts can be made to design molecules to fit them. The compatibility of the potential molecule to a particular receptor can be observed.

QSAR (quantitative structure-activity relationships)

This is used to predict the possible biological effects of a new compound. QSAR equations attempt to define relationships between the structure of chemicals – the shape, size and reactivity of the particular groups of atoms present, and their biological activities. The information collected may indicate ways of changing the structure of a molecule to alter its therapeutic or toxic properties.

DEREK (deductive estimation of risk from existing knowledge)

DEREK interfaces on-screen structural information with a toxicity database so that qualitative predictions about novel structures similar to those on the database, drawn by the toxicologist, can be made and toxicophores identified.

PBPK (physiologically based pharmacokinetic) modelling

PBPK modelling predicts the disposition of xenobiotics and their metabolites by integrating three types of information: species-specific physiological parameters; partition coefficients for the chemical; and metabolic parameters. PBPK can provide information to predict tissue exposure to xenobiotics and their metabolites for various doses and species. PBPK presents a clear potential for refining ADME (absorption, distribution, metabolism and excretion) studies.

Laser/computer model
A new laser/computer model has been developed to simulate orthodontic tooth movement.

Significance of mathematical and computer models
So significant is mathematical and computer modelling to replacement that as far back as 1993 the RSPCA sponsored a research programme at the University of Surrey. Its object was to develop a computer modelling approach for the testing of chemicals. Such methods, however, are even now in an early stage of development. The computer's ability to predict beneficial or toxic effects of chemicals depends on the amount and quality of the information available for use in their programming. In the future it may be possible to assess the biologically useful and toxic effects of untested substances simply from a knowledge of their 3-D structure.

The use of models, films and videos
Some very realistic models of experimental animals have been developed for the replacement of the live animals used in teaching and training. The Japanese silicone rat model has proved useful as a teaching aid. A further advance has been an artificial rabbit with all the necessary characteristics of the live animal. This model is an accurate simulation of a female New Zealand White rabbit weighing 2.4 kg. It has life-like fur and body plasticity. The abdominal wall can be simply opened to show the position of the stomach, while the abdominal cavity conceals small tubes which conduct and drain fluids during practice injections.

The usefulness of films and videos of animal handling and procedures made by experts, for use in teaching and training, as a replacement of live animals, is self evident.

Human beings
The use of humans for replacement of animals includes the use of human tissues and human volunteers as well as post-marketing surveillance and epidemiology. This method of replacement avoids the problem of inter-specific extrapolation from animals to humans and provides more relevant information.

Human tissues have been used to establish organotypic culture models, e.g. skin equivalents. Immortalised human cells have been established to overcome problems of the supply of fresh tissue. This has been done mainly by DNA virus oncogene transfection.

There are problems with obtaining human tissue samples. Logistic problems include safety issues associated with the necessity to screen for HIV, hepatitis and other infections. Furthermore, there will be a need to obtain detailed histories of donors relating to genetic background, drug intake and details of any other exposures, as well as the need for a system to keep track of tissues obtained from each donor, in case of future problems.

In the UK, regulations require prior informed consent from donors/relatives and from local research ethics committees. Morally, there are potential ownership problems and many commercial and legal (e.g. possibly in the future, the patenting of genetic material) implications. The use of foetal tissue needs careful consideration since it has its own complex moral aspects.

Validation

Apart from the time it takes to develop alternative techniques the factor which has emerged as causing the most delay in the acceptance of various proposed methods of replacement has been validation. Validation refers to the process whereby the reliability and relevance of an assay are established for a particular purpose.

The time-consuming aspect of the whole process of achieving validation is due to the need to:

- establish the accuracy of the new technique or approach, e.g. in the case of epidemiology;
- establish the repeatability of the method;
- perform trials using genuine products in real situations;
- obtain acceptability by official bodies who use the result to issue safety certificates.

This last point is perhaps the most time-consuming part of the venture, impeding rapid progress. This is particularly the case when a variety of national attitudes and a mosaic of bureaucratic practices of byzantine complexity need to be taken into account.

The nature and the scale of validation is dictated by the purpose of the assay. If a method is to be used for in-house purposes only, then validation can be conducted on a limited scale. If an assay is designed to replace an animal method and to be used widely for regulatory purposes then validation trials are often conducted at several different laboratories according to specific, internationally harmonised criteria, which are intended to facilitate regulatory acceptance of the alternative method.

ECVAM (European Centre for the Validation of Alternative Methods) is specifically concerned with the drive to increase the role of Replacement of animals in research. Details of this enterprise can be obtained from JRC, Environment Institute, 21020 Ispra (Va), Italy, or e-mail: julia.fentem@jrc.it

Reduction

The ideal method of reducing the number of animals used in research is of course by replacement. In the more restricted sense however reduction includes strategies for obtaining comparable levels of information from the use of fewer animals in scientific procedures, or for obtaining more information from a given number of animals. There are areas of overlap between reduction and replacement. *In vitro* methods may be used in the initial screening of compounds for toxicity, so that the most toxic compounds can be rejected before continuing with further tests on animals. The *in vitro* screening serves both to replace and reduce animal tests.

No doubt the reduction of the number of animals used in research is a number game and the relevant figures given above (see p. 338) indicates progress. There is evidence that although fewer animals are being used, neither scientific progress nor medical research are being seriously curtailed. The call for reduction has come from within the scientific community itself. ICLAS (International Council of Laboratory Animal Science) has in the past called upon regulatory authorities to help reduction still further by revising the number of animals used in toxicity testing and to avoid duplications from one country to another. The 1986 European Convention on animal use in research reflected this spirit in Article 29:

'In order to avoid unnecessary repetition of procedures for the purposes of satisfying national legislation on health and safety each Contracting Party shall, where practicable, recognise the results of procedures carried out in the territory of another party.'

The drive for reduction may sometimes have to be balanced against the comparative severity of proposed procedures. It would appear to be preferable, if the choice needs to be made between using a larger number of animals in milder procedures or fewer animals in more severe procedures, to select the former option. This decision, of course, presumes that other factors are equal and that the principles of good science are observed.

Reduction methods

Communication of information
Proper use of all available data can obviate unnecessary repetition of research using animals and can assure that the best use of the smallest number of animals for a particular purpose can be achieved.

In these days of the 'global village' and rapid extension of electronic means of communication, the dissemination of relevant information is not only possible but should be given priority by those responsible for using experimental animals. Research establishments should provide adequate information and a centralised and efficient retrieval system of useful data. Laboratories ought to publish full results of animal studies to avoid unnecessary repetition of animal procedures. Furthermore, researchers may be made aware when animals are to be killed so that any spare tissue etc. can be shared with other researchers, thus reducing the overall numbers of animals required in other areas.

Individual researchers now have access to on-line databases which give up-to-date lists of published research in all areas of science. Before planning an experimental procedure, a scientist should be aware of any similar work which has already taken place, with either animal or non-animal procedures, so that unnecessary repetition is avoided.

There is no lack of informative literature in this field. FRAME (Fund for the Replacement of Animals in Medical Experiments) publishes abstracts giving information about methods of reducing the number of animals used in experiments.

The ideal model

The significance of using a specialised animal model for a specific type of research has been referred to above. A direct result of this good practice is a reduction in the numbers of animals used because the animals which are used are more suitable for providing the required data in smaller numbers. For example, the use of the mutant strain of nude mice which are athymic and thus immunologically incompetent, means that fewer individuals of this strain are needed than individuals of other mouse strains in cancer research for the passaging of tumours.

In-breeding

The advantage of using in-bred animals in research has been dealt with above (see p. 333). Consequent upon the advantages mentioned, smaller numbers of a chosen inbred strain will be used in the appropriate research because strain variations found within that species will be eliminated.

Transgenic and chimeral animals

In this area of research we have the possibility of producing the ideal model animal rather than merely selecting the best model from those available or developing a suitable one, if we can, by in-breeding for twenty generations. In this way the end product of genetic manipulation can produce the same effect – a reduction of individual animals used. In the wider aspect of genetic manipulation and cloning could lead to the production of groups of animals which lacked even individual variations, at least as regards the genotype. This could open up the opportunity of an even greater reduction in the number of animals used.

Unfortunately, from experience, the number of animals needed for initiating a transgenic programme, starting with the procedure of superovulation, can be very high. Since the early days in this research, methods have been refined and this particular difficulty is diminishing in importance.

Among the many examples of how genetic manipulation can produce the ideal model animal for research and thus reduce the number of animals needed in a procedure, is the case of the Duchene Muscular Dystrophy Mouse. This mouse, ideal for the study of the effects of Duchene on both the skeletal muscle and the heart, was produced by the Washington School of Medicine in St. Louis. The new mouse strain develops muscle wasting and heart disease, dying before adulthood thus mirroring the effect of the disease in humans. The disorder results from a defect in the gene for an enormous protein called Dystrophin which forms on the scaffold in muscle fibres.

Known health status

The use of animals protected from infection and maintained in a healthy condition, as discussed above obviates a potent source of variations between individuals. This ensures that a smaller number of animals is sufficient for producing valid results in research. Disease in animals masks and distorts reactions, leading to a greater demand for experimental animals in order to offset these defects. A further reason why reduction can result from using barrier-maintained or isolator animals is that there will not usually be a loss of animals due to death or disease during a research programme. Such an unfortunate occurrence would necessitate the use of even more animals if the programme is to be successfully completed. In the case of the gnotobiotic animal the complete micro-organic burden of the individual is known. This means that variations between individuals are minimised and data is not affected by pathogenic conditions which are not fully accounted for or understood. Consequently, fewer animals will be needed to achieve the level of statistical precision, or the use of the same number of animals will lead to better experiments with fewer incorrect results. This could obviate the need of repetition which might otherwise be required for confirmation purposes.

Experimental design

It must be a prime principle of research that all animals being used are used economically. 'Economically' is meant to apply to the minimising of the discomfort of the animal not to the cost of the project.

By careful planning, superfluous experiments can be discarded and effective experimental projects using the minimum number of animals can be designed. The number of products going forward for conventional tests using animals has been reduced by trying to predict potential carcinogenic or other hazardous qualities in groups of chemicals. By this type of early investigative work many suspect substances can be screened out at an early stage.

Expert care and thoughtful management of animals is conducive to the accuracy and validity of experimental results. The application of such expertise on the part of researchers can effectively reduce animal use.

Critical appraisal of the worthiness of a proposed project can lead to reduction in the number of animals required for an experiment. It may be possible to carry out small pilot studies using few animals, which can be reviewed before committing larger numbers of animals to a major research programme.

Statistics

Statistics are vital to the proper implementation of the 3Rs – the mandatory study module for obtaining a project licence has to have a statistical content. Proper statistical design, prior to undertaking the study, and appropriate analysis of the resulting data can make it possible to obtain results of comparable or greater precision while using fewer animals. There is evidence that poor experimental design, together with inappropriate statistical analysis of experimental results is leading to inefficient use of animals and of scientific resources in toxicological research and testing, and in other areas of biomedical research. A study of papers in *Index Medicus* carried out on behalf of the Humane Society of the United States in 1961, showed that a saving of 23% to 40% of the animals used could have been achieved if better statistical methods had been employed.

The statistician rather than the moral philosopher has probably been more directly responsible for the greatest amount of reduction in animal use.

Refinement

More effective refinement of procedures has been accomplished by competent anaesthetists than those skilled in ethics. Refinement encompasses those methods which alleviate or minimise potential pain and distress, and which enhance animal well-being. The details of refinement are so varied and numerous that it is only possible in this text to indicate the general areas in which animal suffering can be alleviated and the care of laboratory animals can be improved. Attention must be paid to:

- the expertise employed in experimental work, e.g. as regards surgery and all other relevant skills;

- the proper use of anaesthetics and a readiness to use them on all appropriate occasions, as would be done in the case of humans undergoing similar procedures;
- the use, when called for, of analgesics;
- the provision of sedation to obviate stress or eliminate discomfort;
- post-operative care in all cases in which it would supply alleviation of animal suffering;
- meticulous observance of humane endpoints which ought to be set so as to prevent as much animal suffering as possible. There should be strict adherence to the permitted level of severity which preferably should be set as low as is feasible in the circumstances;
- the most suitable form of euthanasia for the species being used must be available without delay at all times;
- husbandry of the highest order must be the accepted practice throughout the animal unit.

Animal welfare should not only be in keeping with the relevant codes of practice but also the specific biology and behavioural patterns of the experimental animal ought to be considered so that suitable environmental enrichment can be provided. The choice of the form of environmental enrichment will, of course, be influenced by the type of research being practised.

A base line of the provision of refinement as regards animal care must be attention to the five freedoms as formulated by Prof. Brambell in 1979 for the FAWC (Farm Animal Welfare Council).

The five freedoms

(1) Freedom from thirst, hunger or malnutrition by ready access to fresh water and a diet to maintain full health and vigour;
(2) freedom from discomfort by providing a suitable environment including shelter and a comfortable resting area;
(3) freedom from pain, injury and disease by prevention or rapid diagnosis and treatment;
(4) freedom to express normal behaviour by providing sufficient space, proper facilities and company of the animal's own kind;
(5) freedom from fear and distress by ensuring conditions which avoid mental suffering.

Training

In order that projects are properly planned, procedures are correctly performed and the animals are properly cared for it is essential that all those involved in animal experimentation are fully trained. The mandatory Home Office modules are designed to provide a modicum of instruction on these matters to all concerned. However, more extensive and intensive in-house training should be provided so that refinement of animal use in research can be fully accomplished.

Bibliography and references

Association of Veterinary Teachers and Research Workers (1989) *Guidelines for the Recognition and Assessment of Pain in Animals.* UFAW, Hertfordshire, UK.

Barclay, R.J., Herbert, W.J. and Poole, T.B. (1988) *The Disturbance Index: A behavioural method of assessing the severity of common laboratory procedures on rodents.* (UFAW Animal Welfare Research Report No. 2). UFAW, London.

Barley, J.B. (1999) Animal experimentation, the scientist and ethics. *Animal Technology,* **50** (1): 1–10.

Dolan, K. (1999) *Ethics, Animals and Science.* Blackwell Science, Oxford.

FRAME and UFAW (1998) *Selection and Use of Replacement Methods in Animal Experimentation.* UFAW, Hertfordshire, UK.

Home Office (1989) *Code of Practice for the Housing and Care of Animals used in Scientific Procedures.* HMSO, London.

Home Office (1994) Licensing and Inspection under the Animals (Scientific Procedures) Act 1986. HMSO, London.

Home Office (1995) *Code of Practice for the Housing and Care of Animals in Designated Breeding and Supplying Establishments.* HMSO, London.

Home Office (1996) *Code of Practice for the Humane Killing of Animals under Schedule 1 to the Animals (Scientific Procedures) Act 1986.* HMSO, London.

Home Office (1998) *Animals (Scientific Procedures) Act 1986 and Statutory Instruments arising from it 1986–1998.* HMSO, London.

Home Office (2000) *Guidance on the Operation of the Animals (Scientific Procedures) Act 1986.* HMSO, London.

Home Office Animal Procedures Committee. *Annual Reports 1986–2006.* www.homeoffice.gov.uk

Hume, D. (1751) *An Enquiry Concerning the Principles of Morals.* A. Millar, London.

Langley, G. (1989) *Animal Experimentation: The Consensus Changes.* Palgrave Macmillan, Hampshire, UK.

LaFollette, H. and Shanks, H. (1996) *Brute Science: Dilemmas of animal experimentation* (Philosophical Ideas in Science Series). Routledge, New York.

LASA Working Party (1990) The assessment and control of the severity of scientific procedures on laboratory animals. *Laboratory Animals,* **24**: 97–130.

Lembeck, F. (1989) *Scientific Alternatives to Animal Experiments.* Ellis Horwood, Chichester, UK.

Linzey, A. (1999) *Animal Rites: Liturgies of Animal Care.* The Pilgrim Press, Cleveland, OH.

Littlewood Committee (1965) *Report of the Departmental Committee on Experiments on Animals.* HMSO, London.

May, R.M. (1988) Control of feline delinquency. *Nature,* **332**: 392–393.

Marsh, N. and Haywood, S. (1985) *Animal Experimentation.* FRAME. Pamphlet available from frame@frame.org.uk

Morton, D. and Griffiths, P. (1985) Guidelines on the recognition of pain, distress and discomfort in experimental animals and an hypothesis for assessment. *Veterinary Record,* **116**, (20/4/85): 431–6.

Orlans, B. (1993) *In the Name of Science – Issues of Responsible Animal Experimentation.* Oxford University Press, New York.

Paton, Sir W. (1984) *Man and Mouse.* Oxford University Press, New York.

Phillips, M.T. and Sechzer, J.A. (1989) *Animal Research and Ethical Conflict. An Analysis of the Scientific Literature.* Springer-Verlag, Berlin.

Poole T. (1997) Happy animals make good science. *Laboratory Animals,* **31**: 116–124.

Porter, D.G. (1992) Ethical scores for animal experiments. *Nature,* **356**: 101–102.

Regan, T. (1983) *The Case for Animal Rights.* University of California Press, Berkeley.

Rollin, B.E. (1993) *Animal Rights and Human Morality.* Prometheus Books, Buffalo, NY.

RSPCA (1994) *Ethical Concerns for Animals.* RSPCA, Horsham, UK.

Russell W.M.S. and Burch R.L. (1959; reprinted 1992) *The Principles of Humane Experimental Technique.* Universities Federation for Animal Welfare (UFAW)/Methuen, London.

Sapontzis, S.F. (1987) *Morals, Reason and Animals.* Temple University Press, Philadelphia.

Sainsbury, D.W.B. (1986) *Farm Animal Welfare: Cattle, Pigs and Poultry.* Collins, London.

Singer, P. (1992) *Applied Ethics.* Oxford University Press, New York.

Smith, J.A. and Boyd, K.M. (1991) *Lives in the Balance: The Ethics of Using Animals in Biomedical Research.* The Report of a working party in the Institute of Medical Ethics. Oxford University Press, New York.

Smyth, D.H. (1978) *Alternatives to Animal Experiments.* Scolar Press, Yorkshire, UK.

United Kingdom Coordinating Committee on Cancer Research (1988) *Guidelines for the Welfare of Animals in Experimental Neoplasia.* UKCCCR, London. Available from www.ncm.org.uk/csg/animal_guides_text.pdf

37

Good Laboratory Practice

Pilar Browne

Introduction

Drugs or medical appliances cannot be used on human or animal patients until they have been authorised, by licence, by government agencies in the countries they are to be used in. In the UK, the authority is the Department of Health (DoH); in the USA the regulatory authority is the Food and Drug Administration (FDA).

Licences are only issued when the regulatory authorities are satisfied that the risks associated with the new substance are acceptable. In order to make these judgements they require the manufacturers to present results of tests (called non-clinical trials) to determine the safety of the new substance.

Good laboratory practice (GLP) is essentially a set of regulations which ensure the quality and integrity of data and reports submitted for non-clinical studies, in support of applications to carry out clinical trials and the marketing of new drugs and medical appliances.

Clinical trials are those carried out on a sample of the target population, the humans or animals, that the drug is intended to treat.

GLP was first introduced in the 1970s in the USA following an investigation by the Food and Drug Administration (FDA) into a report on a potential new drug, published by a US company which contained 'inconsistencies'. Inspections of hundreds of universities, pharmaceutical and contract research companies across Europe and America followed.

General concerns from these investigations included:

- carelessly conducted studies;
- absence of protocols or, where they existed, they were not followed;

- data which had been incorrectly analysed and reported;
- deliberate falsification of data;
- inappropriate animal and laboratory procedures;
- inappropriate training and supervision of staff;
- omission of adverse findings in reports.

Any of the above could have lead to the FDA inadvertently authorising clinical trials of drugs which were potentially dangerous. As a result they introduced Good Laboratory Practice, a system which required organisations wishing to gain their approval for clinical trials to carry out a specific programme of tests and to report them in a specific way. First introduced by the FDA in the USA, this system has been adopted by many countries in the world. It became law in UK on 1st April 1997.

The scope of GLP

GLP is concerned with the organisational processes and conditions under which laboratory studies are planned, performed, monitored, recorded and reported.

It ensures:

- the proper planning of studies and the provision of adequate means to carry them out;
- the facilitation of proper conduct of studies, promoting their full and accurate reporting, providing a means whereby the integrity of a study can be checked;
- quality and integrity of data generated.

The GLP compliance programme covers laboratory inspections and study audits carried out in accordance with internationally agreed principles of GLP, these include the following.

Planning

Shown by the production of a protocol, detailing all aspects of the study. The protocol sets out the objectives of the study and the methodology. It should be signed by the study supervisor or director (who has overall responsibility for the study) and should be available to all relevant staff (animal unit, pharmacy, necropsy, etc.).

Standard operating procedures (SOPs) should be in place and also available to all relevant staff. These ensure consistent methodologies for all procedures.

Management and performance

Facilities should be available to allow separate procedures to be performed in different areas (e.g. a separate necropsy area).

Personnel should be adequately qualified and trained in the relevant procedures. Records of these details, a job description and a CV should be in place for all members of staff.

Repeatability

It is important that animal technologists appreciate the importance of the ability to reconstruct a study. It is essential that all data is recorded accurately and promptly when a procedure is performed ('raw data'), and that it is signed and dated. This data must be clear, legible and permanent. This means that at a later date, should it be necessary, the study could in theory be reconstructed. It also means that all data is traceable.

Reporting

The report is a written outline of the work performed for a study. This means that all data recorded by the animal technologist will be included in this. It is vital that all data recorded is accurate.

The GLP regulations

The GLP regulations cover:

- animal room preparation;
- environmental monitoring of animal rooms;
- animal care;
- handling of animals found moribund or dead on test;
- identification of animals on test and correct cage allocation;
- cleaning of cages, racks and accessory equipment;
- monitoring of food for analysis and shelf life;
- monitoring of drinking water;
- monitoring of bedding materials;
- adequate documentation of the above.

Monitoring

The DoH inspectorate is part of the Medicines Control Agency (MCA) which forms the GLP monitoring authority (GLP MA). They run the GLP compliance programme in the UK.

Every two years they inspect facilities conducting non-clinical safety studies. If the inspection is successful, they issue the facility with a compliance certificate. Without this, the facility would not be able to claim GLP compliance status. These inspections also take place if a company changes its name or key personnel or if there is any other significant change.

The GLP MA also conducts study specific inspections if data is suspected of being of poor quality, inconsistent or unreliable. They offer advice to industry and provide UK input into international affairs.

All data and significant procedures or time points in a study are also monitored continuously by a quality assurance (QA) unit. QA are also part of the GLP compliance programme and are inspected themselves every two years. They ensure the compliance of the test facility to GLP and in addition all staff to standard operating procedures (SOPs). At the end of a study, QA review the final report for accuracy. QA are also there to provide help and advice to all personnel involved in the study.

Standard operating procedures

As part of the GLP compliance programme, an unambiguous, clear set of instructions, detailing each stage of every procedure from start to finish, should be in place. These standard operating procedures (SOPs) should be step-by-step instructions which can prevent the introduction of systematic errors in data, resulting from variation between individuals performing test procedures. They are required to cover all operations and need to be readily available to all personnel concerned.

When a new SOP has to be prepared, each procedure should be broken down into the smallest components possible. For instance, the procedure for oral gavage of a mouse may be thought of as:

- draw up the dose;
- restrain mouse;
- dose mouse.

An SOP should detail the method for drawing up the dose and to what accuracy, exactly how and where the animal should be restrained, a detailed description of how the cannula/catheter is inserted and what to look for. It would also detail the removal and replacement of the animal from its cage, the identification of the animal and a reference to another SOP detailing any post dose observations which may be observed.

Once the draft SOP is prepared, it should be circulated to personnel who will be using it for comment (this may be restricted to senior members of staff). It should also be circulated to QA and management for approval. Once all comments have been dealt with, the SOP should be redistributed for any further comments. After its return, the SOP can be put forward for issue.

Updated SOPs should replace old SOPs which should be removed from reference files and destroyed (as these will just be copies). Master SOPs are archived for later reference should they be needed. Only up-to-date SOPs should be available and in use.

SOPs are reviewed on a regular basis – usually every two years.

Webliography

Medicines and Healthcare Products Regulatory Agency – www.mhra.gov.uk

38

Experimental Procedures

Bryan Waynforth

Introduction

Administration of compounds and withdrawal of body fluids form a major part of experimental work with animals. The conduct of these procedures is controlled by the Animals (Scientific Procedures) Act 1986 (see Chapter 35) and must be covered by a project licence and a personal licence and take place in a designated scientific procedure establishment. In addition, researchers must undergo mandatory training and keep records to confirm that they have been assessed as competent in the relevant procedures. They must also be aware of the conditions of the project licence, in particular the severity condition, which limits the amount of pain, suffering, distress or lasting harm that they can produce in an animal. Any deviations from these conditions, however slight, must be reported to the Home Office and may constitute an infringement punishable by law! All animals must be monitored at least once a day and if their condition is a cause for concern, appropriate action, as defined in the project licence, must be taken. In these or any circumstances where there is concern, it is always advisable to seek the advice of a veterinary surgeon or the named animal care and welfare officer (NACWO).

Every opportunity must be taken to refine a procedure so that the amount of harm produced by the procedure is the least that can possibly be inflicted in the circumstances. For instance, consider whether an indwelling cannula can be used to accomplish serial administration of substances or collection of blood, which otherwise would be done, to an animal's increasing discomfort, using multiple skin punctures? Can an alternative, less distressful method of blood collection be used than by puncture of

the retro-orbital plexus? It is incumbent upon an establishment's Ethical Review Process to ask these types of questions of every researcher (see Chapter 35).

Only the principles associated with the performance of experimental procedures are given in this chapter. However, details of how to carry out each procedure can be found in the publications in the References and further reading section at the end of the chapter.

The administration of substances

The administration of a substance to an animal is probably the most frequently employed procedure in animal experimentation. Such administration may be done to study the biological activity of a compound or to induce a biological or chemical change in the animal. Whatever the requirement, it is important in the cause of animal welfare, accuracy, precision and reproducibility, that the person carrying out the procedure knows how to do it properly. This will entail knowing something about the characteristics of the substance to be administered, the routes and methods of administration and about the possible reactions of the animal. Consideration of the use of local anaesthetics must be made where appropriate (see Chapter 41, Schedule 2A of the Animals (Scientific Procedures) Act 1986).

Routes of administration – parenteral

Substances which have been administered into any site of the body except the alimentary canal are said to have been administered parenterally.

Common parenteral routes

Route	Description
Intradermal (i.d.)	into the skin layers
Intramuscular (i.m.)	into a muscle
Intraperitoneal (i.p.)	into the peritoneal or abdominal cavity
Intravenous (i.v.)	into a vein
Subcutaneous (s.c.)	immediately under the skin
Topical	onto the skin

Less common parenteral routes

Route	Description
Intra-articular	into a synovial joint
Intracisternal	into the space of the cisterna magna
Intracranial	into the brain
Intrathecal	into the spinal column
Intrathoracic	into the thoracic cavity
Intravesicular	into the bladder
Inhalation	into the lung cavity

Routes of administration – enteral

Substances which have been deposited directly into the stomach, or into the mouth or are given via the rectum are said to have been administered enterally. More specifically, when substances are placed in the mouth, it is called an oral administration, while intra-gastric administration or administration by oral gavage applies to the stomach. In practice these terms are often used synonymously.

Common methods of administration

Subcutaneous (s.c.)

The most common areas of the body used for s.c. administration in all species are the neck and the sides (flanks). The neck skin can be conveniently tented allowing the needle to be pushed easily through it into the subcutaneous space. The skin on the sides of the body may be fairly taut and injection here requires more care. The mechanics of the injection may vary slightly with the species and may depend on the methods used to restrain the animal.

Care must be taken to ensure that the needle is lying subcutaneously and not in the peritoneal cavity, or in a muscle. The tip can usually be felt if the needle is raised within the subcutaneous space.

When making an s.c. injection it is important that the whole needle shaft lies subcutaneously and not just a small part of it. This ensures that the material is deposited well forward of the needle puncture site and leak-back and loss of solution through it are minimised.

Intraperitoneal (i.p.)

The i.p. injection is made into the centre of the lower left or right quadrant of the abdomen. This avoids the bladder which lies in the mid-line. The needle is pushed in almost vertically with only the tip of the needle lying inside the peritoneal cavity, otherwise it is possible to puncture and inject into the intestine where the material may be lost through the rectum.

It is often easier to place the needle s.c. and then to elevate the syringe to a more acute angle and make a short push through the abdominal muscle into the peritoneal cavity. If the animal is correctly held the abdominal skin and muscle can often be made taut, which facilitates passage of the needle through them.

Intramuscular (i.m.)

The muscles of the cranial (quadriceps muscle group) and caudal (semitendinosus m., etc.) part of the thigh, and the gluteal muscles of the rump are the most frequently used sites for i.m. injections. Care must be taken not to touch the bone with the needle as this will be painful for the animal and would require the needle to be pulled back slightly before making the injection. In some cases, an i.m. injection may fail because the needle lies in the fascia or connective tissue surrounding the muscle. Once the needle has entered the muscle, the syringe plunger should be withdrawn slightly to ensure that the needle is not inadvertently lying within a blood vessel. However, the expected show of blood in the hub of the needle which indicates correct placement, and which occurs when injecting into large animals, may not always be seen in smaller animals.

Intravenous (i.v.)

Any vein can be used for i.v. injections, but some are considerably more accessible than others. The most available sites for i.v. injection in the common laboratory species are given in Table 38.1. In some instances the animal must be anaesthetised in order to restrain it before an injection is made. In all species, aseptic technique should be used when entering a vein. However, in practice this is often dispensed with in the small species.

Table 38.1   Common sites for intravenous administration.

Species	Site	Restraint
Mouse	Tail vein	Manual
	Sublingual vein	Anaesthesia
Rat	Tail vein	Manual
	Sublingual vein	Anaesthesia
	Penile vein	Anaesthesia
Syrian hamster	Jugular vein	Anaesthesia
Guinea pig	Marginal ear vein	Manual
	Dorsal metatarsal vein	Manual
	Penile vein	Anaesthesia
Rabbit	Marginal ear vein	Manual
Cat	Cephalic vein	Manual
	Recurrent tarsal vein	Manual
Dog	Cephalic	Manual
	Saphenous	Manual
Mini pig	Ear vein	Sedation
Goat	Jugular vein	Manual
	Cephalic vein	Manual
Sheep	Jugular vein	Manual
	Cephalic vein	Manual
Chicken	Wing (brachial) vein	Manual

There are some important points to consider to ensure a successful injection.

(1) The vein itself, or its outline, must be seen clearly. This will entail removing hair in many cases. The application of 70% alcohol, another antiseptic or a vasodilator (e.g. Vasolate®) to the skin over-lying the vein may help to make the vein more visible. Occluding the vein, depending on the species, by for example digital pressure or the use of a tourniquet, or rubbing the vein vigorously, will also make it dilate and therefore easier to inject.

(2) The vein should be stabilised to prevent it from moving when the needle is inserted. This may involve stretching the skin over the vein with the fingers of the free hand, or with the help of an assistant.

(3) It is important to stabilise the hand when making an injection into a small vein, most often in the smaller species. Any shake in the hand can be minimised by supporting the arm on the bench or by resting the side of the hand or the little finger on the bench while making the injection.

Supporting the needle against the thumb of the other hand which is holding the area containing the vein, e.g. the rabbit's ear or the penis of the rat, can also be effective.

(4) When injecting into very small vessels, the syringe should be held so that the plunger can be depressed after needle insertion without having to reposition the hand. If this is not done then too much movement will be created, with the probability of the needle coming out of the vein.

(5) To ensure the needle is in the vein, the syringe plunger is withdrawn slightly to see if blood enters the hub of the syringe. This is usually only possible with the larger veins. With superficial veins the tip of the needle can generally be seen when raised and disappears when depressed indicating blood flowing under and over the tip respectively. If the needle is inadvertently positioned outside the vein, a bleb appears around the vein on injection of a small amount of the solution and the needle will have to be repositioned. If possible, the needle should be repositioned while remaining within the tissue, otherwise if the needle is first removed, bleeding may occur, reducing visibility and making it more difficult to reinsert the needle, in addition to the extra discomfort caused to the animal.

(6) When it is necessary to enter the same vein a number of times, as for serial injections, the injections should start distally and proceed proximally, towards the heart. This ensures that if an injection damages or blocks the vein, a more proximal site will still be available. Insertion of an in-dwelling catheter may be more appropriate where serial injections have to be made and will reduce the distress to the animal which occurs with multiple needle penetrations.

(7) Where the vein is not easily accessible, or is very small, e.g. the rat or mouse tail vein, placing the animal in a box heated to 40 °C for no more than five to ten minutes, or placing the tail in warm water, will dilate the vein and make it easier to enter.

(8) After completing an i.v. injection, pressure must be applied to the entry point for several seconds to prevent bleeding or the formation of an haematoma.

Intradermal (i.d.)

The most commonly used sites are the lateral areas of the body and the ears. If the area contains hair, this should be clipped short. The needle is advanced about 5–10 mm into the dermis of the skin. This can be quite difficult if the skin is thin. There is considerable resistance to the passage of the needle, in contrast to an s.c. injection, which could be made in error. Usually, injection of a minute quantity of material i.d. will cause a bleb to appear. Also, if the material is coloured, it can be seen through the skin after an i.d. injection, but not after an s.c. injection. The swelling must not be rubbed after an i.d. injection. The use of the footpads is inadvisable under all circumstances as it has major welfare implications.

Topical

The sides of the body are the preferred sites in most cases, but under special circumstances, the ears may be used. If the area has hair, this is removed by clipping and may, if required, be further denuded by careful atraumatic shaving and/or the application of a depilatory. It is advisable to do this twenty-four hours before the test substance is to be applied as there may be a slight inflammatory response after hair removal. It should be noted that depilatories are chemical substances which may have a pharmacological effect on the skin in their own right or may act synergistically with the material to be administered. These possible effects can be minimised if the depilatory is applied the day before the test substance is to be applied. Once the test substance has been applied to the prepared area, it may be necessary to protect it from removal by the animal licking it. A suitable dressing or an Elizabethan collar can be used. Elizabethan collars are available commercially for rodents and larger animals.

Oral (intragastric; oral gavage)

In small rodents, administration of liquids into the stomach can be made using a special stainless steel cannula, of the right gauge (e.g. 16 G for adult rats), with a bulb at its tip. The bulb prevents damage to the oesophagus and reduces the chance of misplacement of the needle into the trachea. The inability to insert the cannula fully is usually diagnostic of misplacement into the trachea. If the bulb is of a size that fills the space of the oesophagus, regurgitation of fluid up into the mouth and possibly into the lungs is prevented

and accuracy of the dose is also maintained. The length of the needle should be just sufficient for the needle to enter the stomach which will lie approximately at the level of the xiphoid cartilage. The animal may 'gag' or become very irritable if the tube passes into the trachea. Any fluid deposited into the lungs may be fatal. While using a metal catheter, great care must be taken with the restraint of the animal. Any possibility of the animal moving unexpectedly must be eliminated so as to avoid oesophageal damage.

An alternative method which can be used in all species, and is particularly suitable for the rat, guinea pig, rabbit, cat, dog and primate, is to employ a rubber or flexible PVC cannula. This is pushed down the side of the mouth and into the oesophagus and stomach while encouraging the animal to swallow. In fractious animals, the cannula can only be inserted with the use of a suitable mouth gag to prevent it being bitten through. Such gags are available commercially. Before the administration is made, the cannula must be filled with the solution so as to eliminate dead space and to give an accurate dose. Alternatively, if this is not done, as is common when dosing the dog for example, a wash-out must be employed after the substance has been given, using water or vehicle, to ensure the animal gets the full dose. Intragastric administration of fluids to animals such as pigs, sheep and goats, is carried out using a special dosing gun or flexible cannula. The oral administration of solids is straightforward in large animals, such as dogs or cats, where tablets or powder-filled gelatin capsules can be placed at the back of the mouth and the animal encouraged to swallow. Alternatively, substances can be mixed with the diet. In rodents and rabbits small gelatin capsules can be filled with the powdered material and placed part way into the oesophagus by using a specially designed cup tipped needle attached to a syringe. The cup holder containing the capsule is placed at the back of the mouth and the capsule is gently blown into the oesophagus by depressing the syringe plunger. Solids can also be fed to small animals by mixing them with their food but accurate dosing is then impossible.

Other methods

The administration of substances into other organs, tissues or body cavities is usually of a specialised nature and is described in appropriate texts (see References and further reading, p. 362).

Restraint

For all methods of administration, proper restraint of the animal is essential and facilitates the procedure. Manual restraint is the method of choice but in some cases, mechanical or chemical restraint may be indicated (e.g. if the animal is large and fractious or is vicious or wild) or if the procedure is painful. However, mechanical and chemical restraint can be more traumatic and stressful to the animal than gentle but firm handling and therefore should be avoided as much as possible. Training animals for the method of restraint before the procedure commences will lessen the adverse effects on them (e.g. placing rabbits in stocks).

Experimental feeding and watering

Three basic principles must be considered when a substance has to be administered mixed in the diet or in the drinking water, or where a novel diet is to be fed:

(1) The diet or water must be palatable.
(2) Any induced nutritive deficiency should be limited to the degree required for the study and should be maintained for as short a time as possible.
(3) Experimental diets – which can be prepared as powders, pellets, gels or liquids – should be introduced gradually if they are in a form which is unfamiliar to the animal. They should be as freshly prepared as possible and rancidity and microbial and fungal contamination must be avoided.

A major problem is uniform mixing of constituents, some of which may be in relatively minute amounts. This may entail mixing one or more constituents in several stages. For example, first mixing in a small aliquot of the diet, then mixing this aliquot with a larger aliquot and finally mixing this with the rest of the diet. If diets are given in powder form, some animals (e.g. rats) are deft at sifting the test compound from the rest of the diet and so avoid being dosed. If this is a problem, diets should be given compacted as gels or pellets. Powdered diets should be given in special containers which minimise scattering of the food and prevent the animal lying or defecating on it. Such containers, which can be weighed, also make it simpler to measure food consumption more accurately. They are available commercially for the smaller animals.

Animals given diets which are nutritionally inadequate are liable to show abnormal behavioural changes (e.g. eating fur, cannibalism, increased fighting, drinking urine, eating faeces) and may also be more prone to incidental diseases and secondary disorders, such as bone distortion and fractures during studies, for example, in experimental rickets.

Appropriate action must also be taken in cases where social order determines who eats first, or at all, if the volume of diet available is reduced (e.g. this occurs especially in rodents, pigs and primates). This will affect the experimental result if it is allowed to occur.

Water containing test substances should be freely available, but if deprivation is required by the protocol this should be permitted only for short periods. The method of delivery of the water to the animal (e.g. bottle, bowl, automatic watering system) should be checked regularly to make sure the animals are not playing with them and thus wasting water. As with diet, social dominance may interfere with an animal's opportunity to drink. If the water supply is inadequate, secondary problems may arise. Rodents in particular seem liable to develop bladder infections and calculi which could invalidate experimental results.

Although weighing food and water containers can give a measurement of consumption and therefore dose, wastage which inevitably occurs to a greater or lesser degree, cannot be accounted for and the dose measured therefore will only be approximate. A much more accurate measurement can be obtained if animals are kept individually in special metabolism cages where the water and food containers are so designed as to minimise wastage and to collect any wastage that occurs, so that it too can be determined. These metabolism cages, for a large number of species, are available commercially.

General aspects of administration

Solvents for administration

Distilled water or physiological saline (0.9% w/v sodium chloride) are ideal for injecting soluble substances. However, some substances are only partly soluble or totally insoluble in water and may need more complex solvents to dissolve them. The maximum tolerated dose of the solvent must also be considered. Ideally, solutions for injection should be isotonic (i.e. have the same osmotic pressure as body fluids, e.g. blood serum).

For insoluble compounds a homogenous suspension in any of the accepted solvents can be made. The smallest particle size possible should be obtained and in some cases this may only be achieved by grinding the material to be injected. Absolute accuracy of the dose cannot be obtained when administering suspensions because of the tendency of particles to sediment and to become compacted when discharged from the syringe.

Lipid soluble compounds can be administered in vegetable oils (e.g. peanut, castor, olive oils) or mineral oils (e.g. paraffin oil), though the former are to be preferred. Such solvents must not be injected i.v. unless they form part of a complex emulsion which has to be specially prepared.

Preparations for topical application may be made in any suitable pharmacologically inert vehicle which should be physically and chemically stable.

Volumes for injection

The volumes which can be injected can be very variable within each species and will also vary proportionally with the size of the animal. Some suggested volumes which can be injected by the common routes are given in Table 38.2. These volumes are generally those which are considered to comply with good practice.

Maximum volumes, i.e. those which might be

Table 38.2   Good practice guidelines for injection volumes (ml/kg).

Species	s.c.	i.p.	i.m. (ml/site)	oral	i.v.
Mouse	10	20	0.05	10	5
Rat	5	10	0.1	10	5
Syrian hamster	5	5	0.1	10	5
Guinea pig	5	5	0.1	10	5
Rabbit	1	5	0.25	10	2
Cat	1	1	0.25	5	2
Dog	1	1	0.25	5	2.5
Marmoset	2	0	0.25	10	2
Mini pig	1	1	0.25	10	2.5
Goat	1	1	0.25	10	2.5
Sheep	1	1	0.25	10	2.5
Chicken	0	3	0.25	0	2

needed in exceptional circumstances, can be much higher but the effects on an animal's well-being will need to be carefully monitored (see References and further reading, p. 362). Injection of large volumes may be at the risk of adverse consequences. For example, administration of more than about 1 ml of fluid by the i.v. route to a young adult rat could result in pulmonary oedema with a fatal outcome. With some routes (e.g. s.c., i.m.) larger total volumes can be administered by employing several injection sites simultaneously but these should not exceed four in number. Large volumes should not be injected i.m. as this causes pain. At all times it is good practice to administer the smallest volume that is compatible with the solubility of the compound and the accuracy of the dose.

The pH of solutions

The pH of solutions for injection should, ideally, be around pH 7.0 but a range of 4.5–8.0 can be acceptable.

The stomach can tolerate more acid conditions since the normal pH there is often in the region of pH 2. Because the blood has the greatest buffering capacity, the widest pH range is tolerated by the i.v. route followed by the i.m. and then the s.c. routes.

The nature of the solution

Substances which cause local irritation or pain are best injected by the i.v. route, though the i.m. route can be used for less severe cases. Substances with an extreme pH value (e.g. a solution of the barbiturate, thiopentone sodium, has a pH of 11) must only be injected i.v. as tissue necrosis and pain can be produced if it is injected elsewhere.

Ideally, solutions for parenteral administration should be sterile but in practice under research conditions, this may be difficult to achieve. Thus the use of sterile solutions will depend on local circumstances. Conventional techniques of sterilisation including filtration, which includes a filter which can be attached to a syringe, may be employed providing they do not affect the active ingredient.

The rate of injection

Most injections should be made slowly, with care and attention, particularly i.v. injections.

The rate of injection depends on the species and experience of the operator. Injections into the peritoneal cavity and the stomach can be made more swiftly but there is a risk with the latter of the material being forced back up the oesophagus into the mouth with consequent loss of accuracy of the dose.

The size of the needle

Hypodermic needles can be obtained in a variety of sizes, lengths and diameters. They are usually described by a gauge number (i.e. standard wire gauge) which is an indication as to their diameter. The higher the gauge number, the smaller will be the diameter. At all times, the needle with the smallest external diameter which is compatible with the viscosity and nature of the substance to be injected and with the size of the animal should be used. If the needle is too large, leak-back through the needle hole will tend to occur with consequent loss of fluid and inaccuracy of the dose. Larger needles increase the discomfort to the animal.

For administration of aqueous solutions to small animals a needle of size 25 G or 26 G should be used for general work, but sizes up to 30 G are useful for i.v. injections (in the mouse for example).

For dogs and larger animals, 21 G or 19 G needles are recommended, but 16 G or 14 G needles may be more suitable in some cases. For fluids which are difficult to inject (e.g. suspensions, oils, emulsions) the larger size needles are needed, and serious consideration should be given to using Luer–Lock syringes for the most difficult fluids, to prevent the explosive separation of the needle from the hub.

The lengths of needles commonly employed are between 25 mm and 50 mm. However for certain routes of administration, in small animals, a length of around 10 mm is more appropriate (e.g. for i.p., and some i.v. routes). In large animals, needles of 100 mm or larger need to be used in cases such as cardiac puncture. Gavage needles of this size are also used for intragastric administration to adult rats. Butterfly needles, which have a plastic, or occasionally a metal, flange and usually come attached to a flexible PVC cannula, can be found in standard sizes. They are extremely useful where it is required to keep the needle in a vein for a period, for example a rabbit ear vein or the dog cephalic vein, where the flange can be taped into place, or for situations where injections are difficult where the flexibility of the butterfly cannula components allows an animal to move without the needle coming out (e.g. a large fractious pig or goat being injected i.m.). The cannula must be filled with the solution before needle insertion, to maintain accuracy of the dose.

For all types of injection the bevel of the needle should be kept pointing upwards. This allows the needle point to 'bite' the tissue easily and also facilitates its passage within the tissue. An exception to this can be made for an i.d. injection where using the needle with the bevel downwards can help in sliding the needle just under the surface of the skin. The Schick needle has a special application for i.d. injection since it has a short bevel.

Special devices

The osmotic mini pump is a fillable capsule which can be implanted s.c. or i.p., under general anaesthesia, and which will allow slow, continuous release of soluble substances at a constant rate for up to four weeks. By suitable adaptation, the pump can also be used for administration i.v. and into other sites. A variety of materials which can be suitably prepared for sustained release applications are also available.

Absorption of substances

The rate and manner in which substances are absorbed from the site of administration and transported via the circulation to the site of action are determined mainly by the physical form of the substance, the route of administration and certain physico-chemical characteristics. There can be a marked species differences in the way a substance is absorbed from the same site. Substances wholly or partly soluble in water are absorbed more rapidly than those dissolved in an oily solvent or those given as suspensions or in a solid form. Every attempt should therefore be made to find a suitable solvent to dissolve the substance for injection. In the body, solids have first to be disintegrated and then become dissolved in the surrounding tissue fluid, before they are available for absorption. Also, chemicals injected in a solution of high concentration may be absorbed more rapidly than those in low concentration.

Choice of route

When selecting a route by which a compound may be administered there are a number of factors to be taken into consideration.

- *The species*: The animal to which the compound is given may effect route selection. Some of the common administration routes can be more difficult in certain species due to problems of restraint or accessibility of the administration site, e.g. intravenous injections in the hamster can be a problem particularly in the absence of an anaesthetic, as superficial vessels are difficult to locate. When dealing with intractable animals, routes requiring more precision, e.g. intravenous, may be more difficult to use because of the difficulty of restraining such animals effectively. Intravenous dosing and oral intubation of the guinea pig are more time consuming and labour intensive than the same procedures carried out on a rat.

- *Physiological condition of the animal*: When the health of an animal is impaired the accessibility of certain routes may be affected. The intravenous route may be made more difficult by a lowered blood pressure. Similar difficulty may be encountered with the intravenous routes in animals that are obese or aged.

- *Nature of the material to be administered*: Some routes may be contra-indicated because of the physical properties of the compound to be given or the method in which the compound has been formulated. For instance, antibodies cannot be administered by the oral route. Highly irritant materials should not be given via the s.c. or i.p. routes where they will cause pain; suspensions must not be administered via the intravenous route as this may cause an embolism; strong or foul-tasting compounds if administered via the diet may be ignored by the animal. Chemical characteristics of the compound may affect the choice of route if the qualitative response varies between routes. For example, magnesium sulphate if given orally can have a laxative effect whereas given intravenously it can act as a CNS depressant or hypnotic.

- *The speed of the transfer to the action site*: Transfer of a compound to the site on which it will have an effect generally takes place via the circulatory system. It follows, therefore, that the sooner the compound enters the system the sooner it will be transported to the action site. Fast methods of administration are characterised by a high initial concentration in the blood, followed by a rapid decline as the compound reaches the action site. If a rapid effect is required, an intravenous injection will be the method of choice. Other routes will first require absorption from the injection site and then passage into the blood stream. The speed of absorption will depend partially on the blood supply network to the particular site but other factors also play an important part. In descending order of absorption rate, the intraperitoneal route is followed by the intra-muscular route which is more rapid than the subcutaneous route. Oral administration is variable but generally the slowest of all. All substances administered by the i.p. or oral route will pass via the mesenteric blood vessels and hepatic portal vein to the liver where they may undergo metabolic change. This may or may not have adverse consequences for the substance's activity.

The advantages and disadvantages of administering compounds by the more common routes are summarised in Table 38.3.

The withdrawal and collection of blood, urine and faeces

Blood

The conditions under which blood is collected can be critical for an experiment and the stress to the animal of collecting blood can cause large increases in several blood constituents. For baseline values it has been suggested that blood collection should be completed within 10–90 seconds of first disturbing the animal. Achieving this in most cases is impractical but it does indicate that competence in blood collection is important and that strict standardisation of the collection method and time should be maintained so as to reduce variability. It should be noted that standardisation of all procedures is the essence of the Good Laboratory Animal Practice which is observed universally throughout the pharmaceutical industry and is therefore a good model to follow.

Blood which is allowed to clot will exude a clear,

Table 38.3   Advantages and disadvantages of using various routes of administration.

Route	Advantages	Disadvantages
Oral (capsule, gavage, diet)	Easily and rapidly administered. Slow, smooth absorption. Unlikely to introduce infection. Large volume may be administered. Painless.	May not be absorbed. Palatability problems (if added to diet). Risk of introduction into trachea (with gavage). Stomach acidity may affect the compound.
Intravenous	Rapid effect. Alkaline solutions may be given (up to pH 11). Irritant materials may be given.	Solution must be sterile and isotonic. Must be in soluble form, no suspensions. Veins may be difficult to locate.
Topical (percutaneous)	Easily and rapidly carried out.	Need to shave. Can be removed by animal licking site and leading to ingestion of compound. May contaminate cagemates, handlers etc. Often requires adhesive dressing or restraint to prevent above, which can be restrictive to the animal.
Subcutaneous	Easy to locate injection site. Large in area and suitable for large volumes. Slow, smooth absorption.	Leakage from site. Solution must be sterile, isotonic and as close as possible to neutral pH.
Intraperitoneal	Easy to perform. Fairly rapid smooth absorption.	Risk of peritonitis. Danger of injecting bladder, intestines and other internal organs. Solution must be sterile and neutral pH. Correct restraint must be used.
Intramuscular	More rapid absorption than intraperitoneal. Small volumes only can be given but with possibility of using multiple sites. Slightly irritating materials may be given by this route.	Some pain. Not suitable for large volumes. Care must be taken to avoid veins, arteries and nerves. Solution must be sterile, near neutral pH and isotonic.

slightly yellow fluid which is the serum. If anti-coagulants are added to the blood when it is freshly drawn, clotting is prevented and the blood will separate into a lower fraction containing the cellular elements and an upper plasma layer. Various anti-coagulants are in common use and although Ethylenediamine tetraacetic acid (EDTA) is the most generally useful, others may need to be used in special investigations. These are lithium heparin, sodium or ammonium oxalate, sodium or lithium citrate and sodium fluoride. The choice of whether to collect serum or plasma may depend on the type of investigation being undertaken.

Methods of obtaining blood

The most useful sites for blood withdrawal from common laboratory animals are shown in Table 38.4. It is difficult to give quantitative aspects of blood collection as both animal welfare and physiological effects will impact on this. Table 38.5 gives some guidelines.

Although the average blood volume varies from species to species, for the sake of standardisation, the Home Office have taken a circulating blood volume of 65 ml/kg body weight as an average for all species.

From this they have recommended that no more than 15% of blood volume (1 ml/100 g body weight) is collected over a twenty-eight-day period. Moreover, it is recommended that a single withdrawal should not exceed 10% of blood volume. After a withdrawal of 10% of blood volume, haemoglobin levels do not return to normal for about two weeks, and after 15% blood withdrawal as a single sample, physiological recovery may not be for four weeks or more. These restrictions do not apply of course to collecting blood as a terminal sample, under general anaesthesia. Variations in these guideline volumes are possible but have to be justified on a case by case basis. After removal of a large amount of blood from a rat or a mouse, e.g. 10% of body weight, it is possible to replace this with blood from an animal of the same type on a single occasion only, with no adverse consequences. This allows an extension of the amount of blood which can be taken and may be useful if large amounts of blood are required, for example for a drug pharmacodynamic study.

Methods such as the ear vein in the rabbit and tail vein in rodents should use a local anaesthetic. In all species, very small samples, adequate to fill a capillary tube can be obtained by puncture of a vein in the ear,

Table 38.4 Common sites for withdrawal of blood.

Species	Site	Restraint
Mouse	Retro-orbital venous plexus	Anaesthesia
	Tail vein/tail tip	Manual
	Axillary pouch	Anaesthesia
	Saphenous venous	Manual
	Heart	Anaesthesia
Rat	Retro-orbital venous plexus	Anaesthesia
	Tail vein/tail tip	Manual
	Axillary pouch	Anaesthesia
	Jugular vein	Manual
	Saphenous vein	Manual
	Heart	Anaesthesia
Guinea pig	Heart	Anaesthesia
	Marginal ear vein	Manual
	Saphenous vein	Manual
Rabbit	Marginal ear vein	Manula
	Central ear artery	Manual
	Heart	Anaesthesia
Cat	Cephalic vein	Manual
	Jugular	Manual
Dog	Cephalic vein	Manual
	Jugular vein	Manual
Marmoset	Femoral vein	Manual
	Saphenous vein	Manual
Mini pig	Femoral vein	Anaesthesia
	Ear veins	Sedation
Goat	Jugular vein	Manual
Sheep	Jugular vein	Manual
Chicken	Wing vein	Manual
	Heart	Anaesthesia
Frog	Veins in foot	Manual
	Jugular vein	Anaesthesia

the foot or the tail as appropriate. Large volumes of blood, even to the point of exsanguination, can be withdrawn from the heart under anaesthesia, but this has the attendant risk of death from technical failure or haemorrhage. Withdrawal from the heart should be considered a terminal procedure only, unless shortage of available sites is a problem, such as in the hamster.

Blood should always be withdrawn slowly and steadily. When ejecting the blood subsequently from a syringe into a container, the needle must be removed otherwise breakage of the red blood cells can occur due to the shearing forces within the needle, this could interfere with the subsequent investigation.

The principles outlined for the administration of substances intravenously (i.v.) (viz. visualisation, stabilisation, venous occlusion and haemostasis) are wholly applicable also to withdrawal of blood (see p. 353). The diameter of the needles used should be the larger of the sizes recommended for injection. For example 23–21 G for rodents and rabbits and 21–14 G for dogs, sheep and other large animals, the sizes depending on the size of vein encountered. Butterfly needles and intravenous cannulae are particularly useful for the temporary catheterisation of blood vessels, by means of which continuous or serial samples can be obtained. This also obviates the need for serial puncture of a vein which can be relatively traumatic to the animal. Some care has to be taken with indwelling needles and cannulae to prevent clotting within them and anti-coagulants such as heparin, will have to be used.

Collection of urine and faeces

Urine

This can be conveniently collected from all species by the use of commercially available metabolism cages. These consist of a cage which sits on top of a funnel or other collecting device which is either itself designed, or has associated with it other constituents which are designed to separate solid faeces from the urine. The completeness of the separation is reflected in the efficiency of the metabolism cage, which also determines the degree of contamination by food or water. However, separation cannot be achieved if animals are excreting fluid faeces (diarrhoea). For collection over twenty-four hours or longer, a preservative, such as a few drops of toluene, is often added. Cooling the urine during collection is good practice, in order to prevent excessive bacterial contamination and decomposition of urinary constituents.

Urine can also be obtained by catheterisation of the bladder via the urethra using sterile flexible rubber or plastic tubing. The method is easiest in female rodents, male rabbits, and in either sex of the dog and larger animals. A few drops of urine can often be obtained from small animals when they are first picked up and urine can also be collected in

Table 38.5 Good practice guidelines for blood collection volumes.

Species	Average blood volume (ml/kg)	Home Office guidelines for average blood volume (ml/kg)	Recommended Home Office maximum volume for blood collection with recovery (ml/kg/28 days)	Maximum volume available by exsanguination (ml/kg)
Mouse	72			30
Rat	64			30
Guinea pig	75			40
Rabbit	56			30
Cat	70			35
Dog	85	65	10	40
Marmoset	70			40
Mini pig	65			25
Goat	65			25
Sheep	80			40
Chicken	85			40
Frog	90			25

larger animals by the patient technician who waits for the animal to urinate naturally!

Faeces

Methods of collecting uncontaminated faeces other than by metabolism cage, involve the use of an anal cup in rodents, usually only applicable to male animals, and by the removal of faeces with a spatula directly from the rectum of large animals. Faeces can also be collected from the floor of the cage or pen or at the time of spontaneous defecation.

Other samples

Non-surgical methods are available for the collection of biological samples other than blood, urine and faeces, such as semen, milk, synovial fluid and cerebrospinal fluid. Collection can also be made of cells and tissues such as bone marrow and peritoneal macrophages and of expired gases. These are specialised techniques, which can be found in the literature (see References and further reading, pp. 362–364).

Safe practices

It is insufficiently appreciated that carrying out experimental procedures incorrectly may give rise to problems regarding the health and safety both of the animals and of the investigator. Examples of some common malpractices will suffice to emphasise the need to take adequate precautions.

(1) Ejecting fluid into the air when removing air bubbles from the syringe and when preparing the measured dose. This creates an aerosol which can disperse throughout the room. If a hazardous chemical is involved (e.g. radioisotope, carcinogen, toxic material) unacceptable contamination of personnel and animals in the vicinity can occur. All fluids should be ejected either back into the original container, preferably a sealed one, or into a wad of cotton wool or gauze which can then be disposed of.

(2) Inoculation of hazardous materials such as radioisotopes, carcinogens and infectious microbes in unprotected areas. Such inoculations should be carried out in isolated areas or at the very least in protected areas with facilities to prevent spillage, such as biosafety cabinets. Personnel protection in all these cases is vital.

(3) Accidental injection of an assistant or oneself. Care should be taken to use a method which reduces this risk. If this is impractical, then appropriate precautions should be taken or an antidote should be available (e.g. the antidote Revivon should be immediately available when using the large animal preparation of the anaesthetic Immobilon, small amounts of which can

be rapidly fatal on injection to human beings). Errors can occur through inexpert handling of animals and therefore attaining competence in handling is crucial.

(4) Inoculations of animals through contaminated skin. Ideally, sterile solutions and sterile transference of these from the container to the syringe, and methods of sterile inoculation into the animal should be employed. If the sterile solution is in a rubber capped vial, it can be withdrawn with a sterile needle and syringe after disinfecting the surface of the cap with 70% alcohol, or other antiseptic, which can then be pierced by the needle. Transference of solutions from open-topped containers should be done with care, avoiding contact with any part of the syringe which may have become contaminated. Before inoculation, the injection site should be clipped to remove hair and wiped with 70% alcohol or other antiseptic to minimise bacterial contamination.

In practice, the use of sterile procedures and solutions is often dispensed with or may be impractical in small animals. In spite of this, overt infection as a consequence, seems only to occur rarely in these animals. Also, any pyrogenic effect of the non-sterile solution does not seem to affect the small animal adversely. In large animals however, it is common practice to observe asepsis during inoculation and withdrawal procedures.

Safe practices in all spheres of work are a legal requirement of the Health and Safety at Work etc. Act, 1974, and it is incumbent upon individuals to take the necessary care in the performance of that work.

References and further reading

Rodents and rabbits

Archer, R.K. and Riley, J. (1981) Standardised method for bleeding rats. *Laboratory Animals*, **15** (25).

Baker H.J., Lindsey, J.R. and Weisbroth, S.H. (Eds) (1980) *The Laboratory Rat*, Vol. 2, *Research Applications*. Academic Press Inc., New York.

Berg, B.M. and Simms, H.S. (1960) Nutrition and longevity in the rat II, longevity and onset of diseases with different levels of food intake. *Journal of Nutrition*, **71** (255).

Besc, E.L. and Chou, B.J. (1971) *Physiological responses to blood collection methods in rats.* Proceedings of the Society for Experimental Biology and Medicine, **138** (1019).

Bickhardt, K., Buttner, D. and Plonait, H. (1983) Influence of bleeding procedure and some environmental conditions on stress-dependent blood constituents of laboratory rats. *Laboratory Animals*, **17** (161).

Bivin, W.S. and Timmons, E.H. (1974) Basic biomethodology. In: S.H. Weisbroth, R.E. Flatt and A.L. Kraus (Eds) *The Laboratory Rabbit*. Academic Press, New York.

Bollman, J.L. (1948) A cage which limits the activity of rats. *Journal of Laboratory and Clinical Medicine*, **33** (1349).

de Brant, V. and Remon, J.P. (1991) A simple method for the intragastric administration of drugs to fully conscious guinea pigs. *Laboratory Animals*, **25** (308).

BVA/FRAME/RSPCA/UFAW Joint working Group on Refinement (1993) Removal of blood from laboratory mammals and birds. *Laboratory Animals*, **27** (1).

Carroll, J.A., Daniel, J.A., Keiser, D.H. and Matteri, R.L. (1998) Non-surgical catheterisation of the jugular vein in young guinea pigs. *Laboratory Animals*, **33** (129).

Claassen, V. (1994) *Neglected Factors in Pharmacology and Neuroscience Research*. Elsevier, Amsterdam.

Coates, M.E. (1995) Feeding and watering. In: A.A. Tuffery (Ed.) *Laboratory Animals: An Introduction for Experimenters* (2nd edn). John Wiley & Sons, Chichester.

Cunliffe-Beamer, T.L. (1983) Biomethodology and surgical technique. In: H.L. Foster, J.D. Small and J.G. Fox (Eds) *The Mouse in Biomedical Research*, Vol. 3: *Normative Biology, Immunology and Husbandry*. Academic Press, New York.

Dalton, R.G., Touraine, J.L. and Wilson, T.R. (1969) A simple technique for continuous intravenous infusion in rats. *Journal of Laboratory and Clinical Medicine*, **74** (813).

EFPIA/ECVAM Technical Subgroup (1999) *A Good Practice Guide to the Administration of Substances and Removal of Blood, Including Routes and Volumes*. Obtained from ECVAM, Institute for Health and Consumer Protection, European Commission Joint Research Centre, 21020 Ispra (VA), Italy.

Flecknell P.A. (1995) Non-surgical experimental procedures. In: A.A. Tuffery (Ed.) *Laboratory Animals: An Introduction for Experimenters* (2nd edn). John Wiley & Sons, Chichester.

Fox, J.G., Cohen, B.J. and Loew, F.M. (1984) *Laboratory Animal Medicine*. Academic Press, Orlando.

Frankenberg, L. (1979) Cardiac puncture in the mouse through the anterior thoracic aperture. *Laboratory Animals*, **13** (311).

Freund, M. (1969) Inter-relationships among the characteristics of guinea pig semen collected by electro-ejaculation. *Journal of Reproduction and Fertility*, **19** (393).

Fullerton, F.R., Hunziher, J. and Bryant, P. (1981) Evaluation of a new rat feeder for use in chemical toxicology and nutrition studies. *Laboratory Animal Science*, **31** (276).

Gartner, K., Buttner, D., Dohler, R. et al. (1980) Stress response of rats to handling in experimental procedures. *Laboratory Animals*, **14** (207).

Gibson, J.E. and Becker, B.A. (1967) The administration of drugs to one-day-old animals. *Laboratory Animal Care*, **17** (524).

Grazer, F.M. (1958) Technique for intravascular injection and bleeding of newborn rats and mice. Proceedings of the Society for Experimental Biology and Medicine, **99** (407).

Grice, H.C. (1964) Methods of obtaining blood and for intravenous injections in laboratory animals. *Laboratory Animal Care*, **14** (483).

Gupta, B.N., Conner, G.H. and Langham, R.F. (1970) A device for collecting milk from guinea pigs. *American Journal of Veterinary Research*, **31** (557).

Haemisch A., Guerra G. and Fyrkert, J. (1999) Adaptation of corticosterone – but not βendorphin – secretion to repeated blood sampling in rats. *Laboratory Animals*, **33** (2): pp. 185–191.

Hammer, C.E. (1974) Semen examination. In: E.C. Melby Jr and N.H. Altman (Eds) *Handbook of Laboratory Animal Science*, Vol. 2. CRC Press, Cleveland, Ohio.

Hem, A., Smith, A.J. and Solberg, P. (1998) Saphenous vein puncture for blood sampling of the mouse, rat, hamster, gerbil, guinea pig, ferret and mink. *Laboratory Animals*, **32** (364).

van Herck, H. (1999) *Orbital puncture: A non-terminal blood sampling technique in rats*. PhD Thesis obtained from: Dr H. Van Herek. Kon. Juliana Straat 26, 4153 Bz Beesd, the Netherlands.

van Hoosier, Jr, G.L. and McPherson, C.W. (Eds) (1987) *Laboratory Hamsters*. Academic Press, Orlando.

Hull, R.M. (1995) Guideline limit volumes for dosing animals in pre-clinical stage of safety evaluation. *Human and Experimental Toxicology*, **14** (305).

Jemski, J.V. and Phillips, G.B. (1965) Aerosol challenge of animals. In: W.I. Gay (Ed.) *Methods of Animal Experimentation*, Vol. 1. Academic Press, New York.

Kaplan, A. and Wolf, I. (1972) A device for restraining and intravenous injection of mice. *Laboratory Animal Science*, **22** (223).

Kaplan, H.M. and Timmons, E.H. (1979) *The Rabbit: A Model for the Principles of Mammalian Physiology and Surgery*. Academic Press, New York.

Karlson, A.G. (1959) Intravenous injections in the guinea pig via veins of the penis. *Laboratory Investigation*, **8** (987).

Karlson, A.G. and Feldman, W.H. (1953) Methods of intravenous injections into guinea pigs. *Laboratory Investigation*, **2** (451).

Kirk, K.W., Latg, G.C., Fausto, G. and Arceijo, G. (1997) Customised rat restraint. *Laboratory Animals*, **36** (75).

Kurien, B.T. and Schofield, R.H. (1999) Mouse urine collection using clear plastic wrap. *Laboratory Animals*, **33** (83).

Kusumi, R.K. and Plouffe, J.E. (1979) A safe and simple technique for obtaining cerebrospinal fluid from rabbits. *Laboratory Animal Science*, **29** (681).

Lane, D.R. (1985) *Jones' Animal Nursing* (4th edn). Pergamon Press, Oxford.

Lax, E.R., Militzer, F. and Trauschel, A. (1983) A simple method of oral administration of drugs in solid form to fully conscious rats. *Laboratory Animals*, **17** (50).

Lewis, R.E., Kynz, A.L. and Bell, R.E. (1966) Error in intraperitoneal injection in the rat. *Laboratory Animal Care*, **16** (505).

Manning, P.J., Ringler, D.H. and Newcomer, C.E. (Eds) (1994) *The Biology of the Laboratory Rabbit* (2nd edn). Academic Press, San Diego.

Minasian, H. (1980) A simple tourniquet to aid mouse tail venepuncture. *Laboratory Animal*, **14** (205).

Moreland, A.F. (1965) Collection and infusion techniques. In: W.I. Gay (Ed.) *Methods of Animal Experimentation*, Vol. 1. Academic Press, New York.

Morrisey, R.E. and Norred, W.P. (1984) An improved method of diet preparation for toxicological feeding experiments. *Laboratory Animals*, **18** (271).

Mouza, G. and Weiss, J.B. (1960) A survival technique for obtaining large volumes of blood from rodents. *Journal of Clinical Pathology*, **13** (264).

National Research Council (1996) *Rodents* (Laboratory Animal Management Series). Pergamon, Washington, DC.

Nelson, W.L., Kaye, A., Morre, M. et al. (1951) Milking techniques and the composition of guinea pig milk. *Journal of Nutrition*, **44** (585).

Nobunga, T., Nakamura, K. and Imamichi, T. (1966) A method of intravenous injection and collection of blood from rats and mice without restraint and anaesthesia. *Laboratory Animal Care*, **16** (40).

Pansky, B., Jacobs, M., House, E.L. and Tassoni, J.P. (1961) The orbital region as a source of blood samples in the golden hamster. *Anatomical Record*, **139** (409).

Petty, C. (1982) *Research Techniques in the Rat*. C. C. Thomas, Springfield.

Phalen, R.F. (1984) *Inhalation Studies: Foundations and Techniques*. CRC Press, Cleveland, Ohio.

Poole, T. (ed.) (1999) *UFAW Handbook on the Care and Management of Laboratory Animals* (7th edn) Vol. 1. *Terrestrial Vertebrates*; Vol 2. *Amphibious and Aquatic Vertebrates and Advanced Vertebrates*. Blackwell Science, Oxford.

Postnikova, Z.A. (1960) A method of intracardiac injection in newborn rats and mice. *Folia Biologica* (Prague), **6** (59).

Reiber, H. and Schunch, O. (1983) Suboccipital puncture of guinea pigs. *Laboratory Animals*, **17** (25).

Rosenhaft, M.E., Bing, D.H. and Knudson, K.C. (1971) A vacuum-assisted method of repetitive blood sampling in guinea pigs. *Laboratory Animal Science*, **21** (598).

Ruckledge, G.J. and McKenzie, J.D. (1980) A new metabolism cage suitable for the study of mice. *Laboratory Animals*, **14** (213).

Smith, C.J. and McMahon, L.B. (1977) Methods of collecting blood from fetal and new born rats. *Laboratory Animal Science*, **27** (112).

Sorg, D.A. and Butcher, B.A. (1964) Simple method of obtaining venous blood from small laboratory animals. *Proceedings of the Society for Experimental Biology and Medicine*, **115** (1131).

Steffens, A.B. (1969) A method of frequent sampling of blood and continuous infusion of fluids in the rat without disturbing the animal. *Physiological Behaviour*, **4** (833).

Sundberg, D. and Hodgson, R.E. (1949) Aspiration of bone marrow in laboratory animals. *Blood*, **4** (557).

West, R.W., Stanley, J.W. and Newport, G.D. (1978) Single mouse urine collection and pH monitoring system. *Laboratory Animal Science*, **28** (343).

White, P.K. and Miller, S.A. (1975) Design of a metabolism cage for infant rats. *Laboratory Animal Science*, **25** (344).

Waynforth, H.B. (1969) Animal operative techniques. In: P.N. Campbell and J.R. Sargent (Eds) *Techniques in Protein Biosynthesis* Vol. 2. Academic Press, London.

Waynforth, H.B. (1995) General aspects of the administration of drugs and other substances. In: A.A. Tuffery (Ed.) *Laboratory Animals: An Introduction for Experimenters* (2nd edn). John Wiley & Sons, Chichester.

Waynforth, H.B. and Flecknell, P.A. (1992) *Experimental and Surgical Technique in the Rat* (2nd edn). Academic Press, London.

Wolfensohn, S. and Lloyd, M. (1998) *Handbook of Laboratory Animal Management and Welfare* (2nd edn). Blackwell Science, Oxford.

Zeller, W., Weber, H., Panoussis, B. et al. (1998) Refinement of blood sampling from the sublingual vein in rats. *Laboratory Animals*, **32** (369).

Dogs, cats and other species

Bennet, B.T., Abee, C.R. and Henrickson, R. (1995) *Non-human Primates in Biomedical Research. Biology and Management.* Academic Press, San Diego.

Conner, G.W., Gupta, B.N. and Krehbiel, J.D. (1971) A technique for bone marrow biopsy in the cat. *Journal of the American Veterinary Medical Association*, **158** (1702).

Flecknell, P.A. (1995) Non-surgical experimental procedures. In: A.A. Tuffery (Ed.) *Laboratory Animals: An Introduction for Experimenters* (2nd edn). John Wiley & Sons, Chichester.

Hall, A.S. and Knezavic, A.L. (1965) Bone marrow sampling in monkeys. *Journal of the American Veterinary Medical Association*, **147** (1075).

Horton, M.L., Harris, A.M., Van Stee, E.W. and Back, K.C. (1975) Versatile protective jacket for chronically instrumented dogs. *Laboratory Animal Science*, **25** (500).

Karl, A. and Kissen, A.T. (1978) Durable jackets for non-human primates to protect chronically implanted instrumentation. *Laboratory Animal Science*, **28** (103).

Lennox, M.S. and Taylor, K.G. (1983) A restraint chair for primates. *Laboratory Animals*, **17** (225).

Lin, S. and Chen, Y.W. (1997) A rapid and simple technique for serial or continuous collection blood samples and intravenous administration of drugs to conscious swine. *Laboratory Animal Science*, **36** (58).

Lloyd, M. (1999) *Ferrets. Health, Husbandry and Diseases*. Blackwell Science, Oxford.

Mann, W.A. and Kinter, L. (1993) Characterisation of maximal intravenous dose volumes in the dog (*canis familiaris*). *General Pharmacology*, **24** (357).

Metandos, K. and Franz, D.R. (1980) Collection of urine from caged laboratory cats. *Laboratory Animal Science*, **30** (562).

Muirhead, M.R. (1981) Blood sampling in pigs. *In Practice*, **3** (16).

National Research Council (1994) *Dogs* (Laboratory Animal Management Series). Academic Press, Washington DC.

Phillips, P.A., Newcomer, C.E. and Schultz, D.S. (1983) A technique of saliva collection in dogs. *Laboratory Animal Science*, **33** (465).

Poole, T. (Ed.) (1999) *UFAW Handbook on the Care and Management of Laboratory Animals* (7th edn) Vol. 1: *Terrestrial Vertebrates*; Vol. 2: *Amphibious and Aquatic Vertebrates and Advanced Vertebrates*. Blackwell Science, Oxford.

Pryce, C., Scott, L. and Schnell, C. (Eds) (1998) *Handbook: Marmosets and Tamarins in Biological and Biomedical Research*. DSSD Imagery, Salisbury.

Terris, J.M. and Simmonds, R.C. (1987) Description of a service metabolism unit for long term studies. *Laboratory Animal Science*, **32** (302).

Wolfensohn, S. and Lloyd, M. (1998) *Handbook of Laboratory Animal Management and Welfare* (2nd edn). Blackwell Science, Oxford.

General

Archer, R.K. and Jeffcott, L.B. (Eds) (1977) *Clinical Haematology*. Blackwell Science, Oxford.

Baggot, J.D. (1977) *Principles of Drug Disposition in Domestic Animals*. W.B. Saunders Co., Philadelphia.

Baker, R. (Ed.) (1980) *Controlled Release of Bioactive Materials*. Academic Press, New York.

Davidson, M., Else, R. and Lumsden, J. (1998) *Manual of Small Animal Clinical Pathology*. British Small Animal Veterinary Association, Cheltenham.

Goettsch, W., Garssen, J., De Gruijl, F.R. et al. (1999) Methods of exposure of laboratory animals to ultraviolet radiation. *Laboratory Animals*, **33** (58).

Hawk, C.T. and Leary, S.L. (1999) *Formulary for Laboratory Animals* (2nd edn). Iowa State University Press, Ames, (now Blackwell Publishing).

HMSO (1974) *Health and Safety at Work etc. Act*. HMSO, London.

Kaplan, S.A. (1973) Biopharmaceuticals in pre-formulation stages of drug development. In: J. Swarbrick (Ed.) *Dosage Form Design and Bioavailability*. Lea & Febiger, Philadelphia.

McGuill, M.W. and Rowan, A.N. (1987) Biological effects of blood loss: implications for sampling volumes and techniques. *Institute of Laboratory Animal Resources*, **31** (5).

Milruka, B.M. and Rawnsley, H.M. (1981) *Clinical, Biochemical and Haematological Reference Values in Normal Animals and Normal Humans* (2nd edn). Manson Publishing USA Inc, New York.

Schermer, S. (1965) *The Blood Morphology of Laboratory Animals* (3rd edn). F.A. Davis Co., Philadelphia.

Schurr, P.E. (1969) Composition and preparation of intravenous fat emulsions. *Cancer Research*, **29** (258).

Woodard, G. (1965) Principles of drug administration. In: W.I. Gay (Ed.) *Methods of Animal Experimentation*, Vol. 1. Academic Press, New York.

Videos

The following videos were prepared by the Institute of Technology:

Handle with Care; *Procedures with Care*; *Farm Animals with Care* – Vols 1 and 2.

These videos can be obtained from:

Mr C. Chambers, University of Bristol, Department of Clinical Veterinary Science, Langford House, Langford, Bristol, BS18 7DU, UK.

39

An Introduction to Telemetry in Laboratory Animals

Jeremy N. Smith and Victoria L. Savage
© Crown Copyright Dstl, 2004

Introduction

Data capture options from living animals have been greatly advanced by the continued development and use of remote monitoring methods. Electronic systems which allow information to be gleaned from the animal without it having to leave its home environment, or be affected by the researcher's physical presence, are a significant refinement of research techniques – traditional methods relied upon chemical restraint. The main method of choice in remote monitoring methods employed over the past twenty-five years has included the use of video cameras to record both individual animal behaviour and the dynamic interactions of groups. Video footage taken remotely still remains an excellent way of analysing learned or spontaneous behaviour. It can be replayed at any time, and acts as a powerful adjunct to the data gleaned by other methods.

The remote measurement of physiological parameters is currently achieved via thermometry transponders installed within the animal, often subcutaneously, or via data logging or radio transmitter devices, which may be either implanted within the animal or fitted externally. Utilisation of all of these methods must be by trained and qualified personnel, as they could have the potential to cause harm or distress to the animal, both in the short term and in the future, if incorrectly placed. A full cost/benefit analysis has to be made to assess the value of the data derived against the costs to the animals, particularly as implantable methods are invasive. The specialist techniques required to perform the surgery associated with the implantation of recording or transmitting devices must be learned from those who have extensive previous experience (Hawkins et al. 2004). The use of all these methods of capturing data remotely is generally referred to as telemetry.

Areas within which telemetry is used

Telemetry is used to measure a range of physiological functions, including:

- blood pressure (BP);
- heart rate (HR);
- core body temperature (CBT);
- surface body temperature (SBT);
- electrocardiogram (ECG);
- motor activity (MA);
- blood flow in specific vessels (BF);
- electroencephalogram (EEG);
- intra-ocular pressure (IOP).

Data logging

Data logging devices worn externally on animals such as marmosets, allow individuals to be monitored within a given group. The small device is worn around the neck of each animal by the aid of a small chain which contains a piezoelectric accelerometer and a 16 kb memory chip. The Actiwatch™ (Cambridge Neurotechnology®, Cambridge, UK) as used by Mann et al. (2001) is capable of recording all types of movement in all directions. The battery life varies depending on the duration of each pre-set measurement of movement, and may last up to thirty days. At the end of a particular recording period the data is downloaded to a PC for final analysis and interpretation.

Transmission devices

Radio transmitters may be worn on the animal via special back-packs or jackets, or installed either subcutaneously or within the abdominal cavity and attached to certain tissues via aseptic surgery. The transmitter, battery and electronics are enclosed within a sealed biocompatible plastic case designed to minimise disruption to the tissues and organs of the animal. Two types of transmitter measure either pressure (Figure 39.1), or electrical activity (Figure 39.2). The electrode wires emanate from the transmitter unit and may either be glued or stitched to specific tissues of interest. Each area to be measured has two wires attached, so multiple readings require more pairs of wires to achieve this. More than

one physiological parameter may be measured at any one time, but both this and greater transmission distances result in larger transmitters. Once the transmitter has been programmed and installed, it is able to transmit real-time data to the receiver(s) which are strategically placed around the cage at a distance which must always be within range.

The care and welfare of animals in studies

Animals chosen for telemetry studies must be of the highest quality and best health standards. Only the most appropriate subjects are chosen and those with a poor temperament should be deselected. If necessary, close liaison with the breeding establishment should be made to ensure that the husbandry practices of both institutes are comparable. All newly arrived animals should be allowed sufficient time to recover from their journey and to habituate to their new environment. Animals should always be pair or group housed as part of best practice principles, but the current limitations of implantable telemetry devices make simultaneous transmission impossible.

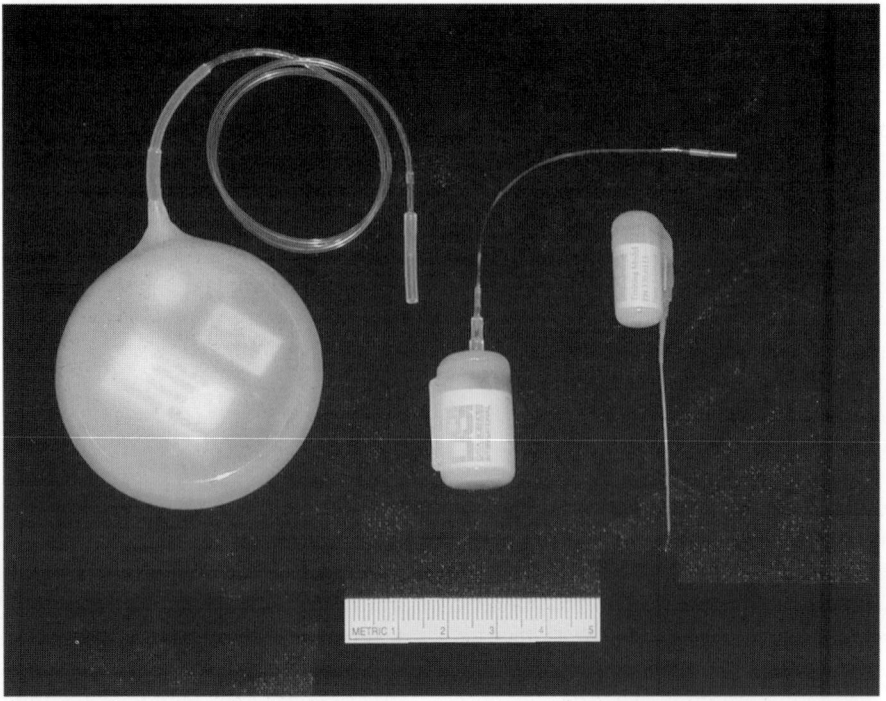

Figure 39.1   Telemetry devices (from left to right) that are implanted within: a dog, a rat and a mouse (Data Sciences®).

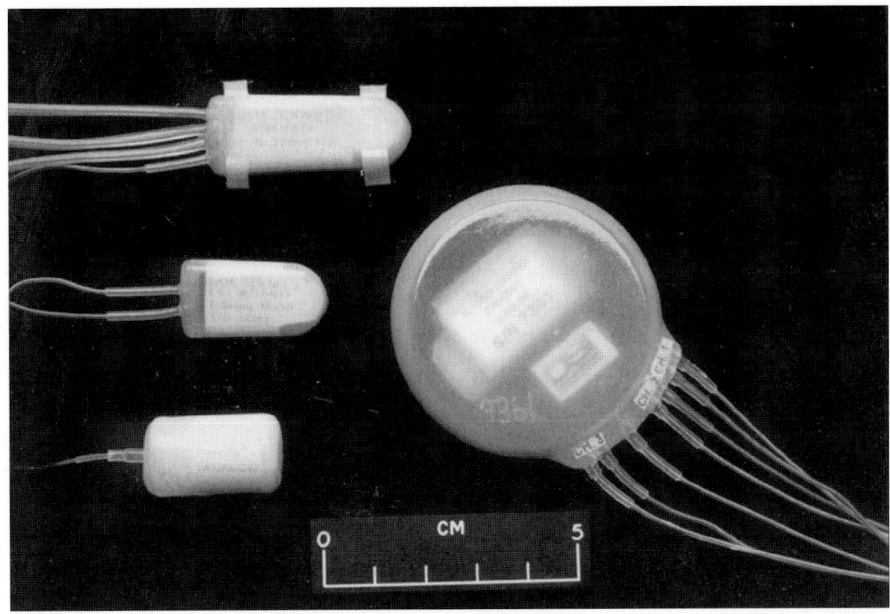

Figure 39.2   Top left: 3 channel device suitable for EGG; middle: 1 channel device suitable for EMG & GI movements; bottom right: 3 channel device suitable for EEG in pharmacology, seizure and sleep studies (Data Sciences®).

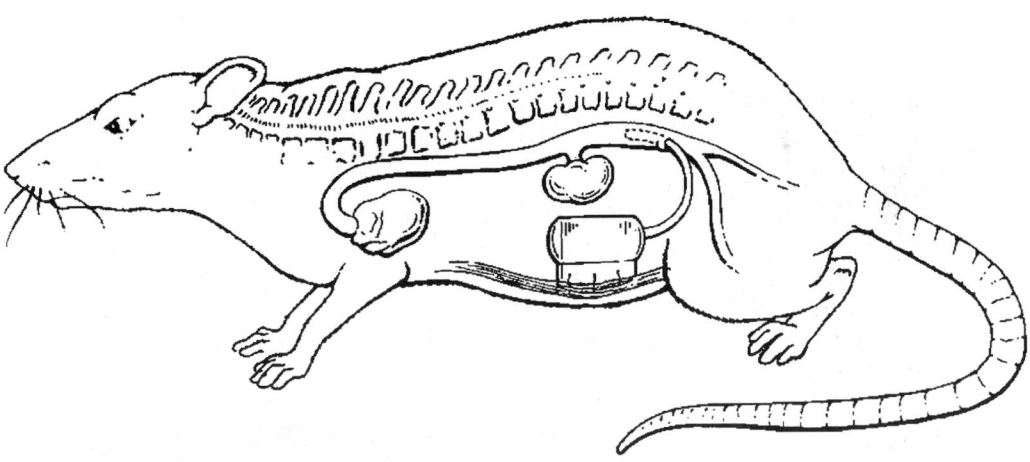

Figure 39.3   Telemetry implantation within the rat recording from the abdominal aorta.

Most implantable telemetry systems operate on the same frequency so data transmission has to be staggered from pair- or group-housed animals.

Before implanting any device, careful consideration must be made to its size, shape and the location it is to be put (Figure 39.3). It is crucial that the animal may conduct a full behavioural repertoire without interference or discomfort. A device that is either too large, badly positioned or the wrong shape, could interfere with the correct function of internal organs, connective tissues or blood vessels.

Experimental design, surgical protocols, antibiotic and analgesic treatments are made in conjunction with a veterinary surgeon and research workers very experienced in telemetry techniques, in accord with best practice principles. The designated facilities within which the surgery is to be conducted must be clean, fit for purpose and must include areas for both pre- and post-operative care. Surgery is conducted under strict asepsis and all animals are closely monitored throughout each stage, until they have regained consciousness and are placed within a recovery or home cage. Recovery periods will vary depending on the species being used and the degree of anaesthesia and surgery that they have experienced. Close observations are made throughout the study to ensure that implantations are functioning correctly and do not cause the animal any unnecessary problems.

Battery life and duration of studies

The timing of when data is taken and transmitted will allow the battery life to be preserved for longer. In addition, devices may be repeatedly turned on or off by passing a magnet over the animal close to the implantation site. Good experimental design and sound knowledge of the particular species will enable data sets to be taken at the optimum times thereby allowing batteries to last for six months or more. At the end of a particular study the telemetry device can be removed and sent back to the manufacturers to

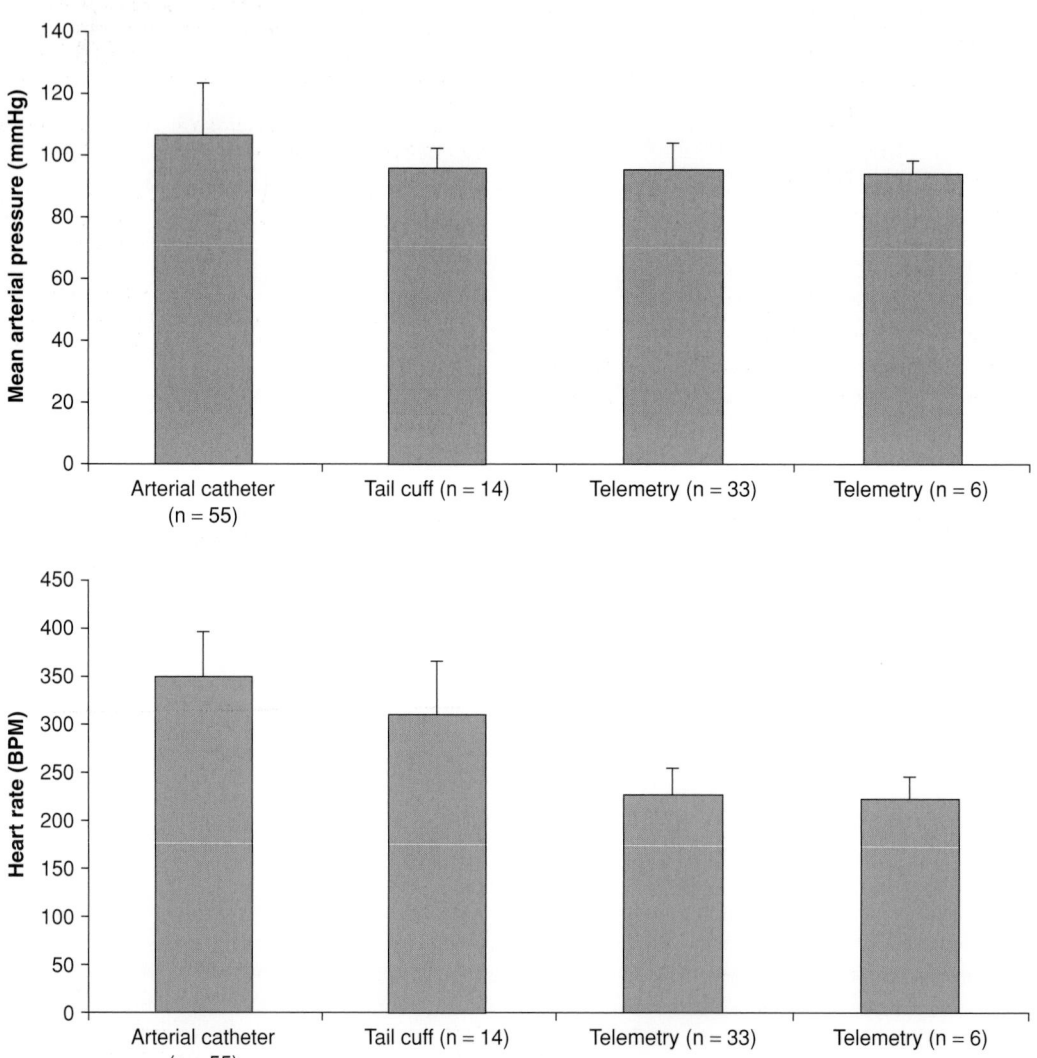

Figure 39.4   Graphs to show arterial blood pressure and heart rate of conscious marmosets using four different means of measurement: 1. Arterial catheter plus physical restraint; 2. Tail cuff plus physical restraint; 3. Telemetry plus physical restraint; 4. Telemetry plus no restraint (Schnell & Wood 1993, dstl; personal communication, P. Pearce 2004).

have its battery replaced. The system is then sterilised, re-packaged and returned for further use.

Benefits of telemetry to good animal welfare

The two graphs show the clear benefits of telemetry as an accurate method of real-time heart and blood pressure data capture in the marmoset (Figure 39.4). The lowered blood pressure and heart rate using telemetry in free-moving animals strongly suggests that it causes the animal less discomfort and is therefore an important refinement technique (Schnell & Wood 1993). Distanced data capture of this type allows the researcher to gather data which is less influenced by the variables associated with more traditional techniques. Telemetry allows us a greater understanding of animal behaviour, which Russell and Burch (1959) identified as providing a new dimension of experimental control. They went on to say that within the study of animal behaviour lie the richest prospects of reduction (Russell & Birch 1959). With this increasing body of knowledge, animal care staff are able to bring the best practices in husbandry to their animals, thereby enhancing the animals' welfare through improved environments.

Ways forward and new equipment

The manufacturers of telemetry equipment are planning to make smaller devices for rodents which have improved contours and profiles, especially for subcutaneous installations. It is also planned to provide multiple-channel transmitters for use in rodents, with improved transmitting distances. In addition to the improved data capture options, experimental design will allow animals to be kept in experimental groups reducing the need to house them individually while on test.

References

Hawkins, P. et al. (2004) *Husbandry refinement for rats, mice, dogs and non-human primates used in telemetry procedures.* Seventh report of the BVAAWF/FRAME/RSPCA/UFAW Joint Working Group on Refinement, Part B. *Laboratory Animals*, Vol. 38 (1): 1–10.

Mann, T., Williams, K.E., Pearce, P.E. and Scott, E.A.M. (2001) Actimetry for marmosets. *Journal of Psycho. Pharmacology*, **Suppl. 15** (A64).

Russell, W.M.S. and Burch, R.L. (1959) *The Principles of Humane Experimental Technique* (pp. 105–133). In: Universities Federation for Animal Welfare (UFAW), Special Edition (1992).

Schnell, C.R. and Wood, J.M. (1993) Measurements of blood pressure and heart rate by telemetry in conscious, unrestrained marmosets. *Am. J. Physiol. (Heart & Circ. Physiol.)*, **264** (33): H1509–H1516.

Further reading

Morton, D.B., Hawkins, P., Bevan, R. et al. (2003). *Refinements in telemetry procedures.* Seventh report of the BVAAWF/FRAME/RSPCA/UFAW Joint Working Group on Refinement, Part A. *Laboratory Animals*, 37: 261–299.

40

Surgical Techniques

Bryan Waynforth

Introduction

The basic principles observed for surgery of all experimental animals are the same as that for human beings. The two main considerations are that surgery is carried out skilfully and that it is performed using aseptic technique. The use of aseptic technique for small animals such as mice and rats has been controversial, with earlier suggestions that asepsis was unnecessary, based on ideas that such animals were resistant to infection. The work of Bradfield et al. (1992) contradicts this and, together with the recommendations in the *Guidance on the Operation of the Animals (Scientific Procedures) Act 1986* (Home Office 2000), these make it very clear that rodent surgery must be carried out aseptically.

Procedures to be carried out before surgery

Planning

Since most experimental surgery is carried out by people who are relatively inexperienced in surgery, the surgical protocol should be planned in detail to ensure that surgery is carried out in a confident and competent manner. This will produce a better surgically prepared animal and as a consequence a better experimental outcome. Until sufficient experience is gained, the novice should prepare a checklist of requirements before undertaking a surgical procedure. This would include the animals to be used, facilities and accommodation required, instruments and apparatus needed, the appropriate anaesthetic schedule to be used, the drugs, antiseptics and other chemicals required, any assistance needed and an outline of the surgical technique and procedure,

which must include the pre- and post-operative care that will be necessary. Such a checklist helps in focusing attention precisely on what is to be done, as well as keeping anyone who is assisting informed.

Time of surgery

Operations should always be carried out so that the animal has recovered before staff go home. It follows that such operations should not be done late in the day or at the end of the week. However, this would not necessarily apply to simple procedures using short-acting anaesthetic management techniques where animals are up and about very shortly after the completion of surgery and will require little monitoring thereafter. If animals have not recovered before the end of the day, provision must be made for post-operative care to continue into the evening and night period, as necessary. This applies as much to a mouse as to a dog for example, and must be mandatory.

Practice

An operative procedure which is new to the investigator, whether a novice or a fully trained surgeon, should first be practised on a freshly killed animal. Although dead animals do not show the effects of respiratory movements, tissue tension and copious bleeding, practice will alert the surgeon to problems which might be encountered.

Before practising, or carrying out the surgery, as much information as possible on such things as the anatomy and physiology of the animal, as well as how to carry out the procedure must be obtained. This will help in locating precisely and quickly the anatomical area of the surgical intervention and also help in avoiding unnecessary manipulation of tissues which could result in unwanted bleeding, nerve and other tissue damage. The best way to obtain this information is first to discuss the surgery with the named veterinary surgeon (NVS). This is an indispensable step, as the NVS will have general, if not specific knowledge of the surgery and will be able to advise on a suitable course of action. Secondly, try to find a colleague who has first-hand experience in the technique and is willing to tutor the investigator. This can save hours of effort and result in better, easier surgery. Failing these, the relevant literature must be consulted. It should be noted that many specialist techniques appear in individual scientific papers rather than in text books and the appropriate search must be conducted.

Adaptation of animals to their surroundings

Animals which need to be transported to the operating area, whether from room to room or from an external supplier, will be stressed. There is evidence of the occurrence of widespread physiological disturbances even when moving animals a short distance, and these take a variable time to return to normal. This will probably be of little consequence in room-to room movement, but animals brought in from outside will be affected by unfamiliar food, staff, husbandry practices and surroundings, in addition to the effects of transport by air, sea or land.

Stressed animals make poor experimental and surgical subjects. It should therefore be routine practice to allow a period of acclimatisation so that the animals can adapt to their new surroundings and have their anxiety allayed by regular contact with the staff. The length of this period will vary with the species and the degree of distress. It may be a few hours for room-to-room movement, days for rats and mice brought in from outside and several months for primates brought into the laboratory from the wild. There are few hard and fast rules and experience and common sense need to be applied. There are often local rules in the animal facility which should be followed.

It seems to be common practice in some cases to disregard the need for acclimatisation for animals destined for non-recovery experiments. Since such animals do not differ from others in the degree of distress and physiological disturbance that they initially experience, this practice must be discouraged on the grounds that the validity of some experimental results could be questioned.

Good management of animal facilities requires that animals brought into an establishment from external sources should undergo a period of quarantine so that any hidden tendency to clinical disease is exposed. Acclimatisation for surgery can therefore be considered as an extension of what, in other circumstances, is epitomised as good laboratory animal practice.

Keeping records

Accurate detailed records of pre-operative, operative and post-operative procedures on individual animals are invaluable in evaluating the course and outcome of an investigation. It also allows precise repetition of the procedure if required at some future date.

With large animals it is common practice to keep such detailed information. For small animals however, this information, if it is kept at all, tends to be collected for groups rather than individuals. There are several reasons for this, most without just cause, but since it results in a considerable loss of possibly valuable data, keeping individual records on these small animals is to be recommended and should be seriously considered. A clinical file for each animal should be opened as soon as the animal is designated for surgery. Initially, personal details such as breed, strain, substrain, colour, sex, body weight, age, source of acquisition and method of identification should be written up. Further entries can then be made as circumstances demand.

Clinical examination

It is usual to give large animals an examination when they are first brought into an animal establishment. Ideally, a full examination by a veterinary surgeon should be performed if possible. Failing this, a good idea of the animal's condition can be gained by a simple check of its behaviour and of the skin, eyes, ears, nose, mouth, feet, tail and other external surfaces. Signs of diarrhoea and abnormal urinary function may indicate an underlying disease condition and careful observation must be made subsequently External and internal parasites, superficial bruising and cuts can usually be easily treated but more serious signs of disease will require consultation with a veterinary surgeon.

Small animals should be acquired, whenever possible, from reliable sources or accredited dealers which are known to have a good health record. Only a very superficial examination is then required. Any animals showing signs of diarrhoea, respiratory disease or other abnormality should be isolated for observation or humanely killed. Immediately before surgery, a second clinical examination should be given to ensure the animal's suitability for the operation.

Some investigators insist on a detailed examination for large animals including clinical chemistry and haematology. This will reveal abnormalities of a serious nature affecting such organ systems as the heart, lungs, liver and kidney and such a thorough examination may be crucial to the investigation. Where the facilities for such an examination are not available or the investigation or species (e.g. rodent) does not normally require it, the animal should nevertheless be shown to be overtly healthy. For large animals, it may be necessary to bath the animal if its skin or fur is soiled. The results of clinical examinations should be written up in the animal's file.

Food and water

Withholding food from at least the night before the operation and for up to twenty-four hours is recommended for large animals. This reduces the risk of regurgitation of stomach contents during the induction of anaesthesia and the potentially lethal effect of entry of vomit into the lungs. The stomach of herbivorous animals such as sheep and cattle will not be empty even after twenty-four hours and they therefore require careful management. It is rarely necessary to withhold food from rodents, rabbits, birds or other small animals but a check should be made that no food pellets are present in the mouth before anaesthesia is administered. If the particular operative procedure requires fasting then this should be for no longer than overnight and for the mouse no longer than four or five hours because of its high metabolic activity. Recently, evidence has been produced that a rat's stomach is virtually empty of food by about six hours after the animal has been fed and that fasting an animal overnight is detrimental to its welfare and therefore unnecessary (see References and further reading, p. 380). Generally, there is no

need to withhold water from animals, which should come to surgery fully hydrated.

Premedication

Tranquillisers

Animals which are usually nervous or just difficult to handle can be given a tranquilliser such as diazepam or xylazine to calm them. The routine use of tranquillisers as part of the anaesthetic regimen is invariably recommended for large animals. Apart from enabling a smaller amount of anaesthetic to be administered, tranquillisers allow a much smoother induction of and recovery from anaesthesia (see Chapter 41).

Atropine

Excessive salivation due to the effect of the anaesthetic can be a problem in all animals. This can usually be reduced or inhibited by the use of atropine sulphate given at the appropriate dose, fifteen to thirty minutes before the induction of anaesthesia. Atropine is contraindicated for certain species such as sheep, goats and cattle.

Antibiotics

If good surgical technique is used it is unnecessary to give antibiotics to combat possible surgical infection in the majority of cases. In fact inappropriate use of antibiotics can defeat a good but uninformed intention by allowing resistant bacteria to emerge and possibly cause a fatal outcome! If antibiotics are required by the protocol, where, for instance, the operation may allow faecal contents to contaminate the body or if a long, bloody operation is envisaged, then the treatment should be a short one.

Two types of treatment are appropriate. A high dose of antibiotic can be injected just before surgery is to begin, or during surgery if the operation is of relatively short duration. This allows peak levels to build up in the circulation at the time that any major infection of the wound is likely to occur. Antibiotics given at the end of a long operation, of about four hours duration or longer, may be ineffective. The second schedule which can be used, especially for long operations, is to give the antibiotic as a split dose, before, during and immediately after the operation. Further administration of antibiotics should not be given. However, an infection contracted pre- or post-operatively and not as a result of the surgery, should be treated with daily antibiotics for a full course, usually of five to seven days.

The choice of antibiotic is best determined by testing the sensitivity of the pathogenic organism involved in an infection, to a panel of antibiotics. Failing this, treatment can be given with a broad-spectrum antibiotic. It should be remembered that some animals react adversely to some antibiotics and the outcome may even be fatal (e.g. penicillin given to conventionally maintained guinea pigs).

The operating area

This can vary from a purpose-built surgical suite to a specially prepared space on a laboratory bench. The latter is suitable only for minor procedures and a room(s) set aside only for performing surgery should be seriously considered. Moreover, if only a single room is available, it should be divided into two areas. One will be 'dirty' and used to prepare and anaesthetise the animal and the other will be 'clean' and used for clothing the surgeon and performing the surgery. All surfaces should be kept clean and preferably wiped over with a detergent/disinfectant to reduce contamination with dust and micro-organisms.

The minimum amount of apparatus should be kept in such rooms though the nature of some forms of experimentation which require bulky equipment sometimes makes this difficult. All such apparatus and any room fittings should be wiped clean regularly.

Equipment for surgery

Instruments

There are certain specialist instruments for veterinary surgery, but in general the instruments used are those available for human surgery. For small animals, these are mainly selected from instruments used in paediatric, ophthalmic and neurosurgery. For large animals, veterinary textbooks describe the instruments which are appropriate for different types of operations. For small animals a basic set used on the majority of occasions comprising a pair of blunt-ended Mayo scissors, a pair of pointed dressing scissors, three pairs of curved or straight forceps, one with rat-toothed tips and the other two with serrated ends, and a skin-clip applicator and forceps, or an automatic stapling device. Specialised instruments will be required in addition for some operations.

In many instances ingenuity is required to fashion home-made instruments, unobtainable elsewhere, for experimental work in both large and small animals. Where instruments are required sterile this is achieved most usually by steam autoclave under pressure. This can be simply done using a domestic pressure cooker at 15 lbs/sq. in. for at least fifteen minutes, or by using a purpose-built autoclave. It is important to allow the steam to come into contact with the instrument for sterilisation to occur. The method of packaging instruments and accessories for autoclaving and for their presentation for aseptic surgery is described in standard textbooks (see References and further reading, p. 380). Alternatively metal and glass instruments can be heated to 160 °C for one hour, in a hot-air oven, to achieve sterilisation but sharp instruments may be blunted to a small degree by this method. Chemical methods are also available to procure complete sterilisation (e.g. ethylene oxide vapour) but their use is specialised. Clean rather than sterile instruments may have to be used for small animal surgery where sterilising apparatus is unavailable. In this case, these can best be prepared by boiling in water for at least ten minutes. Alternatively, instruments can be placed in a disinfectant for at least thirty minutes. Disinfectants such as 70% ethyl or isopropyl alcohol, 0.5% aqueous chlorhexidine or 0.1% aqueous banzalkonium chloride are often used. Both boiling and chemical treatment kill bacteria but not bacterial spores and therefore some potential for producing infection is retained.

Apparatus

These are usually difficult or impossible to sterilise by steam or heat, both of which could cause damage. In such cases, a disinfectant wiped over the surface will achieve a reasonable degree of cleanliness. Some plastics, e.g. PVC cannulae and syringes can only be sterilised satisfactorily by irradiation or by exposure to the vapour of ethylene oxide. However, soaking a plastic cannula in an appropriate disinfectant may suffice in some cases to enable it to be inserted into a body cavity, for example, and minimise the possibility of infection. However, this is not recommended as a routine procedure and should only be carried out if no better sterilising method is readily available. Plastic instruments and apparatus such as hypodermic needles, as well as some metal components, are generally obtainable ready packaged and sterilised.

The operating table

Special veterinary tables are available for use with large animals (Figure 40.1). They can also be used as a flat surface for small animals but tables specifically for small animals are available commercially and are generally to be preferred. For simple operations, a cork or rubber-covered wooden board may suffice but particular care should be taken to keep these clean and disinfected and a sterile drape should be placed over them during surgery. Extremely useful accessories in the form of various retractors, tooth and leg holders and other accessories are very worthwhile but availability is limited.

Lighting

In simple cases, in small animal surgery, an anglepoise lamp with a 100 w bulb may be enough. However, good lighting is essential if mistakes are not to be made and a portable cold-illuminating light system which gives high intensity diffuse or pin-point light is relatively inexpensive and to be preferred. The ideal attainment, essential in a purpose-built surgical suite,

is a proper operating light which can be fitted even in very small areas.

Other accessories

Many accessories may be required for surgery. Their precise nature will depend on the form of the operation. Such accessories include drapes or towels prepared from paper, plastic or cotton, swabs, cotton wool, bandages and adhesive tape. These can be sterilised, or disinfected, or cleansed by appropriate methods as necessary.

Aseptic technique

This can be defined as removal of micro-organisms (antisepsis) followed by measures aimed at preventing contamination or re-contamination. Full asepsis is the objective of all surgery on large animals (cats, dogs, sheep, goats, pigs, cattle and horses) but for small animals such as rodents, birds, reptiles and amphibia the type of surgery that is often carried out, particularly sequential surgery on a batch of animals,

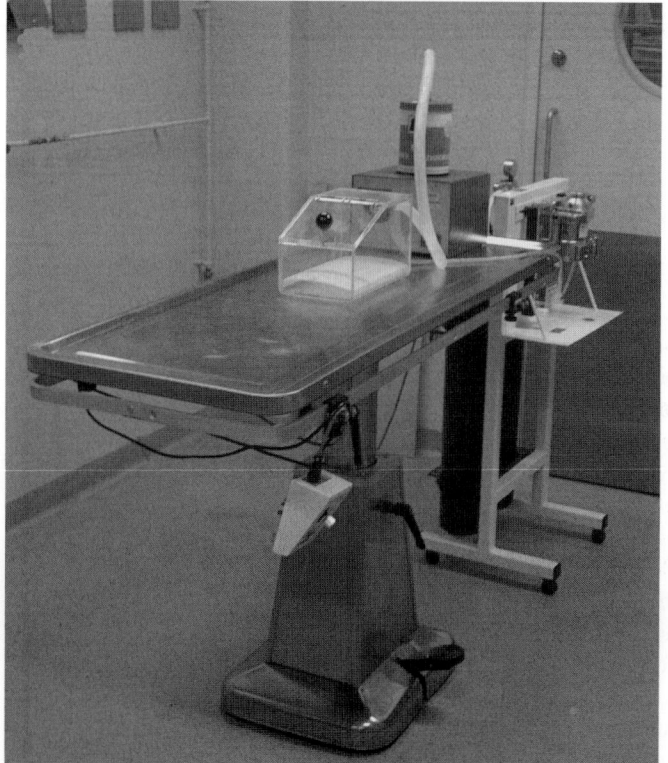

Figure 40.1 Operating table with anaesthetic apparatus.

may make the attainment of full asepsis difficult. Nevertheless, it should be attempted at all times.

Preparation of the surgical site

For large animals, hair, if present, must be removed with clippers. Further removal if required can be carried out by shaving, but care must be taken not to cut or abrade the skin. The skin is then washed with a germicidal detergent such as 3% aqueous hexachlorophene or 1% aqueous cetrimide and rinsed and dried with a paper towel. An antiseptic is then applied generously with a gauze sponge, starting along the incision site and working outwards for a reasonable distance. Antiseptics in common use are 0.5% chlorhexidine in 70% alcohol, 0.1% aqueous benzalkonium chloride, tincture of iodine containing 2.5% iodine and potassium iodide in 90% alcohol, and 10% aqueous or alcoholic providone-iodine. The latter is popular since unlike iodine it is non-irritant and non-staining. It is also highly effective against bacteria, viruses and fungal organisms. Following the application of antiseptic, sterile drapes are attached to the skin with skin clips so that only the incision site and a small area around it is exposed, while most of the body is covered. This helps to reduce contamination of the wound from bacteria residing deep within the skin of the surrounding area which are not affected by the surface application of antiseptic solutions. This also implies that the term 'asepsis' is relative, since in reality all surgical wounds become contaminated to at least a small degree by deep-seated bacteria exposed at the edges of the wound created by the incision. Drapes are also useful for maintaining instruments placed on them in a sterile condition.

Removal of hair, fur and feathers should also be carried out as appropriate, in rodents, rabbits and other small animals. Care must be taken to avoid getting hair into the wound where it may cause irritation and delay wound healing. An antiseptic is applied by liberally dousing the surgical area and wiping off the excess with sterile gauze. Antiseptics generally used are those already mentioned. In addition 70% ethyl or isopropyl alcohol can also be used alone. However, when the alcohol has evaporated, the skin is no longer protected and alcohol alone should therefore be used only for short operations.

The use of drapes is now normal practice in all species, however small. Drapes can be made from paper or cloth, appropriately sterilised, and with a small opening cut into the drape which is aligned with the surgical area. As already pointed out, the drape allows sterile instruments to be placed on it during surgery, which are therefore maintained as sterile throughout.

Preparation of the surgeon and assistants

Where full aseptic technique is being used, it is necessary for the surgeon to wear a gown and surgical gloves, both of which must be prepared sterile by appropriate means. Gloves normally come sterile and ready packaged with a supply of lubricant talcum powder to ease entry of the hands into the gloves. In addition, a non-sterile but clean face-mask and head covering must be worn to prevent spread of micro-organisms from these sources. Clean boots or overshoes can be worn if desired. Assistants who are involved in the technical aspects of the surgery or who need to handle sterile instruments must be prepared in a similar way to the surgeon.

Where less than full aseptic technique is being used, the wearing of clean gowns, mask, head coverings and sterile gloves can be at the discretion of the surgeon but it is a matter of good hygiene to wear at least a clean gown or laboratory coat and sterile gloves. At all times hands and forearms should be washed and this sequence is of particular importance if carrying out aseptic procedures.

Procedures required to be carried out during surgery

Surgical routine

Aseptic technique must be continued during surgery. Ideally, the antiseptic preparation of the skin site and the induction of anaesthesia should be carried out in a separate room preferably adjoining the surgical theatre. When this is done, the animal is transferred to the surgical table. Meanwhile, the surgeon and assistants prepare themselves for the operation. If assistants are available they unwrap the instrument packs, taking care not to touch the contents. The surgeon then places the sterile drapes on the animal, just before which he may want to apply another coat of antiseptic. The incision is made and the operation gets under way. In most surgical procedures, the

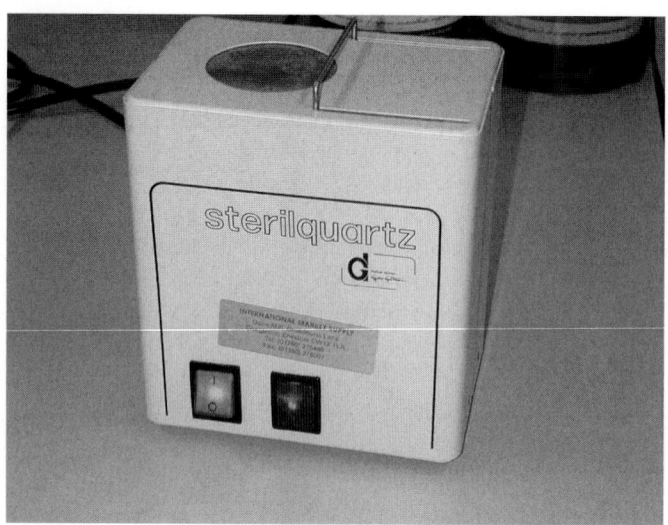

Figure 40.2 Hot bead steriliser.

hands are used as very effective 'blunt instruments' which can separate tissues and organs gently. In certain specialised operations (e.g. in orthopaedic surgery) at no time is the operation area touched by the surgeon's hands, all procedures being carried out by the use of sterile instruments only. This is called a 'no-touch' technique and is an attempt to achieve a minimal amount of bacterial contamination. During the operation the instruments should be kept on a clean paper or cotton towel or placed on the drapes. In practice, for small animals, the same set of instruments may be used to operate sequentially on a large number or batch of animals. However, it is very important to keep the tips of the instruments sterile and this is most conveniently achieved by use of a hot bead steriliser (Figure 40.2). Two sets of instruments used alternately, allows batch surgery to be carried out most effectively using this type of sterilisation method.

The surgery itself will proceed smoothly only if the surgeon is skilled, competent and well prepared. There are often many pitfalls of which the surgeon needs to be knowledgeable.

Temperature

Animals undergoing surgery lose heat by evaporation of tissue fluid and inhalation of anaesthetic which cools surfaces. Since the metabolic activity of an anaesthetised animal is reduced and heat loss further compromises it, the animal is unable to counteract the loss of heat effectively. Since loss of heat can jeopardise surgery, heat must be supplied to maintain normal body temperature. A mouse for example can, in certain cases, have its body temperature reduced by several degrees within ten minutes from the start of the operation, and this therefore has the potential to seriously compromise it. The smaller the animal, the greater is the rate of the heat loss. Heat can be supplied by a heating blanket placed under the animal or by a lamp placed above it or by increasing the room temperature. Some small animal operating tables have a heating facility incorporated in them. During the operation it is useful to monitor the body temperature, several devices, some very sophisticated, are available to do this. In many cases, a simple oral thermometer placed in the rectum will suffice.

Fluid balance

Animals lose substantial amounts of fluid and minerals during surgery by evaporation of tissue fluid, loss of blood and during respiration. Dehydration puts the animal at risk and fluid must be replaced in operations of more than short duration. Fluid balance is a complex matter and advice may have to be sought from a veterinary surgeon. As an interim measure, particularly for small animals, physiological saline or a 4% dextrose/0.18% saline solution can be administered at a rate of 4% of body weight per twenty-four hours. Continuous i.v. infusion is commonplace for large animals but fluids can be given by any other route, the s.c. and i.p. routes are more easily managed in small animals.

Bleeding

Excessive loss of blood will induce shock. Bleeding will also obscure the surgical area making surgery difficult. Blood loss must therefore be minimised by practising good surgery and haemostatic technique. Bleeding can be stopped by several methods including manual pressure, clamping with haemostatic forceps, ligation and electrocautery. Any surplus blood and blood clots must be removed since these provide an ideal growth medium for bacteria.

Trauma

Bad surgical technique, such as excessive retraction of tissues and inexpert handling of instruments, results in tissue damage and necrosis. This delays wound healing and necrotic tissue provides nutrient for the multiplication of bacteria with consequent infection. Tissue trauma is also a significant cause of postoperative pain. It is important therefore that tissues are handled gently, and that blunt dissection is carried out as much as possible, using correct instruments or hands and fingers, unless contraindicated. If necrotic or damaged tissue is encountered, such as in infected wounds, it must be cut away so that only healthy tissue remains.

Monitoring

Anaesthesia must be continued satisfactorily during surgery. Monitoring the heat rate, blood pressure and rate of respiration are means of ensuring that the correct plane of anaesthesia is being maintained. Equipment, generally of a sophisticated nature is available to perform these and other monitoring functions (see Chapter 41). Although they find most use with large animals, they can successfully be adapted for rodents, rabbits and birds. However, they do require a thorough knowledge of how they work and are applied and of how to interpret the results, training in their use is therefore advisable. It may be much better to employ a veterinary technician or surgeon to assist, if available.

Wound health

During surgery, tissues must not be allowed to dry and it will sometimes be necessary to apply warm saline or proprietary compounds to prevent this. This will include the eyes. At the completion of the operation all foreign material, such as swabs, must be removed as well as blood clots and damaged tissue. Sometimes it may be necessary to wash out or irrigate a body cavity such as the peritoneal cavity and this can be done with 0.01% aqueous chlorhexidine or 10% aqueous providone-iodine both of which at these concentrations are relatively non-irritant. In addition, they have some germicidal activity. If an antibiotic is to be placed in the wound, it is preferable to give it as a solution rather than as a powder, which will cake and its absorption will then be delayed.

Wound closure

Suturing together the edges of a wound is an art which is achieved properly only after practice. There are a number of components to consider.

Apposition of wound edges
When closing a wound it is necessary to bring the two edges together properly. How they are brought together will depend on the type of tissue. When joining components of the intestine for example, the outer surfaces should come together with the wound edges being inverted. For skin, the inside of wound edges should be apposed resulting in their slight eversion. Incorrect apposition could result in delayed wound healing or even a failure to heal.

Needles
These come in a variety of sizes and in various semi-circular forms or are straight. They are generally round bodied when they are used for soft tissues such as muscle, and triangular or cutting when they are required to pierce through tissue such as skin. Semi-circular needles require to be applied with a needle holder, which needs practice. If a needle has an eye it will have to be threaded manually, but many needles are bonded to the thread, this reduces the bulk of thread which has to pass through the tissue. Bonded needles are often described as atraumatic needles (Figure 40.3).

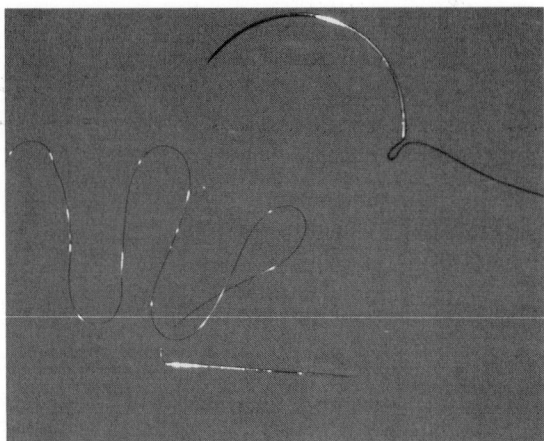

Figure 40.3   Straight and curved bonded needles.

Thread

Suture thread comes in different thicknesses and lengths and is usually coded from 11/0 or higher, which is the finest, down to 0 and then from 1 up to 5 which is the thickest. Sizes 2/0 and 3/0 are generally the most useful for operations on small animals while sizes 0, 1 or 2 are often used in large animals. There may be considerable variation, however, depending on the delicacy of the tissue and purpose for which the thread is used.

Suture material can be made of silk, cotton, catgut, plastic or stainless steel. It will be either non-absorbable in the body, e.g. silk, cotton, some plastics and stainless steel, or it will be absorbed, e.g. catgut (chromic catgut is a variation in which the rate of absorption is delayed) and some plastics. All types of thread material can be used anywhere in the body. Non-absorbed material produces no major adverse reactions and is accepted by the body tissues. However, there are technical reasons for preferring one type of thread over another depending on the type of operation being done. Each thread material has its own characteristics as regards such things as degree of flexibility, strength, rate of absorption, how much inflammation of the tissues it produces, and so on. Silk is very widely used in all animals and is relatively inexpensive.

Suture material can be purchased already packaged and sterile, in various lengths, and bonded to a needle, or it can be sterilised or disinfected by such means as autoclaving, irradiation, chemical disinfection and boiling in water.

The stitch and suturing

Many types of stitches can be used depending on what is required to be done. However, for general purposes continuous and interrupted stitches are the ones most often employed. The continuous or running stitch goes through and over the wound edges in a continuous sequence from one end of the wound to the other. Its disadvantage is that if it breaks it will unravel, allowing the whole wound to open. However, this is a very rare occurrence if a thread of the right calibre has been selected. It is considerably faster to apply than interrupted stitches. The latter are individual stitches placed a few millimetres apart along the wound. The interrupted stitch has several suturing patterns such as simple, mattress etc. and the appropriate pattern is selected depending on how it is intended to appose or suture the two edges of the wound. In large animals there are often more layers of tissue in the wound edges to close individually than in an animal such as a rat and it is often the case that a continuous stitch may be used to stitch the peritoneum and abdominal muscle while the outermost layer(s) are closed with interrupted stitches. In small animals a continuous stitch alone is usually quite adequate for all areas, though this really is a matter of preference.

Rodents and rabbits can and frequently do use their teeth to remove stitches which have been placed in accessible parts of the skin. It may therefore be more appropriate to use special metal wound clips (e.g. Michel clips) to close the skin. These clips

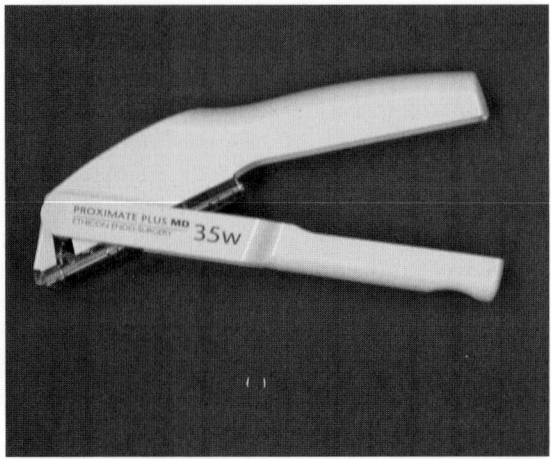

Figure 40.4   Automatic stapling device.

are applied 5–8 mm apart with special application forceps. They can easily be sterilised by steam or heat. Special staple sutures, applied by an automatic device are also readily available (Figure 40.4). They have the advantage that unlike the Michel clip, they cannot be applied too tightly, thereby avoiding the possible formation of local necrosis and pain. Although they are more expensive than Michel clips, they are considerably finer, less obtrusive and probably less painful for the animal and are thus to be recommended as a refinement.

The knot

The knot in wound closure, or for ligation, is the reef knot, or variations on it such as the surgeon's knot which has an extra twist in the first half-hitch. Often two or three reefs are incorporated in the knot to reinforce it and prevent it unravelling. The art of making knots with forceps, particularly at the end of a continuous stitch has to be practised and it is useful to seek the advice of a veterinary surgeon.

Dressings

Some wounds may require to be protected by a dressing or bandage. This is rarely practised in rodents which tend to remove them with their teeth. Rabbits are usually more manageable. Dressings can be used most successfully in large animals but even here, in the dog for example, problems of getting the dressing to stay in place may be encountered. Wounds can be covered by application of a plasticised aerosol dressing if thought necessary, to help prevent ingress of dirt and micro-organisms.

Procedures to be carried out after surgery

The immediate post-operative period

The period immediately after surgery is often the most difficult one for the animal. Not only does it have to recover from the physiologically depressive effects of the anaesthetic but it has to cope with the success or failure of the surgery. It represents a period where there is a high likelihood of death if either the anaesthetic management and/or the surgical expertise are faulty. The post-operative period is one to which novice surgeons may pay scant attention,

often to their cost and to the well-being of the animal. Good practices in the management of post-operative recovery are described in Chapter 41.

Mechanical restraint

There are occasions when animals carry indwelling vascular and other cannulae or other appliances such as radiotelemetry sensors, infusion pumps, electrodes etc. These must be protected mechanically from the vigorous efforts of the animal to remove them. Many methods are available to restrain the animal, both for small and large animals, and under a variety of conditions (see References and further reading, p. 380). Animals may wear Elizabethan collars, protective jackets, with or without swivel spring tethering devices, they can be restrained in a sling or in a purpose-built chair or be kept in a box-like holder. The period of restraint can vary from a few minutes to days and weeks as required. All restraint is distressing for the animal. It will result in both and physiological and psychological disturbances, which at the very least could affect experimental results. It is essential that the welfare of the animal under restraint is carefully considered. The best method of restraint to use is the one which allows the animal the greatest freedom of movement and which produces the least disturbance and which is compatible with the protection of the experimental device. For example, for rats, the Bollman apparatus is available, but it almost totally restricts the freedom of movement of the animal. It is extremely easy to use but it is likely to cause marked psychological and physiological disturbances. An alternative restraint procedure which can be considered, is a special jacket worn by the animal and which is attached to a light spring which itself is attached outside a normal cage and contains a swivel device. The spring can protect an indwelling cannula. The animal has considerable freedom of movement and normal function is affected relatively little. This method of restraint would be the method of choice, if it is possible to use it.

For all restraint procedures a reduction in the degree of disturbance to the animal can be achieved by familiarising the animal to the apparatus. Three or four days of training will often find the animal showing little resistance to the application of the restraint procedure.

Choosing the right restraint procedure, as well as prior training, is known to ameliorate physiological changes in many instances. During restraint, the animal must be kept under frequent observation and this may require overnight supervision. The animal's needs and comfort must be cared for and are paramount. It should be encouraged to urinate and defecate normally if the restraint is prolonged. Its immediate environment must be kept clean. Any untoward effects of prolonged restraint, for example in a primate chair, must be relieved or treated. There may be signs of abnormal bowel and bladder function, weight loss, bruising and muscle dysfunction. Appropriate action must be taken at the first signs of any of these. If adequate relief and treatment cannot be given then the animal must be released from the restraint. The period of restraint must be the minimum compatible with the requirements of the experiment, and if an animal is to be returned to its normal environment after the period of restraint, it must be carefully observed to ensure it returns to normal functioning in all respects.

References and further reading

Bickhardt, K., Buttner, D., Muschen, U. and Plonait, M. (1983) Influence of bleeding procedure and some environmental conditions on stress-dependent blood constituents of laboratory rats. *Laboratory Animals*, **17** (161).

Bleicher, N. (1965) Care of animals during surgical experiments. In: W.I. Gay (Ed.) *Methods of Animal Experimentation*, Vol. 1. Academic Press, New York.

de Boer, J., Archibald, J. and Downie, H.G. (Eds) (1975) *An Introduction to Experimental Surgery: A Guide to Experimenting with Laboratory Animals*. Excerpta Medica, Amsterdam.

Bojrab, M.J., Crane, S.W. and Arnoczky, S.P. (1989) *Current Techniques in Small Animal Surgery* (2nd edn). Lea & Febriger, Philadelphia.

Bradfield, J.F., Schachtman, T.R., McLaughlin, R.M. and Steffan, E.K. (1992) Behavioural and physiological effects of inapparent wound infection in rats. *Laboratory Animal Science*, **42** (572).

British Laboratory Animal Veterinary Association (1992) Experimental surgery slide programme, slide sets and notes. Obtained from P.A. Flecknell, Comparative Biology Centre, Medical School, Framlington Place, Newcastle Upon Tyne, NE2 4HH, UK.

College of Animal Welfare (1997) *Veterinary Surgical Instruments. An Illustrated Guide*. Butterworth Heinemann, Oxford.

Condon P.E. (Ed.) (1974) Symposium on surgical infections and antibiotics. In: *The Surgical Clinics of North America*, **55** (6). W. B. Saunders Co., Philadelphia.

Cravener, T.L. and Vasilatos-Younken, R. (1989) A method for catheterisation, harnessing and chronic infusion of undisturbed chickens. *Laboratory Animals*, **23** (270).

Cunliffe-Beamer, T.L. (1983) Biomethodology and surgical technique. In: H.L. Foster, J.D. Small and J.G. Fox (Eds) *The Mouse in Biomedical Research* (Vol. 3). Academic Press, New York.

Cunliffe-Beamer, T.L. (1989) Surgical techniques. In: H.N. Guttman (Ed.) *Guidelines for the Well-being of Rodents in Research*. Scientists Center for Animal Welfare, North Carolina.

van Dongen, J.J., Remie, R., Rensema, J.W. and van Wannik, G.H.J. (Eds) (1990) *Manual of Microsurgery on the Laboratory Rat. Part 1. General Information and Experimental Techniques*. Elsevier, Amsterdam.

Flecknell, P.A. (1984) The relief of pain in laboratory animals. *Laboratory Animals*, **18** (147).

Flecknell, P.A. (1996) *Laboratory Animal Anaesthesia* (2nd edn). Academic Press, London.

Flecknell, P.A. and Liles, J.H. (1991) The effects of surgical procedures, halothane anaesthesia and nalbuphine on locomotor activity and food and water consumption in rats. *Laboratory Animals*, **25** (50).

Gartner, K., Buttner, D., Dohler, P. et al. (1980) Stress response of rats to handling and experimental procedures. *Laboratory Animals*, **14** (267).

Green, C.J. (1987) Microsurgery in the clinic and laboratory. *Laboratory Animals*, **21** (1).

Green, C. and Simpkin, S. (1990) *Basic Microsurgical Techniques. A Laboratory Manual*. Obtained from the surgical Research Group, MRC Clinical Research Centre, Northwich Park Hospital, Harrow, Middlesex, UK.

Harkness, J.E. and Wagner, J.E. (1983) *The Biology and Medicine of Rabbits and Rodents* (2nd edn). Lea & Febiger, Philadelphia.

Hickman, J. and Walker, R. (1980) *An Atlas of Veterinary Surgery* (2nd edn). John Wright & Sons, Bristol.

Hillyer, E.V. and Quesenberry, K.E. (1997) *Ferrets, Rabbits and Rodents. Clinical Medicine and Surgery*. W.B. Saunders Co., Philadelphia.

van Hoosier, G.L. Jr and McPherson, C.W. (Eds) (1987) *Laboratory Hamsters*. Academic Press, Orlando.

Home Office (2000) *Guidance on the Operation of the Animals (Scientific Procedures) Act 1986*. HMSO, London.

Horton, M.L., Harris, A.M., Van Stee, E.W. and Beck, K.C. (1975) Versatile protective jacket for chronically instrumented dogs. *Laboratory Animal Science*, **25** (500).

Hurov, L. (1978) *Handbook of Veterinary Surgical Instruments and Glossary of Surgical Terms*. W.B. Saunders Co., Philadelphia.

Kaplan, H.M. and Timmons, E.H. (1979) *The Rabbit. A Model for the Principles of Mammalian Physiology and Surgery*. Academic Press, New York.

Karl, A. and Kissen, A.T. (1978) Durable jackets for non-human primates to protect chronically implanted instrumentation. *Laboratory Animal Science*, **28** (103).

Kirk, R.M. (1978) *Basic Surgical Techniques*. Churchill Livingstone, Edinburgh.

Kohn, D.F., Wixson, S.K., White, W.J. and Benson, G.J. (1997) *Anaesthesia and Analgesia in Laboratory Animals*. Academic Press, San Diego.

Laber-Laird, K., Swindle, M.M. and Flecknell, P.A. (Eds) (1996) *Handbook of Rodent and Rabbit Medicine*. Pergamon Press, Oxford.

Lambert, R. (1965) *Surgery of the Digestive System of the Rat*. C.C. Thomas, Springfield, IL.

Lane, D.R. (1985) *Jones' Animal Nursing* (4th edn). Pergamon Press, Oxford.

Lennox, M.S. and Taylor, K.G. (1983) A restraint chair for primates. *Laboratory Animals*, **17** (225).

Leonard, E.P. (1968) *Fundamentals of Small Animal Surgery*. W.B. Saunders Co., Philadelphia.

Liles, J.H. and Flecknell, P.A. (1993) The influence of buprenorphine or bupivacaine on the post-operative effects of laparotomy and bile-duct ligation in rats. *Laboratory Animals*, **27** (374).

Lumley, J.S.P., Green, C.J., Lear, P. and Angell-James, J.E. (1990) *Essentials of Experimental Surgery*. Butterworth Heinemann, London.

Manning, P.J., Ringler, D.H. and Newcomer, C.E. (Eds) (1994) *The Biology of the Laboratory Rabbit* (2nd edn). Academic Press, San Diego.

Morris, T. (1995) Antibiotic therapeutics in laboratory animals. *Laboratory Animals*, **29** (16).

Petty, C. (1982) *Research Techniques in the Rat*. C.C. Thomas, Springfield, IL.

Schlingmann, F., Vermeulen, J.K., de Vries, A. et al. (1996) *Food deprivation: how long and how?* Proceedings of the Sixth FELASA Symposium on the Harmonisation of Laboratory Animal Husbandry. Royal Society of Medicine Press, London.

Strachan, C.J.L. and Wise, R. (Eds) (1979) *Surgical Sepsis*. Academic Press, London.

Swaim, S.F. (1980) *Surgery of Traumatized Skin: Management and Reconstruction in the Dog and Cat*. W.B. Saunders Co., Philadelphia.

Swindle, M.M. and Adams, P.J. (1988) *Experimental Surgery and Physiology*. Williams & Wilkins, Baltimore.

Taylor, R. and McGehee, R. (1995) *Manual of Small Animal Post-operative Care*. Williams & Wilkins, Baltimore.

Tuli, J.S., Smith, J.A. and Morton, D.B. (1995) Stress measurements in mice after transportation. *Laboratory Animals*, **29** (132).

Waynforth, H.B. and Flecknell, P.A. (1992) *Experimental and Surgical Technique in the Rat* (2nd edn). Academic Press, London.

Waynforth, H.B. (1995) Basics of surgery. In: A.A. Tuffery (Ed.) *Laboratory Animals. An Introduction for Experimenters* (2nd edn). John Wiley & Sons, Chichester.

Williams, D.J. and Harris, M.M. (1975) *Fundamental Techniques in Veterinary Surgery*. W.B. Saunders Co., Philadelphia.

Wingfield, W.E. and Rawlings, C. (1979) *Small Animal Surgery. An Atlas of Operative Techniques*. W.B. Saunders Co., London.

Wolfensohn, S. and Lloyd, M. (1998) *Handbook of Laboratory Animal Management and Welfare* (2nd edn). Blackwell Science, Oxford.

41

Anaesthesia and Peri-operative Care

Paul Flecknell

Introduction

An understanding of the principles and practice of anaesthesia is important in many areas of research which involve the use of animals. Anaesthesia is used not only to allow surgical or other painful procedures to be carried out humanely, but also to immobilise animals which would otherwise become distressed during periods of physical restraint. Anaesthesia can be produced by a variety of means, either by injection or inhalation of drugs, or by injection of local anaesthetic agents. In some instances only a single anaesthetic agent is used, but more frequently a combination of drugs is administered whose combined effects produce anaesthesia.

Definitions

- Anaesthesia is defined as a state of controllable, reversible insensibility in which sensory perception and motor responses are both markedly depressed. This state can be either general anaesthesia, when animals lose consciousness, or local anaesthesia, when the loss of sensory and motor function is confined to a specific region, for example one limb.
- Analgesia is the temporary abolition or diminution of pain perception.
- Sedatives produce drowsiness and appear to reduce fear and apprehension in animals.
- Tranquillisers produce a calming effect without causing sedation, and at high doses they produce ataxia (unsteady, uncoordinated movement) and depression, but animals are easily roused. There is considerable overlap in the action of many agents, and different animal species often respond differently.

- Muscle relaxant usually describes neuromuscular blocking agents, which produces paralysis of the skeletal muscles.

Aims of anaesthesia

Anaesthesia aims to eliminate pain and to immobilise the animal so that surgical and experimental procedures can be carried out safely, humanely and accurately. It is usually advantageous to produce relaxation of skeletal muscles to reduce or eliminate reflex responses and muscle spasm. In addition to preventing movement in response to surgical stimuli, elimination of pain also reduces the risk of shock. In many laboratory species, it is often preferable to use general anaesthesia, and produce loss of consciousness, so that the animal is unaware of its surroundings and of the procedures being undertaken. It is therefore likely to experience less distress than when local anaesthetic techniques are used (see below, p. 386).

Selecting an anaesthetic regimen

Anaesthesia can be produced by injectable anaesthetics (e.g. pentobarbital), by inhalation (e.g. isoflurane), or by local anaesthetics (e.g. lidocaine). Although regimens are often selected on this basis, it is often beneficial to use two or more techniques in combination, for example isoflurane by inhalation to produce loss of consciousness and some muscle relaxation, and an analgesic such as fentanyl, to block the perception of pain. This approach is called 'balanced anaesthesia'. Although it might appear at first to be an unnecessary complication, by reducing the dose of the individual agents used, it reduces their undesirable side-effects (such as hypotension – a reduction in arterial blood pressure), and can also result in more rapid recovery. For convenience, the different groups of anaesthetics are described separately below, but it is important to remember that they can be combined, at lower dose rates, to produce balanced anaesthesia.

The choice of a particular technique will depend on a variety of factors – for example the species of animal, the depth and duration of anaesthesia required, the availability of equipment such as anaesthetic machines, and the experience and skills of the operators should all be taken into consideration. It is often helpful to discuss your proposed anaesthetic technique with veterinary staff, and with colleagues who have relevant experience with the species concerned.

There remains one further important objective when anaesthetising laboratory animals, which is to select an anaesthetic technique which interferes as little as possible with the particular experiment which is being undertaken.

Injectable anaesthetic agents

A number of different injectable anaesthetic agents are used in laboratory animals, and extensive descriptions of these can be found in anaesthesia texts (e.g. Flecknell 1994; Kohn et al. 1997). Recommended dose rates for all of the common species are given in Tables 41.1 (a) and 41.1 (b). Injectable anaesthetics can be administered by a variety of routes. Intravenous administration is usually preferable, since this produces the most predictable and rapid onset of action. This enables the drug to be administered 'to effect' so that just sufficient is given to provide the desired depth of anaesthesia. Practical considerations, such as the absence of suitable superficial veins or difficulty in providing adequate restraint of the animal, may limit the use of this route in many smaller laboratory species. Administration by intramuscular (i.m.), intraperitoneal (i.p.) or subcutaneous (s.c.) injection is relatively straightforward in most species, but the rate of drug absorption, and hence its anaesthetic effects, may vary considerably.

It is important to appreciate the very great variation in response to anaesthetics which occurs between different strains, ages, and sex of animals. When using an anaesthetic regimen for the first time, especially when it is not possible to administer the agent intravenously, it is essential to assess its effects in one animal, before beginning to anaesthetise the remainder of the group. This will enable the recommended doses to be adjusted to suit the responses of the particular animals being used.

As mentioned above, this variability in response can be a particular problem in small rodents, since most injectable anaesthetics are administered to these species by the i.p. route as a single dose. When administering anaesthetics in this way it is impossible to adjust the dose according to the individual animal's response, so inadvertent over and under dosing will frequently occur until experience is gained with a particular strain, age and sex of animal. Variation in response also occurs with changes in environmental factors, and standardisation of all these variables will not only simplify anaesthetic dose calculations, but also constitutes good experimental design. When selecting anaesthetics for intramuscular, intraperitoneal or subcutaneous administration, it is also advisable to select those which have a wide safety margin.

An additional consideration with i.m., i.p. or s.c. injection is that injection of an irritant compound can cause unnecessary pain or discomfort to the animal. This is a particular concern with intramuscular injection in small rodents, and there are a number of reports of tissue reactions such as myositis, for example, after use of ketamine. Pain on injection can also result because of the large volume of injectate required. In many instances, the dose per kg of body-weight of anaesthetic increases as body size decreases. For example the induction dose of ketamine is 10–15 mg/kg in a pig, but 75–l00 mg/kg in rodents. An adult (100 g) hamster would require a dose of 0.l ml intramuscularly – equivalent to 70 ml in an adult human. It seems advisable to avoid intramuscular injection, and use the subcutaneous or intraperitoneal routes when possible – provided that the agent is not irritant.

If the intravenous route can be used, then a number of short-acting anaesthetics can be used to provide five- to ten-minute periods of anaesthesia (e.g. propofol, thiopental, methohexital). When carrying out venipuncture in animals, the use of EMLA™ cream (Astra Pharma Inc.) to produce local anaesthesia of the skin should be considered.

Induction of anaesthesia following intravenous administration is usually rapid. In most circumstances

Table 41.1 (a)   Anaesthetic drugs for use in small laboratory animals. Note that considerable between-strain variation occurs, so that these dose rates should only be taken as a general guide. Note also that the safety of different anaesthetic agents varies considerably (see text).

Anaesthetic and related agents	Gerbil	Guinea pig	Hamster	Mouse	Rabbit	Rat
Atipamezole	1 mg/kg s.c., i.m., i.p., i.v.	1 mg/kg s.c., i.m., i.p., i.v.	1 mg/kg s.c., i.m., i.p., i.v.	1 mg/kg s.c., i.m., i.p., i.v.	1 mg/kg s.c., i.m., i.p., i.v.	1 mg/kg s.c., i.m., i.p., i.v.
Fentanyl/fluanisone and diazepam	0.3 ml/kg i.m. + 5 mg/kg i.p.	1.0 ml/kg i.m. + 2.5 mg/kg i.p.	1.0 ml/kg i.m. + 5 mg/kg i.p.	0.3 ml/kg i.m. + 5 mg/kg i.p.	0.3 ml/kg i.m. + 2 mg/kg i.p. or i.v.	0.3 ml/kg i.m. + 2.5 mg/kg i.p.
Fentanyl/fluanisone and midazolam*	8 ml/kg i.p.	8 ml/kg i.p.	4 ml/kg i.p.	10 ml/kg i.p.	0.3 ml/kg i.m. + 2 mg/kg i.p. or i.v.	2.7 ml/kg i.p.
Ketamine + medetomidine	?	40 mg/kg + 0.5 mg/kg i.p.	100 mg/kg + 0.25 mg/kg i.p.	75 mg/kg + 1 mg/kg i.p.	15 mg/kg + 0.5 mg/kg i.p.	75 mg/kg + 0.5 mg/kg i.p.
Pentobarbitone	60–80 mg/kg i.p.	37 mg/kg i.p.	50–90 mg/kg i.p.	40–50 mg/kg i.p.	30–45 mg/kg i.v.	40–50 mg/kg i.v.

Table 41.1 (b)   Anaesthetic drugs for use in larger laboratory animals. Note that considerable between-strain variation occurs, so that these dose rates should only be taken as a general guide. Note also that the safety of different anaesthetic agents varies considerably (see text). Combinations marked * will generally produce only light anaesthesia, those marked ** will usually produce a surgical plane of anaesthesia.

Anaesthetic and related agents	Cat	Dog	Pig	Sheep
Atipamezole (antagonist to medetomidine)	0.1–1 mg/kg i.m., i.v., s.c. depending upon dose of medetomidine used	0.1–1 mg/kg i.m., i.v., s.c. depending upon dose of medetomidine used	0.1–1 mg/kg i.m., i.v., s.c. depending upon dose of medetomidine used	0.1–1 mg/kg i.m., i.v., s.c. depending upon dose of medetomidine used
Alphaxalone/alphadolone	9–12 mg/kg i.v.** or 18 mg/kg i.m.**	–	6 mg/kg i.m. followed by 2 mg/kg i.v.**	2–3 mg/kg i.v.**
Ketamine/midazolam	10 mg/kg i.m. plus 0.2 mg/kg i.m.**	–	10–15 mg/kg i.m. plus 0.5–2 mg/kg i.m.*	10–15 mg/kg i.m. plus 2 mg/kg i.m.* or 4 mg/kg i.v. plus 1 mg/kg i.v.*
Ketamine + medetomidine	7 mg/kg i.m. plus 0.08 mg/kg i.v.**	2.5–7.5 mg/kg i.m. plus 0.04 mg/kg i.m.**	10 mg/kg i.m. plus 0.08 mg/kg i.m.*	1 mg/kg i.m. plus 0.025 mg/kg i.m.**
Thiopentone	10–15 mg/kg i.v.**	10–20 mg/kg i.v.**	6–9 mg/kg i.v.**	10–15 mg/kg i.v.**
Pentobarbitone	20–30 mg/kg i.v.**	20–30 mg/kg i.v.**	20–30 mg/kg i.v.**	20–30 mg/kg i.v.**
Propofol	5–8 mg/kg i.v.**	5–7.5 mg/kg i.v.**	2.5–3.5 mg/kg i.v.**	4–5 mg/kg i.v.**

half the calculated dose of anaesthetic is given rapidly (typically over a five- to ten-second period), then additional anaesthetic is given to produce the desired effect. The institute's veterinary surgeon will be able to provide further advice on this technique, and will also be able to help with all other aspects of anaesthesia. When anaesthetics are given by intraperitoneal or subcutaneous injection, the onset of action is slower, and the animal will pass through a phase in which it becomes progressively ataxic ('wobbly'), may exhibit some excitation and hyperactivity, then lose its ability to right itself, and eventually lose consciousness. Anaesthesia then becomes progressively deeper until the pedal withdrawal response is lost (see below, p. 396). At this stage painful procedures can be carried out without the animal being aware of them.

In summary, the main advantage of injectable anaesthetics is the ease with which they can be administered, without the use of specialised equipment. In addition, the wide variety of different agents which are available allows careful selection of a regimen to suit a particular species or purpose. The main disadvantages are the difficulty of controlling anaesthetic depth when some agents are used and the prolonged recovery times. Both of these disadvantages can often be overcome by use of newer anaesthetic agents such as propofol, administered by intravenous injection.

Injectable anaesthetics

Neuroleptanalgesic combinations
Fentanyl/fluanisone (Hypnorm®, VetaPharma Ltd), when administered alone, produces sedation and sufficient analgesia for superficial surgery in most small rodents, rabbits and in dogs (Tables 41.1(a) and (b), see p. 384). The degree of muscle relaxation is generally poor, and the high doses needed for more major surgery produce marked respiratory depression. In small rodents and rabbits, combining this regimen with a benzodiazepine (midazolam or diazepam) produces surgical anaesthesia with only moderate respiratory depression. The combination has the advantage that it can be partially reversed with a mixed opioid agonist/antagonist such as butorphanol or a partial agonist such as buprenorphine. This reverses the respiratory depression caused by the fentanyl, but maintains post-operative analgesia. The benzodiazepine antagonist flumazenil can be used to further speed recovery, but repeated doses are needed to avoid re-sedation.

In small rodents, a mixture of midazolam and Hypnorm™ can be given as a single intraperitoneal injection. In rabbits it is preferable to give the Hypnorm™ first, by intramuscular injection. The midazolam or diazepam can then be administered intravenously to effect as described above.

Other neuroleptanalgesics
Fentanyl/droperidol (Innovar-Vet®) when used alone produces effects similar to Hypnorm™ but with a greater tendency to produce limb rigidity. In combination with midazolam its effects are unpredictable and it is best used alone to provide immobility, sedation and analgesia for minor procedures.

Ketamine
When used alone, ketamine produces immobility but little analgesia in most species. In cats, primates and ferrets its effects are greater and sufficient analgesia is provided for minor procedures to be carried out.

In these and other species it is often best given in combination with other agents which increase the degree of analgesia and muscle relaxation. In dogs it should not be given alone, as it can produce seizures.

When combined with acepromazine, midazolam or diazepam, ketamine produces light to moderate surgical anaesthesia in non-human primates, cats, sheep, pigs, ferrets and rabbits. In small rodents the effects of these combinations are less predictable, and usually only light planes of anaesthesia, insufficient even for minor surgery, are produced. In contrast, administration of ketamine in combination with medetomidine or xylazine results in surgical anaesthesia in most mammals. Its effects are slightly less uniform in guinea pigs and pigs, and some individuals may not become sufficiently deeply anaesthetised for major surgery. In these circumstances, it is preferable to deepen anaesthesia using an inhalational agent, or to provide additional analgesia using local anaesthesia. Since ketamine alone has limited effects in many species, reversal of medetomidine or xylazine with atipamezole greatly speeds recovery. Since ketamine appears to have limited analgesic effects in small mammals, if atipamezole is used following surgery, then an analgesic should be administered to provide post-operative pain relief (see below, p. 398).

Barbiturates
Pentobarbital has been used for many years but it has a narrow margin of safety, since the anaesthetic dose is close to the lethal dose in many species. When given by intravenous injection, the dose can be adjusted carefully, but in the rabbit, even careful administration of a diluted solution (6 mg/ml) is hazardous, and respiratory arrest may occur before surgical planes of anaesthesia are attained. In smaller animals, when it is usually administered by intraperitoneal injection, it is best used in low doses to provide light planes of anaesthesia, with inhalational agents used to deepen anaesthesia if required.

Thiopental, methohexital and thiamylal can all be used to produce short periods of anaesthesia when administered intravenously. This can be useful both for short surgical procedures, and to allow intubation followed by maintenance with volatile agents.

Propofol
Propofol, when administered intravenously, produces short periods of surgical anaesthesia in most

species, and additional doses can be given to prolong the period of anaesthesia, without unduly prolonging recovery. In rabbits, it can provide sufficient depth of anaesthesia for intubation, but respiratory arrest usually occurs before the onset of surgical anaesthesia. In sheep, relatively high doses are needed to induce and maintain anaesthesia.

Alphaxalone/alphadolone

In most species, intravenous administration of alphaxalone/alphadolone produces surgical anaesthesia, which can be prolonged with additional doses. It has been recommended for intramuscular injection in guinea pigs, but the high dose required to produce anaesthesia requires administration of large volumes of drug (3.3 ml to a 1 kg animal). The commercial preparation of alphaxalone/alphadolone contains Cremophor® EL, a solubilising agent which produces histamine release in cats and dogs. In the dogs, the effects can be serious, and the drug should not be used in this species. In rabbits, its effects are similar to propofol, with respiratory arrest occurring before surgical anaesthesia is attained, although sufficient depth of anaesthesia for intubation can be produced.

Local anaesthetics

Local anaesthesia is most often used in larger species, when the animal has become accustomed to handling and can be safely restrained. Either physical restraint can be used, provided that this can be achieved safely and without causing distress to the animal, or a sedative or tranquilliser can be administered. Local anaesthetics, such as lidocaine, can then be infiltrated into the area which needs to be rendered insensitive (for example to allow a skin biopsy to be taken) or the drug can be injected around nerve trunks to produce larger areas of anaesthesia. Local anaesthetics can also be administered into the epidural space, or into the cerebrospinal fluid (intrathecal administration) to produce anaesthesia of the hind limbs and lower abdomen.

Use of local anaesthetics to provide analgesia as an adjunct to the use of other anaesthetics which produce unconsciousness, is a technique which can be used in a wide range of different species. However, when using drugs such as lidocaine in small animals, it is important to reduce the volume so that toxicity is avoided. The local anaesthetics are no more toxic in small animals than in larger species, but the small body weight of rodents makes inadvertent overdose easier.

Inhalational anaesthesia

Anaesthetics which are given by inhalation are either:

- volatile liquids, which are vaporised before delivery to the animal (e.g. halothane and isoflurane); or
- gases (e.g. nitrous oxide).

Halothane and isoflurane are the two most widely used volatile anaesthetics in both animals and man. They are liquids at room temperature, and because of their potency, they must be delivered in a carefully controlled way, using an anaesthetic machine fitted with a calibrated vaporiser (Figure 41.1).

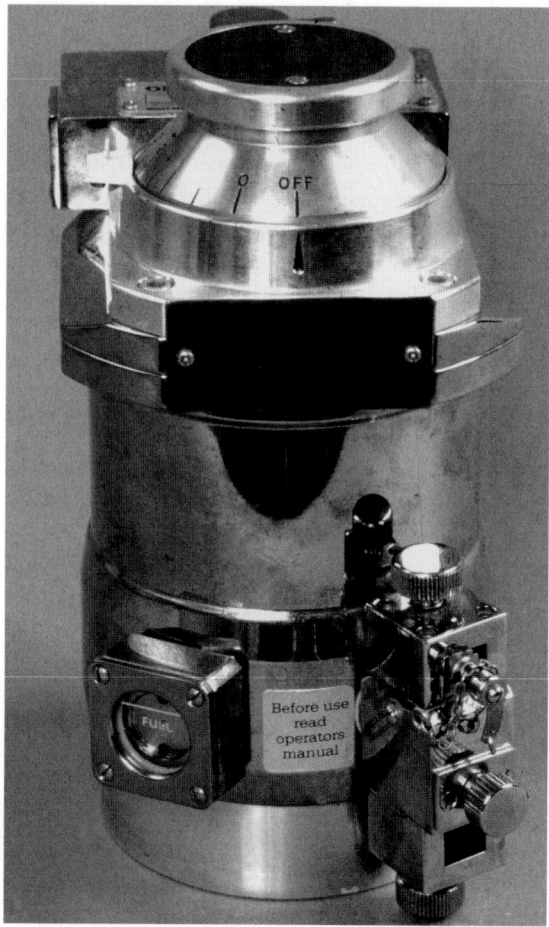

Figure 41.1   Anaesthetic vaporiser (Isotec Mk 3, Cyprane).

Table 41.2 Concentrations of volatile anaesthetics for induction and maintenance of anaesthesia. The concentrations required can be reduced by administration of pre-anaesthetic medication or concurrent use of injectable anaesthetics (adapted from Flecknell, 1966).

Anaesthetic	Induction concentration	Maintenance concentration
Enflurane	3–5%	1–3%
Ether	10–20%	4–5%
Halothane	3–4%	1–2%
Isoflurane	3–4%	1.5–3%
Methoxyflurane	3–3.5%	0.4–1%

Anaesthetic vapour of known concentration is produced by blowing oxygen through the vaporiser. The vaporiser setting can be adjusted easily to provide an appropriate concentration for induction of anaesthesia, or for maintenance (see Table 41.2). If an animal is too lightly anaesthetised, then the depth of anaesthesia can be quickly and easily changed by changing the vaporiser setting. If anaesthesia appears too deep, the vaporiser setting can be reduced. Usually adjustments of only up to +/− 0.5–1.0% are needed.

The depth of anaesthesia can be assessed fairly easily when using volatile agents. Light anaesthesia is indicated by the presence of withdrawal responses (see p. 399). As anaesthesia deepens, these responses are lost and respiration becomes progressively more shallow. At dangerously deep planes of anaesthesia, respiration may cease, or gasping respiratory movements may occur.

Anaesthetic machines

It is usually most convenient to deliver volatile anaesthetics using an anaesthetic machine. At first sight these appear complex, but all share several common features (Figure 41.2):

- a source of compressed gas, either from a cylinder or piped from a central supply;
- a regulator which reduces the pressure of the gas;
- a pressure gauge which indicates how much gas remains in the cylinder;
- a flow-meter, which controls the rate of gas flow to the animal;
- a vaporiser, which adds anaesthetic at known concentration to the gas.

Most machines also have an emergency oxygen button which allows the vaporiser to be by-passed and a high flow of 100% oxygen to be delivered to the animal. The majority of these features can be provided by constructing a simple work-station, which although lacking some of the sophisticated features of commercially produced anaesthetic trolleys, is adequate for simple procedures in rodents.

The yokes for attaching the gas cylinders to anaesthetic trolleys, or for attaching tubing from a piped

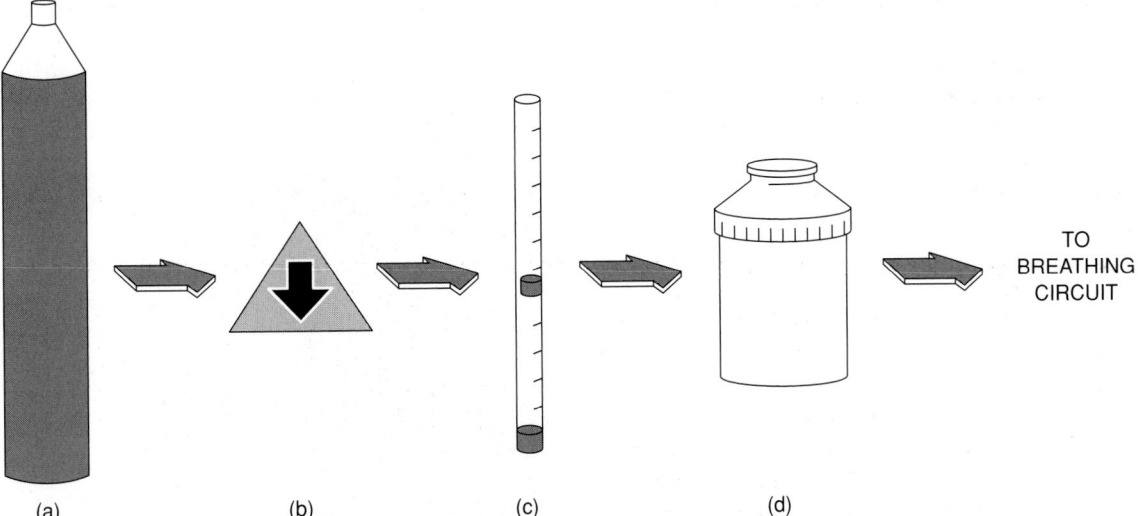

(a)	(b)	(c)	(d)

Figure 41.2 Diagrammatic representation of the components of an anaesthetic machine. A source of compressed gas (e.g. oxygen) (a) is passed via a pressure-reducing valve (b) to a flow meter (c), then through an anaesthetic vaporiser (d) to a breathing circuit.

gas supply, are fitted with small metal pins, with different configurations for oxygen, nitrous oxide and other gases. This helps prevent inadvertent attachment of a cylinder or pipe to the wrong inlet and flow-meter. The cylinders are also colour coded – nitrous oxide cylinders are blue in the UK, and oxygen cylinders are black with a white top; carbon dioxide cylinders are grey.

It is important that anaesthetic machines are serviced regularly, so that they continue to function efficiently. Faults in machines can have serious consequences to the animals which are being anaesthetised, and can also pose a health hazard to the operator. Other apparatus used, such as anaesthetic circuits and endotracheal tubes, must also be properly maintained. Endotracheal tubes may be plain tubes, or may have an inflatable cuff which seals the gap between the wall of the tube and the trachea. The cuff can be inflated either with a syringe (2.5 ml) or with a specially designed inflator. The cuff is prevented from deflating either by means of a non-return valve (present on some disposable tubes) or by clamping with a pair of haemostats. Tubes may be re-usable or be intended only for single use. Re-usable tubes are generally constructed of rubber and are opaque. They deteriorate gradually, becoming brittle and easily kinked. The cuff often becomes distorted and may leak. It is preferable to purchase single-use tubes and allow a limited amount of re-use. Tubes should be inspected carefully before use to ensure they have not begun to deteriorate. If apparatus for pasteurisation is available, tubes can be pasteurised. Many types do not withstand autoclaving, although some may be autoclaved a limited number of times at lower temperatures (121 °C for fifteen minutes), or sterilised using ethylene oxide. Anaesthetic circuits and reservoir bags should be washed in hot soapy water and either pasteurised or rinsed with chlorine disinfectant. Metal components can be autoclaved after washing. If a laryngoscope has been used, the handle should be separated from the blade and wiped clean. The blade should be washed in hot soapy water and dried thoroughly.

Administration of anaesthetics by inhalation

In small animals such as rats and mice, the anaesthetic can be administered easily using an anaesthetic chamber. With all agents, animals first become slightly ataxic (wobbly), may then go through a period of involuntary excitement, then lose their righting reflex and become immobile. With agents such as isoflurane, induction can be very rapid, so that animals pass almost immediately from a state of full alertness to complete unconsciousness. This can be achieved without using dangerously high concentrations of anaesthetic, providing the concentration of anaesthetic agent in the chamber is raised rapidly. Simply calculate the volume of the chamber (usually about 5–10 litres) and aim to fill the chamber in less than a minute by using flow rates of 5–10 litres/minute. Chambers should have transparent sides or lid, so that the animal can be observed during induction of anaesthesia. The chamber should have an inlet for anaesthetic gases, preferably situated at the base of the chamber, and an outlet for surplus gas near the top (Figure 41.3). Always fill the chamber from the

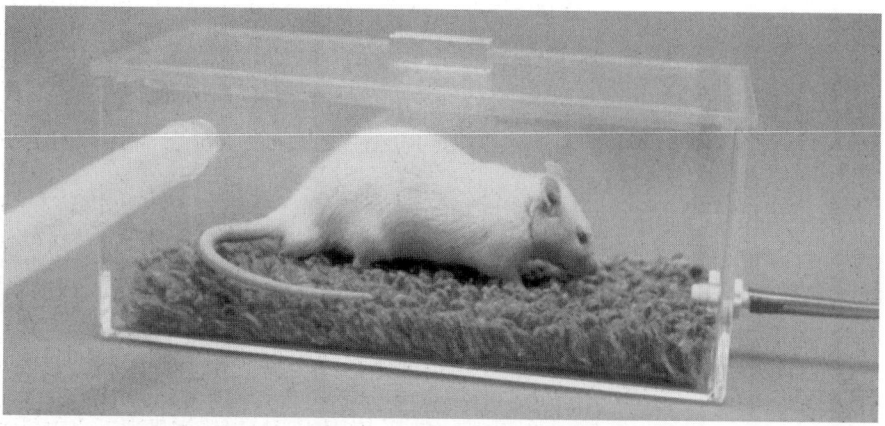

Figure 41.3   Anaesthetic chamber for use in small mammals.

bottom, and remove excess gas at the top, as these anaesthetic vapours are all denser than air.

Once the animal is unconscious, it can be removed from the chamber and administration continued (at a lower concentration, e.g. 2% isoflurane, see Table 41.2, p. 387) using a face-mask. Exposure of personnel to anaesthetic gases is considered hazardous, and Health and Safety Executive requirements include the need to minimise exposure. This is most easily achieved in small animals by using a double-mask system (e.g. the apparatus manufactured by IPS Ltd). Fresh anaesthetic gases are delivered through the inner mask, and waste gases extracted through the outer mask, which is attached to an extraction fan (Figure 41.4). This system can also be used to scavenge surplus gas from an anaesthetic chamber.

Practical considerations usually limit the size of animal which can be placed in an anaesthetic chamber. If larger animals have become accustomed to handling and restraint, it may be possible to induce anaesthesia using a face mask, but many animals resent the procedure and struggle. It is often preferable to use an injectable agent either to heavily sedate the animal, or to induce anaesthesia (see below).

In the rabbit, exposure to halothane or isoflurane is associated with breath holding, which may be prolonged (>2 minutes). Animals may struggle violently during induction and seem to resent the procedure. When placed in an anaesthetic chamber, they attempt to avoid inhaling the vapour. If mask induction is to be used, the mask should be briefly removed if apnoea occurs, and replaced when the animal breathes. Alternatively, a sedative or tranquilliser can be administered. Although this prevents struggling, breath holding may still be seen, and the mask may need to be removed temporarily. Administration of oxygen is not associated with breath holding, and it is advisable to allow the animal to breath 100% oxygen for one to two minutes before adding halothane or isoflurane to minimise the risk of hypoxia. It is generally preferable to induce anaesthesia with an injectable agent, intubate the rabbit, then maintain with a volatile agent.

In certain circumstances, use of an anaesthetic machine may present major practical difficulties (for example when anaesthetising wild-caught animals or birds 'in the field'). In such circumstances, if an injectable anaesthetic cannot be used, it may be necessary to anaesthetise small animals by placing them in a chamber containing a pad of gauze or cotton wool soaked in liquid anaesthetic. Direct contact with the liquid anaesthetic is extremely unpleasant for the animal, as it is irritant to mucous membranes. Even if the gauze is separated from the animal by a metal

Figure 41.4 Gas scavenging system for use in small animals (IMS Ltd).

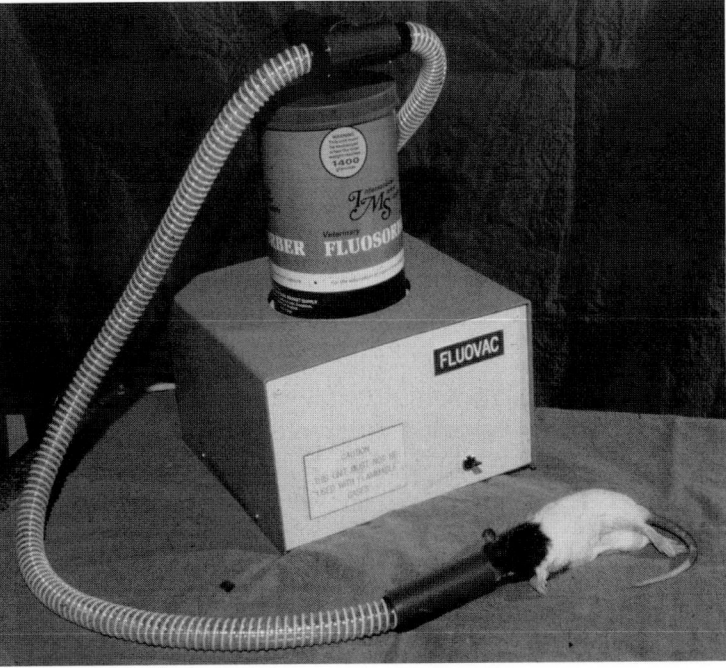

grid, liquid anaesthetic is often spilt on to areas which are in contact with the animal. The concentration of anaesthetic achievable in such containers is unpredictable and is invariably dangerously high if potent, easily vaporised anaesthetics, such as halothane or isoflurane, are used. For example, the concentration of halothane produced at 20 °C is 32%, more than six times the safe induction concentration. In these circumstances the only currently available agent that can be used is ether. This can no longer be purchased as an anaesthetic in the UK, but can be obtained through suppliers of laboratory reagents. Ether is flammable and forms explosive mixtures with air and oxygen, so when used, there will be a significant risk of fire or explosion. It is also frequently impossible to prevent contamination of the environment with anaesthetic vapour and this may present a hazard to the anaesthetist if the technique is used in a confined space. It is important to note that many gas-scavenging devices are not 'spark proof' and so cannot be used with ether.

Administering anaesthetics by inhalation has the advantage that it is relatively easy to control the depth of anaesthesia, when using a calibrated vaporiser, and induction and recovery from anaesthesia are usually rapid (unless anaesthesia has been maintained for prolonged periods e.g. > 1 hour). The most commonly used agents, halothane and isoflurane, can be administered to a wide range of different species. Nitrous oxide has very little anaesthetic effect in animals, so it can only be used in combination with other anaesthetics. Its potency in animals is low, and for simple rapid procedures, adding nitrous oxide to the anaesthetic gases used offers little benefit.

Anaesthetic circuits

Irrespective of whether an animal has been anaesthetised with inhalational or injectable agents, it is often advisable to deliver oxygen or anaesthetic gases by means of an anaesthetic breathing circuit, rather than simply using a face mask. The majority of circuits function most effectively when they are attached to the animal using an endotracheal tube or a close-fitting face mask. The shape of the muzzle in most animals often makes finding a suitable mask difficult, so endotracheal intubation is often preferable, especially if it becomes necessary to assist ventilation (see below, p. 395). A wide range of different anaesthetic circuits are available, and they are described in detail in standard anaesthetic text books. Those most widely used in laboratory species are the T-piece, the Bains circuit, the Magill circuit (Figure 41.5) and the circle system (Figure 41.6).

Use of an appropriate anaesthetic circuit reduces the volume of fresh gas and volatile anaesthetic agents which need to be used, and provides a means of assisting ventilation, should this be necessary. During normal respiration, oxygen and anaesthetic gases are required only during inspiration, but they are delivered from the anaesthetic machine for the whole of the respiratory cycle. This leads to wastage of a high proportion of the gas supplied. In addition, if gas is supplied by using a face mask, the gas flow must be rapid enough to meet the peak needs during inspiration. As a result, three times the animal's minute volume (the volume of gas inhaled in one minute) must be supplied. Minute volume is calculated by multiplying the volume of one breath (the tidal volume) by the respiratory rate. Tidal volume ranges from 7–15 ml/kg, so it can be seen that for a small animal, such as the mouse, the flow rates needed on a face mask are not large. However, large animals require very high gas flow rates, for example a 30 kg pig would need a flow of around 18 litres per minute.

Using a Bains circuit or T-piece reduces this to 12 litres (approximately twice the minute volume), or to 6 litres if a Magill circuit is used. Circuits such as the Bain or T-piece are most suitable for small (<10 kg) animals, when the gas flow rates needed are not very high, as these circuits offer very little resistance to breathing. In larger animals, a Magill circuit can be used or the animal can be connected to a circle system. This type of circuit differs in that it includes a soda-lime absorber, to remove exhaled carbon dioxide allowing expired gas to be recycled and returned to the animal, rather than vented out of the circuit. This arrangement allows very low, fresh gas flow rates (100–500 ml) to be used, so making the system very economical. A disadvantage of the circuit is that it offers some resistance to breathing, and so it is less suitable for small animals, although newer designs have very low resistance valves, which allow them to be used in small animals (e.g. 2–3 kg). It is also important to be aware that when using a low, fresh gas flow, the concentration of anaesthetic vapour in the circuit may be much lower than the vaporiser

Figure 41.5   Anaesthetic circuits.

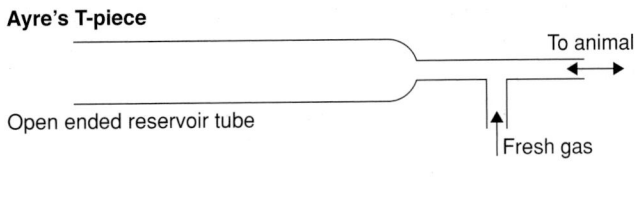

Ayre's T-piece

To animal

Open ended reservoir tube

Fresh gas

Jackson-Rees modified T-piece

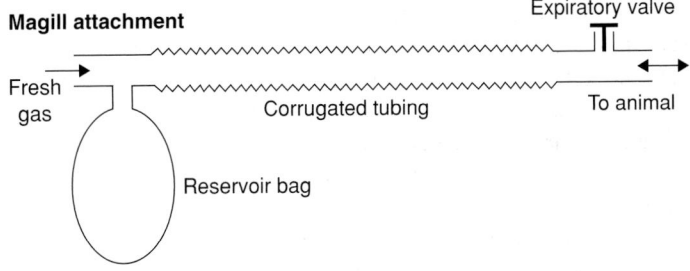

To animal

Open ended
reservoir bag

Fresh gas

Magill attachment

Expiratory valve

Fresh
gas

Corrugated tubing

To animal

Reservoir bag

Modified Bain circuit (Penlon Ltd)

Expired
gas

Valve

To animal
From animal

Fresh
gas

Corrugated tubing

Reservoir bag

Figure 41.6   Circle system. The direction of gas flow is controlled by two one-way valves (a), the circuit incorporates a soda lime canister to absorb carbon dioxide (b) and a reservoir (c).

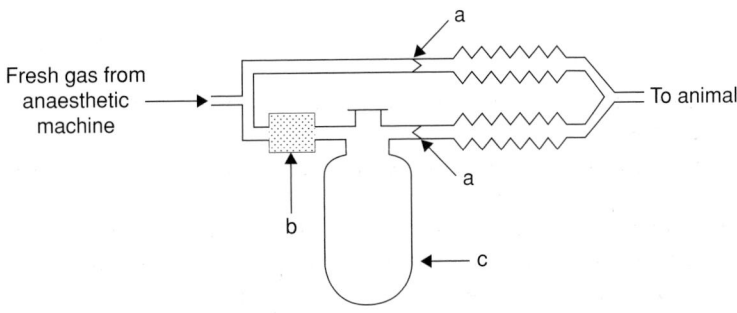

a

Fresh gas from
anaesthetic
machine

To animal

a

b

c

setting. This can easily result in the animal becoming too lightly anaesthetised. To avoid this, an anaesthetic agent analyser can be placed in the circuit. If an agent analyser is not available, great care must be taken to monitor the depth of anaesthesia regularly. It is also advisable, irrespective of the monitoring apparatus available, to seek assistance from an experienced anaesthetist when first using a circle system.

Pre-anaesthetic preparations

Before anaesthetising an animal, it is important to establish that all of the equipment needed is in working order and readily available and that any personnel involved are familiar with its operation. In the UK it is necessary to check that the particular anaesthetic technique to be used is authorised on the relevant project and personal licences. The animals to be anaesthetised should have been examined for signs of ill-health, and a period of acclimatisation allowed so that they could recover from the stress of transportation and adapt to their new environment. A period of acclimatisation also enables training of the animal, for example to familiarise it to physical restraint, and to record basic pre-operative data such as body weight (and growth rate) and food and water consumption.

Dogs, cats, ferrets, and non-human primates may vomit on induction of anaesthesia, so it is advisable to withhold food for twelve to sixteen hours, and water for three to four hours, before induction of anaesthesia. Pigs rarely vomit when anaesthetised, although withholding food for twelve hours is usual. Sheep and other ruminants regurgitate stomach contents irrespective of whether they have been fasted or not. In animals kept on grass, housing indoors and withdrawal of food overnight may reduce the degree of gas accumulation in the stomach during anaesthesia. Withholding food from ruminants which are housed indoors has relatively little effect. In both instances it is advisable to pass a stomach tube after induction of anaesthesia to reduce the build-up of gas.

Pre-anaesthetic fasting of small rodents and rabbits is unnecessary since vomiting during induction does not occur in these species. In addition, in small rodents fasting may result in a depletion of glycogen reserves and the development of hypoglycaemia, and in rabbits and guinea pigs it may lead to the development of gastro-intestinal disorders in the post-operative period. If fasting is required for a particular research protocol, it is important to remember that these species are coprophagic so removing the animal's food may not result in an empty stomach. Problems are most unlikely to be encountered when allowing free access to both food and water until immediately prior to anaesthesia in both rodents and rabbits.

Pre-anaesthetic medication

It may be helpful to include pre-anaesthetic medication as part of the anaesthetic protocol. The advantages of this are:

- use of sedatives and tranquillisers can reduce aggression and fear or apprehension;
- use of analgesics can reduce pain and provide 'pre-emptive analgesia' (see below, p. 399);
- atropine or glycopyrollate can be given to reduce bronchial and salivary secretions, and to protect the heart from vagal inhibition caused by some surgical procedures (e.g. manipulation of the viscera);
- use of sedatives, tranquillisers and analgesics can reduce the amount of anaesthetic needed to produce desired level of anaesthesia.

Some of the commonly used pre-anaesthetic agents are listed in Tables 41.3 (a) and (b).

Animal handling

Whichever method of anaesthesia is chosen, careful and expert handling of the animal is important. The fear and stress associated with movement from the animal holding room to the operating theatre or procedure room should also be considered. In some instances, a balanced anaesthetic regimen may be used which includes administration of a tranquillising drug to calm an animal before it is moved from holding room to theatre.

Anaesthetic management

Many of the problems which may arise during anaesthesia can be minimised by ensuring that the animal is both in overt good health and free from sub-clinical disease. Whenever possible, animals of defined health status should be obtained, so that the occurrence of conditions such as respiratory infections can be minimised.

Anaesthetic monitoring

Even during brief periods of anaesthesia, it is important to give attention to supporting the animal's vital body functions. Onset of surgical anaesthesia usually results in the loss of all protective airway reflexes, and

Table 41.3 (a) Sedatives and tranquillisers for use in small laboratory animals.

	Gerbil	Guinea pig	Hamster	Mouse	Rabbit	Rat
Acepromazine	3 mg/kg i.p.	5 mg/kg i.p.	5 mg/kg i.p.	5 mg/kg i.p.	1–2 mg/kg i/m	2.5 mg/kg i.p.
Diazepam	5 mg/kg i.m.	5 mg/kg i.m.	5 mg/kg i.m.	5 mg/kg i.m.	2 mg/kg i.m.	2.5 mg/kg i.p.
Hypnorm® (fentanyl/ fluanisone)	0.5–1.0 ml/kg i/m	0.5 ml/kg i.m.	0.5 ml/kg i.m.	0.5 ml/kg i.m.	0.3–0.5 ml/kg i.m.	0.5 ml/kg i.m.
Medetomidine	–	–	100 µg/kg s.c.	30–100 µg/kg s.c.	100–500 µg/kg s.c.	30–100 µg/kg s.c.
Midazolam	5 mg/kg i.m.	5 mg/kg i.m.	5 mg/kg i.m.	5 mg/kg i.m.	2 mg/kg i.m.	2.55 mg/kg i.p.
Xylazine	2 mg/kg i.p.		5 mg/kg i.p.	10 mg/kg i.p.	2.5 mg/kg i.m.	10 mg/kg i.p.

Table 41.3 (b) Sedatives and tranquillisers for use in larger laboratory animals.

	Cat	Dog	Pig	Sheep
Acepromazine	0.05–0.2 mg/kg i.m.	0.1–0.25 mg/kg i.m.	0.2 mg/kg i.m.	0.05–0.1 mg/kg i.m.
Diazepam	(unpredictable effects)	(unpredictable effects)	1–2 mg/kg i.m.	2 mg/kg i.m. or 1 mg/kg i.v.
Ketamine	5–20 mg/kg i.m.	–	10–15 mg/kg i.m.	20 mg/kg i.m.
Medetomidine	0.05–0.15 mg/kg i.m. or s.c.	0.01–0.08 mg/kg i.m. or i.p.	–	0.025 mg/kg i.m.
Midazolam	(unpredictable effects)	(unpredictable effects)	1–2 mg/kg i.m.	0.5 mg/kg i.v.
Xylazine	1–2 mg/kg i.m. or s.c.	1–2 mg/kg i.m.	–	0.2 mg/kg i.m.

the animal should be placed in a position with its head and neck extended, to help ensure its airway remains clear and unobstructed. During longer periods of anaesthesia, if inhalational agents are not used, it is often advisable to provide oxygen by face mask to prevent the animal becoming hypoxic. Anaesthetised animals also lose their protective blink reflexes, and the eyes should be protected both from physical damage and from drying. Ophthalmic ointment can be placed in the eyes, or the lids can be taped closed with micropore tape.

Careful monitoring of the patient is important to allow early detection and correction of any problems which may arise. In all species, respiratory and cardiovascular function are of primary importance, but in small rodents in particular, maintenance of body temperature is of critical importance.

Small mammals have a higher surface area to body weight ratio than larger species such as the pig and the dog, and so lose heat more rapidly. For example, significant falls in body temperature (5–10 °C) can occur in mice within fifteen minutes of induction of anaesthesia. Monitoring and maintenance of body temperature is of particular importance. Most anaesthetics depress thermoregulation, and this effect, coupled with use of cold fluids, shaving and preparation of the surgical site, and use of cold anaesthetic

gases can rapidly result in severe hypothermia. Small mammals should be placed on a heating pad, and if necessary covered in insulating material (e.g. bubble packing or aluminium foil). Body temperature should be monitored, and although this is difficult without specialist equipment in mice, suitable inexpensive thermometers for larger species can be obtained easily (RS Components Ltd, Corby, Northants, UK) (Figure 41.7).

Respiratory function

Respiratory rate can be monitored relatively easily in animals weighing over 200 g using inexpensive respiratory monitors which use a thermistor to detect the temperature change associated with each breath. A better indication of respiratory function can be gained by using a pulse oximeter. These instruments measure the percentage saturation of haemoglobin in the blood, and so indicate the adequacy of oxygenation. These generally function well in animals weighing more than 200 g. Probes can be placed on the feet of rats and guinea pigs, and across the tail in rabbits and cats or on the tongue or toe pad in rabbits, ferrets, cats and dogs (Figure 41.8). In pigs the probe can be placed across the tail or on the ear. The probes generally function well, but in smaller animals they are particularly susceptible to signal loss caused by

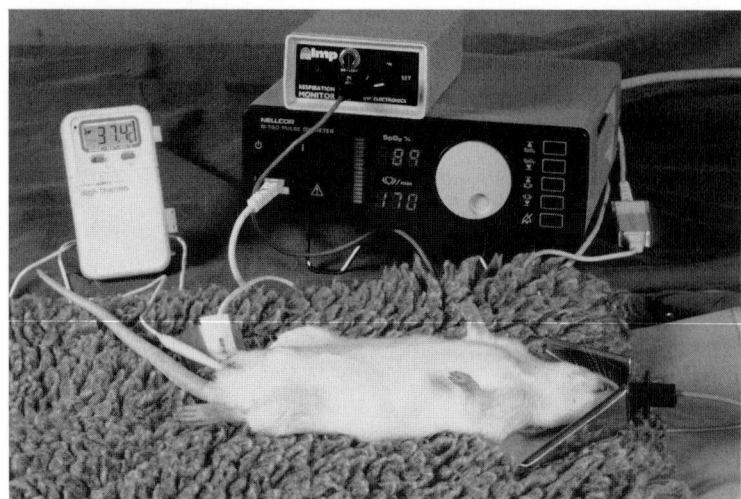

Figure 41.7 Rat on a heating pad. Body temperature is monitored via a rectal probe from an electronic thermometer. The rat is also being monitored using a respiratory monitor (with a thermistor sensor at the animal's nose) and a pulse oximeter (with a probe placed on the hind foot).

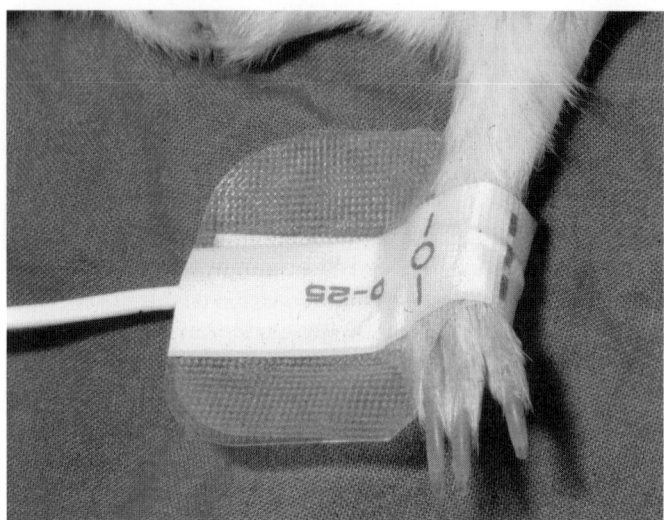

Figure 41.8 Pulse oximetry probe placed on the hind-foot of a guinea pig.

peripheral vasoconstriction. This is a common problem when anaesthesia is produced using ketamine/medetomidine or ketamine/xylazine. Many instruments designed for use in man will have an upper heart rate limit of 250 beats per minute (bpm). This is frequently exceeded in many small mammals. Some instruments will continue to register an accurate oxygen saturation, but others may fail at high heart rates. If possible it is helpful to assess an instrument before purchase, and in many instances instruments designed for veterinary use are to be preferred. Several of these have upper heart rate limits of 300–350 bpm or greater, and so can be used to their full potential with small mammals.

Respiratory depression

If respiratory depression occurs, it can be treated by assisted ventilation and use of respiratory stimulants such as doxapram. It is advisable to administer oxygen immediately following induction of anaesthesia with injectable anaesthetics, since all of the agents used produce some degree of respiratory depression. In many instances, severe hypoxia occurs, and if uncorrected this can lead to cardiac failure.

Assisting ventilation is considerably easier if the animal has been intubated, and this is an easy technique to master in the dog, cat, sheep, pig, non-human primate and rabbit. Endotracheal intubation of small rodents is more difficult, but can be carried out with practice. Assisting ventilation, by manually compressing the thorax and providing oxygen by face mask, can be effective, but attempts to ventilate the lungs using a face-mask are often relatively ineffective. In small rodents such as the rat, ventilation can be assisted temporarily by positioning the animal with its head and neck in extension, and placing the barrel of a plastic syringe over the nose. Gently blowing down the tube will usually enable the lungs to be inflated.

Detailed descriptions of endotracheal intubation are given in Flecknell (1996). In general, intubation is made easier if an appropriately sized laryngoscope blade is obtained, so that the larynx can be visualised clearly. In species in which the oropharyngeal opening is relatively small (e.g. the pig and the rabbit), it is often easier to use an introducer to straighten the endotracheal tube and guide it into the larynx. A similar technique can be employed using an otoscope to visualise the larynx in smaller species such as rats. An introducer is passed down the speculum into the trachea, the otoscope is removed and the endotracheal tube passed over the introducer and into the trachea. The introducer is then removed and the tube tied in place.

In all species it is advisable to administer 100% oxygen for one to two minutes before attempting intubation. Insertion of the tube should always be carried out gently. If difficulty is encountered, the tube can be withdrawn, repositioned and a further attempt made. When learning the technique, it is helpful to monitor the animal with a pulse oximeter during this process, so that attempts can be discontinued and oxygen administered if the animal becomes hypoxic (oxygen saturation < 80%).

Cardiovascular function

Circulatory function can be assessed clinically by palpating the peripheral pulse in larger species, and by observing the colour of mucus membranes and the capillary refill rate. This is assessed by pressing gently on the gums with a forefinger, then observing the rate at which the blanching of the mucus membranes is reversed after removal of finger pressure. This should occur in less than one second.

Pulse oximetry can provide some indication of cardiovascular function, but more information can be obtained by measuring arterial blood pressure. Invasive blood pressure monitoring, which requires cannulation of an artery, is relatively straightforward in larger species, and femoral arterial cannulae can be placed through the skin in dogs, pigs and sheep. In smaller animals (e.g. cat) arterial cannulation requires surgical exposure of the vessel, although in the rabbit the central ear artery can be used. Non-invasive monitoring, using an inflatable cuff and a detector, is useful in the dog, but is less reliable in other species, and not often used. The electrical activity of the heart can be monitored using an electrocardiogram (ECG). This will allow assessment of both cardiac rate and rhythm, and allow detection of any abnormal electrical activity. Apparatus is usually designed for larger (>2 kg) animals, with heart rates of below 250 bpm. Some equipment is available which can be used successfully in very small mammals at high heart rates (up to 800 bpm, EC60, Silogic Inc.)

Circulatory failure

Methods for supporting the circulation or treating cardiac arrest are similar in most species, but correct use of these techniques requires considerable experience. It is always preferable to try to anticipate impending problems, and to try to prevent them. If some blood loss is likely, then setting up an intravenous infusion of fluid is advisable. Initially, a balanced electrolyte solution should be given, at a rate of approximately 10 ml/kg/h, and if blood loss occurs, whole blood or plasma volume expanders (e.g. Haemaccel®) can be given. Whole blood should be collected from a donor animal and immediately mixed with acid-citrate-dextrose (ACD), at a rate of one part ACD to four parts blood. Blood from most species can be stored at 4 °C for several days until required. Cross-matching of blood is advisable, but in an emergency, an initial transfusion can usually be given safely in several species.

If intravenous administration of fluids is considered impractical or technically too demanding, then some circulatory support can be provided by administering intraperitoneal or subcutaneous electrolyte solutions. This is ineffective in cases of severe haemorrhage, but is of value in providing fluid supplementation post-operatively.

Stages of anaesthesia, monitoring depth of anaesthesia

It is clearly important to ensure that an animal is at an appropriate depth of anaesthesia. If animals are too deeply anaesthetised, there is a higher risk of complications or death. In addition, since the effects of anaesthetics on the different body systems are dose-dependent, there is a greater likelihood of anaesthesia interfering with a research protocol if unnecessarily high dose rates are used. Conversely, of course, if animals are too lightly anaesthetised, they may experience pain or distress.

A number of reflex responses can be assessed in order to judge the depth of anaesthesia. In some species, for example dogs and cats, the position of the eye can be monitored – with many anaesthetics the globe rotates downwards as anaesthesia deepens, and then returns to a central position at very deep planes of anaesthesia. Very light and very deep anaesthesia can be distinguished by testing for the presence of a blink reflex, when the corner of the eye is lightly touched – this is absent at deeper planes of anaesthesia. A further indication of anaesthetic depth can be obtained by assessing the degree of relaxation of the jaw – as anaesthesia deepens, the jaw relaxes so that it can be opened easily. It is important to note that these responses do vary between species, and perhaps the most useful technique is assessment of a response to a brief painful stimulus. This is usually carried out by extending one hindlimb, and pinching the skin in the interdigital space, or pinching a toe. If there is no reflex withdrawal of the leg, or a barely perceptible response, then the animal has reached a depth of anaesthesia sufficient to allow surgery to be carried out. In larger species, such as sheep and pigs, applying a clamp across the coronary band of one digit is often used as the painful stimulus. The response to pinching the ear or tail is also of use.

Detailed descriptions of the order in which reflex responses are lost have been published (Thurmon et al. 1996), in an attempt to classify particular stages and planes of anaesthesia. Since anaesthesia is a dynamic process, and animals may rapidly move between different planes, such a rigid classification is not often particularly useful in many laboratory species. A second problem is that changes such as eye position, loss of the blink reflex, and changes in the pattern and depth of respiration vary depending

upon the anaesthetic regimen used. It is important, then, to become familiar with an animal's responses to a particular anaesthetic protocol, so that the depth of anaesthesia can be assessed.

Neuromuscular blocking (NMB)

Many of the assessments described above rely on changes in skeletal muscle tone, or the ability to make voluntary muscle movements. If a neuromuscular blocking drug, such as pancuronium, is administered, then all of these responses are immediately abolished. It then becomes very difficult to assess the depth of anaesthesia, for this reason the use of NMB requires specific Home Office authority (see Chapter 36).

At present, if a procedure involving the use of neuromuscular blocking agents is to be carried out, the following points should be considered:

- The procedure should first be undertaken without the use of a neuromuscular blocking drug, so that the adequacy of the anaesthetic protocol can be assessed.
- If the animal appears to be anaesthetised to an appropriate depth, then the NMB agent can be added to the regimen. It is strongly recommended that a familiar anaesthetic regimen is used, and that the NMB agent be administered by intermittent injection, rather than as a continuous infusion. This enables somatic reflex responses to be reassessed periodically in order to judge the adequacy of anaesthesia.
- During the period of neuromuscular blockage, it is advisable to monitor cardiovascular autonomic responses to surgical stimuli. Although a lack of response does not guarantee adequate anaesthesia, a large increase (15–20%) in heart rate or blood pressure is a strong indication of inadequate anaesthetic depth.

Finally, it is worth noting that neuromuscular blocking agents are *not* required simply to mechanically ventilate an animal.

New methods for monitoring depth of anaesthesia

Currently, work is in progress to evaluate the use of the electroencephalogram and evoked potential as means of assessing the depth of anaesthesia. These monitoring techniques are likely to remain suitable only for specialist applications for some time, but may be of particular value in long-term, non-recovery neurophysiological studies, where the required apparatus may already be readily available.

Post-anaesthetic care

Since all animals will require some degree of special attention in the post-operative period, it is preferable to provide a separate recovery area. This not only enables more appropriate environmental conditions to be maintained but also encourages individual attention and special nursing.

During recovery from anaesthesia, care should be taken that respiratory obstruction does not occur, and that animals are kept warm. In most instances small animals can be allowed to recover in their normal cages, placed either in a recovery room (maintained at a high ambient temperature, with supplemental heating of the cage as necessary) or inside an incubator. A temperature of 25–30 °C is needed for adult animals, 35–37 °C for neonates. If an incubator is unavailable, heating pads and lamps should be provided. Care must be taken not to overheat the patient, and a thermometer should be placed next to the animal to record its surface temperature. If groups of small mammals are anaesthetised, and allowed to recover together, care must be taken that semi-conscious animals are not suffocated by cage mates lying on top of them.

Small rodents and rabbits should not be allowed to recover from anaesthesia in cages which contain sawdust or wood shavings as bedding. This type of bedding will often stick to the animal's eyes, nose and mouth so should be replaced by more suitable materials. A synthetic bedding with a texture similar to sheepskin (Vetbed®, Alfred Cox Ltd.) has proven particularly useful for all species of animal. It is washable, autoclavable, extremely durable and appears to provide a comfortable surface for the animal. If such material is unavailable, towelling or a blanket should be used. Tissue paper is often provided as bedding for small rodents, but it is relatively ineffective as animals usually push it aside during recovery from anaesthesia and end up lying in the bottom of a plastic cage soiled with urine and faeces. Rabbits and guinea pigs should not be placed in grid-bottomed cages to recover from anaesthesia, but should be placed either directly in an incubator or in a temporary plastic or cardboard holding box.

Animals should be provided with water, but care must be taken that they do not spill water bowls – if the animal becomes wet it will lose heat rapidly. Small rodents are usually accustomed to using water bottles, so this is rarely a problem, but it can present difficulties with rabbits, guinea pigs, ferrets and larger species. It is often advisable to administer fluid therapy postoperatively. In larger animals, this can be given by intravenous infusion, but in small rodents it is most convenient to give warmed (37 °C) subcutaneous or intraperitoneal dextrose/saline at the end of surgery. Animals should be encouraged to eat as soon as possible after recovery from anaesthesia. If necessary, highly palatable foods should be offered. Providing soaked pelleted diet is often beneficial for small rodents.

Animals should be checked regularly until they have completely recovered from anaesthesia, and individual records should be kept of the nature of the procedure. Even minor procedures can be associated with a reduction in food and water consumption and body weight, and obtaining pre-operative measurements of these variables will allow them to be used to monitor the animal's recovery.

If animals have undergone an invasive procedure, then they may experience post-operative pain and this must be controlled using analgesics. Further information on pain assessment and analgesic use are provided below.

The effective alleviation of post-operative pain in laboratory animals should be considered an important goal in all research establishments. Despite the emphasis given to humane treatment of laboratory animals in the national legislation of many countries, analgesics may still not be administered routinely in the post-operative period. This omission is particularly common when the animals concerned are small rodents. When analgesics are administered, assessment of their efficacy is usually based on highly subjective criteria. The lack of an objective means of pain assessment may account in part for the relatively infrequent use of analgesics in animals, in comparison to their use in man. A variety of methods for assessing pain have been described (see Flecknell & Waterman-Pearson 2000), including numeric scoring systems based on the methods described by Morton and Griffiths (1985), or use of visual analogue scales. Alternatively, assessment may be by clinical assessment, without using a formal scoring system. In all circumstances, pain assessment will be facilitated by a good knowledge of the species-specific behaviours of the animal being assessed, and preferably a knowledge and comparison of the individual animal's behaviour before and after the onset of pain. In some circumstances, palpation or manipulation of the affected area and assessment of the responses obtained can be useful, as can administration of an analgesic regimen or dose rates which have been shown to be effective in controlled clinical studies, and evaluation of the change in behaviour this brings about. When trying to identify signs of pain, it is also important to be aware of the non-specific effects of any analgesic, anaesthetic or other drugs which have been administered

Pain relief

Although we would wish to alleviate pain because of concerns for animal welfare, a number of counter-arguments have been advanced to justify withholding analgesics.

(1) 'Alleviation of post-operative pain will result in the animal injuring itself': provided that surgery has been carried out competently, administration of analgesics which allow resumption of normal activity, rarely results in problems associated with the removal of pain's protective function. Claims that analgesic administration results in skin suture removal are unsubstantiated, and contrary to findings in our laboratory. In certain circumstances, for example after major ortho-paedic surgery, additional measures to protect and support the operative site may be required, but this is preferable to allowing an animal to experience unrelieved pain. All that is required in these circumstances is to temporarily reduce the animal's cage or pen size temporarily, or to provide additional external fixation or support for the wound. It must be emphasised that these measures are very rarely necessary, and in our institute, administration of analgesics to laboratory animals after a wide variety of surgical procedures has not resulted in any adverse clinical effects.

(2) 'Analgesic drugs have undesirable side-effects such as respiratory depression': the side-effects of opiates in animals are generally less marked than in humans and should rarely be a significant consideration when planning a post-operative care regimen.

(3) 'We don't know the appropriate dose rates and dosage regimens': this is primarily a problem of poor dissemination of existing information. Virtually every available analgesic drug has undergone extensive testing in animals. Dose rates are therefore available for a range of drugs in many common laboratory species (Flecknell 1984; Liles & Flecknell 1992). Although these dose rates are likely to be safe, they are dose rates which are effective in experimental analgesiometry. Determining doses which will be effective for clinical use requires use of a method of pain assessment. Nevertheless, in most instances they provide a reasonable guide as to a suitable, and safe, dose rate.

(4) 'Pain relieving drugs might adversely affect the results of an experiment': although there will be occasions when the use of one or other type of analgesic is contraindicated, it is extremely unlikely that there will be no suitable analgesic which could be administered. More usually, the reluctance to administer analgesics is based upon the misconceived idea that the use of any additional medication in an experimental animal is undesirable. The influence of analgesic administration in a research protocol should be considered in the context of the overall response of the animal to anaesthesia and surgery. The responses to surgical stress may overshadow any possible adverse interactions associated with analgesic administration. An additional consideration is that many arrangements for intra-operative care fail to control variables such as body temperature, respiratory function and blood pressure. It seems illogical to assume that changes in the function of the cardiovascular or respiratory systems are unimportant, but that administration of an analgesic will be of overriding significance. It should be considered an ethical responsibility of a research worker to provide a reasoned, scientific justification if analgesic drugs are to be withheld. It is also important to realise that the presence of pain can produce a range of undesirable physiological changes, which may radically alter the rate of recovery from surgical procedures.

Table 41.4 (a)   Analgesics for use in small laboratory animals. Note that these are only suggestions based on clinical experience and the limited published data which is available. Dose rates should be adjusted depending upon the clinical response of the animal. (Data adapted from Flecknell & Waterman-Pearson, 2000.) bid = twice daily.

Analgesic	Gerbil	Guinea Pig	Hamster	Mouse	Rabbit	Rat
Buprenorphine	0.1 mg/kg s.c.	0.05 mg/kg s.c.	0.1 mg/kg s.c.	0.1 mg/kg s.c.	0.01–0.05 mg/kg s.c.	0.05 mg/kg s.c.
Butorphanol	?	2 mg/kg s.c.	?	1–5 mg/kg s.c.	0.1–0.5 mg/kg s.c.	2 mg/kg s.c.
Carpofen	?	?	?	?	1.5 mg/kg *per os* bid	5 mg/kg bid
Flunixin	?	?	?	2.5 mg/kg s.c. bid	1.1 mg/kg s.c. bid	2.5 mg/kg s.c. bid
Ketoprofen	?	?	?	?	3 mg/kg i.m.	5 mg/kg i.m.
Morphine	?	2–5 mg/kg s.c. or i.m. 4 hourly	?	2.5 mg/kg s.c. or i/m 4 hourly	2–5 mg/kg s.c. or i.m. 4 hourly	2.5 mg/kg s.c. or i.m. 4 hourly
Pethidine	?	10–20 mg/kg s.c. or i.m. 2–3 hourly	?	10–20 mg/kg s.c. or i.m. 2–3 hourly	10 mg/kg s.c. or i.m. 2–3 hourly	10–20 mg/kg s.c. or i.m. 2–3 hourly

Table 41.4 (b)   Analgesics for use in larger laboratory animals. Note that these are only suggestions based on clinical experience and the limited published data which is available. Dose rates should be adjusted depending upon the clinical response of the animal. (Data adapted from Flecknell and Waterman-Pearson, 2000)

Analgesic	Cat	Dog	Pig	Sheep
Buprenorphine	0.005–0.01 mg/kg i.m., s.c. or i.v. 6–12 hourly	0.005–0.02 mg/kg i.m., s.c. or i.v. 6–12 hourly	0.005–0.02 mg/kg i.m. or i.v. 6–12 hourly	0.005–0.02 mg/kg i.m. or i.v. 4 hourly
Butorphanol	0.4 mg/kg s.c. or i.v. 3–4 hourly	0.2–0.4 mg/kg s.c. or i.m. 3–4 hourly	?	?
Carprofen	4 mg/kg s.c. or i.v. (once)	4 mg/kg s.c. or i.v. (once daily)	2–4 mg/kg s.c. or i.v., once daily (?2–3 days)	1.5–2 mg/kg s.c. or i.v., once daily (?2–3 days)
Flunixin	1 mg/kg s.c. (once)	1 mg/kg i.v. or i.m. 12 hourly (up to 3 days)	1 mg/kg i.v. or s.c. once daily	2 mg/kg i.v. or s.c. once daily
Ketoprofen	2 mg/kg s.c. daily (up to 3 days)	2 mg/kg s.c. daily (up to 3 days)	3 mg/kg s.c. (once)	?
Morphine	0.1 mg/kg i.m., 4 hourly	0.5–5 mg/kg i.m., 4 hourly	0.2–1 mg/kg i.m., 4 hourly	0.2–0.5 mg/kg i.m., ?4 hourly
Pethidine	2–10 mg/kg i.m. or i.v. 2–4 hourly	10 mg/kg i.m. or i.v. 2–4 hourly	2 mg/kg i.m. or i.v. 2–4 hourly	2 mg/kg i.m. or i.v. 2–4 hourly

Pain relief agents

Analgesics can be broadly divided into two groups, the opioids or narcotic analgesics and the non-steroidal anti-inflammatory drugs (NSAIDs) such as aspirin. Local anaesthetics can also be used to provide post-operative pain relief by blocking all sensation from the affected area. Suggested dose rates of analgesics are given in Tables 41.4 (a) and (b).

Pre-emptive analgesia

During anaesthesia, although the animal is unconscious and so unaware of any pain, nerve impulses from the surgical site continue to be generated and are transmitted to the central nervous system (CNS). These nerve impulses trigger changes in the CNS which increase the degree of pain that is perceived when the animal recovers consciousness. If analgesics are administered before any potentially painful stimuli occur, then they are generally more effective in preventing post-operative pain. For this reason, it is now widely recommended that analgesics should be administered pre-operatively, as this provides more effective pain relief, and also may reduce the dose of anaesthetic required. For example, experience in small rodents and rabbits has shown that use of buprenorphine in this way enables the concentration of isoflurane or halothane needed for surgical anaesthesia to be reduced by 0.25–0.5%. When using neuroleptanalgesics, the opioid component will provide analgesia during surgery, and this can conveniently be partially reversed with buprenorphine or butorphanol at the end of the procedure. If the latter opioid is used, although it provides better reversal, it has a short duration of action, so either additional doses should be given, or it should be combined with a potent NSAID.

In some circumstances, it may not be possible to administer analgesics pre-emptively, nevertheless, administering analgesics as soon as is practical is of significant benefit. The longer pain is established, the greater will be the degree of central hypersensitivity, and the more difficult pain management becomes.

'Multi-modal' pain therapy

Clinical pain arises from a combination of central and peripheral hypersensitivity involving a multiplicity of pathways, mechanisms and transmitter systems. So it is unlikely that a single class of analgesic will completely alleviate pain, irrespective of the dose used. In order to provide the most effective clinical pain relief, drugs of different classes will be required, each acting on a different part of the pain system. This concept is easy to apply, for example by combining the use of opioids with NSAIDs. The opioid acts centrally to limit the input of nociceptive information into the CNS and so reduces central hypersensitivity. In contrast, the NSAID acts both centrally, to limit the central changes induced by the nociceptive information which does get through, and also peripherally to decrease inflammation during and after surgery, and thus limit the nociceptive information entering the CNS as a result of the inflammation. By acting on different points of the pain pathways, the combination is more effective than either drug given alone. Adding a local anaesthetic to this regimen can provide additional analgesia by blocking specific nerve pathways, and so further improve the degree of pain control.

Problems with analgesics

A number of problems arise when analgesics are administered to control post-operative pain in laboratory species. The most important problem is the short duration of action of most of the opioid analgesics. Maintenance of effective analgesia with, for example, pethidine, may require repeated administration every one to three hours, depending upon the species. Continuation of such a regime overnight can cause practical problems. One method of avoiding this difficulty is to use buprenorphine as the analgesic, since there is good evidence in humans, rodents, rabbits and pigs that it has a duration of action of six to twelve hours. Its duration of action in the sheep appears to be considerably less, although still of longer duration than pethidine and morphine.

An alternative approach is to adopt the well-established human clinical technique of administering analgesics as a continuous infusion. Infusions of analgesics have the advantage of maintaining effective plasma levels of the analgesic, so providing continuous pain relief. This is in contrast to intermittent injections, where pain may return before the next dose of analgesic is administered. This technique obviously poses some methodological difficulties in animals, but if an indwelling catheter and harness and swivel apparatus are available, then this can be arranged quite simply. In larger species (>3–4 kg bodyweight), a lightweight infusion pump can be bandaged directly to the animal and continuous infusion made simply by means of a butterfly-type needle anchored subcutaneously or intramuscularly.

Epidural and intrathecal opioids

Epidural and intrathecal opioids have been shown to have a prolonged effect and to provide effective analgesia in several different species. Epidural morphine administration is now widely used by veterinary anaesthetists for providing post-operative analgesia in dogs, and the technique could usefully be applied in the larger laboratory species. The necessary techniques of epidural or intrathecal injection have been described in the rabbit (Kero et al. 1981) and the cat, dog, sheep and pig (Thurmon et al. 1996; Dobromylskyj et al. 2000).

Oral administration

The need for repeated injections of analgesics is time consuming and may be distressing to the animal, particularly in smaller species which require firm physical restraint to enable an injection to be given safely and effectively. In addition, the need for repeated injections requires veterinary or other staff to attend the animal overnight. Administering analgesics in the food or drinking water might therefore be of value, but several practical problems limit the use of this technique. Some animals eat and drink relatively infrequently or may only do so at night. Food and water intake may be depressed following surgery, and this, coupled with wide individual variation in consumption make routine application of the technique difficult. Finally, the high first-pass liver metabolism of opioids administered by the oral route requires that high dose rates are given, and this can represent a significant cost if all of the animal's drinking water or food is medicated. Administration of small quantities of medicated food does not avoid the need for repeated attendance overnight, but does remove the need for repeated subcutaneous or intramuscular injections in small rodents. Provision of analgesia with buprenorphine in flavoured gelatine, buprenorphine jello, seems to be an effective means of providing post-operative pain relief.

Additional considerations in pain relief

Although the use of analgesic drugs remains the most important technique for reducing post-operative pain, the use of these drugs must be integrated into a total scheme for peri-operative care. Pain relief in the immediate recovery period can be provided by including an analgesic drug in any pre-anaesthetic medication. Good surgical technique which minimises tissue trauma and the prevention of tension on suture lines can considerably reduce post-operative pain. The use of bandages to pad and protect traumatised tissue must not be overlooked and forms an essential adjunct to the use of analgesic drugs. Aside from measures directed towards alleviating or preventing pain, it is important to consider the overall care of the animal and the prevention of distress.

Supply of anaesthetic and analgesic agents

All of the drugs discussed above are subject to some control with regard to their supply in most countries. In the UK, all are prescription only medicines (POMs) and their supply is controlled by the Medicines Act, 1968. In addition, many anaesthetics and all of the opioid (morphine-like) analgesics are subject to additional controls. Records of their purchase and use must be maintained in a specified manner, and they must be stored in a locked receptacle. Although a number of health-care professionals can supply or dispense some of these agents for use in man, in the UK the institute's named veterinary surgeon is the only person who can supply these drugs for use in the laboratory animals which are under his or her care.

References

Dobromylskyj, P., Flecknell, P.A., Lascelles, B.D. et al. (2000) Management of post-operative and other acute pain. In: P.A. Flecknell and A. Waterman-Pearson (Eds) *Pain Management in Animals*. W.B. Saunders Co., London.

Flecknell, P.A. (1984) The relief of pain in laboratory animals. *Laboratory Animals*, **18**: 147–60.

Flecknell, P.A. (1994) *Laboratory Animal Anaesthesia*. Academic Press, London.

Flecknell, P.A. and Waterman-Pearson, A. (2001) *Pain Management in Animals*. Academic Press, London.

Kero, P., Thomasson, B. and Soppi, A.M. (1981) Spinal anaesthesia in the rabbit. *Laboratory Animals*, **15**: 347–348.

Kohn, D.F., Wixson, S.K., White, W.J. and Benson, G.J. (1997) *Anaesthesia and Analgesia in Laboratory Animals*. Academic Press, New York.

Liles, J.H. and Flecknell, P.A. (1992) The use of non-steroidal anti-inflammatory drugs for the relief of pain in laboratory rodents and rabbits. *Laboratory Animals*, **26**: 214–255.

Morton, D.B. and Griffiths, P.H.M. (1985) Guidelines on the recognition of pain, distress and discomfort in experimental animals and an hypothesis for assessment. *Veterinary Record* **116**: 431–436.

Thurmon, J.C., Tranquilli, W.J. and Benson, G.J. (1996) *Lumb and Jones' Veterinary Anaesthesia* (3rd edn). Lea & Febiger, Baltimore.

42
Euthanasia

Jasmine B. Barley

Introduction

Euthanasia is an unpleasant but necessary task which has to be performed by people working in designated scientific procedure establishments. There are several reasons why laboratory animals have to be killed and these fall into three main groups:

- to alleviate unnecessary suffering, e.g. ill health, injury or where there might be continuing adverse effects;
- the animal is surplus to requirements, e.g. not exhibiting a required characteristic (age, type or sex are not needed);
- as part of an experiment or for other scientific purposes, e.g. at the end of an experiment, to provide tissues or blood for a scientific purpose.

The term euthanasia means 'bringing about an easy death'. To achieve this, all personnel involved in the use and care of laboratory animals must be capable of killing an animal with care and compassion and without causing the animal any unnecessary pain, stress or discomfort.

Legal control

The Animals (Scientific Procedures) Act 1986 considers methods of euthanasia in two ways. One group of methods, listed in Schedule 1 of the Act, are not considered regulated procedures. All other methods, performed on an animal for scientific purposes, are regulated procedures and must therefore be authorised by project and personal licences. In certain circumstances the Home Secretary may permit non-Schedule 1 methods to be added to a certificate of designation as a special condition, in which case the method has the effect of being a Schedule 1 method in that establishment.

Although Schedule 1 methods are not regulated procedures they are subject to specific controls:

- they can only be carried out by those who have demonstrated their competence in the technique and whose name therefore appears on a register of competent people kept on behalf of the certificate holder;
- methods involving the use of captive bolt guns can only be used by veterinary surgeons and holders of a licence granted under the Welfare of Animals (Slaughter or Killing) Regulations 1955;
- methods involving the use of free bullets can only be used by veterinary surgeons.

The responsibility for ensuring euthanasia is carried out proficiently is given to several people by the Animals (Scientific Procedures) 1986 which requires:

(1) The certificate holder:
   — to ensure that a person competent to kill animals not subject to a project licence is available (Standard Condition 17, designated scientific procedure establishments); and
   — to keep a register of people competent in Schedule 1 methods of euthanasia.

(2) The Named Animal Care and Welfare Officer (NACWO):
   — to be familiar with the methods listed in Schedule 1 under the 1986 Act and other methods used in the establishment and either be competent in their use or know how to contact someone who is.

(3) The Named Veterinary Surgeon (NVS):
— to be familiar with the methods listed in Schedule 1 under the 1986 Act and other methods used in the establishment and be competent in their use.

Factors affecting choice of method of euthanasia

The most suitable method of euthanasia must be selected for each set of circumstances. Factors which need to be considered include the following.

Species

Some species are more difficult to handle, may not have readily available veins or may react adversely to particular methods or agents, e.g. rabbits may react adversely to gases and show signs of excitation, therefore other methods are preferable (Green 1979).

Age and size of the animal

Beyond a certain age and size some physical methods (e.g. cervical dislocation) become more difficult and the likelihood of the animal suffering increases. Difficulties may also be experienced with very young animals, e.g. the use of carbon dioxide is considered unsuitable for neonate animals due to their higher tolerance of CO_2 and the consequential increase in the time it takes for them to die.

Numbers of animals to be killed

It is unusual for species other than small mammals or birds to be required to be killed in large numbers, but killing large numbers of any animal is stressful for the operator. Where large numbers are to be killed the use of physical methods may be precluded due to operator fatigue/distress and consequent risk of reduced efficiency of the method.

Fate of the cadaver

The scientific study an animal is involved in will often dictate the method of euthanasia which must be used. Every effort is made to prevent animal wastage so even if an animal is killed because it is surplus to stock or too old for breeding, its tissues are often recovered for *in vitro* studies and this future use will influence the method of euthanasia used. Examples include:

- physical methods will be unsuitable if the brain or spinal cord tissues are required or the carcass is to be used for dissection;
- chemical methods are unsuitable for hysterectomy rederivation due to their effect on the unborn young.

Other factors determining the choice of method of euthanasia

- *Temperament of individual animals*: Particularly larger species, aggressive or excitable animals may be difficult to restrain, thus making the use of injectable agents difficult.

- *Skill of the operator*: As has been mentioned above, individuals must undergo a course of instruction and a form of assessment to prove their competence in each method they will need to use and each species they will use it on. The methods which can be used in any establishment will be restricted to the methods staff are competent to use.

- *Availability of the necessary apparatus*: Most methods of euthanasia require simple apparatus and can be carried out in most circumstances (e.g. injection of anaesthetic or cervical dislocation of a small mammal) but some methods require more elaborate or unusual apparatus (captive bolt gun or anaesthetic machine). Clearly if the apparatus is not available methods which need them cannot be used.

- *Safety of other animals and operator*: Any operation involving animals has a risk associated with it, for instance, the risk of bites and scratches. Euthanasia involves some extra elements, e.g.:
  - unless a suitable scavenging system is available the risk to human health posed by some inhalational anaesthetics may be precluded;
  - free bullets can leave the body at any angle and can injure animals or people standing by.

- *Economic considerations*: Economics must never be the overriding consideration in the choice of methods of euthanasia, but it is a valid reason to select between two or more appropriate methods, e.g. the cost of anaesthetic agents, especially if large numbers of animals are to be killed, may render their use undesirable.

In addition to the factors mentioned above the following points should be considered:

- the method must be reliable and non-reversible;
- the time taken to produce loss of consciousness must be as short as possible;
- the time required to produce death must be as short as possible.

Euthanasia techniques

Euthanasia only provides an easy, painless death if:

- the animal is treated with appropriate care before the procedure begins;
- the method is appropriate for the circumstances and efficiently carried out (hence the need for training and proof of competence);
- death is definitely confirmed at the end of the procedure.

Before the procedure

Although most people find killing animals an unpleasant and distressful procedure this must not be communicated to the animal. They must be handled in the same way as any other time or they will sense something unusual and will become stressed. Similarly they will become disturbed if they have to travel to the place they are to be killed (as might be the case with farm animals), if this is unavoidable the use of sedation should be considered.

Animals should never be killed in the vicinity of other animals. Distress can be communicated by sight, sound and odours. Equipment must be thoroughly cleaned between each batch of animals to remove all signs of the previous occupants and previous activity.

Methods of euthanasia

Euthanasia methods may be categorised into physical or chemical methods.

Table 42.1 Physical methods of euthanasia.

Manual	Other Physical
Dislocation of the neck Concussion	Decapitation Stunning by captive bolt, electricity or percussion gun Refrigeration

Physical methods

These descriptions are not intended to be a training manual. Nobody should use a method of euthanasia unless they have been appropriately trained and assessed as competent.

Physical methods are further divided into manual methods and other physical methods (Table 42.1).

Physical methods may be distasteful to the operator, but when applied efficiently often appear less distressing to the animal than other techniques. All of the physical methods of euthanasia involve rapid production of massive trauma to the brain and/or the spinal cord. This trauma results in immediate loss of consciousness and death. Physical methods generally require a greater of level of competence on the part of the operator than does the use of chemical agents. Competence should be achieved by practising on cadavers.

Physical methods have the advantage of avoiding the use of chemical agents which may obscure or interfere with experimental results but conversely may cause damage to the organ of interest.

When using physical methods of euthanasia the operator must always bear in mind the weight restrictions for some species established by Schedule 1 of the Animals (Scientific Procedures) Act 1986.

Cervical dislocation
This method results in rapid disruption of the cervical spinal cord and also usually disruption of the blood supply to the brain. The method is suitable for most of the smaller species, larger animals may present difficulties due to more extensive musculature in the neck region.

Small rodents
The animal is placed on a surface that allows it to grip. A pencil or similar blunt edged object is placed firmly across the back of the neck, a firm grasp is taken around

the hindquarters or the base of the tail which are then pulled back sharply. The neck will dislocate and the animal will die instantly.

Guinea pigs and small rabbits

These animals should be held firmly around the rear of the body or hind legs with one hand and by the head with the other hand. Simultaneously the head is bent sharply backwards and the legs and body pulled downwards. It may help to rotate the head as it is bent backwards.

Alternatively, guinea pigs may be placed on a flat surface facing the operator. One hand is then placed over the top of the head with the first and second fingers on either side of the neck. Pressure on the fingers is increased and the animal is swung so that the body is vertical then let the arm drop swiftly to the side. The weight of the falling guinea pigs body will cause dislocation.

Poultry

The legs of the chicken are taken in one hand and the head between the first two fingers of the other hand with the thumb over the beak. A sharp stretching movement, pulling the head backward over the neck will part the spinal cord in the cervical region.

Chicks in small numbers may be killed by pressing the neck against the sharp edge of a table or similar surface in order to part the vertebrae.

In all cases a gap between the vertebrae of the cervical region should be felt.

Concussion

In small animals, a forceful blow on the back of the head, for example by striking them on the edge of a laboratory bench, can cause rapid and severe injury to the brain resulting in immediate death. The animal should be held firmly around the body, not by the tail. Technical expertise is required to carry out this method humanely.

Decapitation

This method is often used for killing embryonic and foetal forms. Its use for adults may be necessary in some experiments in order to avoid interference with physiological parameters due to other methods or agents. Ideally only a purpose-made guillotine should be used and the animal must be securely immobilised during the procedure. Severance of the neck causes immediate failure of the cerebral circulation and disruption of the cervical spine. This results in immediate loss of consciousness.

Stunning – captive bolt, electrical and percussion

Use of these methods should only be under qualified supervision, and is limited under Schedule 1 of the Animals (Scientific Procedures) Act 1986 to veterinary surgeons and holders of a licence granted under the Welfare of Animals (Slaughter or Killing) Regulations 1955. Other people intending to use these methods must have them listed on their personal licence.

Captive bolt gun

People who possess captive bolt guns must hold a firearms licence. The equipment must be kept in a secure cabinet according to conditions attached to the licence.

A penetrating captive-bolt pistol (see Figure 42.1) resembles a normal pistol in appearance and is fired by a blank cartridge. The muzzle of the pistol has a castellated face to reduce involuntary movement of the pistol when in the firing position. The cartridge is detonated by the hammer when the trigger of the pistol is squeezed. When fired, a captive bolt is projected into the brain. Cartridges come in differing strengths, the greater the charge, the deeper the bolt will penetrate into the brain. It is important to use the correct strength cartridge for the species and size of animal to be killed.

This method does not kill the animal outright, it stuns. After stunning with the pistol, the brain of the animal should be destroyed by a pithing rod, which is passed into and out of the hole made by the bolt several times. Alternatively, the animal may be

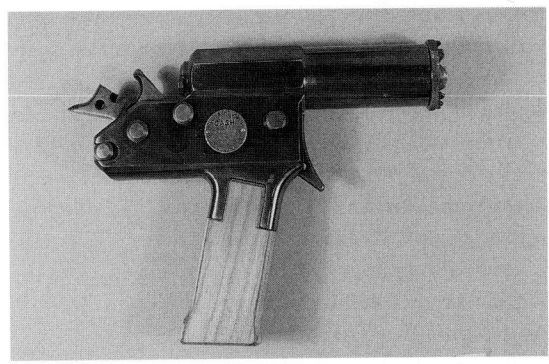

Figure 42.1 Captive bolt gun.

exsanguinated. Animals often show strong involuntary movements following stunning and great care must be taken by the operator when approaching the animal to complete the killing process.

Electrical and percussion stunning

Electrical and percussion (or compressed-air) stunning are methods used in commercial slaughterhouses and are unlikely to be used within the usual animal laboratory environment.

Free bullet humane killers

This is an efficient method of killing horses, mules, donkeys and old or hard-headed animals. It is not as safe as the captive bolt and therefore great care must be taken. All personnel must be trained in the method to ensure correct positioning of the weapon and that the correct calibre is used. The animals tend to slump forward when shot and therefore the operator must take care to avoid injury. In addition, the bullet may pass out of the animal at unexpected places so people standing nearby could be in danger. The method is only considered acceptable under field conditions. These guns, like the previous one mentioned in this section are subject to firearms controls.

Refrigeration

This method is only suitable for embryonic and foetal forms. Animals should be placed in a refrigerator at approximately four degrees Celsius rather than at sub-zero temperatures. The process will be aided by placing the foetus on wet tissue, thus increasing the 'chill' factor and thereby speeding death.

Chemical methods

Chemicals used to induce euthanasia are most often administered to animals by injection or inhalation.

Overdose of anaesthetic via injection

The administration of an overdose of anaesthetic is generally one of the simplest and most effective means of carrying out euthanasia. However, the development of modern anaesthetic agents with their wide safety margins may mean that large volumes of the drug is needed and this may restrict their use both on the grounds of practicality and economy.

The most common injectable agent used for euthanasia of animals is sodium pentobarbitone.

A concentrated solution of 200 mg per millilitre for this purpose is available commercially. A dose of 60 mg/kg intravenously or 80–150 mg/kg intraperitoneally may be used. Animals which are difficult to handle or restrain should first be given a sedative or a tranquilising agent, e.g. acetylpromazine, xylazine, medetomidine (Flecknell 1995). Sodium pentobarbitone causes death, after the initial loss of consciousness by cardiac and respiratory arrest.

Other anaesthetic agents can also be used for euthanasia, and in an emergency most will be suitable. In general, two or three times the anaesthetic dose will cause cardiovascular and respiratory depression and death.

Overdose of anaesthetic through inhalation

Euthanasia agents administered by inhalation should be non-irritant and inhaled readily by the animal. The animal must be placed in a suitable induction chamber and the vapour introduced in a controlled manner. Waste gases should be removed by scavengers to reduce the risk to human health. The commonly used volatile anaesthetic agents, such as halothane, isoflurane and enflurane, can all be used for euthanasia purposes. These produce rapid unconsciousness followed by cardiac and respiratory arrest. Because of its slower onset of action methoxyflurane is not recommended for euthanasia purposes. All of these agents are non-flammable, non-explosive and the vapour is non-irritant.

The safest method both for the operator and the animal is to deliver the anaesthetic agent into an anaesthetic chamber from an anaesthetic machine. However, it is also possible to place an absorbent pad soaked with the liquid anaesthetic agent in an airtight container such as a laboratory desiccator. A grid or other device must be used to prevent the animal from coming into contact with the liquid anaesthetic, which is highly irritant. It is important to ensure that animals die from an overdose of anaesthetic rather than from hypoxia, therefore a sufficient level of air or oxygen should be provided during the induction period (Andrews et al. 1993). Since many of the anaesthetic agents used pose a human health risk, even at low concentrations, it is essential that an effective gas-scavenging system be used. Some animals, particularly rabbits, may exhibit prolonged periods of breath-holding and may be distressed by this method of euthanasia.

Exposure to carbon dioxide

At concentrations above 50%, carbon dioxide acts as an anaesthetic agent and causes rapid loss of consciousness. It is effective and humane for euthanasia of most small animals above 70% concentration. Schedule 1 of the Animals (Scientific Procedures) Act 1986 states that a rising concentration of CO_2 must be used. This ensures that unconsciousness is produced before asphyxia. The concentration should rise rapidly over a five- to ten-second period, since exposure to low concentrations of carbon dioxide stimulates respiratory activity and this may be distressing to the animal. Animals may also pass through a period of involuntary excitement, which makes the method unsuitable for the larger species such as rabbits, cats, dogs and above.

The euthanasia chamber (Figure 42.2) must be designed to prevent injury and should be easy to clean. In between each animal the chamber should be emptied of previously used gas, since CO_2 is heavier than air this can be easily achieved by simply tipping the chamber on its side. The chamber should also be cleaned between animals. The gas should be supplied in a controlled way from a gas cylinder. The use of a fire extinguisher or 'dry ice' is not acceptable. It is acceptable to euthanise small groups of rodents together. Providing the gas can flow freely into the cage it is also acceptable to euthanise groups of animals by placing their home cage in the chamber, thus reducing any stress due to handling.

Carbon dioxide is only suitable for the euthanasia of juvenile and adult animals. Neonatal animals, i.e. less than ten days old, are resistant to the effects of CO_2 and very prolonged exposure is necessary to kill these animals. For this reason, alternative methods should be used.

Research has been carried out examining the possible advantageous effects of combining CO_2 with oxygen during euthanasia as a means of ensuring that animals die from CO_2 narcosis, rather than hypoxia (Iwarsson & Rehbinder 1993). In some species there appears to be a reduction in stress and anxiety, but this is accompanied by a longer induction time (Blackmore 1993). Hewett et al. 1993 felt that there was no welfare advantage in using CO_2/O_2 mixtures.

Exposure to nitrogen/argon

Nitrogen or argon displace oxygen and produce death by hypoxia, and it has been suggested that both gases are suitable for euthanasia. It has been shown that at concentrations of 39% it takes at least three minutes for rats to become unconscious and that they show signs of panic and distress.

These gases are therefore not acceptable as euthanasia agents unless the animal is anaesthetised.

Confirming death

The Animals (Scientific Procedures) Act 1986 states that 'an animal continues to live until permanent cessation of circulation or destruction of the brain' so these factors have to be identified before an animal can be considered dead. The Home Office *Code of Practice on Humane Killing* (1997) says that destruction of the brain means permanent loss of function not necessarily physical destruction and points out that it can be difficult to identify a pulse or heart beat in some laboratory species, particularly the small ones. Confirmation of death which must be done before a carcass is disposed of can, therefore, be troublesome.

A number of signs can indicate that an animal is dead:

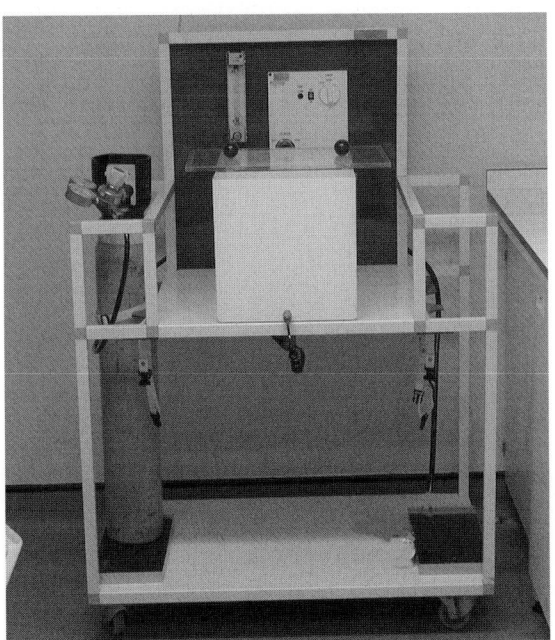

Figure 42.2 CO_2 euthanasia apparatus.

- pale or cyanosed mucus membranes;
- lack of breathing;
- lack of heartbeat;
- relaxation of anal and urinary sphincters;
- *rigor mortis.*

Of these only the last one is a sure sign, the others are indications.

A number of actions which can ensure an animal is dead before it is disposed of are listed as part of Schedule 1 of the Animals (Scientific Procedures) Act 1986, they are:

(1) confirmation of cessation of the circulation;
(2) destruction of the brain;
(3) dislocation of the neck;
(4) exsanguination;
(5) confirmation of the onset of *rigor mortis*;
(6) instantaneous destruction of the body in a macerator.

Further details of the methods described above can be found in *An Introduction to Animal Technology* (Barnett 2001) and are illustrated in the IAT video, *Euthanasia with Care.*

Schedule 1 to the Animals (Scientific Procedures) Act 1986 has not been reproduced here as it may be amended. The current version can be downloaded, with the Code of Practice for the Humane Killing of Animals under Schedule 1, from the Home Office website (www.homeoffice.gov.uk).

References

Andrews, E.J., Taylor-Bennett, B. and Clark, J.D. (1993) Report of the AVMA Panel on Euthanasia. *Journal of the American Veterinary Medical Association* **202**: 229–249.

Blackmore, D.K. (1993) Euthanasia; not always eu. *Australian Veterinary Journal,* **70** (11): 409–413.

Flecknell, P. (1995) Euthanasia (pp. 375–381). In: A.A. Tuffery (Ed.) *Laboratory Animals: An Introduction for New Experimenters* (2nd edn). John Wiley & Sons.

Green, C.J. (1979) Euthanasia (pp. 237–241). In: *Animal Anaesthesia. Laboratory Animal Handbook 8.* Laboratory Animals Ltd, London.

Hewett, T., Kovacs, M.S., Artwohl, J.E. and Bennett, B.T. (1993) Comparison of euthanasia methods in rats using carbon dioxide in pre-filled and fixed flow rate filled chambers. *Laboratory Animal Science,* **43**: 579–582.

Home Office (1997). *Code of Practice for the Humane Killing of Animals under Schedule 1 to the Animals (Scientific Procedures) Act 1986.* HMSO, London.

Iwarsson, K. and Rehbinder, C. (1985) Euthanasia in laboratory animals. *Zeitschrift für Versuchstierkunde,* **27** (2): 20–26.

Further reading

LASA (1996) Recommendations for euthanasia of experimental animals: Part 1 Laboratory Animals. 30:4 pp. 293–316.

LASA (1997) Recommendations for euthanasia of experimental animals: Part 2 Laboratory Animals. 31:1 pp. 1–32.

Barnett, S.W. (2001) *Introduction to Animal Technology* (2nd edn). Blackwell Science, Oxford.

Appendix
Animal Technology Calculations

Stephen W. Barnett

This chapter covers calculations which have not been dealt with in other parts of the book. Breeding productivity calculations are explained in Chapter 1 and nutritional calculations in Chapter 26.

Note: the most common unit of volume used in science is cubic metres (m^3) or cm^3 for smaller volumes. However the litre (l) and millilitre (ml) are still used in some circumstances and ml is almost universally used when calculating amounts to be administered to experimental animals and so will be used here: $1 \ cm^3 = 1 \ ml$.

Experimental procedure calculations

Administration of therapeutic and experimental substances

The amount of a substance that must be administered to an animal is usually quoted in milligrams per kilogram body weight, e.g. 5 mg/kg. The substance may be in solution or suspension in which case the bottle will be labelled with the concentration, e.g. 2 mg/ml.

To calculate the volume of a substance which needs to be administered the dose required (in mg) must be multiplied by the body weight of the animal (in kg) and, if the drug is in solution or suspension, the answer must be divided by the concentration stated on the bottle.

Example a
A 14 kg dog must be administered substance A at a dose of 5 mg/kg body weight. Substance A is in solution at a concentration of 15 mg/ml. What volume must be injected?

The dog is 14 kg therefore the amount that must be administered is:

$14 \times 5 = 70 \ mg$

To calculate the volume which must be injected, the concentration must be divided into the amount which must be administered.

$70 \div 15 = 4.7 \ ml$

Example b
A 300 g rat must be administered substance B at a dose rate of 15 mg/kg body weight. Substance B is in solution at a concentration of 2 mg/ml. What volume must be injected?

The calculation is the same as in example a except that the body weight of the rat is a fraction of a kg. The rat is 300 g therefore the amount to be administered is:

$$\frac{300}{1000} \times 15 = 4.5 \ mg.$$

The volume to be injected is $4.5 \div 2 = 2.25 \ ml$.

Example c
It may be necessary to administer the required dose in a given volume, e.g. 6 mg/kg body weight in 0.5 ml of water. If the animal to be injected was a 350 g rat the calculation would be as follows:

$$\frac{350}{1000} \times 6 = 2.1 \ mg.$$

This would then be dissolved in 0.5 ml of water.

Withdrawal of blood

It is recommended that 65 ml/kg body weight is taken as the average amount of circulating blood for all species and that no more that 15% of this should be removed over a twenty-eight day period. It is also recommended that a single withdrawal should not exceed 10% of the total blood volume (see

Chapter 39). It may, therefore, be necessary to calculate the value of these figures.

Example d

What would be the maximum single amount of blood which could be withdrawn from a 3 kg rabbit?

Theoretical circulating blood volume of the rabbit would be:

$$3 \times 65 = 195 \text{ ml}$$

Ten per cent can be found by dividing the number by 100 and multiplying the answer by 10 (or by pressing the % button on a calculator):

$$= 19.5 \text{ ml}$$

Example e

What would be the maximum single amount of blood which could be withdrawn from a 600 g guinea pig?

Theoretical circulating blood volume would be:

$$\frac{600}{1000} \times 65 = 39 \text{ ml}$$

Ten per cent of this figure $= 3.9$ ml

Measuring food intake

Assessment of food consumption is carried out routinely in animal facilities. A rough indication can be gauged by judging how the level of food has gone in a hopper but often experimental demands require a more exact measurement.

One approach is to weigh the amount of food given (1) and the amount of food remaining in the hopper after twenty-four hours (2). The amount of food consumed is calculated by taking (2) from (1). Increased accuracy can be given by adding the amount of food wasted (e.g. as crumbs under the hopper) to that left in the hopper but this is usually only possible if animals are kept in grid-bottomed cages. If several animals are kept in a cage the average food consumption can be calculated by dividing the figure for food consumed by the number of animals in the cage.

Example f

Calculate the average individual daily food intake of a group of five rats housed in a grid-bottomed cage.

Two hundred grams of diet is placed in the hopper. Twenty-four hours later 120 g remained in the hopper and 10 g of crumbs were recovered from under the hopper.

200 g given − (120 g left + 10 g wasted)
= 70 g consumed by five rats

Average consumption per rat is $70 \div 5 = 14$ g.

Where greater accuracy is required single animals should be housed in metabolism cages.

Water consumption can be measured in the same way but spills are difficult to measure, unless the animal is housed in a metabolism cage.

Solution calculations

Percentage solutions

Percentage solutions are often referred to as either weight in volume (w/v) or volume in volume (v/v). In the first case it means the solute is a solid and is measured by weight, the solvent is a liquid and is measured in ml. In the second case both solute and solvent are liquid.

Example g

(1) A 5% solution of NaCl in water (w/v) means 5 g of NaCl made up to 100 ml with water.
(2) A 10% solution of chloros in water (v/v) means 10 ml of chloros made up to 100 ml with water.

Dilution of solutions

Calculating the volume of stock solution needed to make up a solution of required strength.

$$\frac{\text{strength required} \% \times \text{volume required}}{\text{strength of stock solution}}$$

Example h

Make up 500 ml of a 1% solution from a 5% stock solution.

$$\frac{1 \times 500}{5} = 100 \text{ ml}$$

Water would then be added to make up the solution to 500 ml.

Breeding calculations

The manager of an animal facility may have a request from a researcher to provide a certain number of animals of a specific strain, every week for a prolonged period. The animals may be required at a specific age, be of one sex only, females supplied with their litters or be supplied at a specific age on a specific day.

In most cases this request would be fulfilled by ordering the animals from a designated breeding establishment, who would have sufficiently large colonies to provide most requirements from stock. However, for the reasons discussed in Chapter 1, the decision may be made to breed them in house (assuming the establishment had a certificate of designation allowing breeding). In these circumstances it is important to ensure enough animals are produced for the researcher to use (too few on one week could jeopardise the project), but it is equally important not to over-produce animals. Producing animals which will be wasted is both unethical and uneconomic. Fortunately there are simple calculations which can be used to establish the size of the breeding colony and the time it will take to start producing them.

The calculation is divided into stages:

(1) The number of females required.
- This is found by dividing the total number of young required by the number of young produced by a female each week.

(2) Variation allowance.
- This is an 'insurance' against some animals failing to breed (e.g. a sterile male). The larger the colony the lower the variation allowance needs to be. An extra 5% is added for colonies of over 1000 breeders, 10% for colonies in the hundreds and 15% for colonies under 100.

(3) Replacement breeding stock.
- If the request for animals is going on for more than six months, extra breeding stock will need to be added so that animals may be replaced as they reach the end of their economic breeding life. Replacement is done gradually, a number every week so that all have been replaced by the time the oldest has reached the end of its economic breeding life.

(4) Set up and time to first issue.
- This calculates how many breeding units are required to be set up each week to satisfy the researcher's request. It is found by dividing the total number of breeders required by the litter interval.
- The time it will take to produce the first animals from the colony is calculated by adding together the length of the oestrous cycle of the females, the gestation period and the rearing time. The first two elements will remain the same in each species but the rearing time will depend on what the researcher has requested. If the request is for mice at weaning age, the rearing time will be three weeks, if the request is for female mice with litters, the rearing time will be much longer because the females will have to be bred, kept until they are old enough to mate and produce a litter.

There is no single correct answer with these calculations, they provide a reasonable assessment of the numbers of animals needed to start up the colony. If experience shows that too many or too few animals are being produced, the colony can be adjusted accordingly.

The following examples will explain the calculation in more detail and will show how values are arrived at.

Example 1

Devise a continuous breeding programme to supply 1000 female mice of weaning age each week.

It is advisable to collect the breeding data together before starting the calculation. In this case average, published data is being used.

Breeding data

Age paired	6 weeks
Oestrous cycle (c)	5 days (round up to 1 week)*
Gestation (g)	3 weeks
Litter size	8
Age at weaning (w)	3 weeks
Economic breeding life 6 litters	

* For ease of calculation it is acceptable to round up some values. It is possible to calculate using days instead of weeks but this makes the calculation slightly more complicated and does not make a significant difference to the answer.

Choice of breeding system and basic assumptions being made must be clear.

- monogamous pairs will be used;
- advantage will be taken of post-partum mating [ppm];
- 1000 females are required so 2000 mice must be produced (assuming 1:1 sex ratio).

Stage 1

Litter interval
This is the time between the production of each litter. As we are using monogamous pairs and taking advantage of ppm, the litter interval should be just the gestation period. However for various reasons (e.g. failure to remate, delayed implantation) ppm is rarely 100% successful in a colony. Success in mice varies with different strains but a reasonable assumption would be 75% successful.

Therefore 75% of the animals in the colony will have a litter interval of just the gestation period. The other 25% will not become pregnant until they cycle again after their young are weaned, therefore their litter interval will consist of weaning (w) + cycle (c) + gestation (g). The average for the colony will be:

$$75\% \,(g) + 25\% \,(w + c + g)$$
$$= 75\% \,(3) + 25\% \,(3 + 1 + 3)$$
$$= 2.25 + 1.75 = 4$$

The litter interval for this mouse colony will be 4 weeks.

Number of young per female per week
If the average litter size is eight and the time between each litter being born is four weeks the average number of young each female produces each week is:

$$= \frac{\text{litter size}}{\text{litter interval}} = \frac{8}{4} = 2$$

Breeding stock required
Two thousand mice are required per week, if each female produces two young per week then:

$$\frac{\text{no. of mice required}}{\text{no. of young produced/female/week}} = \frac{2000}{2}$$

= 1000 breeding females (as monogamous pairs are used this means 1000 breeding pairs).

Stage 2

Variation allowance
The variation allowance for this number of breeders is 5% so:

$$\frac{1000 \times 5}{100} = 50 \text{ pairs}$$

So now 1050 pairs are required.

Stage 3

Replacement of breeding stock
The females have litter intervals of four weeks and an economic breeding life of six litters, therefore every $4 \times 6 = 24$ weeks the entire colony has to be replaced. If this were done at the same time breeding would have to come to a halt every twenty-four weeks and would have to start from scratch again. In order to ensure no breeders go beyond their economic breeding life and that no halt occurs in production, replacement is done in stages.

There are 1050 breeding pairs all of which have to be replaced within twenty-four weeks so:

$$\frac{1050}{24} = 43.75 \text{ (rounded up to 44)}$$

Each week 44 pairs of mice are replaced so that by the time twenty-four weeks has elapsed no pair has exceeded its economic breeding life. Each week an extra 44 pairs have to be added to the colony and therefore these need to be bred.

Forty-four pairs means 88 mice need to be produced. Each female produces two mice per week so 44 extra pairs are needed.

The breeding stock will now be 1050 + 44 = 1094 pairs.

Stage 4

Starting the programme
Assuming all the initial breeding stock are available the first issue of mice will be issued in:

c + g + rearing time (which in this case is the weaning age)

1 + 3 + 3 = 7 weeks.

Setting up the programme

If all the breeding stock were set up at once then all the young animals would be produced at four week intervals. In order to produce them every week they have to be set up over the litter interval:

$$\frac{\text{no. of breeding animals}}{\text{litter interval}}$$

$$= \frac{1094}{4} = 274 \text{ pairs are set up each week}$$

The answer can be checked to see if it is reasonable by multiplying the pairs set up each week by the average litter size, in this case that would $274 \times 8 = 2192$. Which would supply the 1000 females required and the extra needed for replacement breeders and variation.

Adjustments to the calculation for other requests

If older animals were required, say at twelve weeks of age, the calculation would be the same except the rearing time would be increased and the first issue would take fourteen weeks.

If the initial request was for 1000 mice there would be no need to double the initial number of animals.

If females and litters were required, rearing time would need to be increased to take account of time to achieve sexual maturity (6 weeks for mice) + cycle time (1 week) + gestation period (3 weeks) = 10 weeks. This means the first issue would take fourteen weeks.

Example 2

Devise a continuous breeding programme to provide 500 rats a week at six weeks of age.

Breeding Data

Age paired	10 weeks
Oestrous cycle (c)	5 days (round up to 1 week)
Gestation (g)	3 weeks
Litter size	10
Age at weaning (w)	3 weeks
Economic breeding life	6 months (26 weeks)

System used will be harems with boxing out. It will not be possible to take advantage of post-partum oestrus.

Stage 1

Litter interval
weaning + cycle + gestation

$$3 + 1 + 3 = 7 \text{ weeks}$$

Young per female per week

$$\frac{\text{average litter size}}{\text{litter interval}} = \frac{10}{7} = 1.4$$

Females required to supply 500 rats

$$\frac{\text{rats required}}{\text{young/female/week}} = \frac{500}{1.4} = 357$$

Stage 2

Variation allowance
Ten per cent extra for a colony of this size = 35.7 rounded up to 36

new total = 393 females.

Stage 3

Replacement breeding stock
Economic breeding life is twenty-six weeks so each week:

$$\frac{393}{26} = 16 \text{ females must be replaced; these must be bred}$$

To produce 16 females 32 rats must be bred.

$$\frac{\text{rats required}}{\text{young/female/week}} = \frac{32}{1.4} = 23 \text{ extra females needed}$$

Final total = 393 + 23 = 416 females required.

Stage 4

Setting up breeders

$$\frac{\text{total females required}}{\text{litter interval}} = \frac{416}{7} = 60 \text{ females}$$

So 60 females must be set up each week. Fifteen harems of one male to four females would be suitable for rats.

First issue

The first issue could be made c + g + rearing time:

$$1 + 3 + 6 \text{ weeks} = 10 \text{ weeks}.$$

Example 3

Devise a continuous breeding programme to supply 100 guinea pigs of seven weeks of age each week.

Breeding data

Age paired	12 weeks
Oestrous cycle (c)	15 days (2 weeks)
Gestation (g)	10 weeks
Litter size	4
Age at weaning (w)	2 weeks
Economic breeding life	8 litters

Breeding system used will be permanent harems so it will be possible to take advantage of post-partum oestrus. It will be assumed that mating at the post-partum oestrus will have a 75% success rate.

Stage 1

Litter interval

As it will be possible for these animals to mate at the post-partum oestrus and mating at this time is approximately 75% successful, the situation is similar to that described in Example 1. Seventy-five per cent of the females will have a litter interval of just the gestation period and 25% will have to wait until the end of lactation before they can mate.

$$75\% \text{ (g)} + 25\% \text{ (w + c + g)}$$
$$= 75\% \text{ (10)} + 25\% \text{ (2 + 2 + 10)}$$
$$= 7.5 + 3.5 = 11$$

The litter interval for this guinea pig colony will be eleven weeks.

Number of young per female per week

If the average litter size is four and the average time between each litter being born is eleven weeks then the average number of young each female produces each week is:

$$\frac{\text{litter size}}{\text{litter interval}} = \frac{4}{11} = 0.36 \text{ young/week}$$

Breeding stock required

One hundred guinea pigs are required each week, if each female produces 0.36 young per week then:

$$\frac{\text{no. of guinea pigs required}}{\text{no. of young produced/female/week}} = \frac{100}{0.36}$$

= 278 breeding females are required.

Stage 2

Variation allowance

The variation allowance for this number of breeders is 10% so:

$$\frac{278 \times 10}{100} = 27.8 \text{ (rounded up to 28)}$$

So now we require 306.

Stage 3

Replacement of breeding stock

The females have litter intervals of eleven weeks and an economic breeding life of eight litters, therefore every 11 × 8 = 88 weeks the entire colony has to be replaced. As with the previous examples replacement is arranged so that some are replaced each week so that by the end of the 88 weeks all of the breeders have been replaced.

There are 306 breeding females all of which have to be replaced within 88 weeks so:

$$\frac{306}{88} = 3.47 \text{ (rounded up to 4) females must be replaced each week.}$$

Four females means eight guinea pigs have to be produced. Each female produces 0.36 young per week therefore eleven extra breeders are needed.

The breeding stock will now be 306 + 11 = 317 pairs.

Stage 4

Starting the programme

Assuming all the initial breeding stock are available then the first issue of mice will be issued in:

c+ g + rearing time (which in this case is the weaning age)

$$2 + 10 + 7 = 19 \text{ weeks}$$

Setting up the programme

$$\frac{\text{no. of breeding animals}}{\text{litter interval}} = \frac{317}{11}$$

= 28.8 (rounded up to 30 females set up each week)

Ten females can be arranged in harems of ten females to one male.

Example 4

Devise a breeding programme to supply forty, female, seventeen-day-old mice every Wednesday for a year.

There are a number of ways to meet these requirements e.g.:

(1) animals can be bought in, as breeders have large colonies they can select those females that will have young on the required day;
(2) vaginal smears can be used to identify those females in oestrus, at a time to produce young of the required age on the required day, but this also requires a large colony;
(3) hormone injections can be used to ensure female will be in oestrus at the required time. This has the disadvantage of being invasive and therefore is a regulated procedure;
(4) by using the Whitten effect, which needs far smaller colony than (1) and (2) above.

The Whitten effect is explained in Chapter 1. It is based on the fact that if female mice who have been housed in the absence of males are placed where they can see and smell males, but separate from them, 60% will come into oestrus in three days.

The calculation differs from those already considered, in this case oestrus is manipulated.

Relevant data

Average litter size	8
Gestation period	3 weeks
Sex ratio	1:1

Forty females are required to be used so 80 young must be born.

The average litter size is 8 so 80 ÷ 8 = 10 breeding females are needed.

Whitten says if twenty females are placed in stock cages with a male caged within it (but separate from the females) on a Friday, the following Sunday 60% of them will be ready to mate. 60% of 20 is 12, this number includes the 10 breeding females required plus a 20% variation allowance.

On Sunday the primed females are removed and placed in trios. Twelve of the twenty will be expected to mate. The males are removed on Monday so they cannot mate females who were not in oestrus on Sunday.

Once the non-mated females have been seen to be non-pregnant (approximately ten to fourteen days later) they are removed and used for future matings.

The mated females will produce litters in time to reach seventeen days old on a Wednesday.

To set up:

week 1	20 females set up
2	20 females set up
3	12 new females set up + 8 not mated in week 1
4	12 new females set up + 8 not mated in week 2
5	12 new females set up + 8 not mated in week 3
6	12 new females set up + 8 not mated in week 4
7	12 original females set up + 8 not mated in week 5
etc.	

References

Breeding calculation methods are based on:
Millican, K.G. (1963), The use of calculations in the establishment of breeding programmes. In: D.J. Short and S.P. Woodnott (Eds) *The IAT Manual of Laboratory Animal Practice and Techniques*. Granada Publishing. ISBN: 0 2589 6739 0.

Glossary

Ad libitum (ad lib)	At leisure – refers to food, water etc. available to an animal all the time.
Acclimatisation	Period of time allowed for an animal to get used to the sounds, smells, people etc. in a unit before an experiment begins.
Acid	Substance which gives rise to hydrogen ions (H+) when in water. Reacts with bases to produce salts and water; pH < 7.
Aerosol	Fine mist of liquid particles in air.
Alkali	Substances which give rise to hydroxyl ions (OH−) when in water; pH > 7.
Allele	One of the two copies of a gene.
Alopecia	Hair loss (baldness).
Ameliorate	Improvement of condition; reduction in the severity of clinical signs.
Amino acid	Chemical units from which proteins are formed.
Amplexus	Mating in frogs and toads. The word means 'embrace' and refers to the position the male takes on the back of the female holding on by gripping her around the abdomen.
Anabolic	Synthesis, in the body, of complex chemicals from simpler ones (see Metabolic and Catabolic).
Anoxia	Lack of oxygen.
Antibiotic	Chemicals originating from bacteria and fungi which destroy bacteria.
Antigen	Antibody generating; anything in the body which stimulates the formation of antibodies.
Antioxidant	Chemicals which inhibit oxidation reactions, e.g. vitamin E in diets.
Arranged mating	Mating system where a female in oestrus is taken to the male for mating and is removed after mating has taken place.
Artificial insemination	Method of achieving fertilisation by collecting semen from the male and introducing it into a female reproductive tract by means of a catheter.
Asepsis	Free from pathogenic organisms.
Asexual reproduction	Reproduction by a form of cell division; without the need for fertilisation.
Ataxia	Uncoordinated movement.
Axenic	An animal free from all demonstrable forms of life.

Balai	European Union directive which regulates free trade between member states. Under this directive mammals can pass from one member state to another without quarantine, providing they are certified not to have been in contact with rabies.
Basal metabolic rate	The minimum rate of metabolism necessary to keep a resting animal alive.
Catabolic	Breakdown of complex chemicals to simpler ones, with the release of energy, within the body of a living organism. See Anabolic and Metabolic.
Caustic	Having corrosive properties, e.g. alkali such as caustic soda (sodium hydroxide).
Chimera	Organism developed from cells of two different genotypes.
-cide or -cidal	Agent which will kill, e.g. bactericide.
cm^3	Measurement of volume (equivalent to ml).
Coccidiostat	Drug used to control coccidian (Eimeria) infections.
Co-isogenic	Two strains of animals genetically identical except for a single gene.
Collagen	A protein fibre found in connective tissue, which is widespread in the body.
Colony	Group kept together for a particular purpose, usually breeding.
Condensation reactions	Chemical reactions involving the removal of water, e.g. amino acids are joined together to form proteins by the removal of a water molecule between them.
Congenic	Two strains of animal identical except for a short segment of chromosome, bearing a gene of interest.
Conspecifics	Animals of the same species.
Contraindication	A clinical sign which indicates that a drug or treatment should not be used in certain circumstances.
Copulation plug	Secretions from seminal vesicle and coagulating glands of the male which solidify in the vagina of the female following mating. The plugs shrink and fall out after a few hours. Seen in certain mammals, e.g. rodents. They can be used as an indication that copulation has taken place.
Corpus luteum	Temporary endocrine gland which is formed from cells lining the Graafian follicle after ovulation. The yellow tissue produces progesterone. If the animal becomes pregnant the gland persists through the pregnancy, if not it breaks down after a short time.
Crepuscular animals	Animals active at dusk and dawn.
Cross fostering	Technique where young are taken from a number of mothers and re-sorted in some way (e.g. same sex or same number) before being re-allocated to females for rearing.
Crude protein	Assessment of the protein in a food, based on the nitrogen content.
Cytology	Study of the structure and function of cells.

Depilatory	Substance that removes hair.
Endopterygota	Type of lifecycle in insects where the egg hatches into a worm-like form which undergoes several moults and metamorphoses to reach the adult form.
Epididymis	Tube running along the outside of the testis which carries sperm from the testis to the vas deferens.
Essential nutrient	A nutrient which cannot be made in the cells of an animal's body and therefore must be provided in the diet, e.g. essential amino acids.
Eukaryotic	Cells which have a nucleus and organelles bound by a membrane. Found in organisms of all kingdoms except the Prokaryotae.
Excretion	Removal of the waste products of metabolism from a body, e.g. urination, sweating, exhaling.
Exopterygota	Type of lifecycle in insects in which the egg hatches into a nymph (see Nymph). The nymph undergoes several moults to reach adult form.
Fatty acid	Organic acid which is required for various biological functions.
Fertilisation	Fusion of genetic material of the male and female gametes.
Foundation stock	Colony from which an inbred strain originates.
Gamete	Reproductive cell (ova and sperm).
Genetic engineering	Techniques used to alter the genetic make-up of an organism.
Genetic monitoring	Techniques used to establish the genetic identity of animals.
Genetically altered	An organism whose genome has been altered by genetic engineering techniques.
Genetically defined	Animals bred with a particular genetic make-up, e.g. inbred.
Gnotobiote	Animal in which all associated life forms are known.
Gonadotrophic hormones	Hormones which control the functions of the gonads, e.g. follicle-stimulating hormone and luteinizing hormone.
Gravimetric	Analysis based on weighing.
Haemocytometer	Instrument used in conjunction with a microscope for accurately counting blood cells, sperm or other single cells in a known volume of liquid.
Harems	One male with two or more females set up for breeding.
Hermaphrodite	Having both male and female sexual organs.
Hertz (Hz)	Cycles per second. Measurement of the frequency of electromagnetic radiation.
Heterozygous	Organisms which have inherited a different allele for any gene from each parent.
Hexacanth	With six hooks. Refers to tapeworm embryos in which six hooks can be seen.
Homogeneous	A mixture of uniform nature.

Homozygous	Organism which has inherited the same allele for a gene from different parents.
Hybrid vigour	Healthy, robust and productive state associated with animals with a good assortment of genes (heterozygotes).
Hymen	A thin membrane at the opening of the vagina.
Hyper-	Over, above or increase.
Hypertension	Increased blood pressure.
Hyperthermia	Increased body temperature.
Hypo-	Under or lower.
Hypotension	Low blood pressure.
Hypothalamus	Region of the brain immediately above the pituitary gland. It secrets neurochemicals which influence the pituitary and is involved in control of motivated behaviours such as eating, drinking and sex.
Hypoxia	Low level of oxygen.
Impedance	Factors which inhibit the flow of electric current.
In vitro	In glass, e.g. tissue culture.
In vivo	In life, e.g. experiments carried out in living animals.
Inbred	Offspring produced by mating close relatives.
Inbred strain	A strain produced as the result of mating brother × sister or youngest parent × offspring for twenty consecutive generations.
Inbreeding	Mating together of close relatives.
Induction (anaesthesia)	Taking a conscious animal to the anaesthetised state.
Intracytoplasmic sperm injection	Fertilisation achieved by injecting a sperm head directly into an ovum.
Intubation	Introduction of a tube into the trachea (for administration of inhalation anaesthesia).
Ion	Atom or molecule which has gained or lost an electron and is therefore electrically charged.
Isogenic	Animals with the same genetic make-up.
-itis	Inflammation, e.g. enteritis – inflammation of the intestines.
Joule	SI unit of energy.
Keratinised	Process whereby the protein keratin is laid down in tissue making it tough, e.g. in the formation of skin.
Knock-in	Introduction of foreign genetic material by genetic engineering techniques.
Knock-out	Inactivation of genetic material by genetic engineering techniques.
Larva	Juvenile form of an invertebrate organism which is unlike the adult and resembles a maggot (see Nymph).

Laryngoscope	Instrument for visualising the larynx.
Lux	Unit of light intensity.
Maintenance (anaesthesia)	Keeping the animal at the required level of anaesthesia during an operation.
Melamine	A hard plastic used to cover surfaces such as bench tops.
Minimal inbreeding techniques	Breeding techniques used in closed colonies to ensure inbreeding does not take place.
Minute volume	Volume of air breathed in one minute.
Monocyte	White blood cells able to engulf large organisms such as protoctista parasites. Mature into macrophages in the tissues.
Monogamous pairs	One male and one female paired for their breeding life.
Mores	Generally accepted moral standards of groups within society.
Morphology	External appearance.
Mutant	A strain of animal with an altered gene which makes it valuable to study, e.g. obese mouse, nude mouse.
Myositis	Inflammation of muscle.
Necrosis	Localised cell death (death of tissue before death of the whole organism).
Negative feedback	Biological control mechanism where, once the level of a substance (e.g. a hormone) reaches the required level in the body, further production of that substance is switched off.
Neonatal	New born.
Neutrophil	Phagocytic white blood cell which engulfs invading micro-organisms.
Nocturnal	Active at night.
Nymph	Juvenile form of an invertebrate organism which resembles the adult but is smaller and sexually immature (see Larva).
Outbreeding	Breeding colonies where there is a deliberate avoidance of inbreeding.
Ovulation	Release of eggs from the ovary. In some species ovulation is spontaneous where it occurs regularly after each oestrus. In other species it is induced, i.e it is stimulated by mating.
Ovum	Female gamete (plural = ova).
Palpation	Examination of the body by touch.
Pasteurisation	Method of killing bacteria by heating a substance to between 70–90 °C followed by rapid cooling. Originally used to remove TB-causing organisms from milk without affecting the nutritional quality of the milk. Will not kill bacterial spores.
Pathogenic	Disease-causing organism.
pH	Numerical scale indicating degree of acidity/alkalinity.

Phagocyte	Cell which engulfs substances through its cell membrane in order to digest them, e.g. white blood cells, neutrophils and monocytes.
Phase-contrast microscope	Microscope which is able to manipulate light so that differences in the way light is refracted by components in a cell is emphasised. Allows tissues to be observed with a microscope without staining.
Phenotype	Observable and measurable characteristics of an organism.
Pheromone	Chemical released into the air by animals to signal to others.
Pituitary gland	Master endocrine gland, situated at the base of the brain produces a number of hormones which direct the activities of other endocrine glands. Also produces hormones which have a direct action on tissues.
Polygamous mating	Alternative name for continuous harems.
Polymerase chain reaction	Technique used to make many copies of a small piece of DNA.
Polysulphone	Plastic with increased tolerance to high temperature and chemicals. Used for rodent caging.
Positive feedback	Regulating system within the body where the presence of a substance stimulates the production of more of the same substance.
Potable water	Water fit for human consumption.
Primary line	Colony of an inbred strain of animals kept mating in b × s pairings and genetically monitored regularly to ensure they do not become contaminated. Offspring from the primary colony passes to the production or expansion colony. Also known as stem colony or foundation colony.
Progeny testing	Study of offspring to ensure they have inherited desired characteristics from their parents.
Prokaryotic	Primitive cell types with no nucleus or other internal cell membranes. Found in members of the kingdom Prokaryotae (bacteria and blue–green algae).
Prolapse	Slipping out of place of an organ, e.g. prolapsed rectum – a rectum protruding through the anus.
Pronucleus	One of two haploid nuclei found in an egg (one from the male parent and one from the female parent) immediately before fertilisation takes place.
Pubic symphysis	Junction of the two pelvic bones.
Quarantine	A period of time when new animals are housed in isolation from existing ones in a facility. Designed to ensure that they do not introduce infectious organisms into the facility. If animals are from within the UK, a period of three weeks is usual. Where statutory quarantine is required, the period is six months.
Raddle	Head collar or chest harness bearing a coloured marker. Worn by bulls or rams so that it leaves a mark on the rump of the female when they mate.

Random breeding	Selecting animals for mating without any regard to their relationship. To be strictly random, animals should be selected using random number tables or a random number generator. Some of the breeding animals may be related, others will not, at each generation the situation will change.
Rectal palpation	Examination of the internal organs of the abdomen by passing an arm or finger into the rectum, e.g. used for pregnancy diagnosis in cattle and horses.
Resistant bacteria	Strains of bacteria which are not destroyed by one or more disinfectant/antibiotic.
Restricted feeding	Feeding a measured amount of food at certain times of the day.
Rheumatoid arthritis	Widespread inflammation of the joints.
Saline	Mixture of salt in water. Normal saline is 0.9% NaCl in water. Normal saline is isotonic to mammalian tissue fluid.
Sequelae	Consequences of disease; 'what follows'.
Shock	Cardiovascular failure. Inability of the circulatory system to provide tissues with nutrients etc. in order to fulfil their functions. Can be caused by several conditions, e.g. blood loss, injury.
Sibling	Offspring from the same parents.
-stat or -static	Prevent multiplication, e.g. bacteriostat.
Stereotypy	Repetitive behaviour pattern with no obvious purpose, e.g. pacing, tumbling. Sign of stress in an animal.
Substrate	An under layer, e.g. the bedding material, in an animal cage.
Super ovulation	A larger number of eggs than normal released from the ovary. Usually in response to hormone treatment.
Swayback	Disease of new-born lambs typified by lack of co-ordination as a result of damage to the nervous system. Caused by the ewe taking in insufficient copper during pregnancy.
Thermistor	Electronic means of measuring temperature. Consists of a semi-conductor whose electrical resistance decreases with increasing temperature.
Thermoregulate	Control of body temperature.
Tidal volume	The volume of air an animal breathes in and out with each breath.
Transgenic organism	Organism whose genetic make-up has been altered by the introduction of foreign genetic material.
Ultrasound	Sound waves with a frequency above 20 kHz.
Vaginal impedance	Technique use to identify oestrus in animals by measuring electrical resistance in the vagina.
Vasodilator	Drug or procedure which causes a superficial vein to enlarge, making it easier to see.

Venipuncture	Insertion of a needle into a vein.
Vestibular apparatus	Part of the ear which is responsible for balance.
Viscosity	Thickness of a liquid.
Vomeronasal organ	Supplementary odour detector in the roof of the mouth of many animals. Concerned with detection of oestrus.
Xiphoid cartilage	The lowest part of the centre of the sternum.
Zona pellucida	Membrane surrounding the ovum in a mammal.
Zygote	The result of fertilisation.

Index